Immune Mechanisms in Renal Disease

Immune Mechanisms in Renal Disease

Edited by

Nancy B. Cummings, M.D.

Kidney, Urologic, and Hematologic Diseases
National Institute of Arthritis, Diabetis, and
Digestive and Kidney Diseases
Bethesda, Maryland

Alfred F. Michael, M.D.

University of Minnesota Medical School
Minneapolis, Minnesota

and

Curtis B. Wilson, M.D.

Scripps Clinic and Research Foundation
La Jolla, California

PLENUM MEDICAL BOOK COMPANY
New York and London

Library of Congress Cataloging in Publication Data

Main entry under title:

Immune mechanisms in renal disease.

Includes bibliographical references and index.

1. Kidneys—Diseases—Immunological aspects. I. Cummings, Nancy B. II. Michael, Alfred F., 1928– III. Wilson, Curtis B.

RC903.I42 1982 616.6′1079 82-15135

ISBN 0-306-40948-8

First printing 1983

Plenum Medical Book Company is an imprint of
Plenum Publishing Corporation
233 Spring Street, New York, N.Y. 10013

Printed in the United States of America

Contributors

Christine K. Abrass, Division of Nephrology and Hypertension, Los Angeles County Harbor/UCLA Medical Center, Torrance, California 90502

Boris Albini, Department of Microbiology, State University of New York, Buffalo, New York 14214

Giuseppe Andres, Departments of Microbiology, Pathology, and Medicine, State University of New York, Buffalo, New York 14214

Jean-Francois Bach, INSERM U 25, Hôpital Necker, 75015, Paris, France

Marie-Anne Bach, INSERM U 25, Hôpital Necker, 75015, Paris, France

W. W. Bakker, Department of Pathology, State University, Groningen, 9713EZ Groningen, The Netherlands

Atul K. Bhan, Departments of Pathology, Massachusetts General Hospital and Harvard Medical School, Boston, Massachusetts 02115

Roland C. Blantz, Department of Medicine, School of Medicine, University of California, San Diego, and Veterans Administration Hospital, San Diego, California 92161

Wayne A. Border, Division of Nephrology and Hypertension, Los Angeles County Harbor/UCLA Medical Center, Torrance, California 90502

Barry M. Brenner, Laboratory of Kidney and Electrolyte Physiology and Departments of Medicine, Brigham and Women's Hospital and Harvard Medical School, Boston, Massachusetts 02115

David M. Brown, Department of Laboratory Medicine and Pathology and Department of Pediatrics, University of Minnesota, Minneapolis, Minnesota 55455

Peter M. Burkholder, Department of Pathology, University of Wisconsin Medical School, Madison, Wisconsin 53706

Kathleen M. Carmody, Department of Pediatrics, University of Minnesota Medical School, Minneapolis, Minnesota 55455

Charles B. Carpenter, Immunogenetics Laboratory, Renal Division, Department of Medicine, Brigham and Women's Hospital, Boston, Massachusetts 02115

Thomas M. Chused, Section on Cellular Immunology, Arthritis and Rheumatism Branch, National Institute of Arthritis, Metabolism and Digestive and Kidney Diseases, National Institutes of Health, Bethesda, Maryland 20205

Charles G. Cochrane, Department of Immunopathology, Scripps Clinic and Research Foundation, La Jolla, California 92037

Barbara R. Cole, Edward Mallinckrodt Department of Pediatrics, Washington University School of Medicine, and Division of Nephrology, St. Louis Children's Hospital, St. Louis, Missouri 63178

Robert B. Colvin, Departments of Pathology, Massachusetts General Hospital and Harvard Medical School, Boston, Massachusetts 02115

Ramzi S. Cotran, Departments of Pathology, Harvard Medical School and Brigham and Women's Hospital, Boston, Massachusetts 02115

William G. Couser, Division of Nephrology, University of Washington, Seattle, Washington 98195

Frank J. Dixon, Department of Immunopathology, Research Institute of Scripps Clinic, Scripps Clinic and Research Foundation, La Jolla, California 92037

Marilyn Gist Farquhar, Section of Cell Biology, Yale University School of Medicine, New Haven, Connecticut 06510

H. M. Fillit, The Rockefeller University, New York, New York 10021

Alfred J. Fish, Department of Pediatrics, University of Minnesota Medical School, Minneapolis, Minnesota 55455

G. J. Fleuren, Department of Pathology, State University, Groningen, 9713 EZ Groningen, The Netherlands.

Michael M. Frank, Laboratory of Clinical Investigation, National Institute of Allergy and Infectious Diseases, National Institutes of Health, Bethesda, Maryland 20205

J. Friedman, Departments of Pediatrics and Pathology, Harvard Medical School, Boston, Massachusetts 02115

Peter S. Friend, Balboa Internal Medicine Group, 306 Walnut Avenue, Suite 38, San Diego, California 92102

Richard J. Glassock, Division of Nephrology and Hypertension, Los Angeles County Harbor/UCLA Medical School, Torrance, California 90502

Ira Green, Section on Cellular Immunology, Arthritis and Rheumatism Branch, National Institute of Arthritis, Metabolism and Digestive and Kidney Diseases, National Institutes of Health, Bethesda, Maryland 20205

J. Grond, Department of Pathology, State University, Groningen, 9713 EZ Groningen, The Netherlands.

Fusao Hirata, Section on Cellular Immunology, Arthritis and Rheumatism Branch, National Institute of Arthritis, Metabolism and Digestive and Kidney Diseases, National Institutes of Health, Bethesda, Maryland 20205

P. J. Hoedemaeker, Department of Pathology, State University, Groningen, 9713 EZ Groningen, The Netherlands.

Phillip E. Hoffsten, Department of Internal Medicine, Washington University School of Medicine, St. Louis, Missouri 63110

Thomas H. Hostetter, Laboratory of Kidney and Electrolyte Physiology and Departments of Medicine, Brigham and Women's Hospital and Harvard Medical School, Boston, Massachusetts 02115

John R. Hoyer, Departments of Pediatrics and Pathology, Harvard Medical School, Boston, Massachusetts 02115

Yashpal S. Kanwar, Section of Cell Biology, Yale University School of Medicine, New Haven, Connecticut 06510

Morris J. Karnovsky, Department of Pathology, Harvard Medical School, Boston, Massachusetts 02115

W. Keane, Department of Medicine, University of Minnesota Medical School, Minneapolis, Minnesota 55455

Nicholas A. Kefalides, Connective Tissue Research Institute, University of Pennsylvania and The University City Science Center, Philadelphia, Pennsylvania 19104

David Koffler, Department of Pathology and Laboratory Medicine, Hahnemann Medical College and Hospital, Philadelphia, Pennsylvania 19102

Jeffrey I. Kreisberg, Department of Pathology, Harvard Medical School, Boston, Massachusetts 02115

Shinuchi Kumagai, Section on Cellular Immunology, Arthritis and Rheumatism Branch, National Institute of Arthritis, Metabolism and Digestive and Kidney Diseases, National Institutes of Health, Bethesda, Maryland 20205

Robert G. Lahita, The Rockefeller University, New York, New York 10021

Edmund J. Lewis, Department of Medicine, Rush Medical College, Rush–Presbyterian–St. Luke's Medical Center, Chicago, Illinois

Robert T. McCluskey, Departments of Pathology, Massachusetts General Hospital and Harvard Medical School, Boston, Massachusetts 02115

John J. McPhaul, Jr., Departments of Medicine and Pathology, University of Texas Southwestern Medical School, Dallas, Texas 75235

Mart Mannik, Department of Medicine, University of Washington, Seattle, Washington 98195

S. Michael Mauer, Department of Pediatrics, University of Minnesota Medical School, Minneapolis, Minnesota 55455

Alfred F. Michael, Department of Pediatrics, University of Minnesota Medical School, Minneapolis, Minnesota 55455

Felix Milgrom, Department of Microbiology, School of Medicine, State University of New York, Buffalo, New York

Thomas E. Miller, Department of Pathology and Laboratory Medicine, Hahnemann Medical College and Hospital, Philadelphia, Pennsylvania

W. R. Montgomery, Departments of Medicine, Wilford Hall USAF Medical Center, San Antonio, Texas 75235

Chicao Morimoto, Section on Cellular Immunology, Arthritis and Rheumatism Branch, National Institute of Arthritis, Metabolism and Digestive and Kidney Diseases, National Institutes of Health, Bethesda, Maryland 20205

Terry D. Oberley, Department of Pathology, University of Wisconsin Medical School, Madison, Wisconsin 53706

Bernard Pollara, New York State Kidney Disease Institute, Division of Laboratories and Research, New York State Department of Health, Albany, New York 12201, and Department of Pediatrics, Albany Medical College, Albany, New York, 12208

L. Raij, Department of Medicine, University of Minnesota Medical School, Minneapolis, Minnesota 55455

Helmut G. Rennke, Departments of Pathology, Brigham and Women's Hospital and Harvard Medical School, Boston, Massachusetts 02115

Susan D. Revak, Department of Immunopathology, Scripps Clinic and Research Foundation, La Jolla, California 92037

Jimmy L. Roberts, Department of Medicine, Rush Medical College, Rush–Presbyterian–St. Luke's Medical Center, Chicago, Illinois

Alan M. Robson, Edward Mallinckrodt Department of Pediatrics, Washington University School of Medicine, and Division of Nephrology, St. Louis Children's Hospital, St. Louis, Missouri 63178

Ulrich H. Rudofsky, New York State Kidney Disease Institute, Division of Laboratories and Research, New York State Department of Health, Albany, New York 12201

Tsuyoshi Sakane, Section on Cellular Immunology, Arthritis and Rheumatism Branch, National Institute of Arthritis, Metabolism and Digestive and Kidney Diseases, National Institutes of Health, Bethesda, Maryland 20205

David J. Salant, Evans Memorial Department of Clinical Research and Departments of Medicine and Pathology, Boston University Medical Center, Boston, Massachusetts 02118

Jon I. Scheinman, Department of Pediatrics, University of Minnesota Medical School, Minneapolis, Minnesota 55455

Mark S. Schiffer, Department of Pediatrics, University of Minnesota Medical School, Minneapolis, Minnesota 55455

George F. Schreiner, Departments of Pathology, Harvard Medical School and Brigham and Women's Hospital, Boston, Massachusetts 02115

Peter H. Schur, Division of Rheumatology and Immunology, Brigham and Women's Hospital, Harvard Medical School, Boston, Massachusetts 02115

Marcel W. Seiler, Departments of Pediatrics and Pathology, Harvard Medical School, Boston, Massachusetts 02115

J. Shorey, Department of Medicine, University of Texas Southwestern Medical School, Dallas, Texas 75235

Yigal Shvil, Department of Pediatrics, Hadassah Hospital, Jerusalem, Israel

Katherine A. Siminovitch, Section on Cellular Immunology, Arthritis and Rheumatism Branch, National Institute of Arthritis, Metabolism and

Digestive and Kidney Diseases, National Institutes of Health, Bethesda, Maryland 20205

Josef S. Smolen, Section on Cellular Immunology, Arthritis and Rheumatism Branch, National Institute of Arthritis, Metabolism and Digestive and Kidney Diseases, National Institutes of Health, Bethesda, Maryland 20205

J. F. Soothill, Institute for Child Health, London WC1N 1EH, England

Michael W. Steffes, Department of Laboratory Medicine and Pathology, University of Minnesota Medical School, Minneapolis, Minnesota 55455

Alfred D. Steinberg, Section on Cellular Immunology, Arthritis and Rheumatism Branch, National Institute of Arthritis, Metabolism and Digestive and Kidney Diseases, National Institutes of Health, Bethesda, Maryland 20205

Robert T. Steinberg, Section on Cellular Immunology, Arthritis and Rheumatism Branch, National Institute of Arthrits, Metabolism and Digestive and Kidney Diseases, National Institutes of Health, Bethesda, Maryland 20205

Magda M. Stilmant, Mallory Institute of Pathology, Boston City Hospital, Boston, Massachusetts 02118

Gary E. Striker, Department of Pathology, University of Washington, Seattle, Washington 98195

Norman Talal, Department of Medicine, University of Texas Health Sciences Center, San Antonio, Texas 78284

Eng M. Tan, Autoimmune Disease Center, Scripps Clinic and Research Foundation, La Jolla, California 92037

Emil R. Unanue, Departments of Pathology, Harvard Medical School and Peter Bent Brigham Hospital, Boston, Massachusetts 02115

Manjeri A. Venkatachalam, Department of Pathology, University of Texas Health Sciences Center, San Antonio, Texas 78284

H. Villarreal, Jr., The Rockefeller University, New York, New York 10021

J. J. Weening, Department of Pathology, State University, Groningen, 9713 EZ Groningen, The Netherlands

Roger C. Wiggins, Department of Immunopathology, Scripps Clinic and Research Foundation, La Jolla, California 92037

Curtis B. Wilson, Department of Immunopathology, Scripps Clinic and Research Foundation, La Jolla, California 92037

H. Alexander Wilson, Division of Immunology and Rheumatology, University of North Carolina, Chapel Hill, North Carolina 27514

John B. Winfield, Division of Immunology and Rheumatology, University of North Carolina, Chapel Hill, North Carolina 27514

Z. B. Zabriskie, The Rockefeller University, New York, New York 10021

Contents

Chapter 3

The Molecular Structure of Basement Membranes as It Relates to Function

Nicholas A. Kefalides

Chapter 4

Glomerular Basement Membrane Antigens

Alfred J. Fish, Kathleen M. Carmody, Mark S. Schiffer, and Alfred F. Michael

Chapter 5

Physiologic Approaches to the Mechanisms of Glomerular Immune Injury

Roland C. Blantz

Chapter 6

Physical Interactions between Macromolecules and the Glomerular Filter

Manjeri A. Venkatachalam and Helmut G. Rennke

Chapter 7

Pathologic and Functional Correlations in the Glomerulopathies

Alan M. Robson and Barbara R. Cole

Chapter 8

Glomerular Mesangium: Introductory Remarks

Alfred F. Michael and Yigal Shvil

Chapter 9

The Influence of Hemodynamic Factors upon Mesangial Kinetics of Macromolecules

L. Raij and W. Keane

Chapter 10

Deposition and Removal of Glomerular Immune Complexes: Relationships to the Mononuclear Phagocyte System

Mart Mannik and Gary E. Striker

Chapter 14

Culture of Human Glomerular Cells

Terry D. Oberley and Peter M. Burkholder

Chapter 15

Immunochemical and Biochemical Studies of Human Glomerular Cells in Culture

Jon I. Scheinman

Chapter 18

Autoimmune Disease Induced in Rabbits by Administration of Mercuric Chloride: Evidence Suggesting a Role for Antigens of the Connective Tissue Matrix

Boris Albini and Giuseppe Andres

Chapter 19

Experimental Autoimmune Renal Tubulointerstitial Disease

Ulrich H. Rudofsky and Bernard Pollara

Chapter 20

Experimental and Human Anti-Tubular Basement Membrane Nephritis

Robert T. McCluskey, Atul K. Bhan, and Robert B. Colvin

Chapter 21

Autoimmunity to Tamm–Horsfall Protein

John R. Hoyer, J. Friedman, and Marcel W. Seiler

Chapter 22

Renal Antigens in Experimental Immune Complex Glomerulonephritis

P. J. Hoedemaeker, J. J. Weening, J. Grond, W. W. Bakker, and G. J. Fleuren

Chapter 23

Mechanisms of Proteinuria Induced by Antikidney Antibodies in Noninflammatory Experimental Glomerulonephropathy

William G. Couser, David J. Salant, and Magda M. Stilmant

Chapter 24

The Pathogenesis of Autologous Immune Complex Glomerulonephritis in Rats

Christine K. Abrass, Wayne A. Border, and Richard J. Glassock

Chapter 25

Immunopathogenesis of Murine SLE

Frank J. Dixon

Chapter 26

Studies on Detection of Nephritogenic Immune Complexes

Felix Milgrom

Chapter 27

The Significance of Cryoimmunoglobulinemia in Immunologically Mediated Kidney Diseases

John J. McPhaul, Jr., W. R. Montgomery, and J. Shorey

Chapter 28

Relationship of Serum Cryoglobulins and Their Composition to Glomerulonephritis in Systemic Lupus Erythematosus

John B. Winfield and H. Alexander Wilson

Chapter 29

Cryoprecipitable Immunoglobulins with Native DNA Reactivity in the Glomerulopathies

Edmund J. Lewis and Jimmy L. Roberts

Chapter 30

The Role of Streptococcal and Glomerular Basement Membrane Antigens in Glomerulonephritis

H. M. Fillit, H. Villarreal, Jr., and J. B. Zabriskie

Chapter 31

The Contact (Hageman Factor) System in Inflammation

Charles G. Cochrane, Susan D. Revak, and Roger C. Wiggins

Chapter 32

The Function of the Reticuloendothelial System in Autoimmune Disease

Michael M. Frank

Chapter 33

A Role of Mononuclear Phagocytes in Immunologically Induced Glomerulonephritis

Emil R. Unanue, George F. Schreiner, and Ramzi S. Cotran

Chapter 34

Genetic Structure of the HLA Region and Implication for Function

Charles B. Carpenter

Chapter 35

Genetic Defects of the Complement Pathways: Relationship to HLA and Disease

Peter H. Schur

Chapter 36

Complement Abnormalities in Allergy and the Nephrotic Syndrome

J. F. Soothill

Chapter 37

Immunogenetic Aspects of Glomerulonephritis

Peter S. Friend

Chapter 38

Autoantibodies in Systemic Lupus Erythematosus

Eng M. Tan

Chapter 39

Serological Studies of Antibodies Reactive with RNA and RNA–Protein Antigens

David Koffler, Thomas E. Miller, and Robert G. Lahita

Chapter 40

Modulation of Autoimmunity by Sex Hormones

Norman Talal

Chapter 41

Thymic and T-Cell Function in Murine and Human Lupus

Marie-Anne Bach and Jean-Francois Bach

Chapter 42

Immune Regulatory Abnormalities in Systemic Lupus Erythematosus

Alfred D. Steinberg, Josef S. Smolen, Tsuyoshi Sakane, Shunichi Kumagai, Chicao Morimoto, Thomas M. Chused, Ira Green, Fusao Hirata, Katherine A. Siminovitch, and Robert T. Steinberg

1

Functional Organization of the Glomerulus: Presence of Glycosaminoglycans (Proteoglycans) in the Glomerular Basement Membrane

Marilyn Gist Farquhar and Yashpal S. Kanwar

1. Introduction

Since the first descriptions of the structural organization of glomerular capillaries with the electron microscope in the 1950s, scientists have struggled to understand the structural basis of glomerular filtration. They have attempted to relate the special fine-structural features of the glomerulus to its special filtration function. Similarly, since the original description of the characteristic patterns of changes in glomerular organization seen in various glomerular diseases, described at about the same period, scientists have struggled to understand the structural basis for the abnormal glomerular function found in these diseases. In spite of nearly 30 years of research on this topic, its understanding is still incomplete and relatively rudimentary. However, there has been continual progress in growth of understanding of these problems during that period.

This review assesses that progress indicating the current "state of the art " of the structural basis of glomerular filtration. The approach is to highlight what is known and what is till unknown—what is established and agreed upon, its supporting evidence, and, similarly, what is still unsettled, controversial, or tentative. Eight major summary points have been selected. The treatment will be brief since further discussion of the work cited can be found in the original references or in several recent reviews (Farquhar, 1975,

---

Marilyn Gist Farquhar and Yashpal S. Kanwar · Section of Cell Biology, Yale University School of Medicine, New Haven, Connecticut 06510. The original research summarized in this chapter was supported by NIAMDD Grant AM 17724 (to MGF).

1978, 1979). Other authors may have a slightly different perspective on these problems and this can be found in other contributions to this volume.

The points to be developed are as follows:

1. The structure of the glomerulus is unique among capillaries both in terms of the fine-structural organization of its layers (especially in the existence of foot processes and filtration slits) and in terms of its polarity—i.e., existence of axial and peripheral regions with different structural components.
2. The visceral epithelial cell is endowed with an unusually rich layer of cell surface sialoprotein known as "epithelial polyanion" and this is required for maintenance of the normal foot process and slit arrangement.
3. The glomerular basement membrane (GBM), not the epithelial slits, represents the main filter preventing passage of plasma proteins.
4. The GBM is most likely the structural equivalent of both the size and the charge barrier in the glomerulus.
5. The GBM contains anionic sites which are distinct from those on the surface of the adjoining endothelium and epithelium and which are concentrated in the lamina rara interna and externa.
6. Loss of epithelial polyanion had been shown to occur in several glomerular diseases. Recently, a partial loss of anionic sites from the GBM has also been demonstrated in aminonucleoside nephrosis.
7. The anionic sites in the laminae rarae of the GBM consist of a quasi-regular, lattice-like arrangement of proteoglycans rich in heparan sulfate.
8. The demonstration of sulfated glycosaminoglycans (GAGs) in the GBM provides another macromolecular component to be taken into consideration in explaining the permeability properties of the glomerulus and mechanisms of glomerular injury.

2. *Glomerular Capillary Organization Is Highly Specialized*

The glomerular capillary wall is stratified like other capillaries, but its structure is unique. It consists of three cellular layers: endothelium, epithelium, and mesangium, plus the acellular basement membrane (GBM). This point does not need to be developed since it is now well known and understood. The glomerular capillaries are polarized and their organization is such that the cell bodies of the endothelial cells and mesangial cells are concentrated axially. No cell bodies are seen along peripheral portions which face Bowman's capsule, and the mesangium is not represented peripherally. In diseased states, the mesangium can extend out to encircle the peripheral regions of the capillary for a variable distance, but normally the layers in the peripheral or filtration surface are limited to three: endothelium, basement membrane, and epithelium (Fig. 1). In these regions, the filtrate passes through the endothelial fenestrae, permeates the basement membrane, and passes through the filtration slits and slit membranes to reach the urinary

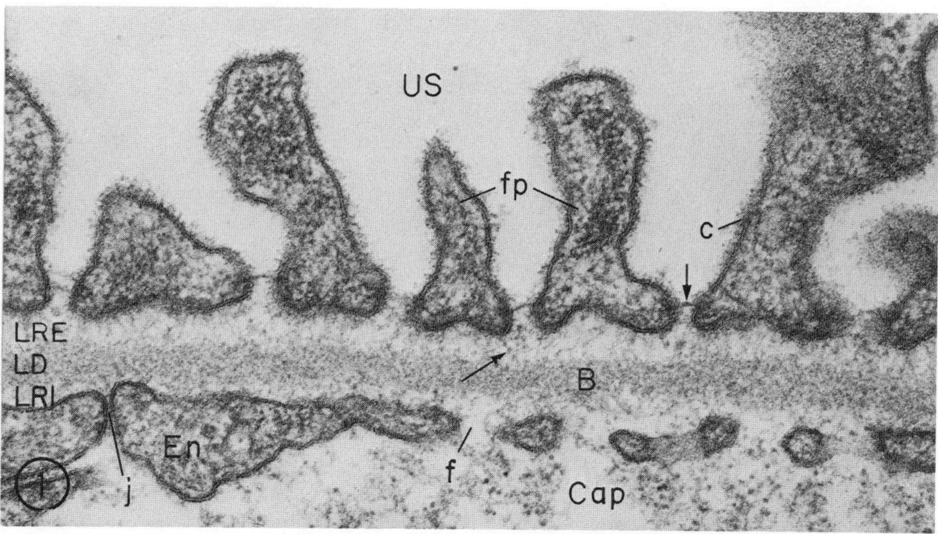

Figure 1. Portion of a glomerulus showing a peripheral region of a capillary loop cut in normal section. The filtration surface consists of the endothelium (En) with its open fenestrae (f) lacking diaphragms, the GBM (B), and the epithelial foot processes (fp) between which are the filtration slits bridged at their base by slit membranes (short arrow). Note that the GBM consists of three layers—a central dense layer, the lamina densa (LD), and two adjoining layers of lower density, the lamina rara interna (LRI) and externa (LRE). A thick cell coat (c) is visible on the membrane of the foot processes. The lamina densa is composed of a fine (~3 nm) filamentous meshwork and wispy filaments are seen extending from the lamina densa to the endothelial and epithelial (long arrow) membranes on either side. Cap, capillary lumen; US, urinary spaces; j, junction between two endothelial cells. × 80,000.

spaces which is the beginning of Bowman's space. Usually, it is assumed that normally the major portion of the filtrate is filtered through the periphery of the loops where the pathway is the shortest but it is clear that at least some of the filtrate must percolate through the mesangial regions before permeating the GBM and epithelial slits. However, there is no information available at present to indicate the precise amount that percolates through the mesangium either in the normal glomerulus or in diseased states. It can be anticipated that the ratio of the peripheral/axial filtrate flow can be affected by pathological alterations in other layers such as the frequency of the endothelial fenestrae, the porosity of the GBM, and especially the junctional arrangements present in the slits (see below). Whichever the route—peripheral or axial—the filtrate encounters only two morphologically continuous barriers during its passage—the GBM and the slit membrane which, therefore, become the only logical candidates for the location of the main barrier serving to retain plasma proteins in the circulation. The details of the organization of these layers are shown in the traditional cross-sectional view in Fig. 1, and in a less traditional, tangential or grazing section in Fig. 2. In such grazing sections, the components of the capillary wall can be seen *en face* which can be very instructive, particularly for delineating the layers of the GBM and defining their components (see Figs. 7, 9, and 28).

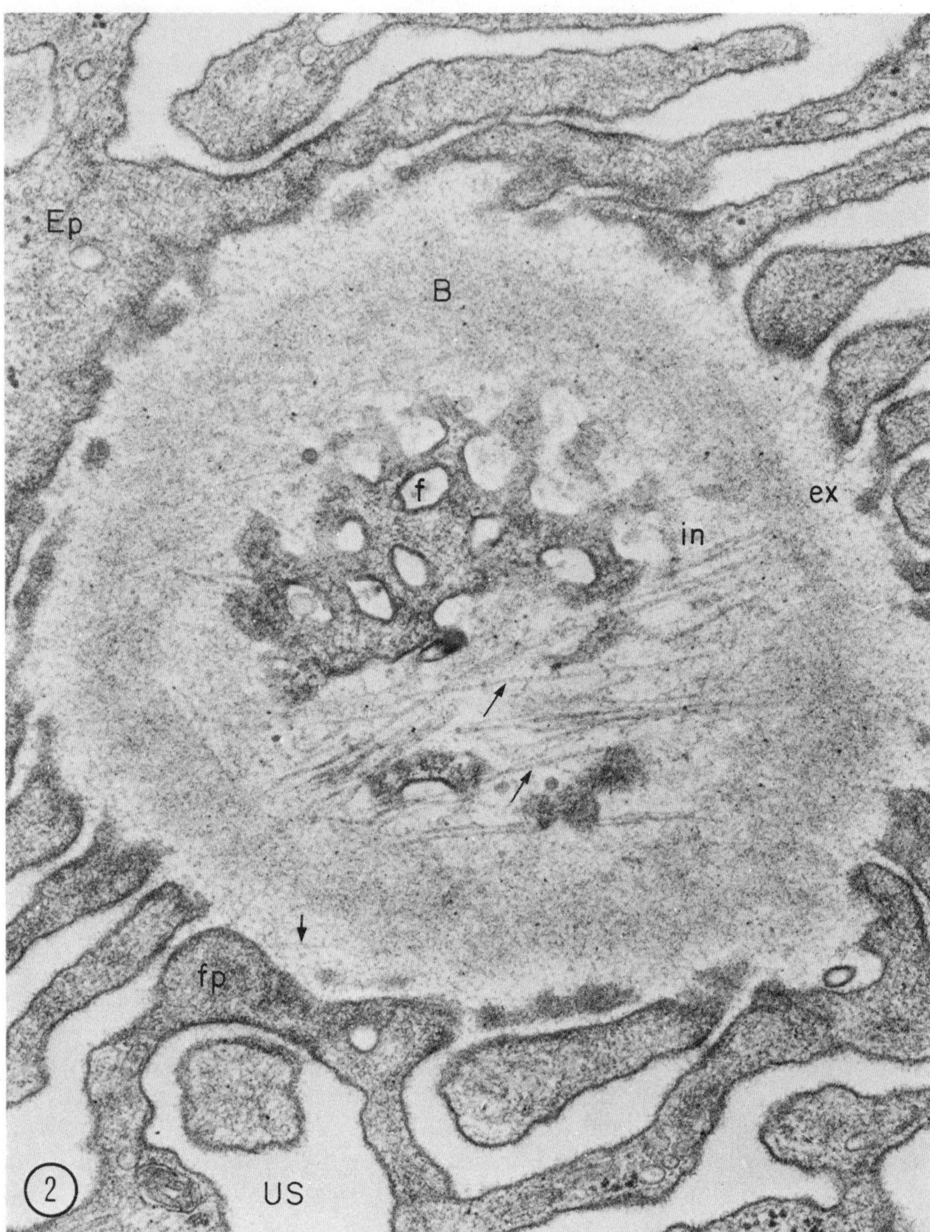

Figure 2. Small field from the periphery of another glomerular capillary loop cut in tangential section, showing the layers of the capillary wall partially *en face*. The endothelial fenestrae (f) appear as irregularly circular, open portholes, and the three layers of the GBM—the lamina densa (B), the LRI (in), and the LRE (ex)—are cut broadly. Two types of fibrils are visible in the basement membrane: (1) a fine (~3 nm) fibrillar meshwork which comprises the main component of the lamina densa (B) and extends across the LRE to the epithelial cell membrane (short arrow), and (2) large (10 nm) tubular fibrils (long arrows) which are located in the subendothelial space between the endothelium and the lamina densa. Ep, epithelium; fp, epithelial foot processes. × 56,000.

3. *Epithelial Polyanion Functions to Maintain Normal Foot Processes and Filtration Slits*

Another special feature of the glomerulus is the existence of a particularly thick cell coat, known as epithelial polyanion, on the plasma membrane of the epithelial cell. Practically all cells have such a sialic acid-rich, cell surface coat which can be stained with any one of a number of cationic dyes, among which the most frequently used are colloidal iron (Jones, 1969; Michael *et al.*, 1970) (Fig. 3), alcian blue (Behnke and Zelander, 1970), and ruthenium red (Latta *et al.*, 1975; Latta and Johnston, 1976). The cell coat of the glomerular epithelium is particularly lush. On a scale of one to four, it would rate + + + +, whereas that on the endothelium (Fig. 3) or on a red blood cell, for example, would rate only a + to + +. The staining of the cell coat

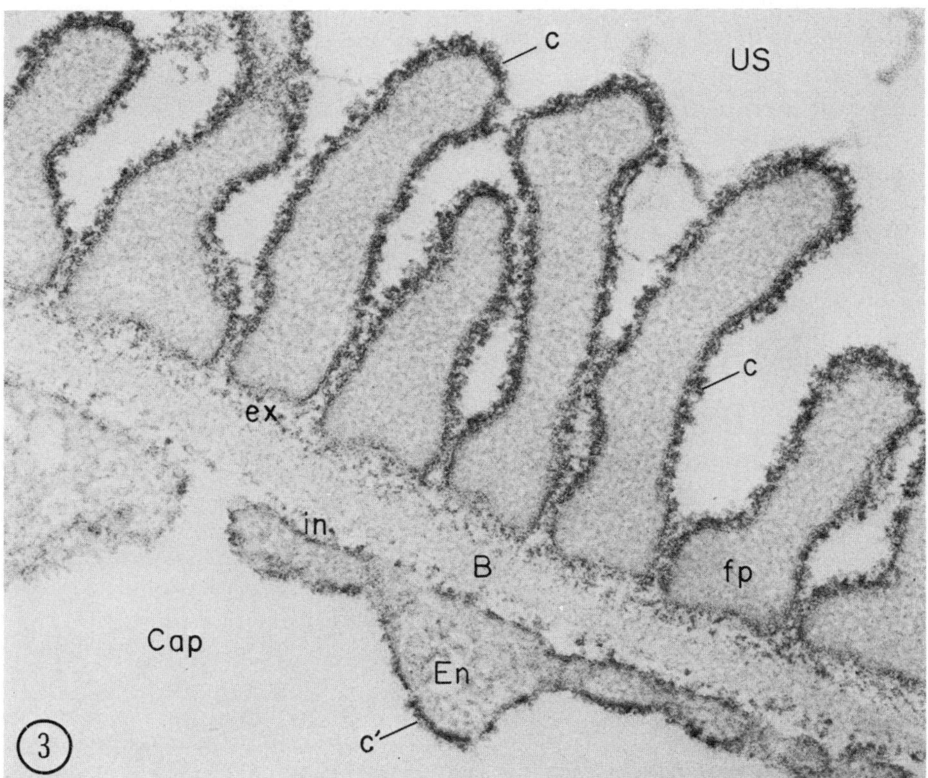

Figure 3. Portion of a glomerular capillary stained with colloidal iron (CI) (at pH 2.0) to demonstrate the epithelial polyanionic cell coat. It consists of a thick layer which stains with CI and is visible all along the cell membrane (c) lining the foot processes (fp) except at their base where the amount of CI deposited is much less. A similar but thinner CI-stained cell coat is also present along the endothelial surface (c′). These surface coats are known to be rich in sialic acid (presumably present in sialoproteins) because they are removed by neuraminidase treatment. Note also the presence of CI staining in the lamina rara interna (in) and externa (ex) of the GBM. Cap, capillary lumen; En, endothelium; US, urinary spaces. × 60,000. (From Farquhar, 1979.)

material, as demonstrated in colloidal iron preparations, appears to be due to the presence of sialic acid, since it is removed by neuraminidase digestion (Jones, 1969; Mohos and Skoza, 1969; Michael *et al.*, 1970). Sialoprotein is present all along the surface of the epithelial cell: on the cell body, the large cytoplasmic processes, and on the foot processes, but along the base of the latter where they face the GBM it is minimal or drastically reduced in amount (Fig. 3).

In regard to function, it is now clear that the presence of epithelial sialoprotein is required for maintenance of the normal foot process and slit arrangement. Concomitantly, loss of eipthelial polyanion leads to a loss of the epithelial foot processes, as shown some years ago in the case of aminonucleoside nephrosis (Michael *et al.*, 1970). The key experiments in demonstrating a direct association between the presence of the negatively charged cell surface polyanion and the maintenance of the normal foot process and slit arrangement were those of Seiler *et al.* (1977). These workers found that when the surface charge is neutralized by infusion of polycations (protamine sulfate, poly-L-lysine), the normal foot process organization is disturbed: there is retraction and flattening of foot processes, narrowing of filtration slits, and formation of occluding junctions between foot processes. Even more importantly, these investigators showed that this effect is reversed upon neutralization of the polycations by reperfusing the polyanion heparin. Therefore, the highly negatively charged, epithelial sialoprotein clearly is necessary for maintenance of the normal foot processes and slit architecture. So far there is a consistent correlation between circumstances in which staining is present and foot processes are normal, and conversely, between circumstances in which staining is missing and foot processes and slits are disturbed. It has been shown, for example, that during glomerular differentiation, initially the epithelium is not organized into foot processes, and no colloidal iron stainable material is present. Staining appears at exactly the same time as foot processes develop (Reeves *et al.*, 1978). It has also been shown (Andrews, 1978) that when glomeruli are placed in culture, the colloidal iron staining disappears along with the foot processes.

Except for its sialic acid content, there is no direct information concerning the chemical nature of the epithelial polyanion. However, extrapolation from what is known on other systems (e.g., the red blood cell, intestinal epithelium) concerning sialoproteins on the cell surface and maintenance of cell shape (Steck, 1974; Singer, 1974; Marchesi *et al.*, 1976), enables one to postulate that the sialic acid represents the peripheral hexoses of intrinsic membrane glycoproteins which completely span the epithelial cell membrane—so-called transmembrane proteins. In other systems, it is clear that such transmembrane proteins can stabilize cell architecture through interaction with other "extrinsic" proteins such as actin, spectrin, or tubulin, which are located on the inner or cytoplasmic membrane surfaces. It is of interest to note that neutralization of cell surface anions by exposure to polycations also has been shown to disrupt the specialized architecture of other epithelia (Quinton and Philpott, 1973).

It should be emphasized that the maintenance of the normal foot process and slit arrangement is the only function of the coat material which is widely accepted and is well-supported by experimental evidence among the various functions proposed for the epithelial polyanion. A direct role for the epithelial polyanion in glomerular filtration of anionic molecules frequently has been postulated (Michael *et al.*, 1970; Mohos and Skoza, 1969; Brenner *et al.*, 1977, 1978) and could be valid but has yet to be directly demonstrated experimentally as will be discussed below.

4. *Epithelial Slits Effectively Ruled Out as the Main Filtration Barrier*

There is now converging evidence from a variety of sources indicating that the GBM, rather than the epithelial slits or slit membranes, constitutes the main filtration barrier serving to retain plasma proteins in the circulation. Although the identity of the filter has been controversial in the past, all groups actively working in this field agree at present that the epithelial slits do not function in this capacity (Farquhar, 1975, 1978, 1979; Rennke *et al.*, 1975; Ryan and Karnovsky, 1976; Latta and Johnston, 1976; Laliberté *et al.*, 1978). The reason for the unanimity on this point at present is that if only results obtained with anionic or neutral tracers of a size equal to or greater than that of albumin are considered and results obtained with positively charged tracers and neutral and anionic tracers of small size are set aside, the data are quite clear and remarkably consistent. In all cases, a sharp drop in the concentration of the tracer is seen along the inner or luminal surface of the GBM, and the tracer fails to penetrate to any great extent beyond the inner, lighter layer of the GBM, the lamina rara interna (LRI). Concomitantly, there is no evidence for retention of any anionic or neutral tracer by the slits or slit membranes. A typical finding is shown in Figs. 4 and 5 for dextran, but the same result applies to a variety of particulate tracers, e.g., ferritin, colloidal gold, thorotrast, and saccharated iron oxide (cf. Farquhar, 1975); to the peroxidatic tracer, catalase (Ryan *et al.*, 1976), which is the only peroxidatic tracer used so far with an isoelectric point <7.0; and to endogenous albumin (Ryan and Karnovsky, 1976) and endogenous IgG (Ryan *et al.*, 1976; Laliberté *et al.*, 1978) localized by immunocytochemistry.

To clarify this point further, the results obtained with electron-dense tracers must be put into historical perspective briefly (see Farquhar, 1978, 1979, for detailed reviews). The first tracer studies, carried out between 1960 and 1966, clearly pointed to the GBM as the main barrier, since it was found that the tracers used (mostly particulate tracers of large size which were either anionic or neutral in charge) did not penetrate to any great extent beyond the inner, less dense region of the GBM or LRI; moreover, these tracers gradually accumulated against the luminal surface of the GBM, expecially in the mesangial regions, and were eventually taken up and disposed of by mesangial cells. In 1966, Graham and Karnovsky used

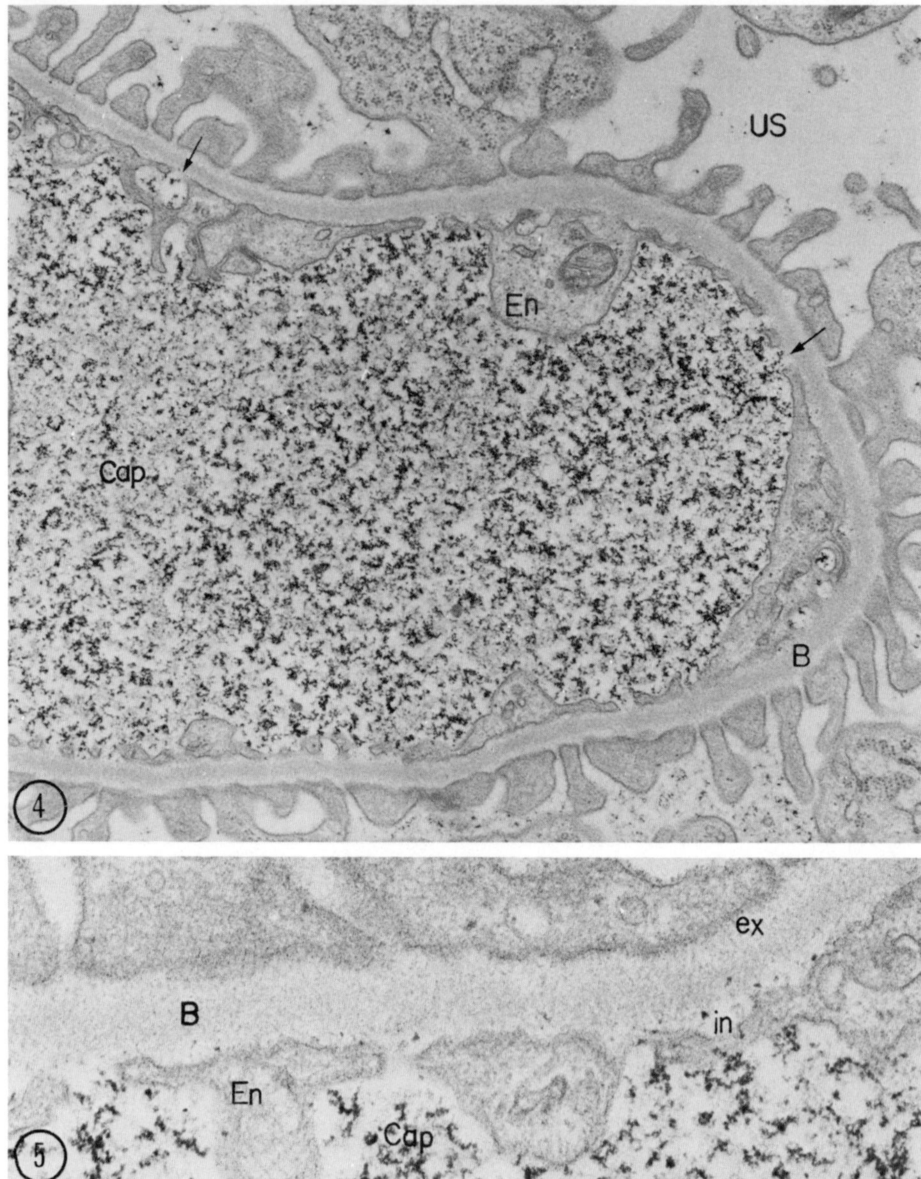

Figures 4 and 5. Portions of a glomerulus from a normal rat sacrificed 3 1/2 hr after the injection of 125,000-MW dextran. The capillary lumina (Cap) are filled with dense-staining dextran particles which appear irregularly aggregated. Particles appear to penetrate the fenestrae of the endothelium (En) (arrows) and can be seen in the lamina rara interna (in) of the GBM. No dextran is seen in the lamina densa (B), the lamina rara externa (ex), or the epithelial slits. Figure 4, × 22,000; Fig. 5, × 87,000. (Figure 4 is from Farquhar, 1979; Fig. 5 is from Caulfield and Farquhar, 1974.)

peroxidatic tracers in an attempt to identify the main glomerular filter and obtained different findings. They observed that these tracers were most concentrated between the GBM and epithelium, i.e., in the lamina rara externa (LRE) and in the filtration slits up to the level of the slit membranes. Based on such images, these workers hypothesized that the GBM acts only as a crude prefilter for large macromolecules, whereas the slits act as the final, fine filter retaining albumin. Data obtained with other peroxidatic tracers were interpreted as corroborating this hypothesis (Karnovsky and Ainsworth, 1973). It is now evident: (1) that the results obtained with peroxidatic tracers were misleading because all of the tracers used (with the exception of catalase) have a net positive charge (pI > 7.0); and (2) that the findings obtained, rather than indicating a restrictive barrier at the level of the slits, were due to binding of cationic tracers to anionic sites on the epithelial cell coat and GBM. This conclusion is supported by the fact that identical results in terms of tracer distribution were obtained with cationic tracers of low molecular weight—such as lysozyme (Caulfied, 1978; Caulfield and Farquhar, 1976) and cationized cytochrome *c* (Kerjaschki *et al.*, 1978), which are small enough in size to be filtered freely. The most informative results were those obtained with lysozyme which originally was infused to test the idea that cationic proteins can bind to the epithelium. Lysozyme was selected as the test protein because of its high net positive charge (pI = 11.0) and small size (MW = 14,000). Because of its small size, it would be expected to be filtered freely so that any accumulation in the glomerulus would be suspected to be due to charge interaction. It proved to bind avidly to the epithelial cell coat (Fig. 6) as well as to sites in the GBM (see below) and to produce images similar to those obtained by Graham and Karnovsky (1966) with peroxidatic tracers, particularly myeloperoxidase (pI = 10.0; MW = 160,000). The lysozyme binding pattern was similar in both fixed and unfixed glomeruli (Caulfield and Farquhar, 1976), and also resembled the staining pattern found in fixed tissues with colloidal iron. That the binding of lysozyme to glomerular components is due to charge interaction was demonstrated conclusively by the following: the lysozyme remained bound when kidney was flushed extensively with saline, binding occurred when isolated glomeruli were incubated with lysozyme, and especially by the fact that when the pI of the lysozyme was modified (by succinylation) to make it anionic, binding no longer occurred (Caulfield and Farquhar, 1976). We and others have found subsequently that virtually any basic protein or dye when administered *in vivo* or perfused *in vitro* will bind to glomerular components. Hence, basic probes are not satisfactory to use as tracers in studies of glomerular permeability since, when they are used, one cannot distinguish between retention due to electrostatic binding to anionic sites and retention due to their size being larger than that of the "pores." However, because of their ability to interact with negatively charged structures, basic dyes and proteins are useful as "stains" for investigating the distribution of anionic sites in the glomerulus, especially those in the GBM, and this laboratory has subsequently used them for this purpose (see below).

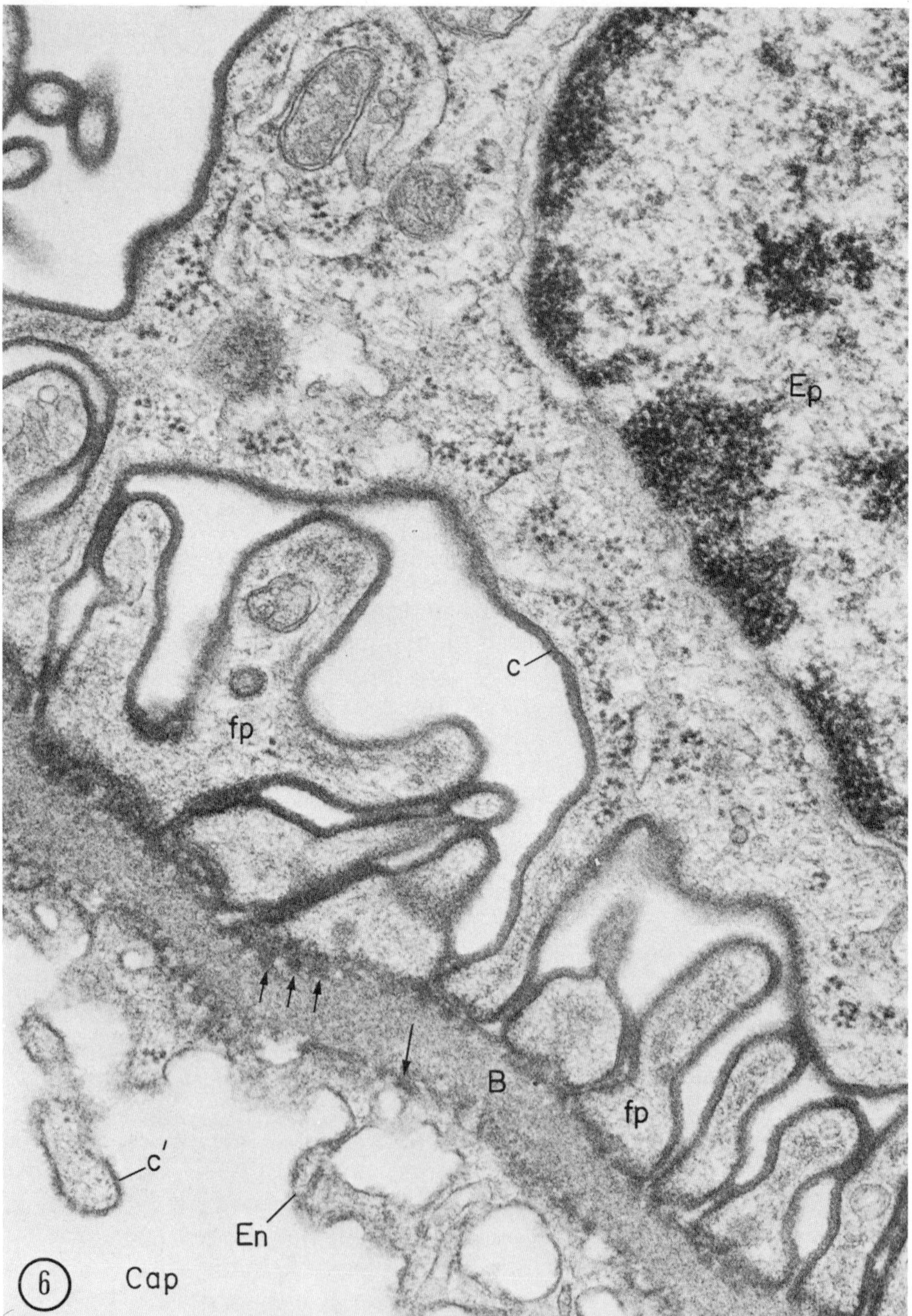

Figure 6. Field from the glomerulus of a normal rat perfused with lysozyme, a highly cationic protein (pI = 11.0). The membrane of the epithelial cell (Ep) is outlined by a thick, dense-staining layer of bound lysozyme. Both those portions of the cell membrane surrounding the epithelial cell body (c) and those surrounding the foot processes (fp) are outlined. The staining

To summarize, data obtained with anionic and neutral tracers are remarkably consistent in that in all cases, restriction of the tracer occurs at the level of the GBM, and there is no evidence of any restriction along the slit membrane. The assumption that the slits represent a barrier more restrictive than the GBM was based on observations using cationic proteins as tracers in which the results obtained were due to electrostatic interaction between the positively charged tracer and the negatively charged structures in the capillary wall.

5. *The GBM Is Both the Size-Selective and the Charge-Selective Barrier in the Glomerulus*

Evidence for this statement is provided by the accumulated tracer data summarized above which demonstrated that all anionic and neutral tracers of the size of albumin or larger fail to penetrate beyond the LRI in significant amounts. The most direct evidence for the GBM as the size-selective barrier comes from the results obtained with neutral dextrans (Caulfield and Farquhar, 1974). These results demonstrated that the GBM serves as the main barrier to dextran molecules over a wide size range (MW = 30,000 to 125,000) since in all cases there was a sharp drop in dextran concentration at the level of the LRI and no accumulation of dextran of any size in the slits or against the slit membranes (Figs. 4 and 5). Since the dextran fractions used were neutral molecules of identical composition varying only in size, variations in behavior of these probe molecules based on other properties (differences in molecular charge, shape, or chemical composition) were eliminated.

The most direct evidence for the GBM as the charge-selective barrier comes from the work of Rennke *et al.* (1975) with differently charged ferritins. These investigators cationized ferritin and produced a number of different ferritin fractions with different isoelectric points (up to 9.0). They found that the permeability of the ferritin to the GBM increases the greater the net charge of the ferritin. Whereas native anionic ferritin (pI = 4.8) fails to penetrate beyond the LRI (Farquhar *et al.*, 1961), cationic ferritin penetrated the GBM in greatly increased amounts. These experiments demonstrated directly: (1) that the charge of a molecule affects its filtration behavior, and (2) that the GBM represents the charge-selective barrier. Since only the charge of the ferritin was altered, differences in behavior of the tracer due to differences in size or molecular configuration were ruled out in these experiments.

---

results from the binding of this basic protein to the highly negatively charged epithelial cell coat. Binding also occurs to the endothelial cell coat (c′) and to the lamina rara interna (long arrow) and externa (short arrows) of the GBM which appear denser than the lamina densa (B). In a few places, the binding sites in the LRE (short arrows) show a regular repeating pattern. × 50,000. (From Caulfield and Farquhar, 1978.)

Another graphic way to directly visualize the barrier function of the GBM is in the acellular perfused kidney preparations of Brendel *et al.* (1978). These workers prepared (by perfusion with detergent) tubes of basement membrane denuded of cells and infused native ferritin. In these preparations in which all the cells were detached, the ferritin can be seen filling the lumen, most of it retained by the GBM.

To conclude that the GBM is the main glomerular filter is not meant to imply that a host of other factors, e.g., glomerular pressure and flow, the composition of the plasma, and the composition of the adjacent cellular layers, cannot modify the behavior of the filter. Of course the layers before and after the filter *can* and *must* play a role in modulating, modifying, and maintaining the filter just as they do in artificial or model membrane systems. In particular, the number of both the endothelial fenestrae* and the epithelial slits would be expected to modify hydraulic fluxes across the glomerulus. (Caulfield and Farquhar, 1975, for further discussion of this point.)† It is also important to keep in mind that in the glomerulus, just as in model systems, there must be a *main* filter. Whether one puts the emphasis on the main role of the GBM as the filter or on the modulating role of the adjacent cellular layers, the conclusion is inescapable that normal filtration behavior requires a normally functioning basement membrane. Conversely, changes in GBM composition and organization can be expected to result in alterations in normal filtration functions.

6. Distinction between Anionic Sites in the GBM and Those on Cell Surfaces

Recent work from this laboratory has demonstrated that the GBM contains anionic sites which can be distinguished from those on the endothelium and epithelium. They are concentrated in the laminae rarae and have a different organization and a different chemical composition (see below) than those on the endothelial and epithelial cell membranes. The first clear indication of the existence of regular organized sites in the laminae rarae of the GBM came from the work done using lysozyme as a cationic stain in which it was found that lysozyme bound not only to the epithelial and endothelial cell coats, but to distinct sites in the laminae rarae of the GBM as well (Caulfield and Farquhar, 1976, 1978). When viewed in normal

* The endothelium probably acts as a "valve" which controls access to the filter by variations in the number and size of its fenestrae (cf. Farquhar, 1978).

† The arrangement of the GBM and associated structures was likened to that of an artificial ultrafiltration membrane composed of a thin membrane which accounts for selective permeability and a "porous support' on which the thin membrane rests. The porous support functions to strengthen the thinner membrane, to increase the effective path length across it, and to limit hydraulic fluxes across the system by reducing the radius or the frequency of the pores in the support. By analogy with a porous support, the epithelium may limit hydraulic fluxes across the glomerular capillary wall as a result of the distribution and width of the filtration slits.

sections, the lysozyme binding showed a regular repeating pattern in both LRI and LRE (Fig. 6). In grazing sections, it took on a discrete reticular pattern (Fig. 7) which was evident in both the laminae rarae but was more prominent and more frequently visualized in the LRE.

More recently, cationized ferritin (CF) and ruthenium red (RR) have been used as cationic probes to further characterize the GBM sites (Kanwar and Farquhar, 1978a, 1979a). A number of CF fractions of narrow pI range were prepared. The most useful proved to be those with a pI of 7.3–7.5.

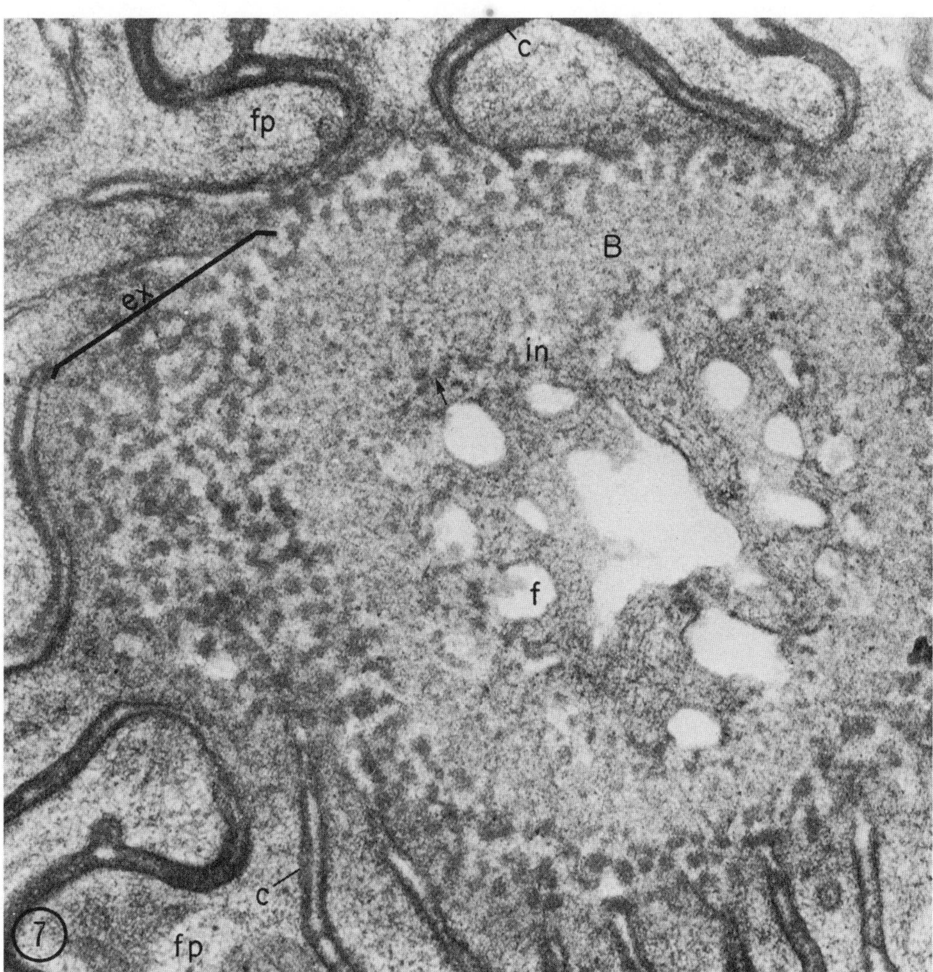

Figure 7. Tangential section through a glomerular capillary from a normal rat perfused with lysozyme. The section grazes through the GBM and shows to better advantage the pattern created by the binding of lysozyme to anionic sites in the lamina rara interna (in) and externa (ex). The sites of heavy binding have a reticular pattern which is particularly striking in the LRE (ex). Lysozyme also binds to the cell membrane (c) lining the epithelial foot processes (fp). f, endothelial fenestrae; B, lamina densa. × 60,000. (From Caulfield and Farquhar, 1978.)

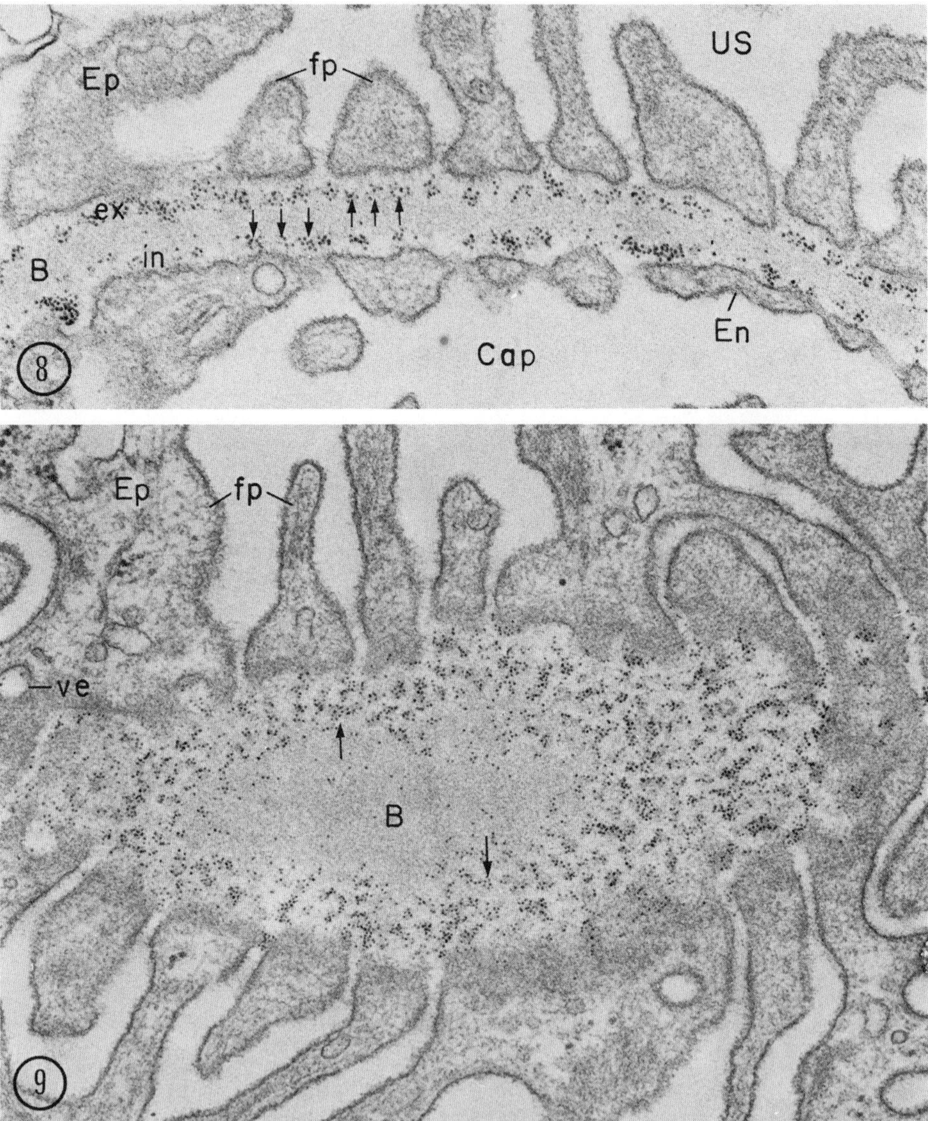

Figures 8 and 9. Figure 8 shows a portion of a peripheral region of a glomerular capillary from a rat given cationized ferritin (pI = 7.3–7.5) by i.v. injection, after which the kidney was briefly flushed with saline and fixed by aldehyde perfusion. CF binds to anionic sites in the lamina rara interna (in) and externa (ex) of the GBM where it is distributed in discrete clusters located at regular ~60-nm intervals (arrows). A few molecules are seen scattered in the lamina densa (B). Note that the CF binds only to the GBM and that no CF is seen binding to the endothelium (En) or epithelium (Ep). Figure 9 shows a grazing section of the same glomerulus as that in Fig. 8, illustrating the reticular pattern of distribution of CF molecules in the LRE (arrows). Very few CF molecules are present in the lamina densa (B), and no binding to the epithelium (Ep) is seen. Several CF molecules are present in a pinocytotic vesicle (ve) in the epithelium. No regular relationship between the clusters of CF molecules and the epithelial slits between the foot processes (fp) is evident: a few slits contain CF aggregates (lower left), a few are free of CF, and a few contain CF at low concentration. Figure 8, × 80,000; Fig. 9, × 60,000. (From Kanwar and Farquhar, 1979a.)

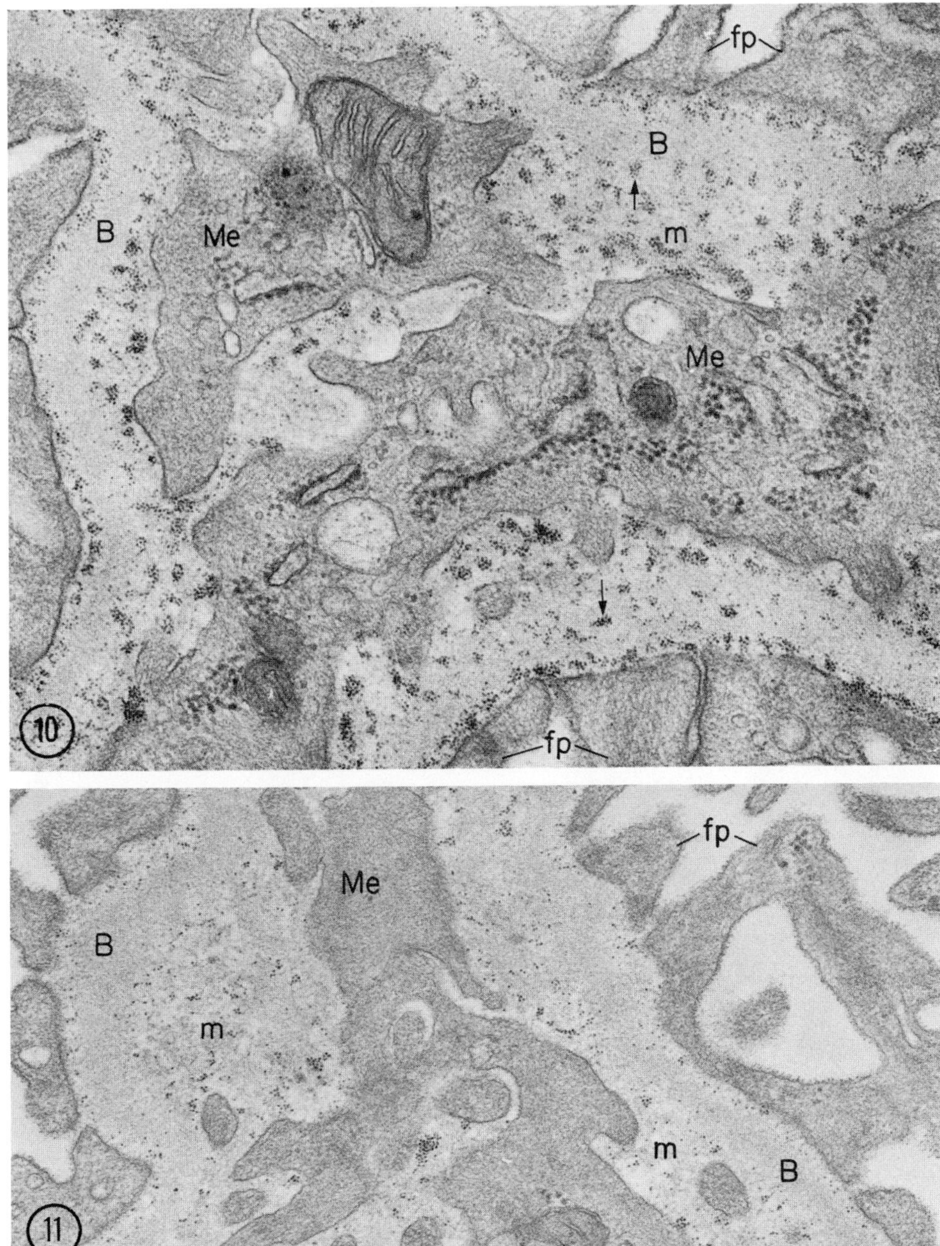

Figures 10 and 11. Figure 10, which is from the mesangial region of a glomerulus from an animal given CF, illustrates CF binding (arrows) to sites in the mesangial matrix (m) between the mesangial cells (Me) and the basement membrane (B) (as well as to sites in the laminae rarae of the GBM). Figure 11 is a field similar to that in Fig. 10 showing part of a glomerulus from a rat given CF followed by kidney perfusion with 0.3 M KCl (as in Fig. 15). Note the reduction in CF binding from anionic sites in the mesangial matrix (m) between the mesangial cells (Me) and the GBM (B) as well as from the laminae rarae after perfusion with buffer of high ionic strength. × 60,000. (From Kanwar and Farquhar, 1979a.)

When such preparations are given *in vivo* (by intravenous injection), CF molecules bind to sites in the GBM (Figs. 8 and 9) and in the mesangial matrix (Fig. 10), but they do not bind to the surfaces of the endothelial cells and circulating blood cells. In normal section (Fig. 8), the CF is seen to be distributed in clusters at regular (60-nm center-to-center spacing) intervals. In grazing section (Fig. 9), the CF is distributed in a reticular pattern similar to that found with lysozyme. Thus, this CF preparation (pI 7.3–7.5) proved to be very useful for studying GBM sites without the complication of background staining due to binding to cell surfaces. CF fractions with a pI > 7.5 were not useful for this purpose since they bind to anionic sites on the surfaces of red blood cells, endothelium, and platelets, forming aggregates which plug the endothelial fenestrae (Fig. 12) and lead to thrombus formation. The fact that CF with a pI of 7.3–7.5 binds to sites in the GBM and not to the cells, indicates that the charge density of the GBM sites is greater than that of the sites on cell surfaces. That binding of CF to the GBM is electrostatic in nature is shown by the fact that it is displaced by treatment (either *in vivo* or *in vitro*) with buffers of high ionic strength or pH (Figs. 11

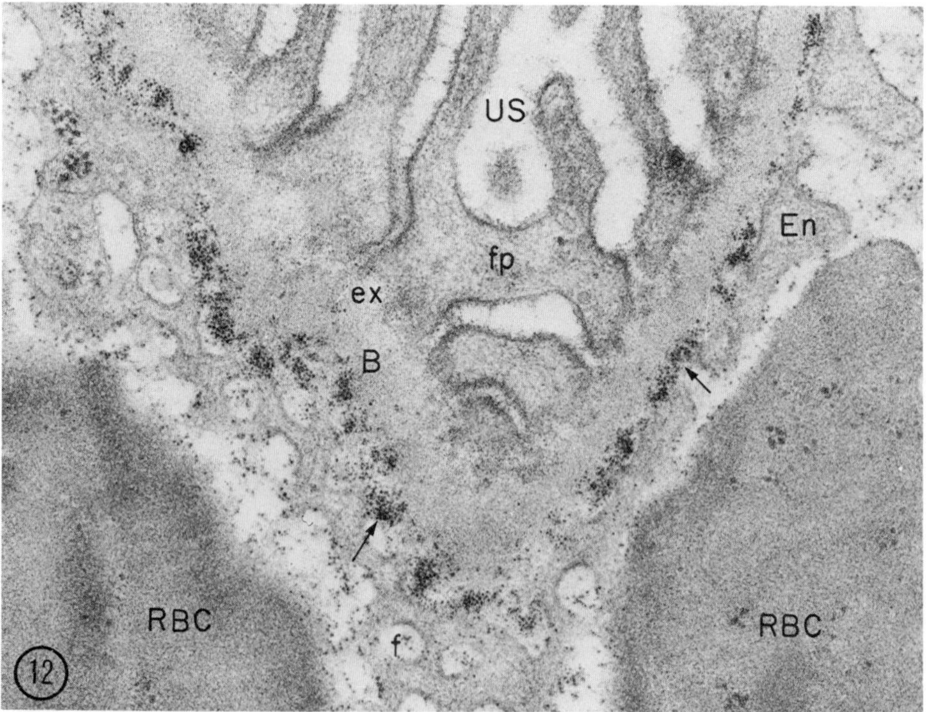

Figure 12. Glomerular capillary from an animal injected *in vivo* with CF (pI > 7.9). This CF is not satisfactory for use as a cationic probe to demonstrate anionic sites in the GBM because (1) CF molecules aggregate into clusters which are concentrated in the LRI (arrows); (2) CF molecules stick to the surface of endothelial cells (En) and red blood cells (RBC); and (3) in contrast to the findings with CF of lower pI (7.3–7.5) shown in Figs. 8 and 9, very few CF molecules are seen in the LRE (ex). × 56,000.

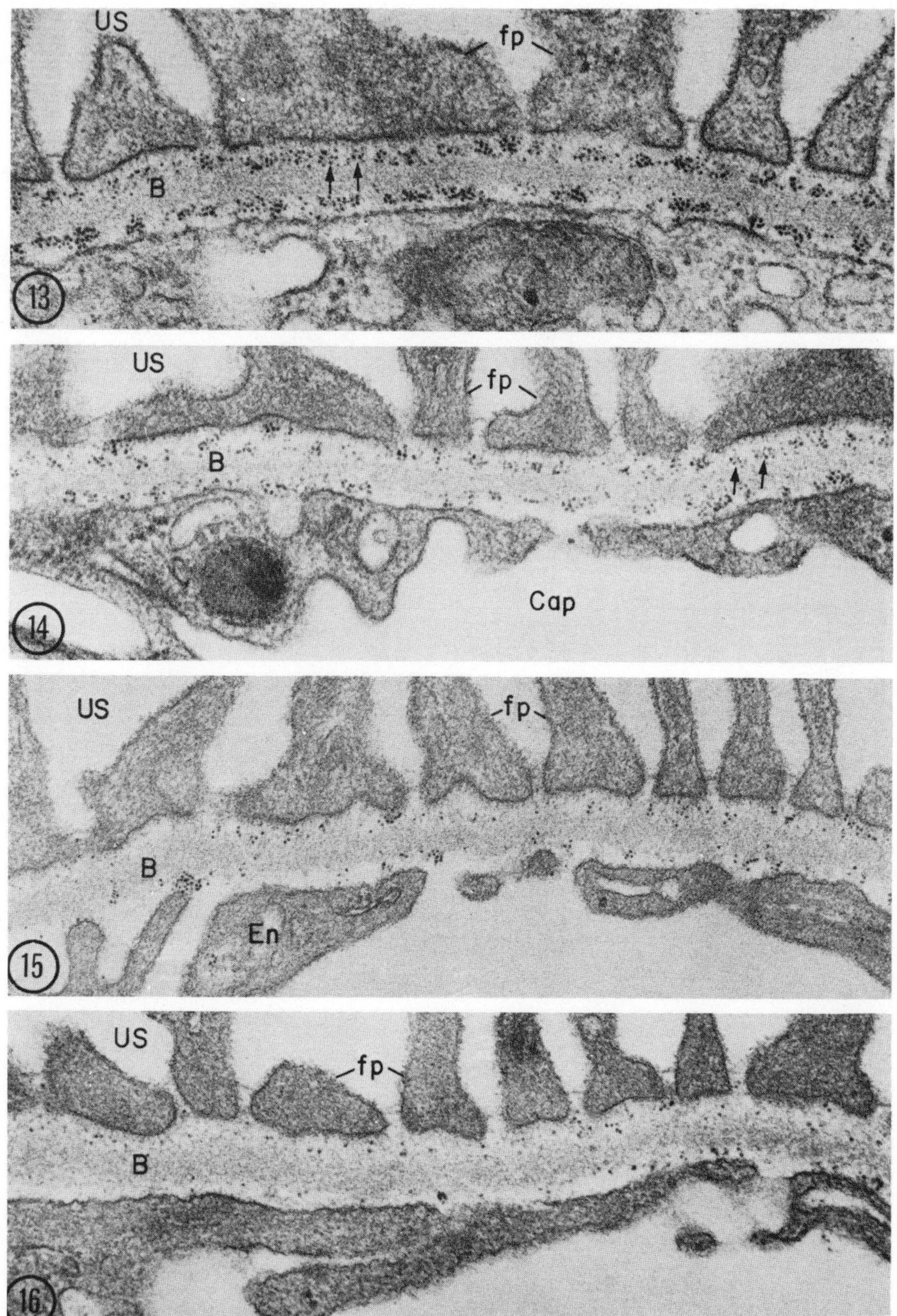

Figures 13–16. Portions of glomerular capillaries from the kidneys of rats which were injected i.v. with CF followed by perfusion of the kidney with 0.05 M Tris buffer (pH 7.4) containing varying concentrations of KCl. After perfusion with 0.1 M (Fig. 13) or 0.2 M (Fig. 14) KCl, most of the CF molecules remain bound to the sites in the LRI and LRE (arrows). However, binding is reduced and largely lost after perfusion with 0.3 M (Fig. 15) or 0.4 M (Fig. 16) KCl. × 80,000. (From Kanwar and Farquhar, 1979a.)

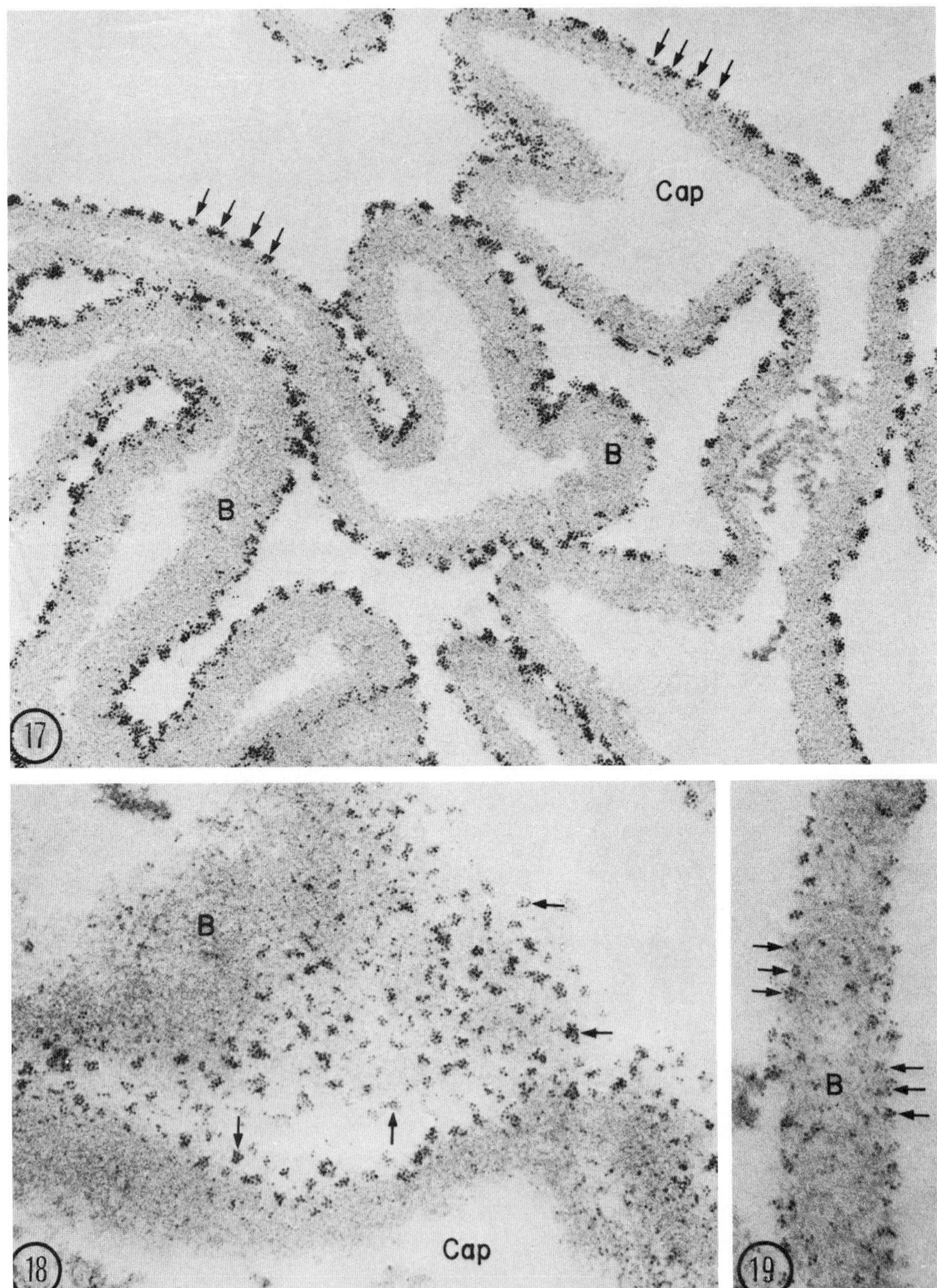

Figures 17–19. Portions of isolated GBMs incubated with CF (pI = 7.3–7.5). Figure 17 shows several loops of intact, isolated GBM (B), demonstrating the binding of CF to the LRE in the same regular pattern as in the intact glomerulus (Fig. 8). CF molecules are located in clusters at regular (~60 nm) intervals on the outer GBM surface (arrows). CF is not seen binding to the LRI or the inside of basement membrane presumably because it does not penetrate the intact loops. Figure 18 is a grazing section through an intact isolated GBM loop showing the regular

and 13–16). CF binding can be demonstrated not only *in vivo*, but also *in vitro* in isolated GBMs (Figs. 17–19) where the binding pattern is identical (clustered at 60-nm intervals) to that seen *in situ*.

The demonstration of the existence of anionic sites in the laminae rarae of the GBM raises the possibility that these sites may contribute to the charge barrier function of the GBM, a possibility that is discussed further below.

7. *Anionic Sites Are Lost from the GBM as well as the Epithelium in Aminonucleoside Nephrosis*

It has been assumed frequently in the past that the epithelial polyanion is responsible for maintaining the glomerular charge barrier function because loss of colloidal iron staining occurs in certain experimental glomerular diseases, such as aminonucleoside nephrosis (Michael *et al.*, 1970) and nephrotoxic serum nephritis (Brenner *et al.*, 1977, 1978) associated with proteinuria. However, at present, this possibility appears unlikely because of the lack of any evidence, based on tracer data, for the existence of any restrictive barrier functioning at the level of the epithelial slits. It seems more likely that the epithelial polyanion has other functions, among which the best established is its role in maintaining normal epithelial architecture as discussed extensively above.

Based on the tracer data summarized above, it would be expected that anionic sites in the GBM are responsible for creation of the charge barrier and, concomitantly, that a loss of anionic sites form the GBM would be expected to occur in renal diseases in which there is proteinuria associated with a loss of the charge barrier function. It is of interest that using lysozyme, a partial loss of anionic sites from the GBM (as well as the well-known loss from the epithelium) recently has been found to occur in aminonucleoside nephrosis (Caulfield and Farquhar, 1978), a disease in which a partial loss of the glomerular charge barrier has been demonstrated both by clearance data (Bohrer *et al.*, 1977) and by tracer studies with native ferritin (Farquhar and Palade, 1961) and catalase (Venkatachalam *et al.*, 1970). This loss of anionic sites from the GBM is manifest as a progressive loss of lysozyme binding to the discrete sites in the laminae rarae. Early in the course of the disease (after 6–8 daily injections), the binding of lysozyme to both the epithelial cell coat and the GBM was reduced. Interruptions and irregularities in the usual binding pattern in the laminae rarae were observed (Figs. 20–22). Later on in the disease (after 9–11 days), lysozyme no longer bound to the epithelium or GBM in most animals (Fig. 23). It should be emphasized

---

pattern of distribution of CF molecules (arrows) which occur in clusters at a distance of ~60 nm (av.) from one another. Figure 19 shows a piece of isolated GBM from a preparation which was subjected to sonication prior to incubation with CF to disrupt the intact loops into short segments. Clusters of CF molecules (arrows) can be seen on both sides of the GBM (B) corresponding to the LRI and LRE. Cap, former capillary lumen. Figures 17 and 18, × 60,000; Fig. 19, × 80,000. (From Kanwar and Farquhar, 1979a.)

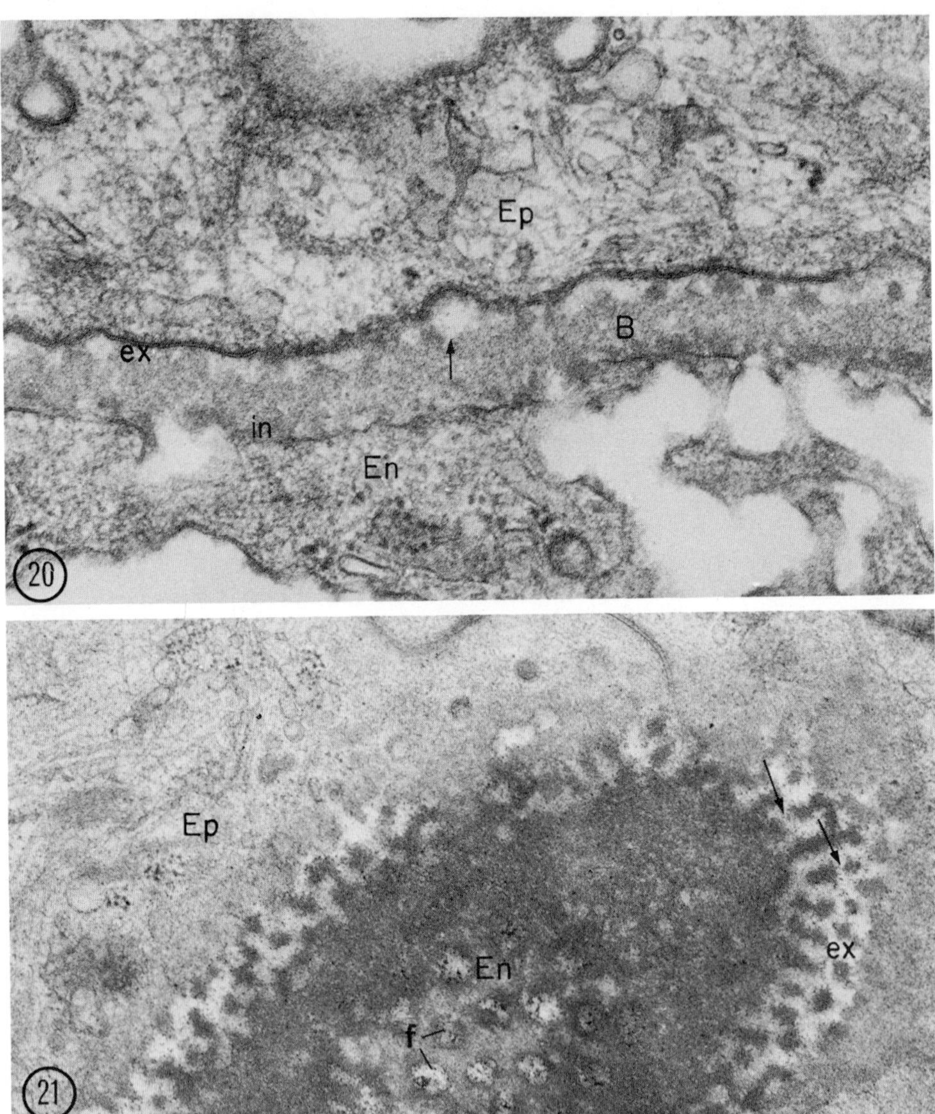

Figures 20 and 21. Figure 20 is a normal section and Fig. 21 is a grazing section of a glomerular capillary from an 8-day nephrotic rat perfused with lysozyme. The pattern of binding to the LRI (in) and LRE (ex) is altered in that the number and distribution of dense deposits appears decreased and more irregular. (Compare with Figs. 6 and 7 from control rats.) In Fig. 21, it can be seen that the usual reticular pattern in the LRE (ex) is disturbed since more of the sites of heavy binding are unconnected (arrows). × 75,000. (From Caulfield and Farquhar, 1978.)

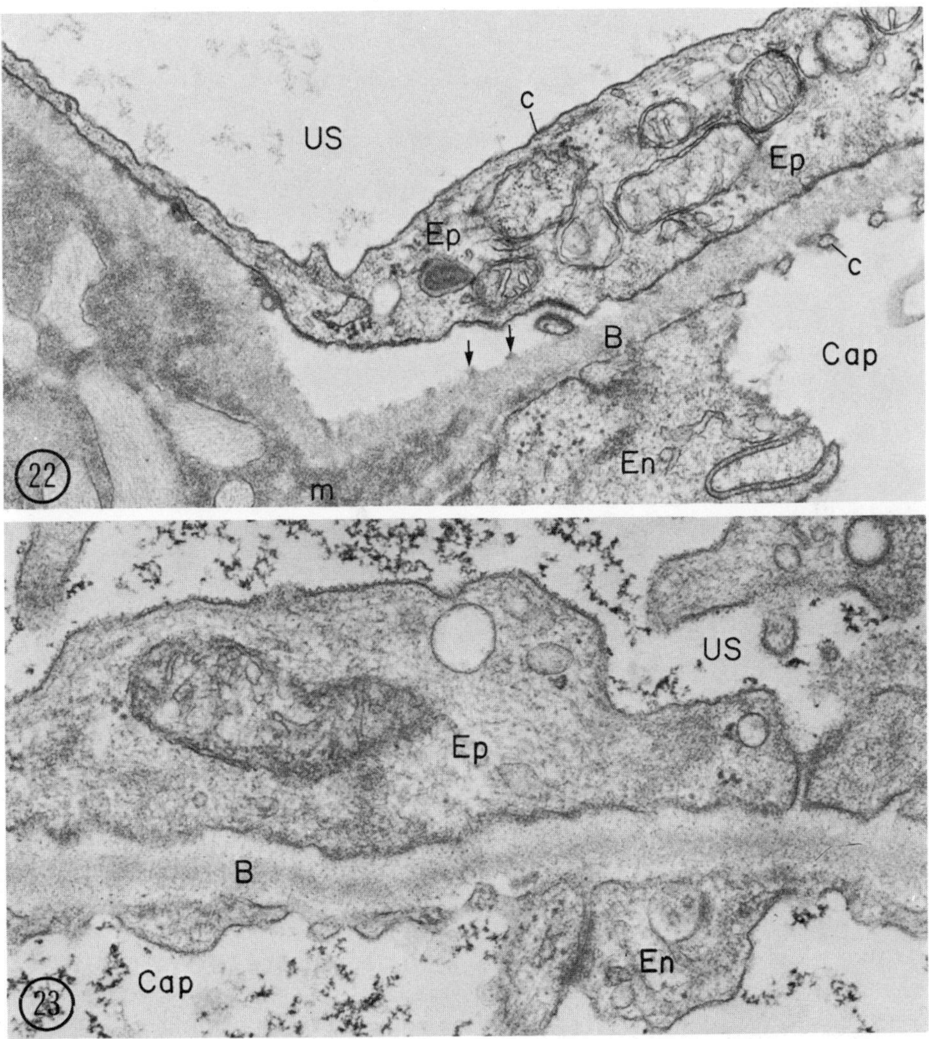

Figures 22 and 23. Figure 22 is another field from the glomerulus of an 8-day nephrotic rat perfused with lysozyme showing a region where the epithelium (Ep) has become detached from the GBM. There is still some binding of lysozyme to the anionic sites in the laminae rarae of the GBM, but it is more irregular than in normals. In places where the epithelium has become partially detached, the lysozyme binding sites remain associated with the GBM (arrows). Some binding to the epithelial and endothelial cell coats (c) and to the mesangial matrix (m) is still seen. Figure 23 is from another nephrotic rat later in the disease (10 daily injections). There is a total lack of binding of lysozyme to any of the layers of the capillary wall. The presence of dextran in the capillary lumen (Cap) and the urinary spaces (US) indicates that the perfusate (which contained both lysozyme and dextran) reached the vessel. Figure 22, × 40,000; Fig. 23, × 60,000. (From Caulfield and Farquhar, 1978.)

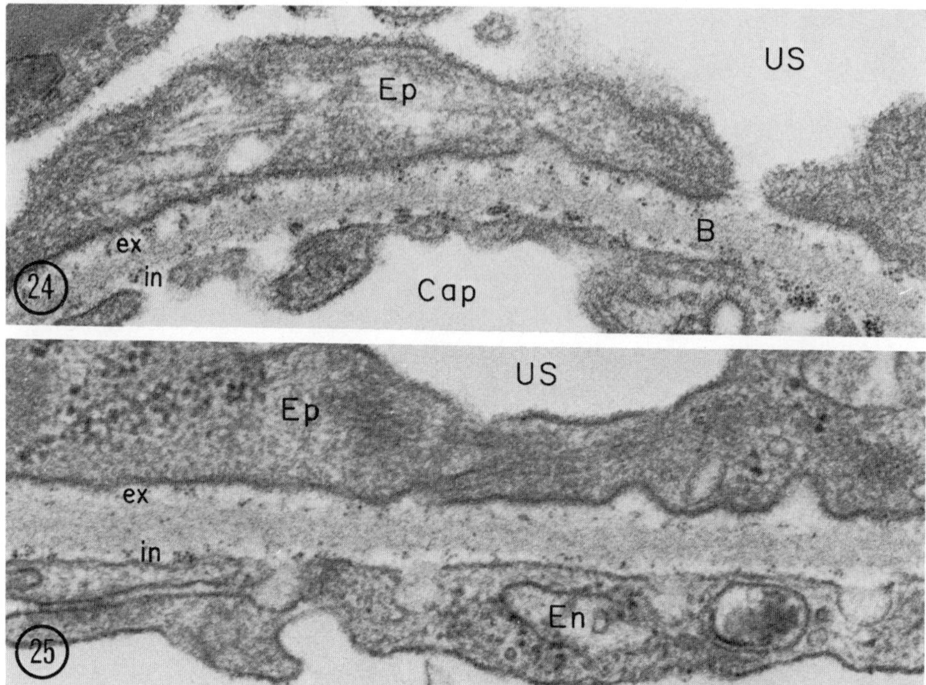

Figures 24 and 25. Glomerular capillaries from 10-day nephrotic rats given CF (pI = 7.3–7.5) by i.v. injection followed by flushing with 0.1 M (Fig. 24) and 0.2 M (Fig. 25) KCl. Much less binding is seen to the sites in the laminae rarae at 0.1 M KCl than is present in normal controls (Fig. 13), and binding is virtually absent at 0.2 M KCl. The fact that CF binding to the sites in the laminae rarae is displaced at lower salt concentration than in normals (0.2 M as opposed to 0.3 M) (Figs. 13–16) indicates that the charge density of the sites in the GBM is decreased in the nephrotic. Note also that in Fig. 24, the lamina densa (B) is thinner than normal, and the LRE (ex) is correspondingly widened. × 80,000.

that the evidence suggests the anionic sites are partially, but not completely lost in this disease as indicated by the fact that most of the native (anionic) ferritin is still restricted from passing beyond the LRI (Farquhar and Palade, 1961), by the results obtained with alcian blue staining of the anionic sites (Caulfield, 1978), and by the findings with CF binding (Kanwar and Farquhar, unpublished data). The results obtained with CF are still preliminary but the data obtained so far indicate that some CF binding occurs in the late (10 day) nephrotic but (1) it is less regular (Fig. 24) and (2) binding is displaced at a lower salt concentration (0.2 as opposed to 0.3 M KC1) (Fig. 25) than in normals. This finding is in keeping with the assumption that there is a definite reduction in the overall charge density of the sites in the GBM, but not a total loss of the anionic sites.

The fact that there is a reduction in charge density of the GBM sites at the same time as the glomerular charge barrier function is impaired, raises the possibility that these sites may be involved in creation of the charge barrier.

8. *Evidence That the Anionic Sites in the Laminae Rarae of the GBM Consist of Proteoglycans Rich in Heparan Sulfate*

Based on what is known about the composition of basement membranes, the most likely candidates for the chemical groups responsible for the binding of cationic probes are the carboxyl groups of the collagenous or noncollagenous peptides, carboxyl groups of sialic acid, or the sulfated groups of sulfated GAGs. That the sites might consist of GAGs, or, more precisely, proteoglycans (i.e., protein–polysaccharide complexes), was first suggested by the findings obtained with the cationic dye RR (Kanwar and Farquhar, 1978a, 1979a). When glomeruli are fixed in the presence of this stain (Figs. 26 and 27), rows of small (~ 20 nm) RR-stained particles were seen throughout the LRI, the LRE, and the mesangial matrix where they were distributed in a quasi-regular, lattice-like arrangement with the same 60-nm repeating pattern as that found with CF binding. Similar, if not identical, particles were also seen in the laminae rarae of other basement membranes in the kidney—i.e., Bowman's capsule, and those of tubules (Fig. 30), and the endothelium of peritubular capillaries (Fig. 30). At high magnifications in favorable preparations, it could be seen that the sites are angular in shape and fine (3 nm) filaments connected the sites (Fig. 26 inset) and radiated between them and the adjoining endothelial and epithelial cell membranes. It could be shown that RR and CF interact with the same sites because when CF was given *in vivo* followed by RR *in vitro*, the distribution of the two cationic probes coincided (Fig. 28).

The results with RR were quite informative and provided the first clue about the chemical nature of the GBM sites because, except for their smaller size (10–20 nm as opposed to 30–50 nm), the particles bear a striking resemblance to proteoglycan particles seen after RR staining in connective tissue matrices, especially in cartilage, tendon, and aorta (cf. Hay *et al.*, 1978). In fact, particles with a similar morphology which were shown (by enzyme digestion) to consist in part of chondroitin sulfate have been described in association with basement membranes in several other locations—specifically, in embryonic tissues (Trelstad *et al.*, 1974; Hay and Meier, 1974) and in aorta (Wight and Ross, 1975). Thus, the findings with RR suggested that the sites in the laminae rarae might consist of proteoglycans.

To obtain further information on the chemical nature of the sites in the laminae rarae, we subjected the GBM to digestion with specific enzymes either by perfusion of glomeruli *in situ* (Figs. 32–37) or by incubation of isolated GBMs *in vitro* (Figs. 38–40) with enzyme solutions (Kanwar and Farquhar, 1978b, 1979b). The results were the same with both *in situ* and *in vitro* preparations: the anionic sites were unaffected by treatment with

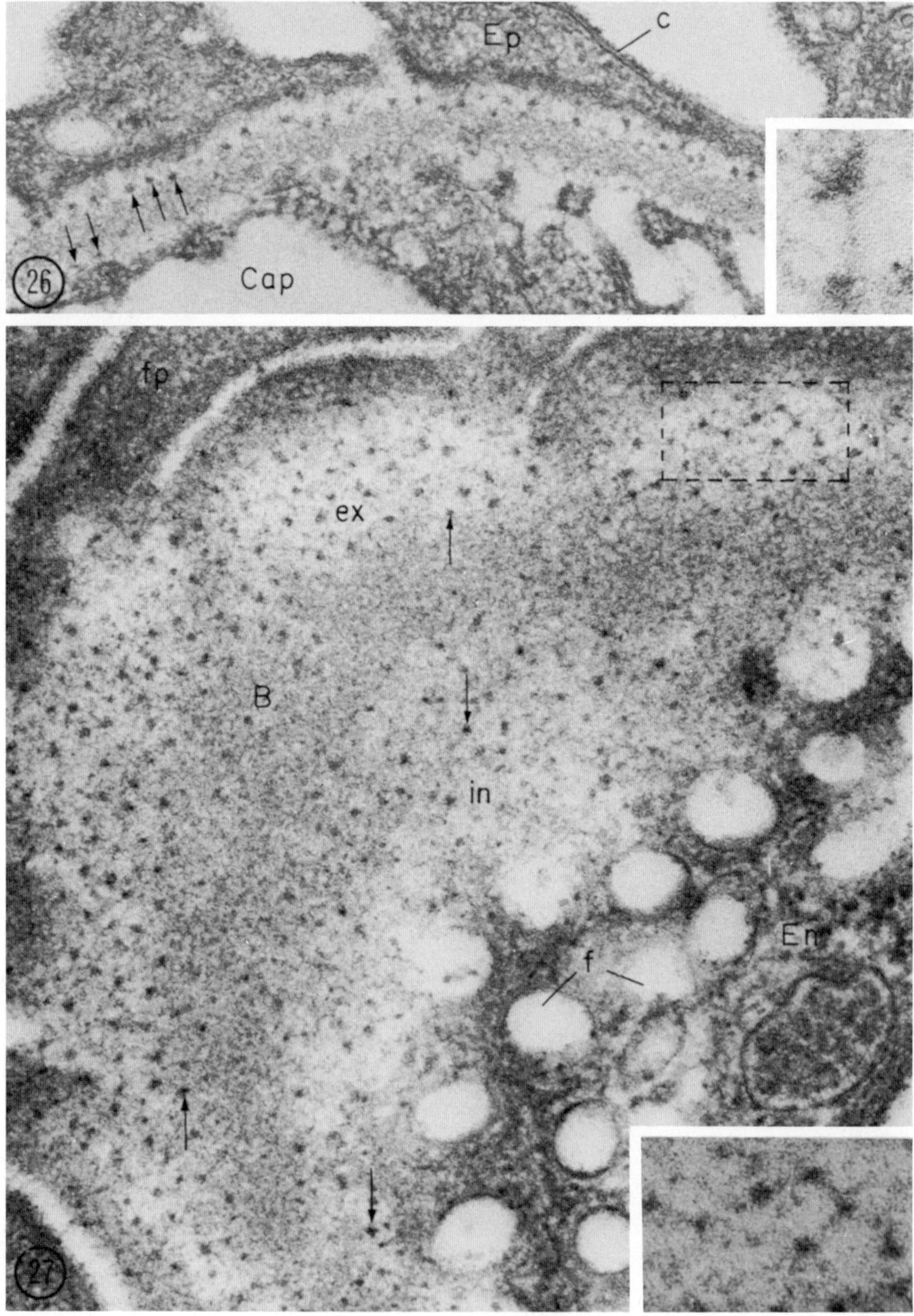

Figures 26 and 27. Portions of glomerular capillaries from a kidney perfused with aldehyde fixative containing the basic dye RR. Figure 26 is a cross section and Fig. 27 is a partially grazing section, illustrating the presence of a network of polygonal, RR-stained particles in the laminae rarae of the GBM. In Fig. 26, the particles are seen to occur in rows distributed at regular ~60 neuraminidase (Figs. 32–34 and 39, chondroitinase ABC (Figs. 35 and 38), and testicular or leech hyaluronidase. However, they could no longer be demonstrated after digestion with crude heparinase, purified heparitinase (Figs. 36, 37, and 40), or Pronase, or after nitrous acid oxidation. The results demonstrate that: (1) the sites contain heparan sulfate since they are removed by treatment with heparitinase and by nitrous acid oxidation, procedures which are specific for heparan sulfate (Linker and Hovingh, 1972); and (2) sialoproteins or other GAGs do not represent major components of these sites since the latter are not affected by digestion with neuraminidase and other GAG-specific enzymes. Identical findings were obtained on basement membranes in other locations [Bowman's capsule, tubule epithelium (Fig. 31), and endothelium of peritubular capillaries]. Thus, the sites in the GBM are chemically as well as morphologically and topographically distinct from the sialoglycoproteins associated with the epithelial and endothelial cell coats.

It is apparent that this represents the first description of sulfated GAGs in the GBM and, in addition, the first description of heparan sulfate in any basement membrane. However, heparan sulfate has been found in association with the surfaces of a variety of cell types (cf. Lindahl and Höök, 1978) including endothelial cells (Buonassisi and Root, 1975).

Implications of the Presence of Sulfated GAGs in the GBM

Besides their high net negative charge, among the well-known physical and chemical properties of sulfated GAGs is their high charge entity which gives them the ability to bind to a variety of macromolecules, and their ability to bind water which gives them their gel-like consistency. Thus, assuming that it is confirmed by biochemical analysis, the demonstration of the presence of sulfated GAGs in the GBM has a number of implications for glomerular physiology and pathology. To begin with, it can be expected that their presence would profoundly affect the permeability properties of the GBM. It has already been shown that GAGs serve to retard transport of macromolecules in connective tissue matrices (see Comper and Laurent, 1978). It follows that the GAGs are prime candidates for at least one type of polyanion responsible for creating and maintaining the glomerular charge barrier function. It can also be expected that any type of glomerular injury which could affect the biosynthesis or distribtuion of GAGs could adversely affect the filtration properties of the GBM.

---

nm) intervals in both the LRI (↓) and the LRE (↑). Fine filaments connect the particles to the adjoining cell membranes of the epithelium (Ep) and endothelium. The epithelial cell coat (c) is also stained by this basic dye. The inset depicts two RR-stained particles with their angular (often triangular profiles) and the fine (~3 nm) filaments which connect them. Figure 27 is a grazing section that cuts broadly through the GBM (B) and shows the meshwork of polygonal granules (arrows) in the LRI (in) and LRE (ex). The inset is an enlargement of part of the LRE showing the quasi-regular, lattice-like arrangement of the RR-stained sites. Figure 26, × 110,000; inset, × 350,000; Fig. 27, × 104,000; inset, × 208,000. (Figure 26 is from Farquhar, 1979; Fig. 27 is from Kanwar and Farquhar, 1979a.)

Other established biological properties of GAGs which are interesting and potentially important for normal glomerular function are their antithrombotic properties, ability to induce conformational changes in proteins, including collagen, and ability to interact with fibrillar collagens to influence the deposition of collagen fibrils (Lindahl and Höök, 1978). Assuming that these last two properties apply to the nonfibrillar, collagenous peptides of basement membranes as well as to fibrillar collagens, the possibility exists that the GAGs associated with basement membranes could affect the depo-

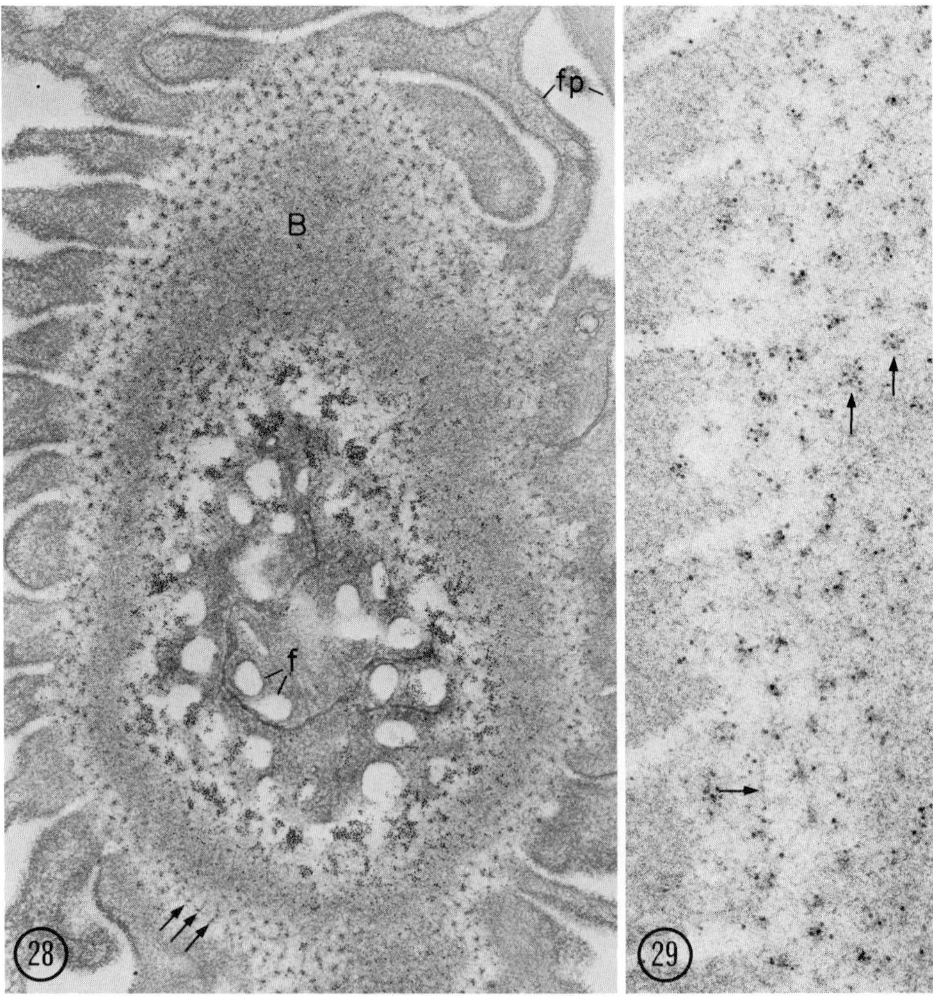

Figures 28 and 29. Grazing section of a glomerular capillary from the kidney of a rat which had been given CF *in vivo* followed by kidney perfusion with RR. Note that the distribution of the clusters of CF molecules and the RR-positive sites in the LRE (ex) coincide (arrows). Figure 29 is an enlargement of a portion of the LRE showing CF molecules clustered on the RR-stained particles. Figure 28, × 60,000; Fig. 29, × 105,000. (From Kanwar and Farquhar, 1979a.)

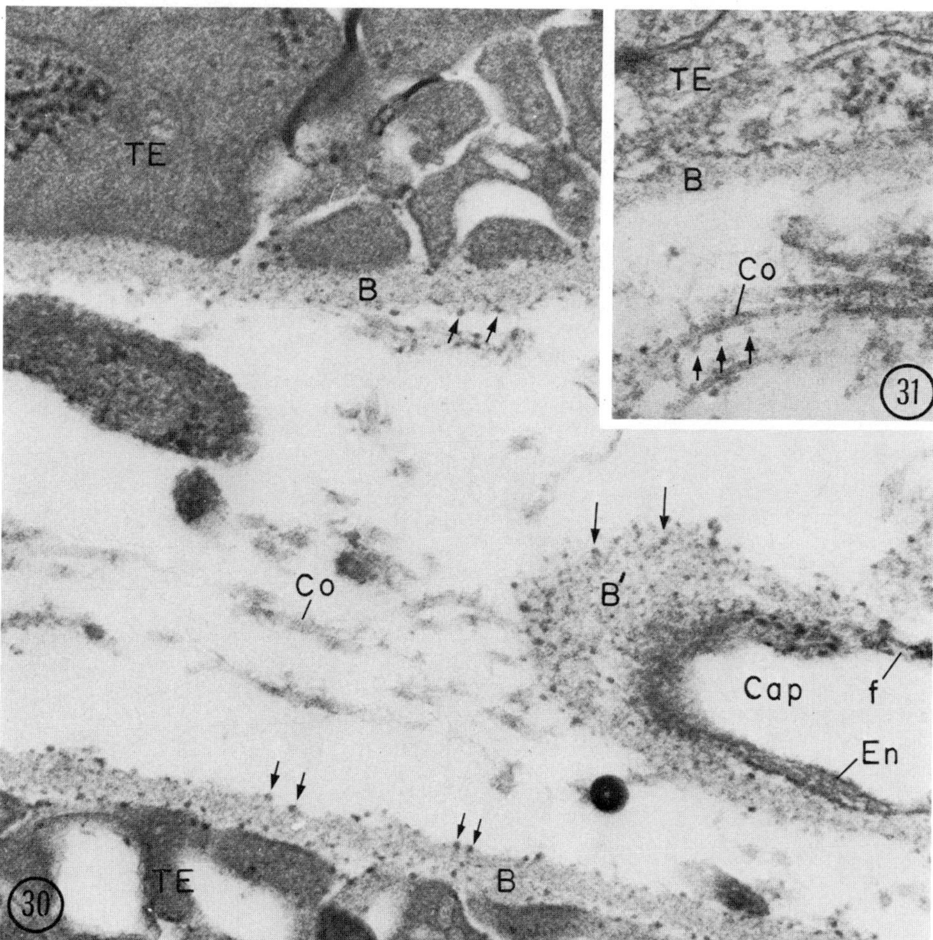

Figures 30 and 31. Peritubular region of a preparation fixed by perfusion with aldehyde fixative containing RR. Figure 30 shows the base of two tubular epithelial cells (TE) with their basement membranes (B), and part of a peritubular capillary (Cap) with its basement membrane (B′), the latter cut in grazing section. RR-stained particles resembling those seen in the GBM are present in both the basement membrane of the epithelium (short arrows) and that of the endothelium (long arrows). Figure 31 is a similar field from a kidney subjected to treatment with purified heparitinase prior to fixation to demonstrate that the particles in the tubular basement membrane (B) as well as those in the endothelial basement membrane (not shown) are removed by this enzyme which is specific for heparan sulfate. Note the RR-stained strands which bind to the collagen at regular ~67-nm intervals (arrows); this material, which is believed to consist of proteoglycans rich in chondroitin sulfate, is not removed by treatment with heparitinase. En, endothelium of peritubular capillary; f, endothelial fenestra with its diaphragm; Co, collagen fibrils in the interstitia. × 70,000.

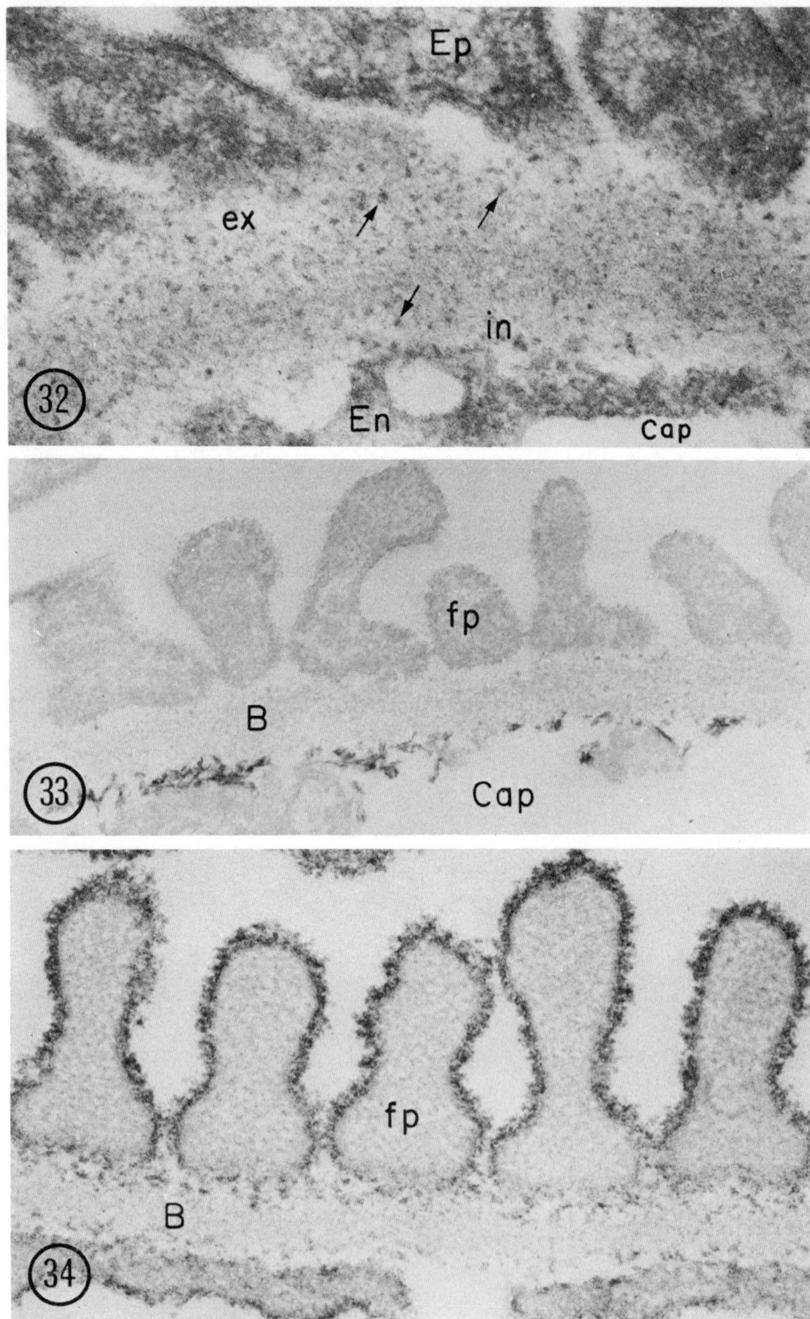

Figures 32–34. Figure 32 is a partially grazing section through a glomerular capillary from a kidney perfused for 30 min with 0.1 M NaCl–acetate buffer, pH 5.4, containing neuraminidase (0.2–0.5 U/ml) followed by perfusion with aldehyde fixative containing RR. RR-stained particles (arrows) can be visualized in both the LRI (in) and the LRE (ex) of the GBM, indicating they

sition and three-dimensional organization of these peptides. It is also of interest to note that in fibrillar (Types I, II, and III) collagens, GAGs are known to bind at regular (67 nm) intervals to specific regions in the collagen molecule (see Fig. 31) where basic groups are clustered (Hay *et al.*, 1978). Thus, the possibility exists that the more or less regular 60-nm spacing of GAGs detected with cationic probes may be reflected in a complementary concentration of basic groups in the adjacent collagenous peptides. It will be of interest in the future to look for such a pattern in basement membranes which have been prepared and stained by appropriate procedures.

The demonstration of GAGs in the GBM provides a new macromolecular component, in addition to collagenous and noncollagenous glycoproteins, to be taken into consideration in explaining the pathogenesis of various glomerular diseases and in contemplating potential mechanisms of glomerular injury. Due to their highly charged and relatively exposed nature, the anionic sites rich in GAGs have the ability to bind, and to thereby concentrate any cationic molecule from the size of RR (MW = 551) up to the size of ferritin (~ 11 nm; MW = 480,000). Moreover, the results obtained following intravenous injection of CF fractions with different isoelectric points show that, providing the surface charge density of the cationic probe is sufficiently great, the net pI of the circulating molecule need not be higher than 7.3–7.5 for binding to take place *in vivo*.* Binding of several cationic molecules (lysozyme, CF, RR, and alcian blue) already has been demonstrated by work from this laboratory and binding of other cationic compounds [polylysine and polylysine–heparin complexes (Seiler *et al.*, 1977), polyethyleneimine (Schurer *et al.*, 1977), cationic horseradish peroxidase and cytochrome *c* (Kerjaschki *et al.*, 1978)] can be inferred from the work by others. Among the molecules of interest which have been suspected or demonstrated to be involved in glomerular injury are various toxic compounds, vasoactive amines, and antigens and antibodies, either individually or as antigen–antibody complexes. It is of interest to note that in connective tissues, precipitation of antigen–antibody complexes already has been demonstrated to be facilitated by the presence of GAGs (Hellsing, 1969). In short, the existence of anionic sites composed of GAGs with a demonstrated ability to bind cationic molecules of varying size and relatively low net positive charge raises the possibility

* In the case of proteins, the extent of binding appears to depend more on the surface charge density of the molecule than the isoelectric point of the protein as evidenced by the fact that lysozyme (pI = 11.0) binding is more easily displaced than CF (pI = 7.3–7.5).

---

are not removed by the enzyme treatment. Figure 33 is also from a kidney perfused with neuraminidase, followed by perfusion with colloidal iron (CI) to demonstrate the absence of CI binding to the epithelial membranes around the foot processes (fp), indicating removal of epithelial sialoprotein by the enzyme treatment. Figure 34 is a control kidney perfused with acetate buffer alone in which there is heavy binding of CI to the cell coat of the epithelial foot processes (fp); a lesser but still detectable binding to the endothelium and the laminae rarae of the GBM is also present. Figures 32 and 34, × 80,000; Fig. 33, × 60,000. (From Kanwar and Farquhar, 1979b.)

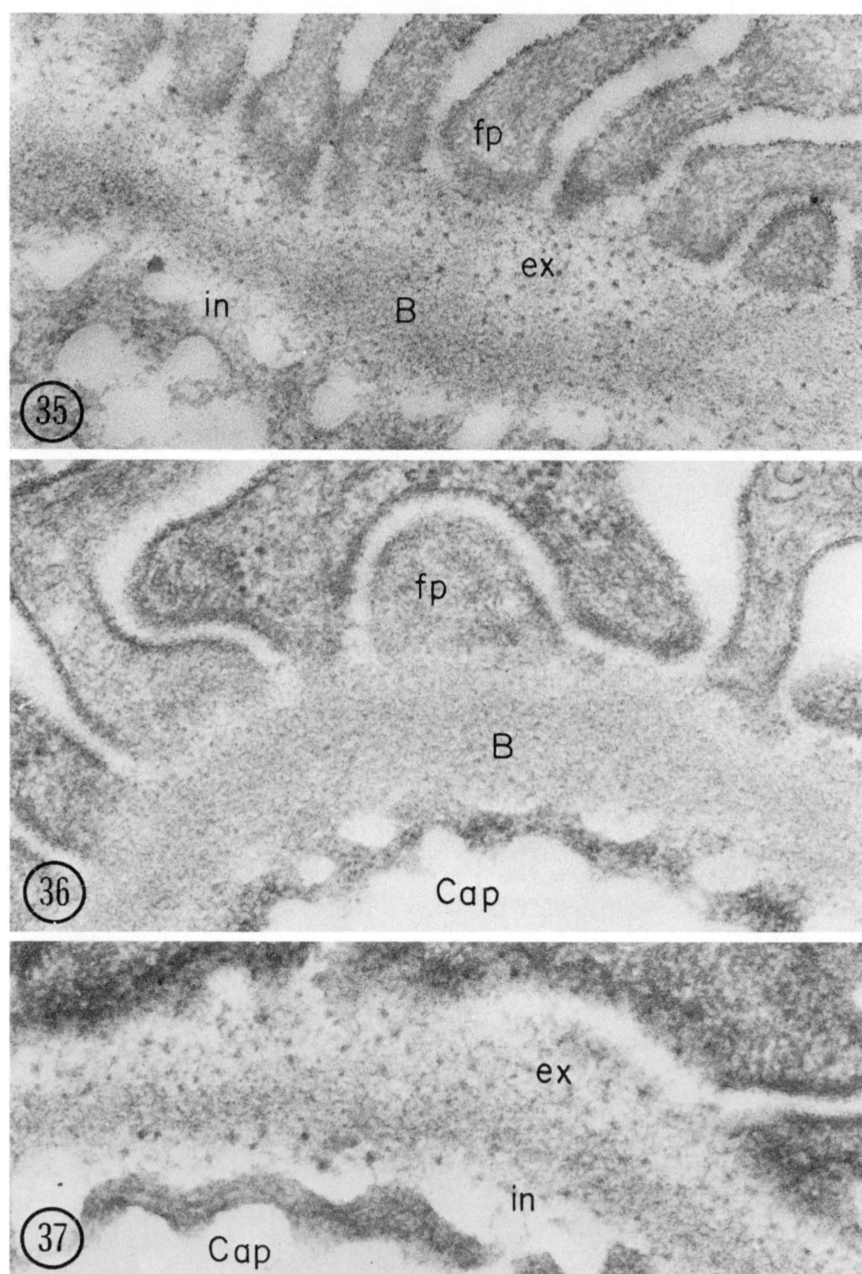

Figures 35–37. Figure 35 is a small field from a glomerular capillary of a kidney perfused with chondroitinase ABC (0.5–2.0 U/ml for 60 min), and Fig. 36 is from a kidney perfused with purified heparitinase (0.2 mg/ml for 20 min) prior to fixation with RR-containing fixative. Note that RR-stained particles were not removed by chondroitinase treatment but were removed by treatment with heparitinase. After treatment with this enzyme, which is specific for heparan sulfate, the RR-stained sites can no longer be visualized in the LRI (in) and LRE (ex) of the basement membrane (B). Figure 37 is from a control kidney perfused with buffer only in which the RR-stained particles in the laminae rarae are prominent. × 60,000. (From Kanwar and Farquhar, 1979b.)

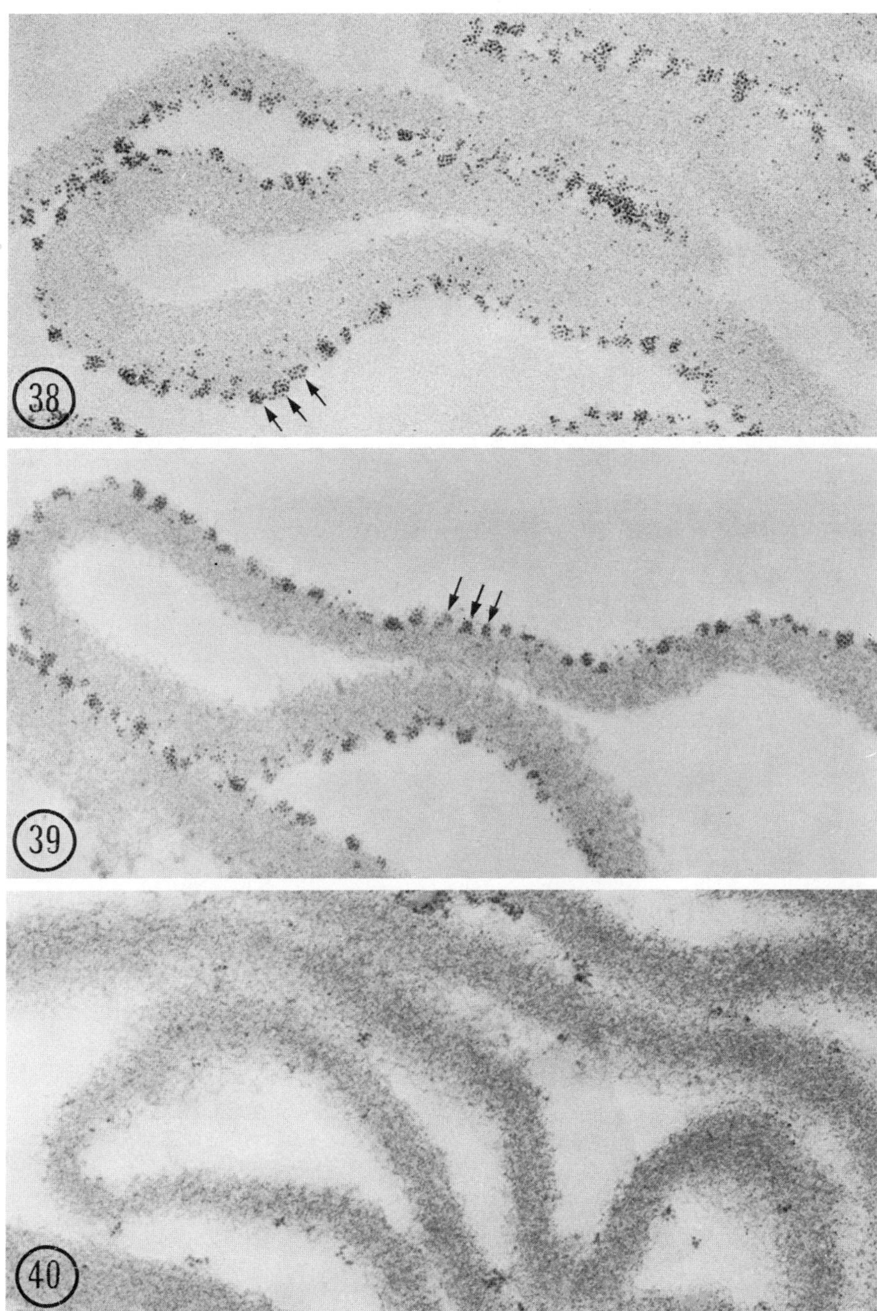

Figures 38–40. These three figures show loops of isolated GBMs subjected to treatment with chondroitinase ABC (Fig. 38), neuraminidase (Fig. 39), and heparitinase (Fig. 40), followed by incubation with CF to label the GBM sites. CF binding (arrows) is not affected by treatment with chondroitinase or neuraminidase, but it is abolished by heparitinase. The specific removal of these sites by heparitinase indicates that they consist of heparan sulfate since the enzyme is specific for this sulfated GAG. CF molecules bind only to the outer or exposed side of the GBM loops because the latter consist of intact, closed tubes, and the tracer does not have access to the inner or unexposed side of the GBM. (See Fig. 19.) × 60,000. (From Kanwar and Farquhar, 1979b.)

that nonspecific trapping of a wide variety of substances could be involved, directly or indirectly, in glomerular injury.

Viewed in the context of this volume with its focus on immune mechanisms of renal disease, the stage is set for the existence of a multiplicity of mechanisms of immune injury involving nonspecific trapping of antigen or antibodies, either alone or as preformed antibody complexes, by ionic interaction with negatively charged sites in the laminae rarae and mesangial matrix. The occurrence of nonspecific, electrostatic binding to GBM components could explain, on the one hand, the variety of pathogenetic mechanisms apparently operating in immune glomerular diseases in humans, and on the other the relatively few common patterns of immune complex localization (mesangial, epimembranous) which have been observed.

9. *Concluding Comments*

Recent work on the functional organization of the glomerulus has been summarized. Results obtained over the last few years allows us to conclude: (1) that the GBM constitutes the main filter which serves to retain albumin in the circulation, and (2) that the cellular elements of the capillary wall serve to modulate, maintain, and cleanse the filter as well as to synthesize and remove its components. In this chapter, evidence indicating the existence in the mesangial matrix and in the laminae rarae of anionic sites which consist of two additional distinctive structural components has been summarized. These two new components (diagrammed in Fig. 41), which are demonstrable after staining with the cationic dye RR, consist of angular, often polygonal (10–20 nm) granules and fine (2–3 nm) filaments which connect the granules one to another and to the overlying endothelial and epithelial cell membranes. Evidence suggesting that the RR-stained granules consist of sulfated GAGs rich in heparan sulfate has been presented. It has been shown that these sites are altered (in terms of charge density) in aminonucleoside nephrosis. Based on these findings it was proposed that the anionic sites in the laminae rarae of the GBM may be responsible, at least in part, for establishing the permeability properties of the GBM.

At the time of the writing of this chapter, there was no direct evidence on this point, and the evidence for the presence of GAGs in the GBM was limited to enzyme digestion studies. In the meantime the available information on this topic has been extended considerably as follows: 1) it has been demonstrated directly that removal of GAGs (by enzyme digestion) leads to an increase in the permeability of the GBM to native ferritin (J. Cell Biol., 1980, **86:**688); 2) the presence of GAGs in the GBM has been confirmed by isolation and biochemical analysis of extracted GAGs (Proc. Natl. Acad. Sci, U.S.A., 1979, **76:**4493); 3) heparan sulfate has been found to be the major (~85%) GAG present in isolated GBMs by both compositional analysis and biosynthetic labeling, but smaller amounts of other GAGs (hyaluronic acid and chondroitin sulfates) are also synthesized and incorporated into the GBM (Proc. Natl. Acad. Sci. U.S.A., 1981, **78:**1726); 4) the proteoglycans

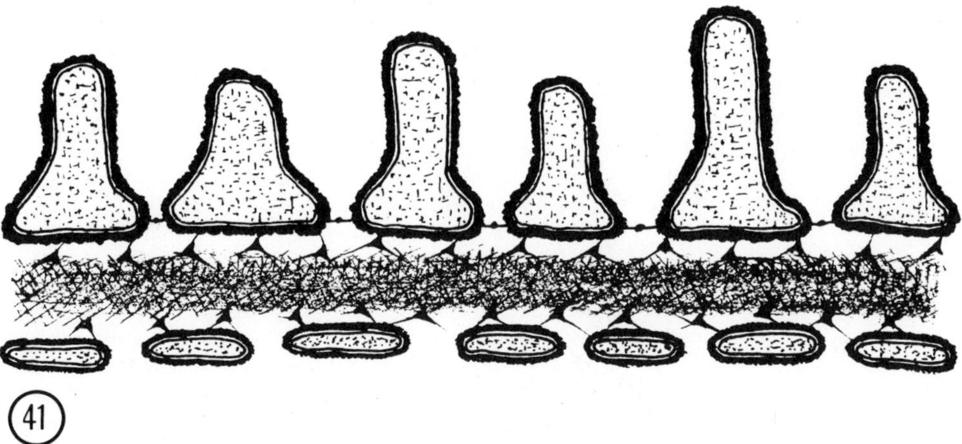

Figure 41. Diagrammatic representation of the proposed distribution of anionic sites in the laminae rarae of the GBM based on results of labeling with cationic probes. The sites are visualized as a network of angular particles (~20 nm) with fine filaments (~3 nm) extending from their points to connect one particle with another, with the membranes of the adjoining endothelial and epithelial cells, and with the lamina densa. (From Kanwar and Farquhar, 1979a.)

(protein plus GAGs) have been isolated from the GBM and partially characterized, and the heparan sulfate and chondroitin sulfate(s) have been shown to be present in different proteoglycans (J. Cell Biol., 1981, **90**:527).*

Finally, it should be mentioned that at present very little is known about the molecular organization of the GBM and the factors which determine its properties as a filter. Four distinctive structural components have been recognized in the GBM—the 3- to 4-nm fibrillar meshwork, the 11-nm tubular fibrils, the 20-nm punctate anionic sites, and their 3-nm connecting filaments; except for the evidence presented here concerning the nature of the heparan sulfide-rich anionic sites, little is known at present concerning the chemical nature or cellular source of these different structural entities. These and many other problems remain to be solved in the future before the molecular basis of normal and abnormal glomerular filtration can be fully understood.

References

Andrews, P. M., 1978, Scanning electron microscopy of the kidney glomerular epithelium after treatment with polycations *in situ* and *in vitro, Am. J. Anat.* **153**:291.

Behnke, O., and Zelander, T., 1970, Preservation of intercellular substances by the cationic dye alcian blue in preparative procedures for electron microscopy, *J. Ultrastruct. Res.* **31**:424.

* For a discussion of more recent work from this laboratory as well as other work in the field, several additional reviews may be consulted: (Farquhar, M. G. in: *Cell Biology of the Extracellular Matrix*, E. D. Hay, ed., Plenum Press, New York, p. 335, 1982; and Farquhar, M. G., in: *New Trends in Basement Membrane Research*, K. Kuhn, R. Timpl, and H. Schone, eds., Raven Press, p. 9, 1982).

Bohrer, M. P., Baylis, C., Robertson, C. R., and Brenner, B. M., 1977, Mechanisms of the puromycin-induced defects in the transglomerular passage of water and macromolecules, *J. Clin. Invest.* **60:**152.

Brendel, L., Meezan, E., and Nagle, R. B., 1978, The acellular perfused kidney: A model for basement membrane permeability, in: *Biology and Chemistry of Basement Membranes* (N. A. Kefalides, ed.), pp. 177–193, Academic Press, New York.

Brenner, B. M., Bohrer, M. P., Baylis, C., and Deen, W. M., 1977, Determinants of glomerular permselectivity: Insights derived from observations *in vivo, Kidney Int.* **12:**229.

Brenner, B. M., Hostetter, T. H., and Humes, H. D., 1978, Molecular basis of proteinuria of glomerular origin, *N. Engl. J. Med.* **298:**826.

Buonassisi, V., and Root, M., 1975, Enzymatic degradation of heparin-related mucopolysaccharides from the surface of endothelial cell cultures, *Biochim. Biophys. Acta* **385:**1.

Caulfield, J. P., 1978, The distribution of anionic sites in the glomerular basement membrane of normal and nephrotic rats, in: *Biology and Chemistry of Basement Membranes* (N. A. Kefalides, ed.), pp. 81–98, Academic Press, New York.

Caulfield, J. P., and Farquhar, M. G., 1974, The permeability of glomerular capillaries to graded dextrans: Identification of the basement membrane as the primary filtration barrier, *J. Cell Biol.* **63:**883.

Caulfield, J. P., and Farquhar, M. G., 1975, the permeability of glomerular capillaries of aminonucleoside-nephrotic rats to graded dextrans, *J. Exp. Med.* **142:**61.

Caulfield, J. P., and Farquhar, M. G., 1976, Distribution of anionic sites in glomerular basement membranes: Their possible role in filtration and attachment, *Proc. Natl. Acad. Sci. USA* **73:**1646.

Caulfield, J. P., and Farquhar, M. G., 1978, Loss of anionic sites from the glomerular basement membrane in aminonucleoside nephrosis, *Lab. Invest.* **39:**505.

Comper, W. D., and Laurent, T. C., 1978, Physiological function of connective tissue polysaccharides, *Physiol. Rev.* **58:**255.

Farquhar, M. G., 1975, The primary glomerular filtration barrier—basement membrane or epithelial slits?, *Kidney Int.* **8:**197.

Farquhar, M. G., 1978, Structure and function in glomerular capillaries: Role of the basement membrane in glomerular filtration, in: *Biology and Chemistry of Basement Membranes* (N. A. Kefalides, ed.), pp. 43–80, Academic Press, New York.

Farquhar, M. G., 1981, Role of the basement membrane in glomerular filtration: Results obtained with electron-dense tracers, in: *Functional Ultrastructure of the Kidney* (A. B. Maunsbach, T. S. Olsen, and E. I. Christensen, eds.), pp. 31–51, Academic Press, New York.

Farquhar, M. G., and Palade, G. E., 1961, Glomerular permeability. II. Ferritin transfer across the glomerular capillary wall in nephrotic rats, *J. Exp. Med.* **114:**699.

Farquhar, M. G., Wissig, S. L., and Palade, G. E., 1961, Glomerular permeability. I. Ferritin transfer across the normal glomerular capillary wall, *J. Exp. Med.* **113:**47.

Graham, R. C., and Karnovsky, M. J., 1966, Glomerular permeability: Ultrastructural cytochemical studies using peroxidases as protein tracers, *J. Exp. Med.* **124:**1123.

Hay, E. D., and Meier, S., 1974, Glycosaminoglycan synthesis by embryonic inductors: Neural tube, notochord and lens, *J. Cell Biol.* **62:**889.

Hey, E. D., Hasty, D. L., and Kiehnau, K. L., 1978, Morphological investigation of fibers derived from various types: Fine sturcture of collagen and their relation to glycosaminoglycans (GAG), in: *Collagen–Platelet Interaction* (H. Gastpar, K. Kuhn, and R. Marx, eds.), pp. 129–151, Schattauer Verlag, Stuttgart.

Hellsing, K., 1969, Immune reactions in polysaccharide media: The effect of hyaluronate, chondroitin sulfate and chondroitin sulfate–protein complex of the precipitin reaction, *Biochem. J.* **112:**475.

Jones, D. B., 1969, Mucosubstances of the glomerulus, *Lab. Invest.* **21:**119.

Kanwar, Y. S., and Farquhar, M. G., 1978a, Partial characterization of anionic sites in the glomerular basement membrane, *J. Cell Biol.* **79**(No. 2, Part 2)**:**150a.

Kanwar, Y. S., and Farquhar, M. G., 1978b, Characterization of anionic sites in the glomerular basement membrane (GBM), *Kidney Int.* **14:**713 (abstract).

Kanwar, Y. S., and Farquhar, M. G., 1979a, Anionic sites in the glomerular basement membrane: *In vivo* and *in vitro* localization to the laminae rarae by cationic probes, *J. Cell Biol.* **81:**137.

Kanwar, Y. S., and Farquhar, M. G., 1979b, Presence of heparan sulfate in the glomerular basement membrane, *Proc. Natl. Acad. Sci. USA* **76:**1303.

Karnovsky, M. J., and Ainsworth, S. K., 1973, The structural basis of glomerular filtration, *Adv. Nephrol.* **2:**35.

Kerjaschki, D., Förster, O., Boltz, G., Scheiner, W., and Albini, B., 1978, Distribution of cationic tracer substances in kidney capillary wall in experimental immunocomplex diseases, in: *Electron Microscopy 1978* (J. M. Sturgess, ed.), Vol. II, pp. 462–463, Microscopical Society of Canada.

Laliberté, F., Sapin, C., Belair, M. F., Druet, P., and Bariéty, J., 1978, The localization of the filtration barrier in normal rat glomeruli by ultrastructural immunoperoxidase techniques, *Biol. Cell.* **31:**15.

Latta, H., and Johnston, W. H., 1976, The glycoprotein inner layer of glomerular capillary basement membrane as a filtration barrier, *J. Ultrastruct. Res.* **57:**65.

Latta, H., Johnston, W. H., and Stanley, T. M., 1975, Sialoglycoproteins and filtration barriers in the glomerular capillary wall, *J. Ultrastruct. Res.* **51:**354.

Lindahl, U., and Höök, M., 1978, Glycosaminoglycans and their binding to biological macromolecules, *Annu. Rev. Biochem.* **47:**385.

Linker, A., and Hovingh, P., 1972, Heparinase and heparitinase from flavobacteria, in: *Methods in Enzymology* (V. Ginzberg, ed.), Vol. 28, pp. 902–911, Academic Press, New York.

Marchsi, V. T., Furthmayr, H., and Tomita, M., 1976, The red cell membrane, *Annu. Rev. Biochem.* **45:**667.

Michael, A. F., Blau, E., and Vernier, R. L., 1970, Glomerular polyanion: Alteration in aminonucleoside nephrosis, *Lab. Invest.* **23:**649.

Mohos, S. C., and Skoza, L., 1969, Glomerular sialoprotein, *Science* **164:**1519.

Quinton, P. M., and Philpott, C. W., 1973, A role for anionic sites in epithelial architecture, *J. Cell Biol.* **56:**787.

Reeves, W., Caulfield, J. P., and Farquhar, M. G., 1978, Differentiation of epithelial foot processes and filtration slits: Sequential appearance of occluding junctions, epithelial polyanion, and slit membranes in developing glomeruli, *Lab. Invest.* **39:**90.

Rennke, H. G., Cotran, R. S., and Venkatachalam, M. A., 1975, Role of molecular charge in glomerular permeability: Tracer studies with cationized ferritins, *J. Cell Biol.* **67:**638.

Ryan, G. B., and Karnovsky, M. J., 1976, Distribution of endogenous albumin in the rat glomerulus: Role of hemodynamic factors in glomerular barrier function, *Kidney Int.* **9:**36.

Ryan, G. B., Hein, S. J., and Karnovsky, M. J., 1976, Glomerular permeability to proteins: Effects of hemodynamic factors on the distribution of endogenous immunoglobulin G and exogenous catalase in the rat glomerulus, *Lab. Invest.* **34:**415.

Schurer, J. W., Hoedemaeker, P. J., and Molenaar, I., 1977, Polyethyleneimine as tracer particle for (immuno) electron microscopy, *J. Histochem. Cytochem.* **25:**384.

Seiler, M. W., Rennke, H. G., Venkatachalam, M. A., and Cotran, R. S., 1977, Pathogenesis of polycation-induced alterations ("fusion") of glomerular epithelium, *Lab. Invest.* **36:**48.

Singer, S. J., 1974, The molecular organization of membranes, *Annu. Rev. Biochem.* **43:**805.

Steck, T. L., 1974, The organization of proteins in the human red blood cell membrane, *J. Cell Biol.* **62:**1.

Trelstad, R. L., Hayashi, K., and Toole, B. P., 1974, Epithelial collagens and glycosaminoglycans in the embryonic cornea: Macromolecular order and morphogenesis in the basement membrane, *J. Cell Biol.* **62:**815.

Venkatachalam, M. A., Karnovsky, M. J., Fahimi, H. D., and Cotran, R. S., 1970, An ultrastructural study of glomerular permeability using catalase and peroxidase as tracer proteins, *J. Exp. Med.* **132:**1153.

Wight, T. N., and Ross, R., 1975, Proteoglycans in primate arteries. I. Ultrastructural localization and distribution in the intima, *J. Cell Biol.* **67:**660.

2

Mechanisms of Glomerular Permselectivity

Barry M. Brenner and Thomas H. Hostetter

1. Introduction

The hydraulic pressure gradient acting across the glomerular capillary wall serves as the principal driving force for the separation of plasma into a nearly ideal ultrafiltrate. In spite of its remarkably low resistance to water flow, however, this capillary network retains within it the plasma proteins, so that only a small fraction of these circulating macromolecules appear in the glomerular urine. The basis for this retention of proteins within the glomerular capillary has been investigated primarily by clearance techniques and by ultrastructural analyses, using various types of tracer macromolecules. These studies have demonstrated that the filtration of macromolecules is influenced both by the intrinsic permeability properties of the glomerular capillary and by the presures and flows determining the filtration rate of water. The intrinsic permeability properties of the various membrane and cell layers of the glomerulus derive from their ability to discriminate on the basis of molecular size and net molecular charge. In this review, the operation of these mechanisms in health and in disease will be explored.

2. The Glomerular Capillary Wall as a Size-Selective Filter

It has been known for many years that large-molecular-weight proteins are denied access to the urine (Bayliss *et al.*, 1933). *In vivo* studies in several species have elucidated the sieving properties of the glomerular wall respon-

Barry M. Brenner and Thomas H. Hostetter · Laboratory of Kidney and Electrolyte Physiology and Departments of Medicine, Brigham and Women's Hospital and Harvard Medical School, Boston, Massachusetts 02115.

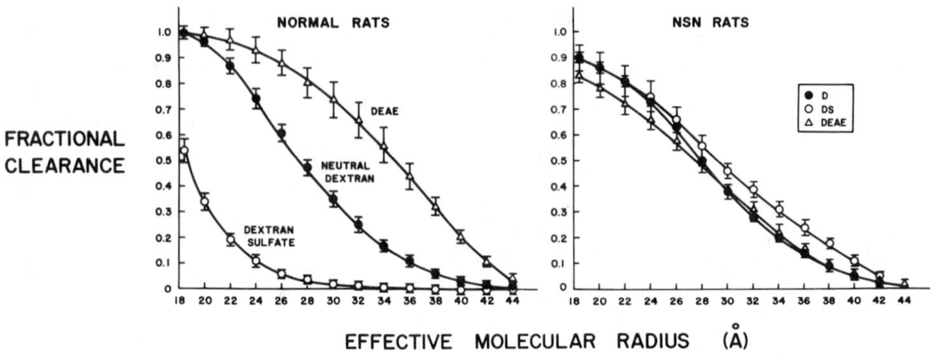

Figure 1. Fractional clearances of DEAE dextran, neutral dextran, and dextran sulfate, plotted as a function of effective molecular radius in normal rats (left) and in NSN rats (right). Values are expressed as means ± 1 S.E.M. (From Bohrer *et al.*, 1978a, with permission.)

sible for this size-selectivity (Arturson *et al.*, 1971; Hardwicke *et al.*, 1970; Rennke and Venkatachalam, 1977; Verniory *et al.*, 1973). These studies generally have relied upon measurements of the clearance of a test macromolecule, relative to some "freely permeable" reference polymer such as inulin. A macromolecular species, such as dextran or polyvinylpyrrolidone, with homogeneous chemical composition but variable molecular weight, and therefore, molecular size, usually is employed as the test solute. Given that the test macromolecule is neither secreted nor reabsorbed (Chang *et al.*, 1975c), and that the excretion of the reference solute is also unmodified by tubule function, but appears in Bowman's space in the same concentration as in plasma water (Chang *et al.*, 1975c), the ratio of urinary clearance of test to reference solute is equal to the ratio of the concentration of the test solute in Bowman's space to its concentration in plasma water. Hence, this ratio of clearances, referred to as the *fractional clearance* of the test solute, becomes a convenient measure of permselectivity, varying from zero, when test molecules are impermeant, to one when they encounter no measurable restriction to filtration.

Employing neutral dextrans ranging widely in chromatographically determined molecular size, it has been shown that molecules with radii equal to or less than that of inulin (~ 14 Å) encounter no measurable restriction to filtration (Chang *et al.*, 1975c). Their concentration in Bowman's space fluid is therefore equal to that in plasma water (i.e., fractional clearance = 1). As dextran radii increase, filtration decreases progressively, reaching low values as the size of serum albumin (~ 36 Å) is approached. Figure 1 illustrates this effect of molecular size, based on measurements of fractional clearances of neutral tritiated dextrans across glomerular capillaries in the Munich-Wistar rat (Brenner *et al.*, 1977). Fractional clearance is plotted as a function of effective dextran radius. Measurable restriction to filtration of neutral dextrans, that is, fractional clearance less than one, does not occur until effective dextran radii exceed approximately 20 Å. Above radii of 20

Å, fractional clearances decrease progressively with increasing size, approaching zero at radii greater than about 42 Å. These values obtained for the Munich-Wistar rat are typical of those reported for dog, man, and other strains of rats using dextrans as well as polyvinylpyrrolidones (Arturson *et al.*, 1971; Hardwicke *et al.*, 1970; Renkin and Gilmore, 1973; Verniory *et al.*, 1973).

3. The Glomerular Capillary Wall as a Charge-Selective Filter

Examination of Table 1 demonstrates that size cannot be the only factor determining the filtration of a macromolecule. Average values for Bowman's space to plasma concentration ratios for serum albumin for the normal rat are clearly much less than for neutral dextran having the same effective molecular radius as albumin, approximately 36 Å. The filtration of albumin is restricted to a much greater extent than is dextran of an equivalent size. Since the difference in clearances of albumin and dextran persists even when fractional clearances are measured using fluid obtained directly from Bowman's space (Gaizutis *et al.*, 1972; Eisenbach *et al.*, 1975), this difference cannot result from albumin reabsorption by the renal tubules. Such an effect would falsely lower the estimate of the fractional clearance of albumin. Thus, factor(s) in addition to molecular size must be invoked to account for the greater restriction to albumin filtration.

Since albumin behaves as a polyanion in physiological solution, Chang *et al.* (1975b) examined the effect of net molecular electrical charge on glomerular filtration of circulating macromolecules by studying the sieving characteristics of dextran sulfate, an anionic polymer of dextran. Figure 1 (left) demonstrates the results of these studies. While the filtration of neutral dextrans is hindered only for molecules with radii greater than approximately 20 Å, the anionic dextrans are restricted in their filtration across the entire range of sizes studied. For any given size, fractional clearance of dextran sulfate is lower than that of neutral dextran. Fractional clearance of dextran sulfate molecules with a radius similar to that of albumin is about 0.01, a value approaching that of albumin. Since dextran and dextran sulfate are

Table 1. Fractional Clearance of Albumin Compared with That of Neutral Dextran, Dextran Sulfate, DEAE Dextran of Similar Molecular Size in the Normal Munich-Wistar Rat

Macromolecule (M)	Molecular radius	C_M/C_I[a]
Albumin	36 Å	<0.01[b]
Neutral dextran	36 Å	0.15 ± 0.02 (15)[c]
Dextran sulfate	36 Å	0.01 ± 0.002 (15)
DEAE dextran	36 Å	0.42 ± 0.06 (9)

[a] Clearance of M/clearance of inulin.
[b] Bowman's space/plasma water ratio of albumin.
[c] Means ± S.E.M.; number of rats shown in parentheses.

neither secreted nor reabsorbed along the nephron (Chang *et al.*, 1975b,c), the observed differences in fractional clearances cannot result from differences in tubular transport (Chang *et al.*, 1975b,c). Furthermore, since glomerular pressures and flows measured in rats given the two test molecules were indistinguishable, these differing clearance profiles could not have been the result of alterations in glomerular hemodynamics (Chang *et al.*, 1975b,c). Thus, molecular charge, in addition to size, influences the filtration of macromolecules across the glomerular capillary wall. This charge selectivity is thought to derive from electrostatic interaction between some fixed, negatively charged component(s) of the glomerular capillary wall and the charged macromolecule.

Though retarding the filtration of circulating polyanions, the highly anionic glomerular capillary wall would be expected to enhance the filtration of circulating polycations. To examine this hypothesis, Bohrer *et al.* (1978a) evaluated the filtration characteristics *in vivo* of diethylaminoethyl (DEAE) dextran, a highly cationic dextran polymer. As shown in Fig. 1, fractional clearances of DEAE dextrans were increased, as compared to neutral dextran and dextran sulfate. The increase relative to neutral dextran was significant for effective molecular radii ranging from 24 to 44 Å. Qualitatively similar findings were obtained recently by Rennke *et al.* (1978) in clearance studies in rats using several horseradish peroxidases with deliberately varied isoelectric points. In this study, the fractional clearance of a cationic form of horseradish peroxidase greatly exceeded values obtained with neutral or anionic forms of the same protein. Thus, these findings of enhanced filtration of polycations add further support for the existence of a functionally significant electrostatic interaction between circulating, charged macromolecules and the anionic components of the glomerular capillary wall.

There is evidence indicating that nonglomerular microvasculature also possesses negative fixed charges and that these charges also serve to retard the transmural passage of circulating polyanions. In a perfusion study of the rabbit ear microcirculation, Areekul (1969) found dextran sulfate molecules to be less readily transported from capillary lumen to interstitial space than were neutral dextran molecules of comparable size distribution. Similar conclusions have been reached for renal peritubular capillaries in the rat (Deen *et al.*, 1976).

Histochemical studies also have supported the existence of highly anionic structural elements of the normal glomerular capillary wall (Jones, 1969; Michael *et al.*, 1970) based on the finding of a pronounced staining by colloidal iron, a so-called "cationic stain," for the glomerular wall. Other cationic stains, including alcian blue, ruthenium red, and lysozyme (Michael *et al.*, 1970; Latta *et al.*, 1975; Caulfield and Farquhar, 1976), also exhibit affinity for all component layers of the glomerular wall. The glomerular epithelial cell and its foot processes are covered with a surface coat of acidic glycoproteins (so-called sialoproteins or glomerular polyanion) which are highly negatively charged. In addition, the epithelial slit diaphragm (a thin membrane lying across channels formed by the interdigitating foot processes) consists, in part, of glycosialoproteins; the glomerular basement membrane (GBM)(Spiro, 1967), as well as the endothelial cell coat have also been shown to contain sialoproteins. Whereas any or all of these highly anionic structural components of the glomerular wall conceivably could contribute to normal electrostatic barrier function, Rennke and Venkatachalam (1977) have recently proposed that the layers closest to the capillary lumen, i.e., the endothelium and the innermost layer of the GBM (lamina rara interna), are likely to provide the primary functional barriers to circulating polyanions. This view also is endorsed by Latta and Johnston (1976).

In addition to molecular size and charge, it is likely that molecular shape (or flexibility) will influence the filtration of macromolecules. Bohrer *et al.* (1978b) have obtained evidence to indicate that, for any given macromolecular radius, Ficoll, an uncharged highly coiled polymer, is filtered to a greater extent than is the less-coiled neutral dextran. Additional studies are required to ascertain the physiological importance of this observation.

4. *Effects of Glomerular Injury on the Size-Selective and Charge-Selective Properties of the Glomerular Capillary Wall*

A variety of glomerular disorders in man and in experimental models of renal disease in animals are associated with alterations in glomerular capillary permselectivity, generally manifested as proteinuria. The effects of immunological injury on the intrinsic selectivity properties of the glomerular capillary wall have been examined using the experimental model of nephrotoxic serum nephritis (NSN) (Bennett *et al.*, 1976; Bohrer *et al.*, 1978a; Chang *et al.*, 1976). Figure 1 compares fractional clearances of neutral dextrans measured in rats with NSN with values obtained in normal rats (Chang *et al.*, 1976). Whereas in normal rats, restriction to filtration of neutral dextrans does not occur until effective radii exceed about 20 Å, in NSN rats, restriction to filtration is evident over the entire range of neutral dextran radii studied. Fractional dextran clearance values at any given molecular size are lower in NSN rats than in normal rats. Differences between NSN and normal rats disappear at effective radii greater than about 40 Å, where fractional clearances for both groups of rats approach zero.

Although not discussed in detail in this brief review, glomerular pressures and flows are themselves capable of strongly influencing fractional dextran clearance profiles (Chang *et al.*, 1975a,c). Values for the glomerular filtration rate of water were near-normal in these NSN rats, while single nephron filtration fraction was lower than that observed in normal rats, despite mean glomerular transcapillary hydraulic pressure differences in excess of normal (Chang *et al.*, 1976). This reduction in filtration fraction resulted from a marked fall in the glomerular capillary ultrafiltration coefficient, the latter on average to a value of about one-third of normal. Hence, the marked reductions in fractional clearances of neutral dextrans in NSN rats must have resulted from changes in the intrinsic properties of the glomerular capillary wall. Since fractional clearances of neutral dextrans in NSN rats decreased, the changes that occurred in effective pore size and/or number of pores would have been expected to decrease, not increase, the filtration and excretion of albumin (Chang *et al.*, 1976). This was not the case since albumin excretion increased about threefold in this model of acute nephritis (Chang *et al.*, 1976).

Because changes in the size-selective properties of the glomerular wall fail to account for the increased filtration of albumin, it was hypothesized that an alteration in glomerular wall charge, and thereby, charge selectivity, could be at fault. Bennett *et al.* (1976) tested this proposal by measuring the filtration of dextran sulfate in another group of proteinuric NSN rats. Figure 1 compares the results in these and normal animals. Animals with NSN had substantially greater fractional clearances of dextran sulfate than normal rats. Histochemical studies revealed that glomerular polyanion content was reduced in NSN rats (Bennett *et al.*, 1976). This supported the conclusion that a loss of fixed negative charge was responsible for the enhanced filtration of circulating polyanions, including both dextran sulfate and albumin.

Such a reduction in fixed negative charges also would be expected to reduce the filtration of polyanionic DEAE dextrans, since the influence of these negative charges on circulating polycations would be lessened. To test this hypothesis, Bohrer *et al.* (1978a) measured DEAE dextran clearances in another group of NSN rats and compared the results to values obtained in normal rats (Fig. 1). In association with the nephrotoxic serum-induced loss of fixed negative charges, there was a pronounced reduction in fractional DEAE dextran clearances, relative to values in normal rats.

Thus, in contrast to the markedly different clearance profiles obtained with the variously charged dextrans in normal rats (Fig. 1, left), in NSN rats, fractional clearances of polyanions such as dextran sulfate, and polycations, such as DEAE dextran, behave much like those of uncharged polymers, such as neutral dextrans (Fig. 1, right). The fractional clearances for all three forms of dextran now assume quantitatively nearly indistinguishable values. With loss of charge discrimination in nephritis, the glomerular barrier becomes essentiall size-selective only, and it processes highly anionic and cationic macromolecules in much the same way as it processes neutral polymers. Since the resulting size-selective barrier is no longer very restrictive for molecules with radii equivalent to that of serum albumin, 36 Å, the presence of substantial amounts of albumin in urine can now be seen as a rather predictable consequence of this form of glomerular injury.

Another model of proteinuria that has been studied in detail is that induced by administration of puromycin aminonucleoside. Morphologically, puromycin leads to changes in glomerular wall structure similar to those seen clinically in patients with minimal change nephrotic syndrome (Vernier *et al.*, 1959). In particular, there is loss of organization of the normally slender, interdigitating glomerular epithelial cell foot processes, or pedicels, which are replaced instead by more or less continuous sheets of epithelial cytoplasm. This is responsible for the term "foot process fusion." Bohrer *et al.* (1977) have recently studied the functional characteristics of this lesion, again by evaluating fractional clearances of dextrans. In these studies, rats were pretreated with puromycin for 6–7 days, utilizing a dose that produces a relatively uniform alteration in glomerular structure, and often dramatic increases in albumin excretion. Nevertheless, fractional clearances of neutral dextrans were found to be decreased, not increased, in puromycin-treated rats, relative to normal controls, over a wide range of molecular radii studied. The results were similar to those obtained with neutral dextrans in rats with NSN, and also in accord with the findings of Robson *et al.* (1974) who noted a decrease, not an increase, in fractional clearances of the neutral molecule, polyvinylpyrrolidone, in children with minimal change nephrotic syndrome. Of note is the fact that fractional clearances of dextran sulfate were found to be higher in puromycin-treated rats than in normal controls (Bohrer *et al.*, 1977), again in agreement with the findings in the NSN model. Enhanced fractional clearances of dextran sulfate, in the absence of a similar change in filtration of neutral dextrans, suggest that, as with nephrotoxic serum, puromycin also reduces the electrostatic barrier to filtration of polyanions. Many workers have observed reduced binding of "cationic stains" to the glomerular wall of animals treated with puromycin (Renkin and Gilmore, 1973; Robson *et al.*, 1974), as well as in patients suffering from a variety of forms of nephrotic syndrome, including, of course, minimal change nephrotic syndrome (Blau and Haas, 1973).

Structural investigations corroborate the role of altered glomerular polyanion content in disease models. Michael *et al.* (1970) documented the coincidence of decreases in glomerular sialoprotein content, proteinuria, and the appearance of foot process fusion in animals with experimental nephrotic syndrome. In regard to this last phenomenon, Seiler *et al.* (1977) have documented the ultrastructural pattern of foot process fusion after perfusion of rat kidneys with polycations (e.g., protamine sulfate). Furthermore, this process reverses upon reperfusion with the strong polyanion heparin. These findings suggest that foot process fusion might result from loss of normal electrostatic repulsive forces between adjacent foot processes, due to the neutralization (or loss) of their anionic coats. Finally, recent evidence indicates that loss of glomerular fixed negative charges also can influence the site and magnitude of immune complex deposition, as well as the deposition of nonimmune circulating aggregates within the glomerular wall and mesangium (Couser *et al.*, 1978; Mauer *et al.*, 1972). One possible, and highly undesirable, clinical consequence of the prolonged presence within the mesangium of such aggregates might be a more or less continuous stimulus to mesangium matrix production, the ultimate result of which might be glomerular sclerosis, either focal or diffuse.

References

Areekul, S., 1969, Reflection coefficients of neutral and sulfate-substituted dextran molecules in the isolated perfused rabbit ear, *Acta Soc. Med. Ups.* **74:**129.

Arturson, G., Groth, T., and Grotte, G., 1971, Human glomerular membrane porosity and filtration pressure: Dextran clearance data analyzed by theoretical models, *Clin. Sci.* **40:**137.

Bayliss, L. E., Tookey-Kerridge, M., and Russell, D. S., 1933, The excretion of protein by the mammalian kidney, *J. Physiol. (London)* **77:**386.

Bennett, C. M., Glassock, R. J., Chang, R. L. S., Deen, W. M., Robertson, C. R., and Brenner, B. M., 1976, Permselectivity of the glomerular capillary wall: Studies of experimental glomerulonephritis in the rat using dextran sulfate, *J. Clin. Invest.* **57:**1287.

Blau, E. B., and Haas, D. E., 1973, Glomerular sialic acid and proteinuria in human renal disease, *Lab. Invest.* **28:**477.

Bohrer, M. P., Baylis, C., Robertson, C. R., and Brenner, B. M., 1977, Mechanism of puromycin-induced defects in the transglomerular passage of water and macromolecules, *J. Clin. Invest.* **60:**152.

Bohrer, M. P., Baylis, C., Humes, H. D., Glassock, R. J., Robertson, C. R., and Brenner, B. M., 1978a, Permselectivity of the glomerular capillary wall: Facilitated filtration of circulating polycations, *J. Clin. Invest.* **61:**72.

Bohrer, M. P., Deen, W. M., Robertson, C. R., Troy, J. L., and Brenner, B. M., 1979, Influence of molecular configuration on the passage of macromolecules, across the glomerular capillary wall, *J. Gen. Physiol.* **74:**583.

Brenner, B. M., Bohrer, M. P., Baylis, C., and Deen, W. M., 1977, Determinants of glomerular permselectivity: Insights derived from observations *in vivo, Kidney Int.* **12:**229.

Caulfield, J. P., and Farquhar, M. G., 1976, Distribution of anionic sites in normal and nephrotic glomerular basement membranes, *J. Cell Biol.* **70:**274 (abstract).

Chang, R. L. S., Robertson, C. R., Deen, W. M., and Brenner, B. M., 1975a, Permselectivity of the glomerular capillary wall to macromolecules. I. Theoretical considerations, *Biophys. J.* **5:**861.

Chang, R. L. S., Deen, W. M., Robertson, C. R., and Brenner, B. M., 1975b, Permselectivity of the glomerular capillary wall. III. Restricted transport of polyanions, *Kidney Int.* **8:**212.

Chang, R. L. S., Ueki, I. F., Troy, J. L., Deen, W. M., Robertson, C. R., and Brenner, B. M., 1975c, Permselectivity of the glomerular capillary wall to macromolecules. II. Experimental observations in the rat, *Biophys. J.* **15:**887.

Chang, R. L. S., Deen, W. M., Robertson, C. R., Bennett, C. M., Glassock, R. J., and Brenner, B. M., 1976, Permselectivity of the glomerular capillary wall: Studies of experimental glomerulonephritis in the rat using neutral dextran, *J. Clin. Invest.* **57:**1272.

Couser, W. G., Hoyer, J. R., Stilmant, M. M., Jermanovich, N. B., and Belok, S., 1978, Effect of aminonucleoside nephrosis on immune complex localization in autologous immune complex nephritis in the rat, *J. Clin. Invest.* **61:**561.

Deen, W. M., Ueki, I. F., and Brenner, B. M., 1976, Permeability of renal peritubular capillaries to neutral dextran and endogenous albumin, *Am. J. Physiol.* **231:**283.

Eisenbach, G. M., Van Liew, J. B., and Boylan, J. W., 1975, Effect of angiotensin on the filtration of protein in the rat kidney: A micropuncture study, *Kidney Int.* **8:**80.

Gaizutis, M., Pesce, A. J., and Lewy, J. E., 1972, Determination of nonogram amounts of albumin by radiommunoassay, *Microchem. J.* **17:**327.

Hardwicke, J., Cameron, J. S., Harrison, J. F., Hulme, B., and Soothill, J. F., 1970, Proteinuria, studied by clearances of individual macromolecules, in: *Proteins in Normal and Pathological Urine* (Y. Manuel, J. P. Revillard, and H. Betuel, eds.), pp. 111–152, University Park Press, Baltimore.

Jones, D. B., 1969, Mucosubstances of the glomerulus, *Lab. Invest.* **21:**119.

Latta, H., and Johnston, W. H., 1976, The glycoprotein inner layer of glomerular capillary basement membrane as a filtration barrier, *J. Ultrastruct. Res.***57:**65.

Latta, H., Johnston, W. H., and Stanley, T. M., 1975, Sialoglycoproteins and filtration barriers in the glomerular capillary wall, *J. Ultrastruct. Res.* **51:**354.

Mauer, S. M., Fish, A. J., Blau, E. B., and Michael, A. F., 1972, The glomerular mesangium. I. Kinetic studies of macromolecular uptake in normal and nephrotic rats, *J. Clin. Invest.* **51:**1092.

Michael, A. F., Blau, E. B., and Vernier, R. L., 1970, Glomerular polyanion alteration in aminonucleoside nephrosis, *Lab. Invest.* **23:**619.

Rennke, H. G., Patel, Y., and Venkatachalam, M. A., 1978, Effect of molecular charge on glomerular permeability to proteins in the rat: Clearance studies using neutral, anionic and cationic horseradish peroxidase, *Kidney Int.* **13:**278.

Rennke, H., and Venkatachalam, M. A., 1977, Glomerular permeability: *In vivo* tracer studies with polyanionic and polycationic ferritins, Vol. 2 *Kidney Int.* 44.

Renkin, E. M., and Gilmore, J. P., 1973, Glomerular filtration, in: *Handbook of Physiology*, Section 8, *Renal Physiology* (J. Orloff and R. W. Berliner, eds.), pp. 185–248, American Physiological Society, Washington, D.C.

Robson, A. M., Giangiacomo, J., Keinstra, R. A., Naqvi, S. T., and Ingelfinger, J. R., 1974, Normal glomerular permeability and its modification by minimal change nephrotic syndrome, *J. Clin. Invest.* **54:**1190.

Seiler, M. W., Rennke, H. G., Venkatachalam, M. A., and Cotran, R. S., 1977, Pathogenesis of polycation-induced alterations ("fusion") of glomerular epithelium, *Lab Invest.* **36:**48.

Spiro, R. G., 1967, Studies on the renal glomerular basement membrane: Preparation and chemical composition, *J. Biol. Chem.* **242:**1915.

Vernier, R. L., Papermaster, B. W., and Good, R. A., 1959, Aminonucleoside nephrosis. I. Electron microscopic study of the renal lesion in rats, *J. Exp. Med.* **109:**115.

Verniory, A., DuBois, R., DeCoodt, P., Gassée, J. P., and Lambert, P. P., 1973, Measurement of the permeability of biological membranes: Application to the glomerular wall, *J. Gen. Physiol.* **62:**489.

3

The Molecular Structure of Basement Membranes as It Relates to Function

Nicholas A. Kefalides

1. Introduction

Any attempt to correlate the chemical structural properties of glomerular basement membrane with those of its apparent functions assumes certain prerequisites. Adequate knowledge of the number and the chemical nature of the macromolecular components as well as of the mode of their interaction is clearly necessary. Knowledge of the immunochemical nature of these components in order to explain a number of immunologic reactions is definitely desirable. Information about the ionic charge of the basement membrane and the fate of molecules and cells brought to it by the circulating blood is an important prerequisite. There are two ways of correlating chemical structure with function: (1) either by assigning possible morphologic and functional properties to known chemical and molecular features, or (2) by attempting to explain a series of apparent functions by the chemical structure of the basement membrane.

Although considerable information on the chemical composition of basement membranes has been published, our knowledge of the macromolecular composition and hence of the structural organization of these extracellular matrices remains incomplete. To attempt to correlate the molecular properties of a given basement membrane, such as the glomerular basement membrane (GBM), with its functional behavior would appear to be a difficult if not an impossible task. However, recent studies in our laboratory (Olsen *et al.*, 1973; Clark and Kefalides, 1978; Minor *et al.*, 1976; Dehm and Kefalides, 1978a,b) and in the laboratories of others (Grant *et al.*,

Nicholas A. Kefalides · Connective Tissue Research Institute, University of Pennsylvania and The University City Science Center, Philadelphia, Pennsylvania 19104. AM 20553, HL 18827, and HL 15061.

1975; Heathcote *et al.*, 1978; Schwartz and Veis, 1978; Timpl *et al.*, 1978) have produced data which allow us to suggest models of the protein macromolecules isolated from basement membranes as well as ways in which these molecules interact to give a supramolecular organization.

It is now well accepted that two general types of protein components constitute the basement membrane complex. One of these exists in the form of a procollagen-like molecule, i.e., a molecule composed of a collagen triple-helix having nonhelical, largely noncollagenous extensions at the carboxy and amino termini. The procollagen-like molecule is thought to interact with one or more glycoproteins which are noncollagenous in nature. The relative proportion of the latter component varies among basement membranes, making up from 0 to 5% of the lens capsule basement membrane and approximately 25% of the GBM (Kefalides, 1975; Minor *et al.*, 1976; Clark and Kefalides, 1978). The information gained from the above studies, when combined with that gained from the studies of Caulfield (1978), Caulfield and Farquhar (1976),Farquhar (1975, 1978), Ryan and Karnovsky (1976), and Venkatachalam *et al.* (1978) about the morphologic and functional properties of GBM, should permit a small venture into the realm of structure–function relationships in basement membranes.

This paper summarizes the morphologic, physicochemical, and immunologic properties of GBM as well as of other basement membranes; presents recent evidence on the structure and biosythesis of their protein components; and suggests a relationship between the molecular properties of basement membranes and their functional behavior.

2. *Morphologic Considerations*

The ultrastructural appearance of GBM as well as of other basement membranes has been established for several tissues and species. The presence of thin filaments, 40–60 Å in diameter, within a homogenous electron-dense matrix has been well documented (Farquhar *et al.*, 1961; Farquhar, 1978; Jakus, 1964).

Unlike the situation in the lens capsule where the basement membrane appears homogeneous in its entire thickness, in the GBM, the subepidermal basement membrane and in the basement membrane of the corneal epithelium an electron-lucid zone appears between the electron-dense zone and the adjacent cell layer. This zone has been termed lamina lucida or lamina rara. In the glomerular capillary, there are two such zones, termed lamina rara interna and lamina rara externa. A loose filamentous structure has been demonstrated in the laminae rarae. Whether the lucid zone is a result of tissue fixation or is a real structural entity, cannot be stated with certainty. It is suggested that the same macromolecular components present in the lamina densa are probably also present in the laminae rarae. However, in the latter, they may not be as completely "condensed" or as crosslinked as in the lamina densa. If this is the case, then one would expect different functional groups on the various molecules of the laminae rarae to be exposed. Conceivably, these might contribute to differences in the net charge and in possible function.

The lack of discernible, specific order of macromolecular organization in GBM and in other basement membranes, as seen with the electron microscope, may very well be a function of the primary, secondary, and tertiary structure of the protein molecules and of their specific interactions within the basement membranes.

3. Physicochemical Properties

The complexity in the composition and structure of basement membranes was recognized rapidly when it was found that these membranes were relatively insoluble in weak solutions of acids and bases or of neutral salts, and that they had an amino acid and carbohydrate composition unlike that of many known proteins. However, the membranes were solubilized readily by reducing agents in the presence of strong denaturants such as 8 M urea of 1% SDS. Bacterial collagenase as well as a number of proteolytic enzymes can solubilize basement membranes at 37°C, degrading them to fragments of various molecular sizes (Kefalides, 1971b, 1973).

Analytical and enzymatic studies indicated the presence of a collagenous component. Since, upon electron microscopy, no typical collagen fibers could be observed, the question was raised as to the nature of the organization of the collagenous molecules. X-Ray diffraction studies of samples of GBM, performed by Dr. I. Corvin of the Illinois Institute of Technology, showed powder diagrams having maximal deflections at 2.85, 4.23, and 10.27 Å which are typical of collagen (Table 1) (Kefalides and Winzler, 1966). The appearance of a powder diagram rather than of a fiber diagram is consistent with the lack of collagen fibers on electron microscopy suggestive of the presence of partially oriented collagen molecules. The persistence of procollagen molecules in basement membranes may explain this structural feature.

The chemical composition of basement membranes has been established

Table 1. X-Ray Diffraction Measurements of Basement Membrane and Interstitial Collagen[a]

Collagen fiber d (Å)		Heat-denatured collagen d (Å)		Dog basement membrane d (Å)	
Arc	11.32	Halo	11.62	Intense halo	10.27
Arc	7.25	Line	7.62		
Arc	7.71	Line	6.02		
Broad halo	4.28	Broad halo	4.18	Intense halo	4.23
Broad halo	2.19	Line	2.86	Line	2.85

[a] Kefalides and Winzler (1966).

Table 2. *Amino Acid Composition of Mammalian Basement Membranes*[a]

	Human[b]		Canine[b] Descemet's membrane
	Glomerulus	Lens capsule	
Hydroxylysine	24.5	34.5	20.0
Lysine	26.4	19.4	24.0
Histidine	18.7	15.2	11.6
Arginine	48.3	39.5	39.5
3-Hydroxyproline	12.0	21.3	6.8
4-Hydroxyproline	53.0	85.0	77.0
Aspartic	70.0	57.0	58.0
Threonine	40.3	31.0	36.4
Serine	54.2	43.4	42.0
Glutamic	101.3	94.4	94.0
Proline	64.1	67.3	95.0
Glycine	225.2	260.0	230.0
Alanine	58.6	40.6	53.0
Half-cystine	22.0	21.0	11.0
Valine	36.0	33.2	45.0
Methionine	7.0	5.0	8.2
Isoleucine	28.6	32.0	28.5
Leucine	60.3	57.7	75.2
Tyrosine	20.5	13.0	21.0
Phenylalanine	28.3	29.8	25.0

[a] Residues per 1000 residues.
[b] Kefalides and Denduchis (1969).

for several tissues and species (Kefalides, 1971a, 1973). Tables 2 and 3 summarize the amino acid and carbohydrate composition of three representative mammalian basement membranes. Characteristic of their amino acid composition is the high content of the amino acids proline and 3- and 4-hydroxyproline, of the nonpolar amino acid glycine, and the basic amino acid hydroxylysine. Although in most mammalian collagens the sum of

Table 3. *Carbohydrate Composition of Mammalian Basement Membranes*[a]

	Human[b]		Canine[b] Descemet's membrane
	Glomerulus	Lens capsule	
Hexose	6.8	11.8	8.2
Glucose	2.5	5.5	3.5
Galactose	2.6	5.6	3.7
Mannose	1.7	0.7	2.0
Glucosamine	1.7	0.8	1.2
Galactosamine	0.3	0.2	0.3
Fucose	0.7	0.6	0.6
Sialic Acid	1.5	0.5	0.7
Hexuronic Acid	—	—	0.05

[a] Grams per 100 g.
[b] Kefalides and Denduchis (1969).

proline plus hydroxyproline accounts for almost 22% of the amino acid residues, the sum of these two amino acids accounts for 14, 17.4, and 17.7% for glomerular, lens capsule, and Descemet's membranes, respectively. Similarly, whereas glycine accounts for one-third of the amino acid residues in interstitial collagens, it accounts for about one-fourth in whole basement membranes. Since hydroxyproline and hydroxylysine are found almost exclusively in interstitial collagen, it was deduced that one of the protein components in basement membranes must be collagenous. The lower hydroxyproline and glycine content indicated that proteins other than collagen are also present. The heterogeneity of the molecular composition of basement membranes was suggested by significant amounts of cysteine and tyrosine, by a low total imino acid content, and by the fact that in addition to glucose and galactose, hexosamine, mannose, fucose, and sialic acid, sugars not present in soluble collagens, are found in basement membranes (Kefalides, 1971a, 1973). Solubility studies and analyses of the solubilized fractions have indicated that basement membranes are composed of dissimilar protein subunits (Kefalides, 1975). The data show that the ratio of hydroxylysine to hexosamine varies according to the conditions of solubilization. Extraction of glomerular basement membrane with 8 M urea alone or by reduction and alkylation alone resulted in a lower hydroxylysine:hexosamine ratio than that found in the intact membrane, whereas with anterior lens capsule, the ratio in the soluble fractions was the same as that in the intact membrane. Reduction and alkylation, in the presence of 8 M urea, of all three types of membranes, solubilized practically the entire membrane. The ratio of hydroxylysine:hexosamine in this fraction was the same as that in the intact membrane. These data support the hypothesis that a noncollagenous protein component or components are associated with the collagenous component via hydrogen and disulfide bonds. Lysine-derived and hydroxylysine-derived cross-links are also present and contribute to the total structural organization and stability of basement membranes (Tanzer and Kefalides, 1973).

Nature of the Protein Components

The Collagenous Component

Further evidence for the presence of collagenous and noncollagenous protein components came from the isolation of a collagen, after basement membranes from various tissues had been treated with Pronase or pepsin at low temperatures (Kefalides, 1968, 1971b; Dehm and Kefalides, 1978a,b). This collagen, designated Type IV collagen, met the chemical and physical criteria for collagens isolated from interstitial connective tissue; proline and hydroxyproline accounted for 20 to 22% and glycine for 33% of all the amino acid residues (Table 4). The isolated collagen molecule had a triple-helical configuration suggested by the high intrinsic viscosity, the high negative specific optical rotation, and the characteristic circular dichroism pattern (Kefalides, 1968, 1973).

Table 4. Amino Acid Composition of α-Chains Isolated from Basement Membrane and Interstitial Collagens after a Single Pepsin Digestion[a]

	Human[b]	Sheep[b]		Canine[c]
	Glomerulus	Anterior lens capsule	Descemet's membrane	Tendon
Hydroxylysine	44.6	57.0	43.0	6.0
Lysine	10.0	10.0	15.2	23.0
Histidine	10.4	8.0	7.8	4.0
Arginine	33.0	27.0	30.0	45.0
3-Hydroxyproline	11.0	12.0	8.0	1.0
4-Hydroxyproline	130.0	120.0	157.0	93.0
Aspartic	51.0	50.0	30.0	46.0
Threonine	23.0	20.0	18.0	18.0
Serine	37.0	38.0	25.0	33.0
Glutamic	84.0	92.0	78.0	73.0
Proline	61.0	67.0	90.0	130.0
Glycine	310.0	330.0	320.0	331.0
Alanine	33.0	32.0	32.0	122.0
Half-cystine	(8.0)[d]	(8.0)[d]	8.0	0.0
Valine	29.0	26.0	25.0	20.0
Methionine	10.0	10.0	9.5	7.0
Isoleucine	30.0	20.0	24.0	110.0
Leucine	54.0	43.0	52.0	21.0
Tyrosine	6.0	2.0	3.0	4.0
Phenylalanine	27.0	30.0	22.0	13.0

[a] Residues per 1000 residues.
[b] Kefalides (1971b).
[c] Kefalides (1973).
[d] Not present in chains obtained after three-step procedure (Dehm and Kefalides, 1978).

When the collagen prepared after the basement membranes had been treated with pepsin was denatured and chromatographed on carboxymethyl-cellulose, only a single major component emerged, eluting in the region of α-chains. Therefore, it was concluded that the basement membrane collagen molecule is composed of three identical α-chains (Kefalides, 1971b). The amino acid composition of the α-chains isolated by carboxymethyl-cellulose chromatography from various basement membrane collagens shows that they are all characterized by unusually high amounts of hydroxyproline and hydroxylysine. The sum of lysine and hydroxylysine is higher than that of interstitial collagens, but the sum of proline and hydroxyproline is closer to the sum observed for interstitial collagens. A significant percentage of the total hydroxyproline is 3-hydroxyproline approaching 9–10 residues per 1000 residues. Glycine accounts for one-third of all the amino acid residues. Alanine and arginine, however, are low and correspond to about 30% and 60% of the values found in interstitial collagens. Another unusual feature was the presence of 4-8 residues and half-cystine. As it will be shown later, this was due to incomplete cleavage of the propeptides by pepsin. The chains from all three types of basement membranes contain from 10.0 to 12.5%

hexoses with equimolar amounts of glucose and galactose (Table 5).About 95% of all the hexose is in the form of the disaccharide unit, glucosyl-galactosyl-hydroxylysine, while the rest is in the form of galactosyl-hydroxylysine. Less than 0.2% of mannose and glucosamine was also found. The presence of small amounts of these two sugars is consistent with the presence of half-cystine and with the persistence of uncleaved propeptides.

The presence of 4–8 residues of half-cystine in the basement membrane collagen isolated after a single pepsin digestion suggested the possibility that persistence of disulfide bonds in the nonhelical carboxy and amino termini of the procollagen molecule of basement membrane may have prevented pepsin from digesting the nonhelical peptide extensions completely. This possibility was strengthened by the fact that the molecular weight of the isolated α-chains was greater than that of interstitial collagen α-chain (95,000 vs. 110,000) (Kefalides, 1971b). Complete cleavage of the propeptides was accomplished in a three-step procedure by Dehm and Kefalides (1978a,b) who succeeded in isolating basement membrane collagen α-chains, from bovine lens capsule and GBM, having a molecular weight of 95,000. The procedure involves an initial treatment of the basement membrane with pepsin at 16°C followed by reduction and alkylation of the resultant product at 16°C, under nondenaturing conditions, and then by another pepsin treatment of the reduced and alkylated material.

Although a single limited proteolysis by pepsin visibly disperses the bovine lens capsule and GBM pieces, it does not cleave all components in the basement membrane to the same extent. This observation could be explained by assuming that the lens capsule and GBM are built from "core units," which are released by pepsin digestion, but are then only cleaved peripherally and remain aggregated because of disulfide bonds. This could explain why essentially identical results are obtained whether basement

Table 5. Carbohydrate Composition of α-Chains Isolated from Basement Membrane Collagens after a Single Pepsin Digestion[a]

	Human	Sheep	
	Glomerulus	Anterior lens capsule	Descemet's membrane
		g/100 g	
Hexose	12.0	12.5	10.0
Glucose	5.5	6.0	5.0
Galactose	6.0	6.3	5.2
Mannose	0.2	0.2	0.2
Fucose	0	0	0
Hexosamine	0.1	0.1	0.1
		μmoles/μmole α-chain	
Glc-Gal-Hly	34	34	26
Gal-Hly	2	2	1.8

[a] Kefalides (1971b).

membranes are subjected first to reduction and alkylation under nondenaturing conditions and then treated with pepsin, or, as described above, are treated with pepsin first and then reduced and alkylated.

The main peptide fragment isolated by gel filtration from the second pepsin digestion was shown by amino acid analysis to be a basement membrane collagen α-chain containing no half-cystine. Gel filtration in 1 M $CaCl_2$ and polyacrylamide gel electrophoresis in the presence of SDS indicated that the fragment has about the same size as the α1-chain of Type I collagen isolated from tendon or skin. Also, it appeared to be a major component of the lens basement membrane as well as of the GBM, in that about 70% of the collagen originally present, determined as hydroxyproline, was recovered after the second pepsin digestion, of which a large portion eluted as the α-chain-size peptide (Dehm and Kefalides, 1978a,b).

Nevertheless, the possibility that there is more than one collagen chain in basement membranes emerged when Dixit (1979) and Gay and Miller (1979) reported on the isolation of two collagenous polypeptide chains from whole glomeruli and anterior lens capsule, respectively. Dixit (1979) digested lyophilized human glomeruli with pepsin at an enzyme substrate ratio of 1:10 for 62 hours at 4°C. The solubilized collagenous protein was purified by salt fractionation. Following molecular sieve filtration, the fraction eluting in the region of α-chains of tendon collagen was chromatographed on a CM-cellulose and the two main fractions, C and D, which emerged were examined by SDS-gel electrophoresis and amino acid analysis. The molecular weight of the C-chain corresponded to 95,000 and that of the D-chain, after reduction of disulphide bonds, to 75,000. On amino acid analysis, both the C and D fractions had features characteristic of basement membrane collagen; however, the D-chain had a lower content of hydroxylysine. Gay and Miller (1979) isolated similar collagenous chains from bovine anterior lens capsules (ALC). Unlike Dixit, they treated the lens capsules with a solution of 5 M urea containing 10 mM 2-mercaptoethanol before digesting with pepsin. Gay and Miller used excessive amounts of pepsin ranging from 1:1 to 1:10 enzyme:substrate ratio.

Dehm and Kefalides (1978a) further demonstrated that if fresh lens capsules containing viable cells were incubated in the presence of ^{14}C-proline and then subjected to the three-step procedure, a hydroxy [^{14}C]proline containing major fraction was obtained which on gel filtration and CM-cellulose chromatography coeluted with the 95,000 m.wt. peptide. Similar results were obtained with GBM (Dehm and Kefalides, 1978b). It was concluded from these studies that basement membranes contain at least one triple helical collagen polypeptide composed of identical chains. Smaller molecular weight fragments containing hydroxy[^{14}C]proline were also present and could have resulted from degradation of the D-chain.

The Noncollagenous Glycoprotein

Soluble glycoprotein fractions which lack hydroxyproline, hydroxylysine, and glucose can be obtained from GBM and Descemet's membrane by extraction with 8 M urea at 40°C for 48 hr followed by gel filtration in Sephadex G-200 with 8 M urea (Denduchis and Kefalides, 1970; Kefalides, 1971a). An alternative method involves solubilization of the membranes by reduction and alkylation without 8 M urea, and isolation of a fraction by gel filtration on Sephadex G-200. These fractions have an amino acid composition unlike that of the collagen component. Consistent with the absence of hydroxylysine is the absence of glucose. Galactose, mannose, hexosamine, fucose, and sialic acid are present in significant amounts. The molecular weight of these fractions is greater than 200,000 (Kefalides, 1972). The sequence and linkage of the sugars in the polysaccharide chains of the high-molecular-weight protein are still unknown although linkage to asparagine has been suggested.

Noncollagenous glycoprotein fractions of low molecular weight were obtained after prolonged digestion of the basement membranes with bacterial collagenase (Denduchis and Kefalides, 1970; Kefalides, 1972). This procedure solubilized 72 to 90% of the membranes and rendered over 90% of the hydroyproline dialyzable. A low-molecular-weight glycoprotein was isolated from the soluble, undialyzable collagenase digest by gel filtration on Sephadex G-200. Amino acid analysis of this fraction showed no hydroxyproline or hydroxylysine but significant amounts of half-cystine. Carbohydrate analysis showed significant amounts of hexose composed mainly of galactose, mannose, hexosamine, fucose, and sialic acid.

The fraction which remains undigested after the basement membrane has been treated with collagenase can be partially solubilized by reduction and alkylation in 8 M urea and further purified on Sephadex G-200 (Kefalides, 1972). On the basis of its amino acid and carbohydrate composition, this fraction contains a noncollagen-type glycoprotein or glycoproteins. Since it is excluded on Sephadex G-200, its molecular weight must be 200,000 or greater and may form a highly cross-linked polymer.

4. Biosynthesis of Basement Membrane Procollagen

Knowledge of the biosynthesis of basement membrane collagen is intimately tied to knowledge obtained from the studies of synthesis of interstitial Type I collagen.

Recent evidence has shown that basement membrane collagen is, like Type I interstitial collagen, synthesized as a procollagen-like molecule (Grant *et al.*, 1972, 1973, 1975; Kefalides, 1973; Kefalides *et al.*, 1976; Minor *et al.*, 1976). The intracellular steps involved in the synthesis of the various procollagens include: (1) transcription of DNA; (2) translation of the specific RNA leading to synthesis of the pro-α chain; (3) hydroxylation of prolyl and lysyl residues to yield hydroxyproline and hydroxylysine as the peptide chain is elongated on the ribosomes; (4) glycosylation of hydroxylysyl residues on the collagenous portion of the chain and of asparagine residues on the propeptide extensions; (5) release of chains from the ribosomes followed by interchain disulfide bond formation giving rise to a triple-stranded molecule which (6) undergoes supercoiling to form a triple-helical procollagen molecule before secretion (Fig. 1).

The molecular structure of basement membrane procollagen is consistent with a triple-helical collagen molecule having non-triple-helical appendages (variably called propeptides or peptide extensions) at the amino and carboxy termini. Although the structure of newly synthesized basement membrane procollagen has not been studied as extensively as that of interstitial Type I procollagen, several experiments have confirmed the following facts. Initial studies (Grant *et al.*, 1972, 1975) employing gel filtration in SDS suggested that the molecular weight of basement membrane pro-α chain was 140,000 but more recent studies by Kefalides *et al.* (1976) and Minor *et al.* (1976) indicate a molecular weight of 155,000 to 160,00. Using the rat parietal yolk sac system, Clark and Kefalides (1978) have shown that the size of basement membrane pro-α chains approaches 185,000 and 170,000. In this respect, basement membrane pro-α chains differ from interstitial Type I pro-α chains

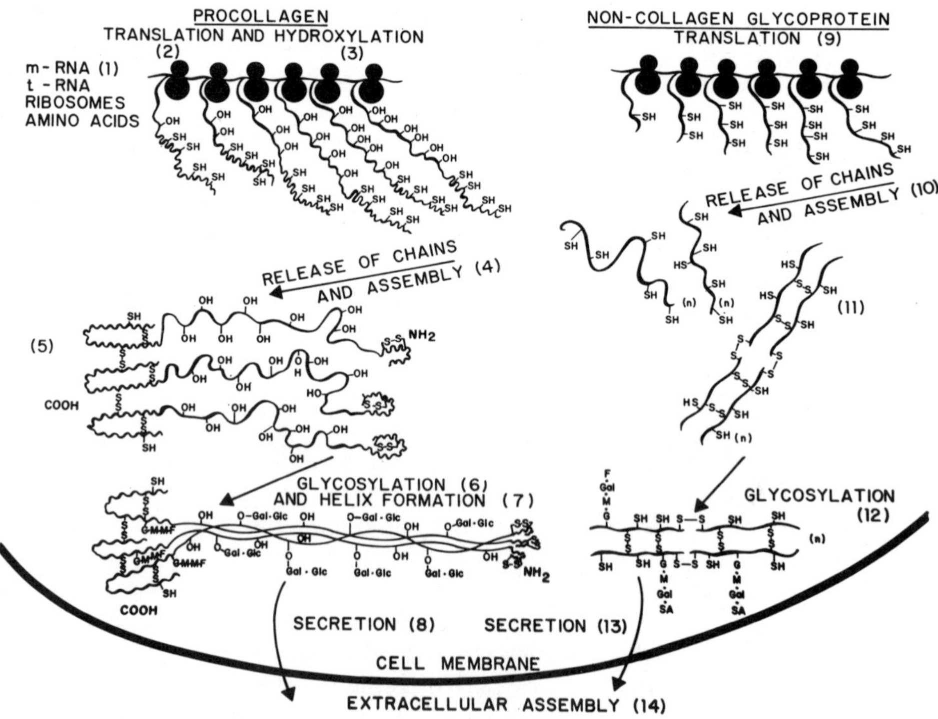

Figure 1. Pathway of the intracellular events in the synthesis of basement membrane procollagen and noncollagen glycoprotein(s). Intracellular event 1 is the transcription, events 2 and 9 depict translation, and events 3–7 and 10–12 are posttranslational. G-M-M-F and G-M-Gal-SA, oligosaccharide units; O-Gal and O-Gal-Glc, hydroxylysine-linked glycosides; G, glucosamine; M, mannose; F, fucose; SA, sialic acid; Gal, galactose; Glc, glucose; NH_2, amino terminus; COOH, carboxy terminus. (Modified from Kefalides, 1975.)

whose molecular weight was recently shown to be 150,00 (Monson *et al.*, 1975).

The basement membrane procollagen secreted into the medium by matrix-free cells isolated from chick lens (Grant *et al.*, 1973) or by parietal yolk sac endoderm (Minor *et al.*, 1976) is highly resistant to pepsin at 15°C. This evidence suggests that it may be in a triple-helical conformation. In contrast, intracellular basement membrane procollagen is digested largely by pepsin at 15°C and therefore is probably in a random coil form. Gel filtration in SDS has shown that when reduction with mercaptoethanol was omitted before chromatography, the procollagen polypeptides in the medium were recovered in aggregates greater than 150,000. In cell fractions, almost all of the procollagen polypeptides eluted with molecular weights of 160,000, regardless of whether or not reduction with mercaptoethanol was used. These observations are consistent with the possibility that the formation of disulfide bonds between the polypeptide chains is of major importance in promotion of the formation of the triple-helix.

This observation may be related closely to the observation that a delay of 60 min is apparent between the incorporation of [^{14}C]proline into protein and the secretion of significant amounts of procollagen as measured by the appearance of 4-hydroxy[^{14}C]proline in the culture medium. This delay is greater than the delay observed in cell systems which synthesize interstitial collagens Type I and II. This delay lasts only 20 and 35 min, respectively. The procollagen molecule must be in a triple-helical conformation to be secreted. This step requires the propr formation of interchain disulfide bonds. Hence, the delay in the secretion of basement membrane procollagen may be due to the delay in disulfide bonding and triple-helix formation (Table 6).

Another important difference in the properties of basement membrane procollagen as compared with the interstitial ones is in the posttranslational modification of the molecule. As is shown in Table 6, the 3-hydroxyproline content is about 10 times higher in basement membrane procollagen (Type IV) than in interstitial procollagens Type I, II, and III. The hydroxyproline content is about 60% in basement membrane procollagen as compared with 44% in Types I and II of interstitial procollagens. The percent glycosylation of hydroxylysine is about 90% and the predominant form is glucosyl-galactosyl-hydroxylysine.

Although it was suggested initially that there was a time-dependent conversion of basement membrane procollagen (Grant *et al.*, 1972), recent studies (Minor *et al.*, 1976; Heathcote *et al.*, 1978) have shown that unlike interstitial procollagens, basement membrane procollagen does not undergo conversion to a smaller molecular species. From these studies and from ultrastructural studies of a sodium citrate-soluble fraction obtained from lens capsule (Olsen *et al.*, 1973), it is apparent that the collagenous component in basement membranes exists in the "procollagen-like" form. This property may be responsible for the failure to observe collagen fibers in basement membranes.

Table 6. Summary of Differences between Newly Synthesized Interstitial and Basement Membrane Procollagens

Collagen Type	3-Hyp: Total Hyp × 100	4-Hyp: Total Pro × 100	Glycosylated Hyl: Total Hyl × 100	Disulfide bond and helix formation	Secretion time	Molecular weight of α-chain after pepsin	Persistence of disulfide bonds: After single pepsin	Persistence of disulfide bonds: After three-step procedure
I	1–3%	44%	21%	5–10 min	20 min	95,000	No	—
II	1–3%	44%	67%	5–15 min	35 min	95,000	No	—
III	1–2%	50%	?	?	?	95,000	Yes	—
IV	10–15%	60%	95%	45 min	60 min	115,000 (95,000)[a]	Yes	No

[a] Molecular weight after three-step procedure involving pepsin digestion followed by reduction and alkylation under nondenaturing conditions and then a second pepsin digestion, all three steps at 16°C (Dehm and Kefalides, 1978a,b).

5. Immunochemical Properties of Basement Membrane

Immunologic studies have demonstrated that basement membranes from various tissues and species possess common antigenic determinants. The nephrotoxicity of antibodies to homologous and heterologous GBM antibodies has been demonstrated (for review see Kefalides, 1971a). Interstitial nephritis has been induced by injecting whole homologous or heterologous tubular basement membrane (Lehman *et al.*, 1974). The antigenic components in the basement membranes responsible for the pathologic reactions have been incompletely characterized (Albini *et al.*, 1978; Johnson *et al.*, 1978; Shibata, 1978). Since all protein moieties in basement membranes are potentially immunogenic, they could cause nephritogenic antisera.

Recent studies on the immunochemistry of collagenous and noncollagenous components isolated from basement membranes, and the use of antibodies against the collagenous components to study the immunochemistry of newly synthesized basement membrane procollagen will be presented below.

Three antigenic components from glomerular and Descemet's membranes (Kefalides, 1971a, 1972) as well as from anterior lens capsule (Denduchis and Kefalides, 1970) have been isolated and characterized immunochemically. One of the antigenic components corresponds to the triple-helical portion of the procollagenous extension of this molecule another to the non-helical propeptide extensions and the third component corresponds to the large-molecular-weight matrix glycoprotein, now referred to as laminin (Timpl *et al.*, 1979) (Fig. 2). Recent studies by Bardos *et al.* (1976) confirm the antigenic complexity of GBM. In tubular basement membrane, three antigenic components also have been demonstrated by Ferwerda *et al.* (1978). One of these components may be represented by the collagen and the other two by noncollagenous glycoproteins.

When whole basement membrane is used for immunization, the antibodies produced are directed against antigenic determinants which reside in noncollagenous peptides. Determinants on the collagenous moiety are masked in the whole membrane and do not stimulate antibody formation to a perceptible degree.

Although antibodies can be produced against either the collagenous or the noncollagenous peptides of GBM or against both, there is not always a direct correlation between the number and the type of antibodies made and the chemical composition of the immunogen. A peptide fraction of GBM may contain both collagenous and noncollagenous regions. The antibody or antibodies may be directed against the collagenous region, against the noncollagenous region, or against both. Kefalides (1972) prepared antibodies not only against whole GBM but also against noncollagenous fractions obtained after digestion of GBM with bacterial collagenase. He showed the presence of at least two antigenic components, both of which were noncollagenous glycoproteins. Antibodies against the collagenous component of GBM and of anterior lens capsule were obtained by Kefalides (1972),

A - Procollagen

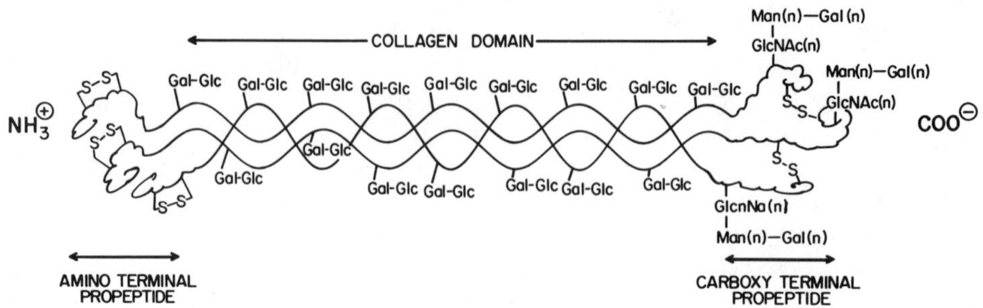

B-Noncollagen Glycoprotein

	A	B
ALC	95%	5%
GBM	75%	25%
DM	70%	30%
PYS	60%	40%

Figure 2. Diagram of basement membrane procollagen and noncollagen glycoprotein molecules. The newly synthesized procollagen molecule is composed of three α-chains having noncollagenous extensions at the amino and carboxy termini. Interchain disulfide bonds stabilize the propeptides at the carboxy terminus while at the amino terminus the disulfide bonds are thought to be intrachain. Disaccharide units are found on the collagen domain of the pro-α chains, whereas oligosaccharide units are thought to be linked to the propeptides. The noncollagen glycoproteins are linked by disulfide bonds and interact with the procollagen molecules via covalent and noncovalent bonds to give the desired ultrastructure at the indicated ratios calculated from analytical data. DM, Descemet's membrane; GBM, glomerular basement membrane; PYS, parietal yolk sac; ALC, anterior lens capsule.

Denduchis and Kefalides (1970), and Gunson and Kefalides (1976). Marquardt *et al.* (1973) solubilized GBM with chaotropes into fractions of varying amino acid composition and demonstrated the presence of at least four distinct antigens.

Antibodies against a human GBM fraction were prepared by Mahieu *et al.* (1974). A radioimmunoassay was developed to detect a peptide fraction of GBM with molecular weight of 70,000. This antigen had an amino acid and carbohydrate composition very similar to that of whole GBM. Glycopeptides containing only either the hydroxylysine-linked glycosides or the heteropolysaccharide were prepared and were used as inhibitors in a radioimmunoassay employing ^{125}I-labeled GBM fractions ([^{125}I]-GBM-Ag). Although both types of glycopeptides inhibited the binding of [^{125}I]-GBM-Ag to anti-GBM antibodies eluted from kidneys of patients with Goodpasture's syndrome, the hydroxylysine-containing glycopeptide was more efficient. However, the purity of these peptides is uncertain as is the interpretation of these data.

The specificity of antibodies against the collagen component of bovine anterior lens capsule, isolated after a single limited digestion with pepsin, was investigated by Gunson and Kefalides (1976). Using a radioimmunoassay, they demonstrated that the above antibodies were type-specific for basement membrane collagen (Type IV) and did not cross-react with interstitial collagens Type I, II, or III. Using the same approach, Gunson *et al.* (1976) demonstrated that basement membrane procollagen synthesized by a variety of cell systems including rat parietal yolk sac endoderm, rabbit Descemet's membrane endothelium or vascular endothelium, could be precipitated with the above antiserum. Antigenic cross-reaction between bovine anterior lens capsule collagen and the procollagen synthesized by bovine aorta endothelial cells in culture was demonstrated by Howard *et al.* (1976). These studies demonstrate the tissue and species nonspecificity of the antibodies.

It can be stated with certainty: (1) that there is immunologic cross-reaction among homologous and heterologous basement membranes, and (2) that the antigenicity of basement membranes resides in glycoprotein components having the composition of collagen, procollagen extension peptides, and noncollagenous glycoprotein molecules. There is some evidence that hydroxylation of proline as well as the integrity of disulfide bonds may influence the antigenicity of the collagen and procollagen components, possibly through their conformational effects on these molecules (Arbogast *et al.*, 1976).

In those tissues where the presence of basement membrane has been demonstrated only by electron microscopy and where the basement membrane isolation has not been accomplished, the demonstration of one or more of its protein components must depend on the use of nonspecific antibodies prepared against basement membrane components of other tissues. This situation is noted particularly in tissues such as skin, aorta, smooth and skeletal muscle fibers, and in developing embryonic tissues.

6. *Supramolecular Organization*

A model for the supramolecular organization of basement membranes is presented in Fig. 3. This model is consistent with most of the available biochemical, biosynthetic, and immunologic evidence.

The main building block is the triple-helical basement membrane procollagen-like molecule depicted in Figs. 2 and 3. The procollagen-like molecules polymerize through the introduction of at least two types of covalent cross-linkage: intermolecular disulfide bonds, and the lysine (and/or hydroxylysine)-derived cross-linkages. The disulfide bonds probably are located within the noncollagenous peptide extensions of the procollagen molecule, whereas the lysine-derived cross-linkages probably are found within the collagenous domain. A third type of covalent linkage also may be present

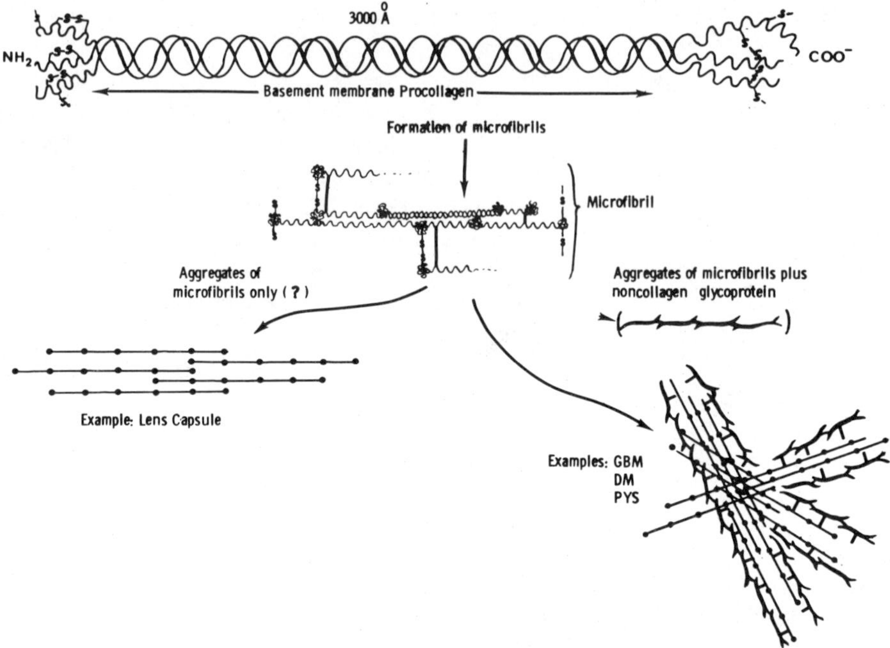

Figure 3. Diagram of a hypothetical model of the supramolecular organization of basement membranes (for details see Fig. 2). Procollagen molecules are thought to form microfibrils which are stabilized by intermolecular disulfide cross-links (-S-S-) and covalent cross-links involving lysine and/or hydroxylysine (solid line). The microfibrils polymerize to form a larger matrix as is the case in lens capsule. The presence of a distinct noncollagenous glycoprotein within the basement membrane matrix has been postulated for certain tissues. This glycoprotein would be linked to the procollagen molecules via disulfide bonds and, possibly, through other types of covalent cross-linkages. It is suggested that the proportion of the noncollagenous glycoprotein varies among basement membranes including glomerular basement membrane (GBM), Descemet's membrane (DM), and rat embryo parietal yolk sac (PYS). (From Kefalides *et al.*, 1979.)

although the chemical nature of this cross-linkage has not been elucidated yet. This linkage probably is located within the noncollagenous portion of the procollagen molecule and may be of importance in the polymerization of basement membrane procollagen.

In addition to the polymerized procollagen, genetically distinct, noncollagenous glycoproteins also may be present within the basement membrane matrix. These molecules would be linked to the procollagen molecule via disulfide bonds and possibly through other types of covalent cross-linkages. It is not clear whether these glycoproteins are present in every basement membrane. It is possible to account for the entire amino acid composition of at least one basement membrane, i.e., the anterior lens capsule, as a polymerized procollagen-like molecule without having to postulate the presence of distinct glycoprotein molecules.

Using the above model, it can be seen that proteolytic enzymes such as pepsin would digest away the noncollagenous glycoproteins and procollagen extension peptides leaving behind the pepsin-resistant, triple-helical collagenous portions of the procollagen chains associated with each other through those disulfide and lysine-derived cross-linkages which were not destroyed during the proteolysis. Similarly, treatment with bacterial collagenase would result in the formation of a series of glycopeptides. One of these would be derived from each of the noncollagenous glycoproteins present within the basement membrane. Others would be derived from the noncollagenous extension peptides present at the ends of the procollagen-like molecules. If the structure of the individual chains of the procollagen-like molecule is analogous to that of Type I procollagen, it would be expected that one peptide would represent the carboxy terminal extension (Fig. 2). The latter peptides would be isolated as triple-stranded units joined by disulfide bonds. Recent studies by Fessler (unpublished data) show that the carboxy terminal propeptides of Type IV collagen are not disulfide linked. Because of the possibility that either or both of the extension peptide fractions could be cross-linked further by nondisulfide, covalent cross-linkages, it has not yet been established that a given glycopeptide fraction isolated after collagenase digestion of a basement membrane is derived from procollagen extension peptides or from a noncollagenous glycoprotein. The cross-linking also complicates the interpretation of immunologic data (Kefalides, 1972) which suggested the presence of at least two immunologically distinct glycoproteins, one of high molecular weight and one of low molecular weight.

It is probable that the multitude of heterogeneous fractions observed after reduction and alkylation of basement membranes is attributable largely to the random nature of the nondisulfide cross-linkages. Finally, it must be recognized that *in vivo*, basement membranes undergo a degree of metabolic turnover. This process may proceed at different rates for different molecular portions of the basement membrane and lead to an increasing heterogeneity.

7. *Molecular Properties of Basement Membranes and Structure–Function Relationships*

The ultrastructural appearance of basement membranes varies with the tissue. Lens capsule appears more fibrillar than GBM. Descemet's membrane shows some degree of ordered structure. Several studies suggest that procollagen molecules constitute the basic ultrastructural unit in basement membranes (Figs. 2, 3). Small or large amounts of noncollagenous glycoprotein laminin may interact with procollagen to give basement membranes a more or less fibrillar appearance. Lens capsule may be considered a prototype of basement membranes composed almost entirely of procollagen (95% by weight) (Figs. 2, 3). GMB is thought to be composed of 75% procollagen molecules and 25% noncollagenous glycoprotein. In Descemet's membrane the proportions are similar. Based on the studies by Clark *et al.* (1975), it is estimated that in Reichert's membrane of the rat embryo the ratio is 60% procollagen and 40% noncollagenous glycoprotein.

The basement membrane procollagen molecule has certain unique structural and compositional features which include the presence of nonhelical propeptide extensions at the amino and carboxy termini (Figs. 1, 2). About 34 glycosylgalactose units per pro-α chain occupy the length of the collagen domain (Figs. 1, 2). Oligosaccharide units are on the propeptide extensions. Newly synthesized basement membrane procollagen is excluded on DEAE-cellulose but is bound to carboxymethyl-cellulose, indicating a net positive (cationic) charge (Clark and Kefalides, 1978).

Based on the above data, one can explain some of the morphologic and functional properties of basement membranes.

7.1. *The Ultrastructural Appearance of Basement Membranes*

"Why are typical collagen fibrils not seen in basement membranes?" is a frequent question. This phenomenon which prevails in vertebrate species can best be explained by postulating that it is due to the persistence of procollagen molecules. It is known that newly synthesized Type I procollagen does not form stable fibers *in vitro* (Goldberg, 1974). A similar situation must occur *in vivo* since electron microscopic studies of skin from dermatosparactic calves show that bundles of collagen fibrils are disorganized (Simar and Betz, 1971).The collagen which is isolated from the skin of these animals has the amino terminal propeptides still in place (Lenaers *et al.*, 1971; Uitto and Lichtenstein, 1976) and exhibits impaired cross-linking (Bailey and Lapiere, 1973). The next question one may ask is, "What is the physiological significance of the above phenomenon with respect to permeability of basement membranes?" An easy assumption is that if the procollagen molecules were allowed to form large aggregates, then much larger molecules would pass through the basement membrane filter than in the usual case (Kefalides, 1969).

The role of the noncollagenous glycoprotein in basement membranes is not clear. It is possible that these molecules interact with procollagen and further diminish its chances of forming fibrils. Another possible function of the noncollagenous glycoprotein may be related to the elastic properties of basement membranes. It is well known that interstitial collagen molecules are inelastic and resistant to stretch. However, when collagen fibers are found in association with other matrix substances, as in tendon, the tissue becomes elastic although stretching (Kuhnke, 1962) has a negligible effect. An analogy could be made to the basement membranes in which the association of the procollagen filaments with noncollagenous glycoprotein may provide elasticity.

7.2. *Permeability Properties of Basement Membranes*

The main function of the glomerular capillaries is considered to be its ability to filter the blood plasma and to yield a protein-free plasma filtrate (Karnovsky, 1968; Farquhar, 1978). The functional components of the capillary wall include: (1) the endothelium which controls the access of plasma filtrate to the GBM, (2) the basement membrane proper which acts as a filter allowing passage of molecules based on size and charge, and (3) the epithelium which helps trap smaller particles which have escaped through the basement membrane.

How do the structural and chemical properties contribute to the filtration properties of basement membranes? In the previous section (7.1), the contribution of the network formed by the interaction of procollagen and noncollagenous glycoprotein to the filtration barrier was discussed. It would be appropriate now to discuss the role and nature of the charge barrier.

Chang *et al.* (1975) and Brenner *et al.* (1976) in a series of studies found that in normal rats the clearance of sulfated dextrans is reduced in comparison to neutral dextrans and postulated that there are fixed negatively charged components in the glomerular capillary wall. Studies by Rennke *et al.* (1975) and Caulfield and Farquhar (1976) have demonstrated that GBM contains anionic binding sites. In their studies, Rennke *et al.* (1975) compared native anionic ferritin with cationized ferritin. It was found that cationic ferritin accumulates in all layers of GBM in amounts far exceeding the anionic ferritin. Caulfield and Farquhar (1976) used lysozyme, a basic protein, and found anionic sites in all layers of GBM. It was concluded that GBM is negatively charged and that the charge on a molecule influences its filtration. The above observations can be correlated with the chemical analyses of intact GBM and its protein components. Table 7 shows the functional group content of whole GBM. There are 0.8 μmole of basic amino acids per milligram of GBM. The acidic amino acids, aspartic and glutamic, account for 1.29 μmoles and sialic acid for 0.06 μmole of the anionic groups, yielding a total of 1.35 μmoles. GBM contains 0.4 μmole of amide nitrogen per milligram which when subtracted from the anionic charge, contributed by the acidic amino acids, gives a net anionic content of 0.95 μmole. When this figure is compared to the 0.8 μmole of cationic amino acids, a net of 0.15 μmole anionic functional group content is obtained for whole GBM. GBM procollagen (collagen plus propeptides) has a net cationic functional group

Table 7. Electrostatic Charge of GBM Based on Amino Acid and Sialic Acid Content

Functional groups	Whole GBM[a]	GBM-collagen[b]	GBM-propeptides[c]	GBM-glycoprotein[c]
			μmoles/mg	
Basic amino acids	0.80	0.68	1.01	0.96
Acidic amino acids	1.29	0.90	1.41	1.41
Sialic acid	0.06	0.00	0.02	0.05
Amide N	0.40[d]	0.30[e]	0.43[e]	0.25[e]
Net ionic charge	−0.15	+0.08	+0.01	−0.25

[a] Kefalides and Winzler (1966).
[b] Kefalides (1971b).
[c] Kefalides (1972).
[d] Determined by microdiffusion.
[e] Estimated from ammonia content.

content of 0.09 μmole/mg (Table 7). This agrees with the observation of Clark and Kefalides (1978) who demonstrated that newly synthesized basement membrane procollagen of rat parietal yolk sac has a net cationic charge since it does not bind to DEAE-cellulose but does so to carboxymethylcellulose. It is obvious from the data in Table 7 that the net anionic charge on whole GBM must be contributed by the noncollagenous glycoprotein which has a net anionic group content of 0.25 μmole/mg. It is of interest to note that sialic acid contributes less than 5% to the total anionic group content of whole GBM.

As more is learned about the structural components of GBM and of other basement membranes, experiments could be devised to help gain an inderstanding of the functional behavior of these substances.

8. *Summary*

The molecular structure of basement membranes has been examined by various approaches which include compositional, immunochemical, physical, and biosynthetic studies. These studies have demonstrated the existence of procollagen-like molecules forming microfibrils composed of no more than 4–5 such molecules. The microfibrils are stabilized by disulfide and lysine- or hydroxylysine-derived bonds. A third, unknown type of covalent bond may be present also. Newly synthesized basement membrane procollagen has a net positive (cationic) charge. The lens capsule is thought to be composed almost exclusively of polymerized microfibrils. The presence of a noncollagenous glycoprotein (laminen) (Timpl *et al.*, 1979) found within the basement membrane matrix, in association with the procollagen-like microfibrils, has been postulated in other tissues including the glomerulus, Descemet's membrane, and the parietal yolk sac of the rat embryo. The percent content of the noncollagenous glycoprotein varies among basement membranes. It is thought to be determined by the functional requirements of the particular tissue. Compositional studies indicate that the net charge of whole GBM is anionic. Aspartic and glutamic acids contribute 95% of the anionic functional groups while sialic acid contributes less than 5%. Immunochemical studies show the presence of at least three antigenic components. One is represented by the collagenous domain and the other by the noncollagenous propeptide extensions of the procollagen molecule. The third antigenic component is represented by the noncollagenous matrix glycoprotein. It is suggested that the persistence of procollagen molecules in GBM as well as in other basement membranes is responsible for the absence of typical collagen fibrils. It is partially responsible for the selective filtration properties of GBM. The association of the noncollagenous glycoprotein with the procollagen microfibrils provides for the supramolecular organization of GBM, its elastic properties, and its net negative charge. These factors together determine the ultimate selective filtration properties of GBM.

References

Albini, B., Brentjens, J., Ossi, E., and Andres, G. A., 1978, The role of tubular basement membrane antigens in renal diseases, in: *Biology and Chemistry of Basement Membranes* (N. A. Kefalides, ed.), pp. 577–587, Academic Press, New York.

Arbogast, B. W., Gunson, D. E., and Kefalides, N. A., 1976, The role of hydroxylation of proline in the antigenicity of basement membrane collagen, *J. Immunol.* **117:**2181.

Bailey, A. J., and Lapiere, C. M., 1973, Effect of an additional peptide extension of the N-terminus of collagen from dermatosparactic calves on the cross-linking of the collagen fibers, *Eur. J. Biochem.* **34:**91.

Bardos, P., Muh, J. P., Luthier, B., Devulder, B., and Tacquet, A., 1976, Immunochemical study of some glycoproteins of the rat glomerular basement membrane, *Comp. Biochem. Physiol.* **53:**49.

Brenner, B. M., Baylis, C., and Deen, W. M., 1976, Transport of molecules across renal glomerular capillaries, *Physiol. Rev.* **56:**502.

Caulfield, J. P., 1978, The distribution of anionic sites in the glomerular basement membrane of normal and nephrotic rats, in: *Biology and Chemistry of Basement Membranes* (N. A. Kefalides, ed.), pp. 81–98, Academic Press, New York.

Caulfield, J. P., and Farquhar, M. G., 1976, Distribution of anionic sites in glomerular basement membranes: Their possible role in filtration and attachment, *Proc. Natl. Acad. Sci. USA* **73:**1646.

Chang, R. L. S., Deen, W. M., Robertson, C. R., and Brenner, B. M., 1975, Permeability of the glomerular capillary wall to macromolecules. III. Evidence for electrostatic repulsion of polyanions, *Kidney Int.* **8:**212.

Chung, E., Rhodes, R. K., and Miller, E. J., 1976, Isolation of three collagenous components of probably basement membrane origin from several tissues, *Biochem. Biophys. Res. Commun.* **71:**1167.

Clark, C. C., and Kefalides, N. A., 1978, Partial characterization of newly synthesized basement membrane procollagen, in: *Cellular and Biochemical Aspects in Diabetic Retinopathy* (F. Regnault and J. Duhault, eds.), pp. 3–13, North-Holland, Amsterdam.

Clark, C. C., Minor, R. R., Koszalka, T. R., Brent, R. L., and Kefalides, N. A., 1975, The embryonic rat parietal yolk sac: Changes in the morphology and composition of its basement membrane during development, *Dev. Biol.* **46:**243.

Dehm, P., and Kefalides, N. A., 1978a, Comparison of α-chain size collagenous peptides isolated from glomerular basement membrane and lens capsule, *Fed. Proc.* **37:**1527.

Dehm, P., and Kefalides, N. A., 1978b, The collagenous component of lens basement membrane: The isolation and characterization of an α-chain size collagenous peptide, and its relationship to newly synthesized lens components, *J. Biol. Chem.* **253:**6680.

Denduchis, B., and Kefalides, N. A., 1970, Immunochemistry of sheep anterior lens capsule, *Biochim. Biophys. Acta* **221:**357.

Dixit, S. N., 1979, Isolation and characterization of two α-chain size collagenous polypeptide chains C and D from glomerular basement membrane, *FEBS Lett.* **106:**379.

Farquhar, M. G., 1975, The primary glomerular filtration barrier—basement membrane of epithelial slits?, *Kidney Int.* **8:**197.

Farquhar, M. G., 1978, Structure and function of glomerular capillaries: Role of the basement membrane in glomerular filtration, in: *Biology and Chemistry of Basement Membranes* (N. A. Kefalides, ed.), pp. 43–80, Academic Press, New York.

Farquhar, M. G., Wissig, S. L., and Palade, G. E., 1961, Glomerular permeability. 1. Ferritin transfer across the normal glomerular capillary wall, *J. Exp. Med.* **113:**147.

Ferwerda, W., van Loon, C. M. I., and Feltkamp-Vroom, T. M., 1978, The specificity of the antigenic determinants of bovine renal tubular basement membrane, in: *Biology and Chemistry of Basement Membranes* (N. A. Kefalides, ed.), pp. 403–419, Academic Press, New York.

Gay, S., and Miller, E. J., 1979, Characterization of lens capsule collagen: evidence for the presence of two unique chains in molecules derived from major basement membrane structures, *Arch. Biochem. Biophys.* **198:**370.

Goldberg, B., 1974, Electron microscopic studies of procollagen from cultured human fibroblasts, *Cell* **1:**185.

Grant, M. E., Kefalides, N. A., and Prockop, D. J., 1972, The biosynthesis of basement membrane collagen in embryonic chick lens. I. Delay between the synthesis of polypeptide chains and the secretion of collagen by matrix-free cells, *J. Biol. Chem.* **247:**3539.

Grant, M. E., Schofield, J. D., Kefalides, N. A., and Prockop, D. J., 1973, The biosynthesis of basement membrane collagen in embryonic chick lens. III. Intracellular formation of the triple-helix and the formation of extracellular aggregates through disulfide bonds, *J. Biol. Chem.* **248:**7432.

Grant, M. E., Harwood, R., and Williams, I. F., 1975, The biosynthesis of basement membrane collagen by isolated rat glomeruli, *Eur. J. Biochem.* **54:**531.

Gunson, D. E., and Kefalides, N. A., 1976, The use of the radioimmunoassay in the characterization of antibodies to basement membrane collagen, *Immunology* **31:**563.

Gunson, D. E., Arbogast, B., and Kefalides, N. A., 1976, Rat parietal yolk-sac basement membrane: An investigation of the antigenic determinants using a radioimmunoassay, *Immunology* **31:**577.

Heathcote, J. G., Sear, C. H. J., and Grant, M. E., 1978, Biosynthesis of rat lens capsule collagen, in: *Biology and Chemistry of Basement Membranes* (N. A. Kefalides, ed.), pp. 335–342, Academic Press, New York.

Howard, B. V., Macarak, E. J., Gunson, D., and Kefalides, N. A., 1976, Characterization of the collagen synthesized by endothelial cells in culture, *Proc. Natl. Acad. Sci. USA* **73:**2361.

Jakus, M. A., 1964, *Ocular Fine Structure*, Little, Brown, Boston.

Johnson, L. D., Warfel, J., and Megaw, J. M., 1978, Synthesis of an epithelial basement membrane glycoprotein by cultured human and murine cells, in: *Biology and Chemistry of Basement Membranes* (N. A. Kefalides, ed.), pp. 299–308, Academic Press, New York.

Karnovsky, M. J., 1968, The ultrastructural basis of transcapillary exchanges, in: *Biological Interfaces: Flows and Exchanges*, pp. 64–99, Little, Brown, Boston.

Kefalides, N. A., and Winzler, R. J., 1966, The chemistry of glomerular basement membrane and its relation to collagen, *Biochemistry* **5:**702.

Kefalides, N. A., 1968, Isolation and characterization of the collagen from glomerular basement membrane, *Biochemistry* **7:**3103.

Kefalides, N. A., 1969, The chemical basis for the structure and function of basement membranes, in: *Diabetes* (J. Östman, ed.), pp. 610–611, Excerpta Medica, Amsterdam.

Kefalides, N. A., 1971a, Chemical properties of basement membranes, *Int. Rev. Exp. Pathol.* **10:**1.

Kefalides, N. A., 1971b, Isolation of a collagen from basement membranes containing three identical α-chains, *Biochem. Biophys. Res. Commun.* **45:**226.

Kefalides, N. A., 1972, The chemistry of the antigenic components of glomerular basement membrane, *Connect. Tissue Res.* **1:**3.

Kefalides, N. A., 1973, Structure and biosynthesis of basement membranes, *Int. Rev. Connect. Tissue Res.* **6:**63.

Kefalides, N. A., 1975, Structural and biosynthetic considerations, *J. Invest. Dermatol.* **65:**85.

Kefalides, N. A., and Denduchis, B., 1969, Structural components of epithelial and endothelial basement membranes, *Biochemistry* **8:**4613.

Kefalides, N. A., Cameron, J. D., Tomichek, E. A., and Yanoff, M., 1976, Biosynthesis of basement membrane collagen by rabbit corneal endothelium *in vitro*, *J. Biol. Chem.* **251:**730.

Kefalides, N. A., Alper, R., and Clark, C. C., 1979, The biochemistry and metabolism of basement membranes, *Int. Rev. Cytol.* **60:**167.

Kuhnke, E., 1962, The fine structure of collagen fibrils as the basis for the functioning of tendon tissue, in: *Collagen* (N. Ramanathan, ed.), pp. 479–492, Interscience, New York.

Lehman, D. H., Wilson, C. B., and Dixon, F. J., 1974, Interstitial nephritis in rats immunized with heterologous tubular basement membrane, *Kidney Int.* **5:**187.

Lenaers, A., Ansay, M., Nusgens, B. V., and Lapiere, C. M., 1971, Collagen made of extended α-chains, procollagen, in genetically-defective dermatosparaxic calves, *Eur. J. Biochem.* **23:**533.

Mahieu, P., Lambert, P. H., and Miescher, P. A., 1974, Detection of antiglomerular basement membrane antibodies by a radioimmunological technique, *J. Clin. Invest.* **54:**128.

Marquardt, H., Wilson, C. B., and Dixon, F. J., 1973, Isolation and immunochemical characterization of human glomerular basement membrane antigens, *Kidney Int.* **3**:57.

Minor, R. R., Clark, C. C., Strause, E. L., Koszalka, T. R., Brent, R. L., and Kefalides, N. A., 1976, Basement membrane procollagen is not converted to collagen in organ cultures of parietal yolk sac endoderm, *J. Biol. Chem.* **251**:1789.

Monson, J. M., Click, E. M., and Bornstein, P., 1975, Further characterization of procollagen: Purification and analysis of the pro-αl chain of chick bone procollagen, *Biochemistry* **14**:4088.

Olsen, B. R., Alper, R., and Kefalides, N. A., 1973, Structural characterization of a soluble fraction from lens capsule basement membrane, *Eur. J. Biochem.* **38**:220.

Rennke, H. G., Cotran, R. S., and Venkatachalam, M. A., 1975, Role of molecular change in glomerular permeability: Tracer studies with cationized ferritins, *J. Cell Biol.* **67**:638.

Ryan, G. B., and Karnovsky, M. J., 1976, Distribution of endogenous albumin in the rat glomerulus: Role of the hemodynamic factors in glomerular barrier function, *Kidney Int.* **9**:36

Schwartz, D., and Veis, A., 1978, Characterization of basement membrane collagen of bovine anterior lens capsule via segment-long-spacing crystallites and the specific cleavage of the collagen by pepsin, *FEBS Lett.* **85**:326.

Shibata, S., 1978, Immunologic and non-immunologic aspects of experimental glomerulonephritis, in: *Biology and Chemistry of Basement Membranes* (N. A. Kefalides, ed.), pp. 535–559, Academic Press, New York.

Simar, L. J., and Betz, E. H., 1971, Dermatosparaxis of the calf, a genetic defect of the connective tissue. 2. Ultrastructural study of the skin, *Hoppe-Seyler's Z. Physiol. Chem.* **352**:13.

Tanzer, M. L., and Kefalides, N. A., 1973, Collagen crosslinks: Occurrence in basement membrane collagens, *Biochem. Biophys. Res. Commun.* **51**:775.

Timpl, R., Martin, G. R., Bruckner, P., Wick, G., and Wiedemann, H., 1978, Nature of a collagenous protein in a tumor basement membrane, *Eur. J. Biochem.* **84**:43.

Timpl, R., Rohde, H., Gehron Robey, P., Rennard, S. I., Foidart, J. M., and Martin, G. R., 1979, Laminin—a glycoprotein from basement membranes, *J. Biol. Chem.* **254**:9933.

Trelstad, R., and Lawley, K. R., 1977, Isolation and initial characterization of human basement membrane collagens, *Biochem. Biophys. Res. Commun.* **76**:376.

Uitto, J., and Lichtenstein, J. R., 1976, Defects in the biochemistry of collagen in diseases of connective tissue, *J. Invest. Dermatol.* **66**:59.

Venkatachalam, M. A., Rennke, H. G., Seiler, M. W., and Cotran, R. S., 1978, Structural and functional effects of glomerular polyanion, in: *Biology and Chemistry of Basement Membranes* (N. A. Kefalides, ed.), pp. 149–164, Academic Press, New York.

4

Glomerular Basement Membrane Antigens

Alfred J. Fish, Kathleen M. Carmody, Mark S. Schiffer, and Alfred E. Michael

1. Introduction

In experimental nephritis produced by the administration of nephrotoxic serum, there is *in vivo* localization of heterologous immunoglobulin antibodies in a smooth linear pattern along the glomerular basement membrane (GBM) (Hammer and Dixon, 1963). Nephrotoxic serum, produced by immunization with isolated GBM, reacts *in vitro* by fixing not only to GBM, but also to tubular basement membrane and to Bowman's capsule as noted by indirect immunofluorescence. The smooth linear staining of these basement membranes is similar to the GBM staining pattern described above in nephrotoxic serum nephritis. The antigenic specificity of nephrotoxic serum has not been defined but it is believed to be due to a reaction with noncollagenous glycoprotein components of GBM, since multiple precipitin lines are formed in Ouchterlony immunodiffusion against collagenase digests of normal GBM (Marquardt *et al.*, 1973). Another experimental model of glomerulonephritis mediated by anti-GBM antibody can be induced in sheep by immunization with heterologous GBM. The proliferative glomerulonephritis, which was first described by Steblay (1962), is associated with linear deposition of host immunoglobulin along the GBM. In this model of experimental anti-GBM nephritis, circulating antibodies to GBM have been detected after nephrectomy (Lerner *et al.*, 1967).

In certain forms of rapidly progressive glomerulonephritis in humans and in patients with Goodpasture's syndrome (severe glomerulonephritis with pulmonary hemorrhage),linear deposition of IgG is present along the

Alfred J. Fish, Kathleen M. Carmody, Mark S. Schiffer, and Alfred F. Michael · Department of Pediatrics, University of Minnesota Medical School, Minneapolis, Minnesota 55455.

GBM by immunofluorescence (Duncan *et al.*, 1965; McPhaul and Dixon, 1970). Acid citrate elution of the bound IgG from the GBM in these patients shows reactivity *in vitro* with normal GBM. Passive administration of this antibody to monkeys has produced fatal glomerulonephritis.

The results of the above studies of experimental and clinical forms of glomerulonephritis have led to the proposal of a common pathogenetic mechanism involving fixation of anti-GBM antibodies to the GBM in a linear fashion. Antigenic specificities of the antibodies are unknown. In the present investigation, it has been demonstrated that heterologous rabbit anti-human GBM (RAHGBM) reacts with separate zones along the inner (endothelial) and outer (epithelial) aspects of the GBM, whereas the central portion of the GBM is nonreactive. Antibodies eluted from Goodpasture (GP) syndrome kidneys fix to the inner layer of the GBM, in a site different from that which reacts with RAHGBM.

2. *Reactivity of Rabbit Anti-GBM with Normal Kidney*

Rabbit anti-GBM antibody using isolated human GBM in Freund's complete adjuvant was prepared by multiple immunizations of rabbits as

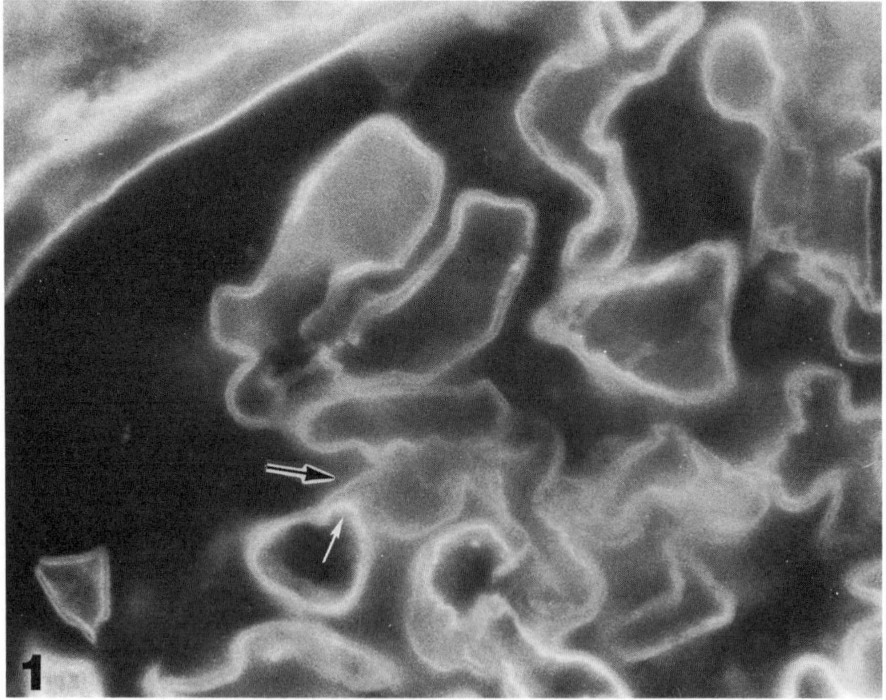

Figure 1. Immunofluorescent photomicrograph of RAHGBM staining of the glomerulus from a normal human kidney showing double linear staining of the GBM; the inner component surrounds the glomerular capillary lumen (white arrow) and the outer component bypasses the mesangial waist (black arrow). × 1600.

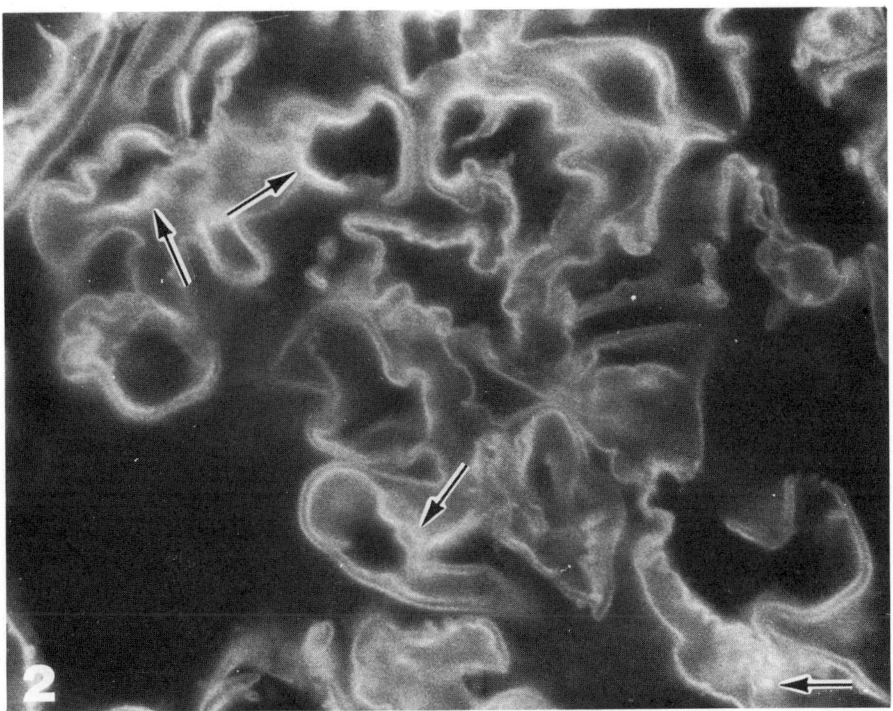

Figure 2. Immunofluorescence of RAHGBM staining of normal human kidney showing blending of the inner antigenic component with mesangial antigens (arrows). × 1600.

previously described (Fish *et al.*, 1979). Indirect immunofluorescence using 1:20 and 1:40 dilutions of RAHGBM and goat anti-rabbit IgG labeled with fluorescein isothiocyanate (FITC) or rhodamine isothiocyanate (RITC) was done by epifluorescence using a Zeiss Universal microscope equipped with Ploem optics (Miller and Michael, 1976).

Within the glomerulus, RAHGBM stains the GBM in two distinct zones (Fig. 1). The first zone has an inner endothelial component which is wide, irregular, and is observed in certain tissue section planes to encircle completely the glomerular capillary loop. This inner component blends with aggregates of mesangial matrix (Fig. 2).The second outer component of GBM staining corresponds to the epithelial side of the GBM, is narrower and more regular than the inner component. The outer zone of GBM staining is continuous and extends across the outer epithelial aspect of the mesangial waist (Figs. 3a and b). These features of the double linear contour of GBM staining, where the two components are clearly separated by a central nonstained area, are delineated most easily by indirect immunofluorescent staining but are discerned less readily using higher dilutions of RAHGBM or by direct staining with RAHGBM labeled with FITC.

Staining reactivity of RAHGBM on normal human kidney was compared with that on kidney from monkey, bovine, rabbit, sheep, goat, and rat sources. RAHGBM did not stain the GBM of rabbit kidney. While double linear

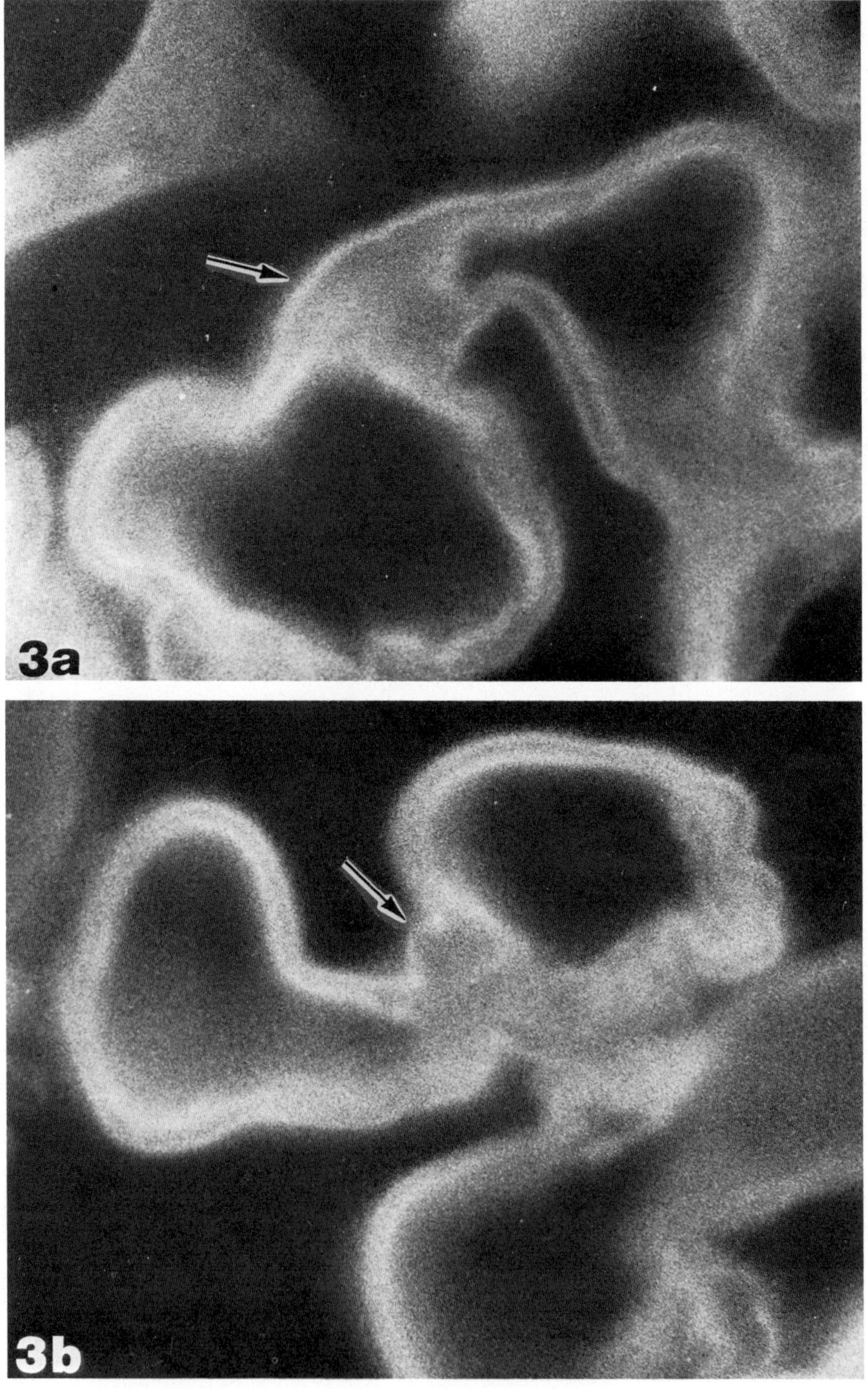

Figure 3. Immunofluorescent photomicrographs of RAHGBM staining of normal human kidney showing the outer GBM component (arrows) bypassing the mesangial waist. × 5550.

reactivity was present on monkey, sheep, bovine, and goat GBM, only single linear staining was evident on rat GBM. Antibody to human GBM also was made by immunization of a sheep (ShAHGBM). This antibody did not react with normal sheep GBM. It was double linear on human and on monkey GBM, but had single linear staining reactivity on bovine, rabbit, and rat kidney. The single linear staining in different species suggests that the immunized animals share antigenic determinants and do not make antibodies to all antigenic determinants of the inner and outer regions of the GBM.

3. Staining of Kidney with GP Renal Eluates

Acid citrate eluates from kidneys of the three patients with GP syndrome were made by the method of Lerner *et al.* (1967). Reactivity with GBM of normal human kidney was produced by indirect immunofluorescence. Unlike the findings described above with heterologous RAHGBM, localization of GP syndrome IgG made a single linear pattern along the GBM. There was minimal reactivity of GP IgG with mesangial antigens as seen by the slight irregularity of staining of the GBM in the mesangial waist area (Fig. 4). Otherwise, there was smooth continuous linear staining from one glomerular

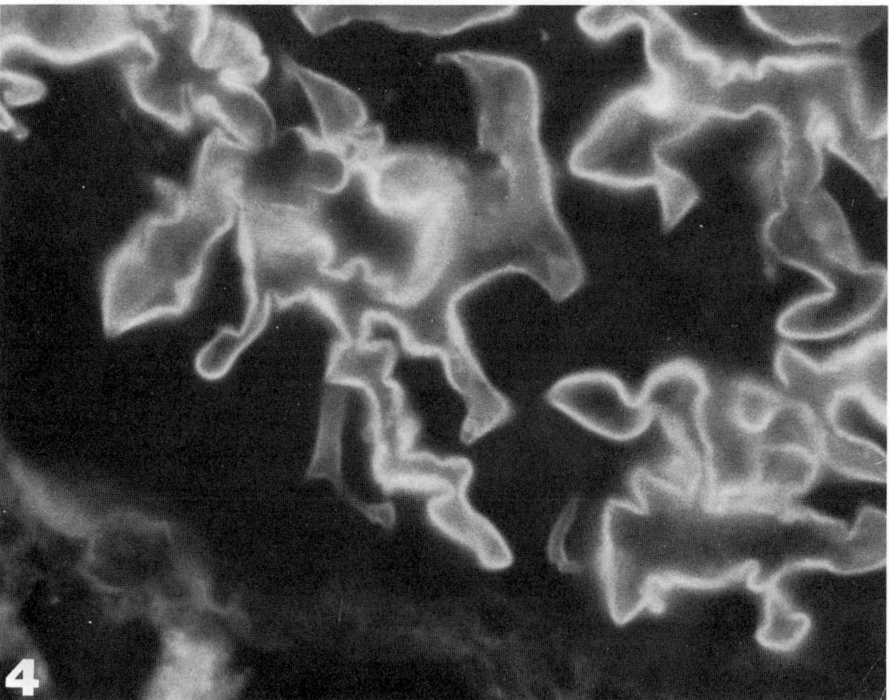

Figure 4. Immunofluorescent photomicrograph of GP antibody staining of normal human kidney showing a continuous smooth single linear fluorescent pattern which has negligible mesangial reactivity and is continuous from one glomerular capillary loop to the next. × 1600.

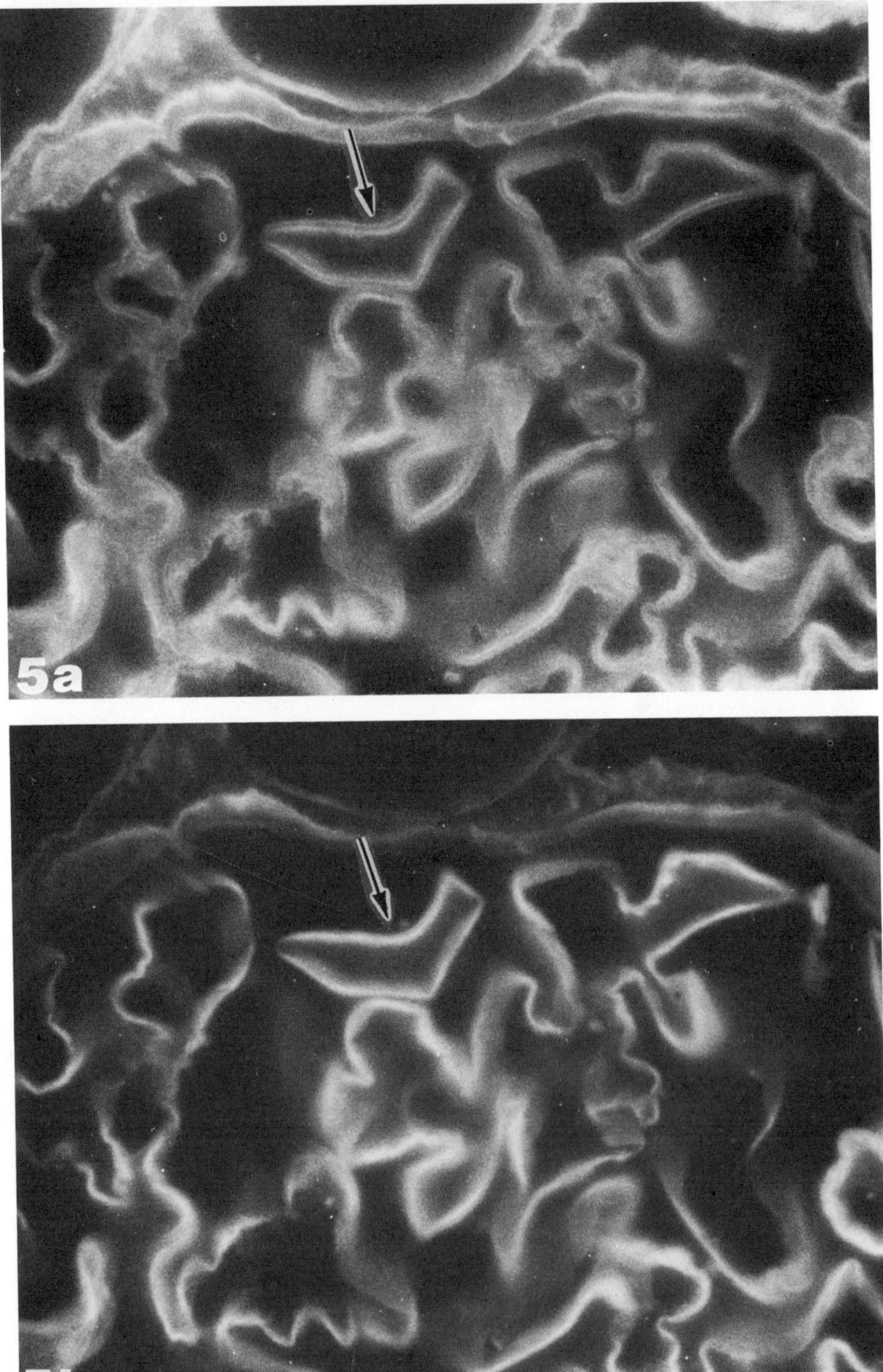

Figure 5. Dual labeled staining by immunofluorescence of human GBM. (a) RAHGBM and GARG rhodamine showing double linear staining of the GBM (arrow). (b) The same field stained simultaneously with GP IgG-GAHIgG-FITC showing a single linear component (arrow) which is on the epithelial side of the inner antigen line observed with RAHGBM. × 1600.

capillary loop to another. Dual staining with RAHGBM and GP IgG revealed that the GP antigen is present along the inner aspect of the GBM, but in a locus that is clearly external and distinct from the inner antigenic site identified by RAHGBM (Figs. 5a and b). GP antibody also reacted with the GBM of monkey, rat, rabbit, bovine, goat, and sheep kidneys. Since this antigen is shared among all of the species examined, it is unlikely that RAHGBM is directed against the GP antigen. This would explain the delineation of these antigen systems by the dual staining described.

4. *Preparations of Isolated GBM*

The immunohistology of isolated GBM fragments was examined after 1,2, and 3 min sonication of whole intact glomeruli. Material was pelleted by centrifugation, incorporated in gelatin, frozen, and sectioned with a cryostat (Fish *et al.*, 1979). There is maintenance of the double linear staining with RAHGBM and single linear GP IgG staining following 1 min sonication. GBM preparations obtained after 2 and 3 min of sonication showed complete loss of the double linear structure and marked decrease in GP antibody reactivity.

5. *Measurements of Linear Widths by Immunofluorescent Staining and Phase Microscopy*

Measurements of staining widths were calculated from fluorescent photomicrographs and phase light micrographs of three normal human kidneys using 63× planapochromate oil immersion objective with magnification of 350×. Photomicrographs (6.58× enlargement) were marked by fine perforations using a 27-gauge needle to delineate the extent of the double linear bands of staining. Three glomeruli were evaluated following indirect staining using RAHGBM 1:20 and 1:160 and GARG-FITC. An average of 10 randomly selected points along the GBM of each glomerulus were measured using a calibrated magnifying eyepiece.

To investigate the observations that the double linear staining of GBM was less apparent and less distinct using higher dilutions of RAHGBM, measurements were made on enlarged photomicrographs (Table 1). Measurements of the outer limits of double linear staining were estimated at 8600 to 8900 Å, using RAHGBM 1:20 as primary antibody. In two of the specimens this decreased to 770 Å with 1:160 dilution of RAHGBM, and in the third no change was detected. The central nonstaining zone was recorded at 2200 to 2500 Å, and decreased to 2200 and 2100 Å with dilution of the RAHGBM in two specimens. In the third specimen, measurements of the inner zone were not possible using a 1:160 dilution of RAHGBM. Measurement of total glomerular capillary wall by phase microscopy was 7300 ± 1200 Å.

Table 1. Measurements of Linear Staining (Å) by Immunofluorescence[a]

	Normal human kidney targets					
	1		2		3	
RAHGBM dilution[b]	Outer	Inner	Outer	Inner	Outer	Inner
1:20	8600 ± 1200[c] (25)[d]	2500 ± 900 (24)	8800 ± 900 (28)	2300 ± 600 (28)	8900 ± 1300 (29)	2200 ± 500 (29)
1:160	7700 ± 1400 (19)	ND	7700 ± 800 (25)	2000 ± 500 (20)	8300 ± 1200 (25)	2100 ± 600 (26)

[a] Width of the outside limits of double linear staining (Outer) and width of the central nonstaining zone (Inner) in Å.
[b] Sections were stained indirectly with RAHGBM ± GARG-FITC.
[c] Mean ± S.D.
[d] Number of measurements.

6. Distribution of RAHGBM and GP Antibody Staining in GBM of Diseased Kidneys

The altered distribution of GBM antigens in disease states has been investigated in this laboratory (Scheinman *et al.*, 1974, 1978). To extend these observations, staining of GBM antigens and GP antigen were performed in disease states where functional and morphologic alteration of the glomerular capillary wall were present (Schiffer *et al.*, 1981). In kidneys from patients with idiopathic nephrotic syndrome and kidneys of patients with focal glomerular sclerosis, the distribution of GBM antigens was the same as that in normal kidneys. In kidneys of patients with membranous glomerulopathy, it was observed that the subepithelial deposits of IgG were related intimately to the outer RAHGBM antigen line. The latter frequently was widened and showed an irregular beaded appearance. Staining for GP antigen was decreased or focally absent. In kidneys of diabetic glomerulopathy, both inner and outer RAHGBM antigen lines were increased in width, as was the central nonstaining zone of the GBM. The distribution of endogenous albumin and of IgG in diabetic nephropathy kidneys (Miller and Michael, 1976) were observed along the inner aspect of the GBM. The endogenous albumin and IgG were distributed more deeply in the basement membrane with diminishing intensity. In type I membranoproliferative glomerulonephritis, the inner RAHGBM line was diminished greatly and focally absent, but the GP antigen was better preserved in most cases. Of interest is the observation that a different distribution of staining is found in type II membranoproliferative glomerulonephritis. RAHGBM shows preservation of the outer antigen component with marked loss of the inner component. Paralleling the "tram track" distribution of C3 around the dense material (Kim *et al.*, 1979), there is double linear staining for GP antigen.

In summary, the various glomerulopathies examined in this study feature increases or decreases in the inner and outer RAHGBM antigens, and GP antigen independent of one or another. This reflects the extent of altered production and turnover of these antigens, depending on which glomerular cell system is altered in each disorder.

7. Discussion

These studies have delineated a bilaminar distribution of reactive antigens on the inner and outer aspects of the GBM. In addition, it has not been appreciated previously that the GP antigen lies along the inner antigen layer and is distinct from other RAHGBM reactive inner antigens. These observations of GBM antigen distribution can be attributed to the superior field illumination of epifluorescent microscopy and to the greater resolution possible under high magnification. There appears to be selective alteration in production and distribution of the GBM antigens in various disease states, also.

As described in detail in Chapters 1, 2, and 6, the filter function of the glomerular capillary wall is related intimately to the fixed negative charges of the lamina rara interna which extends to the fenestrated plasma membrane of the glomerular capillary endothelium and of the lamina rara externa between the foot processes of glomerular epithelial cells and the lamina densa.

The inner and outer antigenic components delineated with RAHGBM antibody in this study are likely present within the laminae rarae. Measurements of the total width of GBM staining on immunofluorescent photomicrographs measured 8600 to 2500 Å. The central inner nonstaining zone was estimated at 2000 to 2500 Å. While these measurements of the double linear staining by immunofluorescence serve to explain why two components can be resolved by the microscopic techniques used in this study, these data should be interpreted as approximate, since variables such as thickness of tissue sections, freezing and diffusion effects, and optical aberrations may affect the absolute measurements. Nevertheless, it is proposed that antigens of the inner linear component may extend from the lamina rara interna toward the capillary lumen and that outer antigens may be distributed from the lamina rara externa outward adjacent to the epithelial cell foot processes. Preliminary immunoperoxidase studies by Drs. R. L. Vernier and N. Dysart in this laboratory, as well as the findings of Hoedemaeker *et al.* (1972)and Druet *et al.* (1972) suggest that anti-GBM antibodies bind to the plasma membranes of the epithelial cell foot processes, as well as to the lamina rara interna aspect of the glomerular capillary endothelium. These findings may explain the extent of GBM staining by immunofluorescence. They suggest also that as GBM antigens are synthesized by the glomerular epithelial and endothelial cells, there is concentration of these antigenic components within the plasma membrane of these cells during the process of extracellular transport to the laminae rarae of the GBM.

In summary, these studies report a heterogeneity and spatial organization of antigens within the GBM which has not previously been appreciated. It is anticipated that with the development of monospecific antisera to GBM antigens, these studies will lead to a new approach to characterization of GBM antigens by mapping their distribution within the glomerular capillary wall.

References

Druet, P., Bariéty, J., Bellon, B., and Laliberté, F., 1972, Nephrotoxic serum nephritis in the rat: Ultrastructural localization of nephrotoxic rabbit antibodies using peroxidase-labeled conjugates, *Lab. Invest.* **27:**157.

Duncan, D., Drummond, K. N., Michael, A. F., and Vernier, R. L., 1965, Pulmonary hemorrhage and glomerulonephritis: Report of six cases and study of the renal lesion by fluorescent antibody technique and electron microscopy, *Ann. Intern. Med.* **62:**920.

Fish, A. J., Carmody, K. M., and Michael, A. F., 1979, Distribution of antigens of human glomerular basement membrane, *J. Lab. Clin. Med.* **94:**447.

Hammer, D. K., and Dixon, F. J., 1963, Experimental glomerulonephritis. II. Immunologic events in the pathogenesis of nephrotoxic serum nephritis in the rat, *J. Exp. Med.* **117:**1019.

Hoedemaeker, P. J., Feenstra, K., Nijkeuter, A., and Arends, A., 1972, Ultrastructural localization of heterologous nephrotoxic antibody in the glomerular basement membrane of the rat, *Lab. Invest.* **26:**610.

Kim, Y., Vernier, R. L., Fish, A. J., and Michael, A. F., 1979, Immunofluorescent studies of dense deposit disease: The presence of railroad tracks and mesangial rings, *Lab. Invest.* **40:**474.

Lerner, R. A., Glassock, R. J., and Dixon, F. J., 1967, The role of anti-glomerular basement embrane antibody in the pathogenesis of human glomerulonephritis, *J. Exp. Med.* **126:**989.

McPhaul, J. J., and Dixon, F. J., 1970, Characteristics of human antiglomerular basement membrane antibodies eluted from glomerulonephritic kidneys, *J. Clin. Invest.* **49:**308.

Marquardt, H., Wilson, C. B., and Dixon, F. J., 1973, Isolation and immunological characterization of human glomerular basement membrane antigens, *Kidney Int.* **3:**57.

Miller, K., and Michael, A. F., 1976, Immunopathology of renal extracellular membranes in diabetes mellitus: Specificity of tubular basement membrane fluorescence, *Diabetes* **25:**701.

Scheinman, J. I., Fish, A. J., and Michael, A. F., 1974, The immunohistopathology of glomerular antigens: The GBM, collagen and actomyosin antigens in normal and diseased kidneys, *J. Clin. Invest.* **54:**1144.

Scheinman, J. I., Fish, A. J., Matas, A. J., and Michael, A. F., 1978, The immunohistopathology of glomerular antigens. II. The glomerular basement membrane, actomyosin and fibroblast surface antigens in normal, diseased and transplanted human kidneys, *Am. J. Pathol.* **90:**71.

Schiffer, M. S., Michael, A. F., Kim, Y., Fish, A. J., 1981, Distribution of glomerular basement membrane antigens in diseased human kidneys, *Lab. Invest.* **44:**234.

Steblay, R. W., 1962, Glomerulonephritis induced in sheep by injections of heterologous glomerular basement membrane and Freund's complete adjuvant, *J. Exp. Med.* **116:**253.

5

Physiologic Approaches to the Mechanisms of Glomerular Immune Injury

Roland C. Blantz

1. Introduction

The technique of renal micropuncture was first devised and utilized by A. N. Richards in the early 1930s (Richards and Walker, 1935), but this method did not come into vigorous use until the early 1960s. Since the early 1960s, renal micropuncture has been utilized primarily in the examination of normal renal physiology, further elucidation of mechanisms of epithelial transport and of the control of volume homeostasis. During this same period and up to the present, there have been major strides in understanding of the role of immune mechanisms as they apply to the pathogenesis of renal disease (Cochrane *et al.*, 1965; Unanue and Dixon, 1965). These investigations have been based both upon models of experimental glomerulonephritis in animals and upon the application of sophisticated techniques to the examination of material from patients with renal disease.

Unfortunately, until the past few years, there was little evidence of collaboration and cross-fertilization of disciplines between these two major fields of scientific investigation in nephrology: the examination of renal physiology by micropuncuture techniques and in-depth analysis of immune mechanisms for renal disease. Only recently have renal micropuncturists turned from the examination of normal control mechanisms in renal physiology and applied the technique to the examination of certain pathophy-

---

Roland C. Blantz · Department of Medicine, School of Medicine, University of California, San Diego, and Veterans Administration Hospital, San Diego, California 92161. These studies were supported by grants from the National Institutes of Health (HL 14914) and the Veterans Administration Medical Research Service.

siologic models of clinical renal disease such as acute renal failure (Blantz, 1975; Baylis *et al.*, 1977; Stein *et al.*, 1975) and to descriptive studies in the later phases of experimental glomerulonephritis (Rocha *et al.*, 1973; Allison *et al.*, 1974; Maddox *et al.*, 1975).

2. An Evaluation of Glomerular Capillary Injury by the Use of Micropuncture Techniques

In collaboration with Dr. Curtis Wilson, Scripps Clinic, La Jolla, this laboratory recently has applied micropuncture methods in a somewhat different manner. The quantitative assessment of the acute phases of glomerular immune injury often has been limited to qualitative methods utilizing histology, immunofluorescence techniques, and electron microscopy. Microtechniques which permit evaluation of the degree to which nephron filtration rate (sngfr) has been altered and the specific mechanisms leading to the reduction in filtration rate (Brenner *et al.*, 1971; Blantz *et al.*, 1972; Blantz, 1974; Deen *et al.*, 1972) have been developed only recently. These techniques have been applied to the evaluation of the filtration process during control periods and within 1 hr of the administration of large doses of anti-glomerular basement membrane antibody (ABGM-Ab) (Blantz and Wilson, 1976; Blantz *et al.*, 1978). These studies were conducted in the Munich-Wistar rat, a strain with glomeruli on the surface of the kidney which are accessible for direct measurement of hudrostatic and oncotic pressures. There are several advantages to this experimental protocol. First, large doses of antibody can be administered. These produce significant reductions in filtration rate while allowing all pertinent pressures, flows, and permeabilities to be measured readily. Second, the filtration response to a given dose of antibody is remarkably uniform in this nearly isogenetic strain of rat. Third, the presence of surface glomeruli permits quantitative evaluation of all of the respective determinants of glomerular ultrafiltration and permits judgments as to the initiating events in the process of immune injury.

Anti-GBM Nephritis

The basic questions that have been examined are as follows:

1. What is the mechanism of acute reduction of nephron filtration rate following the infusion of large doses of AGBM-Ab?
2. If several determinants of glomerular ultrafiltration contribute to reduced single nephron glomerular filtration rate (sngfr), are the mechanisms separable and can they be associated with specific ultrastructural changes?
3. What is the contribution of fixation of complement to glomerular immune injury and reduced filtration rate?

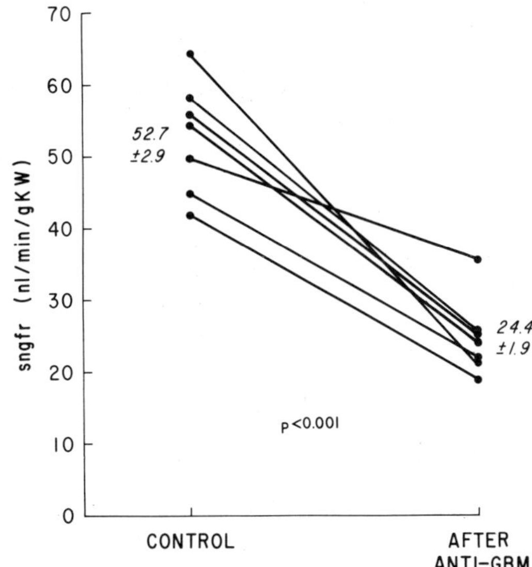

Figure 1. The sngfr in control rats and after the infusion of anti-GBM antibody. Each point represents the mean sngfr for each rat in the respective periods. The sngfr fell consistently in each animal.

There are several potential mechanisms which could reduce filtration rate following acute immune injury.

1. The hydrostatic pressure gradient between glomerular capillary and Bowman's space (ΔP) could be reduced due to
   a. Reductions in glomerular capillary hydrostatic pressure, or
   b. Increases in tubular and Bowman's space pressure.
2. There could be reductions in nephron plasma flow (rpf) due to vasoconstriction.
3. Glomerular filtration could decrease due to loss of filtering nephron units.
4. Reductions in the glomerular permeability coefficient (L_pA) due to either
   a. Loss of capillary surface area (A), or
   b. Reductions in hydraulic permeability of the glomerular membrane (L_p).

Each study was paired with measurements of nephron filtration rate (sngfr), plasma flow (rpf), and hydrostatic and oncotic pressures in a control period and repeated within 60 min of the infusion of large doses of AGBM-Ab. In the initial study, sngfr fell rather uniformly to slightly less than 50% of the control value (Fig. 1).

The several determinants of filtration rate were measured in these same animals permitting precise conclusions as to the specific mechanisms leading to reduced filtration rate. Two of the critical determinants of glomerular filtration are the hydrostatic pressure gradient from capillary to Bowman' space (ΔP) and the rate of nephron plasma flow (rpf) (Fig. 2). The ΔP actually increased following glomerular immune injury, by approximately 12 mm

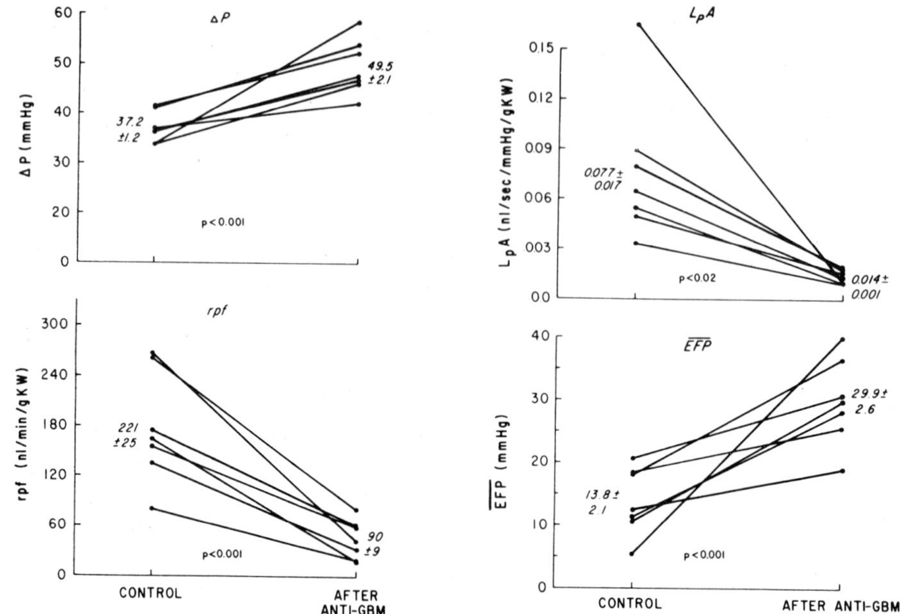

Figure 2. (Left) The effect of anti-GBM antibody upon ΔP (upper) and rpf (lower panel). ΔP increased in each rat and the mean value increased from 37 ± 1 to 50 ± 2 mm Hg. This finding was primarily the result of a large decrease in tubular pressure.The rpf decreased in each rat and the mean value fell from 221 ± 25 to 90 ± 9 nl/min per g kidney wt after antibody infusion. (Right) The glomerular permeability coefficient (L_pA) and mean effective filtration pressure ($\overline{EFP}$) during control and after anti-GBM antibody infusion (sngfr = $L_pA \cdot \overline{EFP}$). L_pA fell from 0.077 ± 0.017 to 0.014 ± 0.001 nl/sec per mm Hg per g kidney wt. In spite of the doubling of $\overline{EFP}$, the sngfr fell as a result of decreased L_pA.

Hg. However, rpt fell to less than 50% of the control values due to vasoconstriction. The effect of the large reduction in rpf was essentially neutralized by the large increase in the ΔP. Therefore, other factors which influence glomerular ultrafiltration must have been operating to reduce sngfr. The mean effective filtration pressure (EFP), or net hydraulic pressure minus oncotic pressure across the glomerular capillary, actually doubled following antibody infusions, which demonstrates that the decrease in sngfr was not the result of reduced net driving pressure (Fig. 2). Therefore, the critical determinant which reduced filtration rate was a large decrease in the L_pA to approximately 20% of the control value.

In these initial studies, an evaluation of glomeruli after AGBM-Ab infusion by light microscopy failed to reveal sufficient infiltration of capillaries by polymorphonuclear leukocytes to explain the large reduction in L_pA solely on the basis of loss of filtering surface area. There were ultrastructural changes observed within the glomerular membrane which could have accounted for a reduction in L_p and produced the reductions in L_pA. These changes were observed primarily upon the endothelial aspect of the glomerular capillary. The normal glomerular membrane is shown in the upper panel in Fig. 3. The normal fenestrated endothelial cell is tightly adherent to the GBM. In the lower panel, the endothelial cell was irregular and detached from the underlying GBM following AGBM-Ab. The creation of this potential space could have lowered L_p by providing a less "well-stirred" compartment, separated from the mixing effect of plasma and cellular flow. Protein concentration could rise to much higher values within this compartment and thereby retard ultrafiltration at the membrane. This effect should result in lower values for L_pA.

The sngfr fell acutely after antibody infusion due to reductions in both rpf and L_pA. Were the respective influences of these determinants of filtration separable or were changes in these factors intimately linked? This issue has been addressed by examining the effect of both low (1.4) and high doses (2.3 μg/g body wt) of AGBM-Ab upon the filtration process. A second AGBM-Ab preparation was utilized for these studies. The sngfr fell significantly at both doses: minimally at the lower dose and rather massively following high doses of antibody (Fig. 4). At the lower dose, vasoconstriction was minimal and the reduction in sngfr was primarily the result of a substantial decrease in L_pA. However, at the higher dose, the large decrease in sngfr was due to major reductions in both rpf and L_pA, both greater in magnitude than with the lower dose.

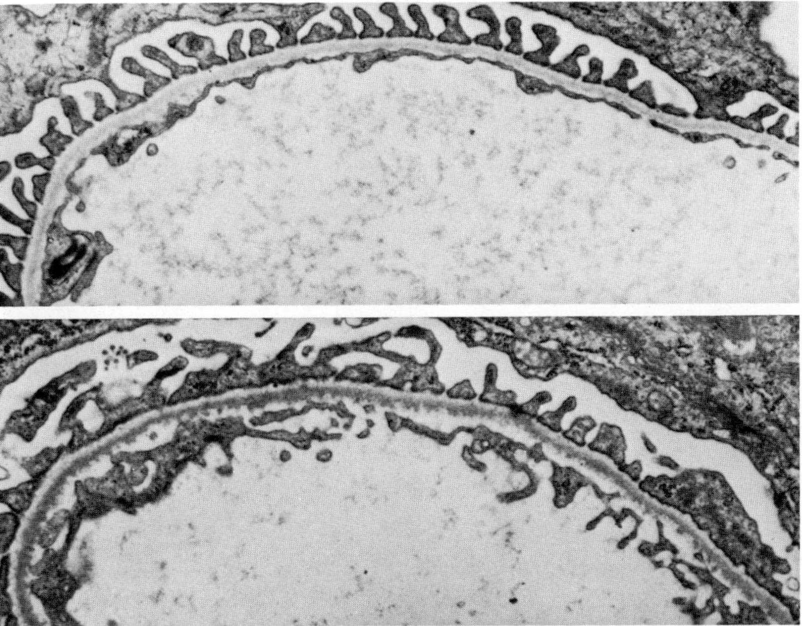

Figure 3. The normal rat glomerular membrane is shown in the upper panel and the structures following anti-GBM antibody in the lower panel. The endothelial cell is swollen, irregular, and separated from the GBM. The subendothelial aspect of the GBM has an irregular appearance consistent with the fixation of antibody. The epithelial cell foot processes show focal areas of fusion.

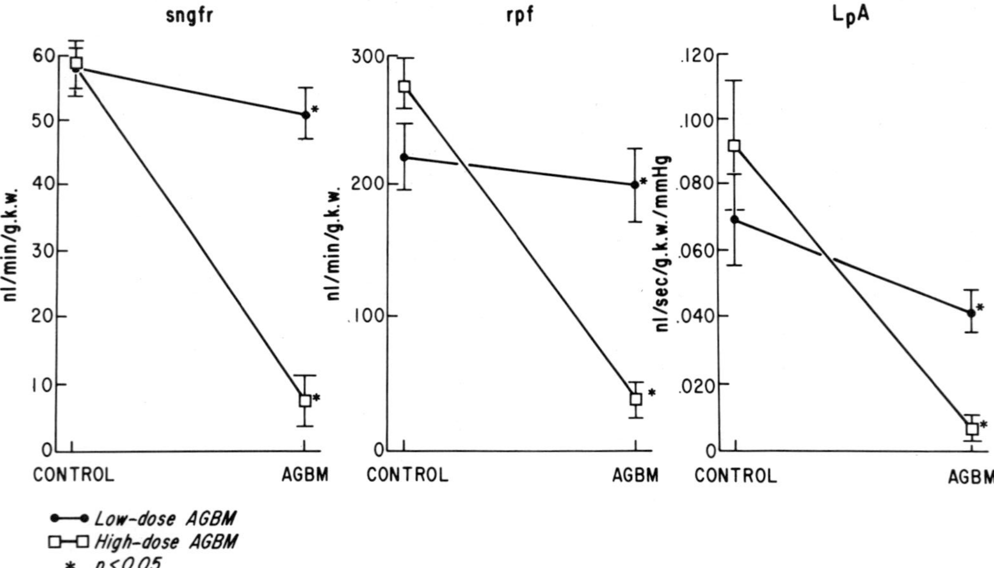

Figure 4. The effect of low- and high-dose anti-GBM antibody infusion on sngfr, rpf, and L_pA. The lesser reduction in sngfr at the low dose was almost entirely the result of decreased L_pA. The large reduction in sngfr after high-dose antibody was the result of major reductions in both rpf and L_pA.

The two major morphologic alterations observed following antibody infusion were: (1) the migration of polymorphonuclear cells into the capillary and the adherence of these cells to the GBM, and (2) the separation of the endothelial cell from the GBM. The major morphologic difference between low- and high-dose groups was that there were considerably more polymorphonuclear leukocytes within capillary lumina at the higher dose. There were no histologic changes or immunoglobulin deposits observed in resistance vessels, suggesting that the vasoconstriction, observed primarily at the higher dose, was of a functional nature.

The role of complement fixation in producing both the physiologic changes in glomerular filtration and the morphologic changes within the glomerulus was examined also. This issue was evaluated by comparing the effects of AGBM-Ab in complement-depleted rats to the findings observed in normal rats. Identical doses of AGBM-Ab were administered to rats pretreated with cobra venom factor, in doses sufficient to reduce C3 to undetectable levels on the day of micropuncture (Ballow and Cochrane, 1969; Gotze and Müller-Eberhard, 1977). Absence of complement was confirmed by immunofluorescence analysis of renal tissue.

The effects of both low and high doses of AGBM-Ab upon the sngfr after complement depletion are shown in Fig. 5. Following complement depletion, low doses of AGBM-Ab no longer resulted in a significant

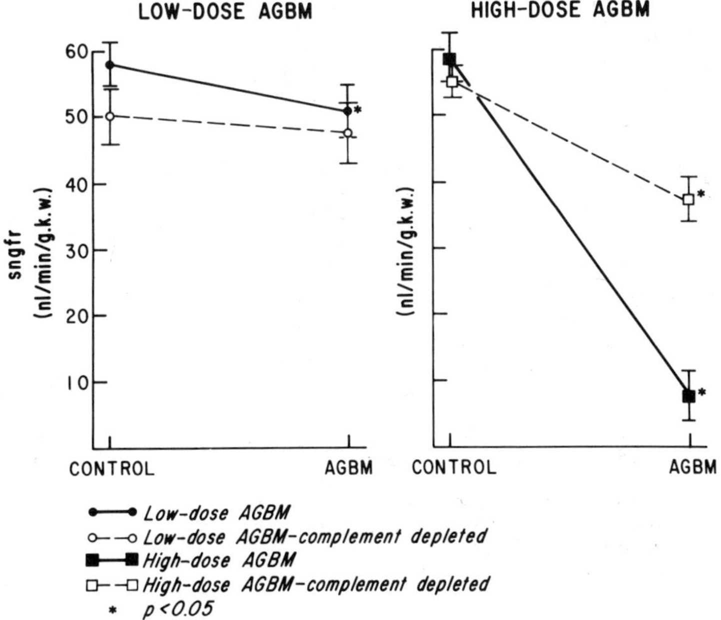

Figure 5. Effect of prior complement depletion upon nephron filtration rate (sngfr) following low- and high-dose AGBM. Complement depletion prevented the small decrease in sngfr observed in normal rats at low doses and greatly reduced the large decrease in sngfr observed in normal rats at the higher dose.

reduction in sngfr. At high doses of antibody, there was an impressive protective effect of prior complement depletion, but sngfr remained affected and fell from 55 to 37 nl/min. This decrease in sngfr which persisted in complement-depleted rats was significantly less than the reduction observed in rats with intact complement systems. The beneficial effects of complement depletion were mediated in part by an effect upon rpf (Fig. 6). Complement depletion totally prevented the small reduction in rpf observed in normal rats at the low dose of antibody. Also, at the higher dose of AGBM-Ab the major reduction in rpf observed in normal rats was prevented largely by prior complement depletion.

The effect of AGBM-Ab on the L_pA in normal and in complement-depleted animals is shown in Fig. 7. At the lower dose, complement depletion had no measurable influence upon the antibody-induced reduction in L_pA. At the higher dose, complement depletion significantly diminished the extent to which L_pA was reduced. However, the L_pA still decreased after AGBM-Ab in the complement-depleted high-dose group. L_pA was not different from the L_pA after the low dose in both normal and complement-depleted rats.

Complement depletion prevented the reduction in sngfr in the low-dose antibody group primarily by preventing vasoconstriction. It had no effect upon the reduction in L_pA. At the higher dose, a decrease in sngfr persisted,

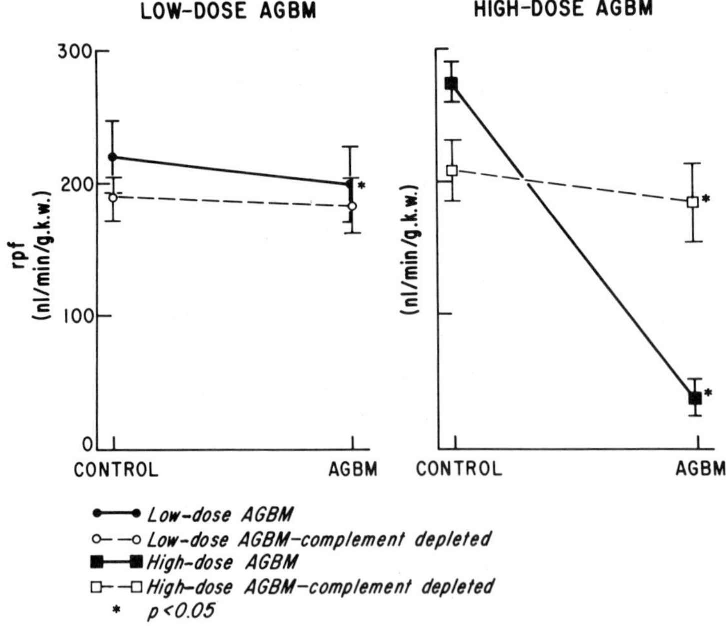

Figure 6. Effect of prior complement depletion upon nephron plasma flow (rpf) following low- and high-dose AGBM. Complement depletion prevented the small reduction in rpf observed in normal rats after low-dose infusion and greatly reduced the major decline in rpf in normal rats after the high dose.

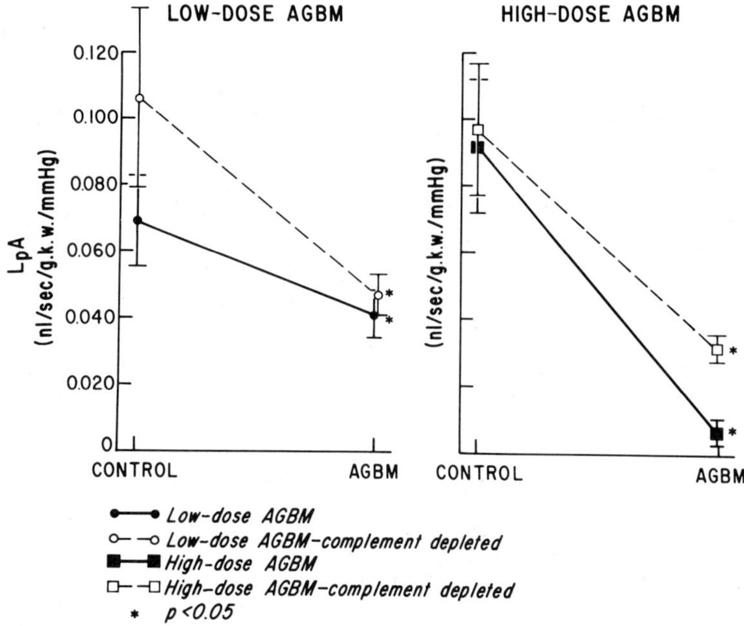

Figure 7. Effect of prior complement depletion upon the glomerular permeability coefficient (L_pA) after low- and high-dose AGBM. Complement depletion had no effect upon the decrease in L_pA noted in normal rats after low-dose antibody, and the experimental values with low-dose AGBM were not different. At the high dose, complement depletion results in a smaller decrease in L_pA in complement-depleted rats.

but to a much smaller degree. Complement depletion largely prevented the vasoconstriction and significantly decreased the magnitude of reduction in L_pA. However, at both doses, there remained a persistent reduction in L_pA that was not dependent upon fixation of complement.

The physiologic consequences of both doses of AGBM-Ab can be correlated closely with the morphologic and ultrastructural changes in normal and in complement-depleted rats. Again, the two major structural abnormalities observed were separation of the endothelial cell from the underlying GBM and infiltration of the capillaries with polymorphs and adherence of these cells to the GBM. In the normal rats with intact complement systems, the greater reduction in sngfr, rpf, and L_pA at the high dose of antibody correlated with greater infiltration of glomerular capillaries by polymorphonuclear leukocytes. This was documented by the large number of polymorphonuclear leukocytes per glomerulus observed by light microscopy. The beneficial effects of complement depletion correlated best with the nearly complete prevention of polymorphonuclear leukocyte infiltration into the glomerulus. The major reduction in L_pA at the higher dose must have been due in part to loss of capillary surface area related to the adherence of polymorphonuclear leukocytes. The prevention of a major portion of the reduction in L_pA by complement depletion must have been due to prevention

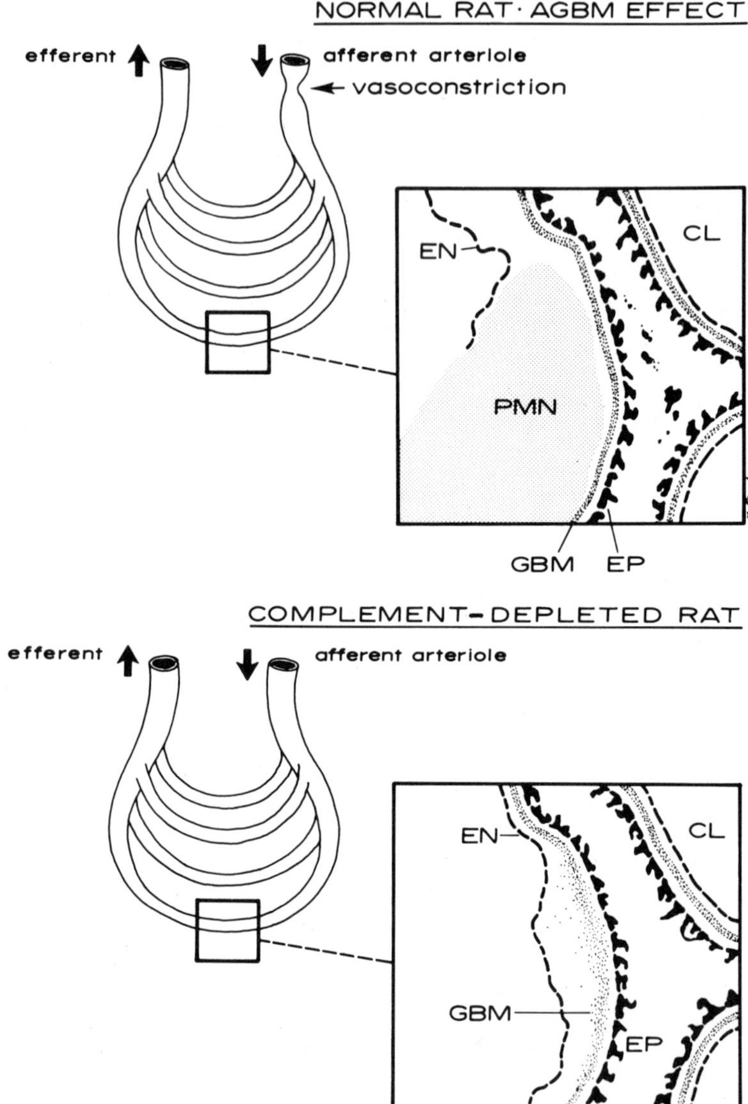

Figure 8. Schematic of physiologic and morphologic results of anti-GBM antibody infusions in normal (upper panel) and complement-depleted rats (lower panel). In normal rats, sngfr fell due to vasoconstriction and decreased rpf and major decreases in L_pA, which resulted from adherence of polymorphonuclear leukocytes to the GBM (loss of capillary surface area) and separation of the endothelial cell from the GBM (decreased L_p). Complement depletion prevented the vasoconstriction and migration of polymorphonuclear leukocytes into the glomerular capillary and thereby affected the antibody-induced changes in sngfr. The endothelial cell changes persisted in spite of complement depletion and contributed to the persistent sngfr reduction which was independent of the complement cascade.

of polymorph migration and to the resultant loss of capillary surface area. The lesser but significant reduction in L_pA which persisted and was not dependent upon an intact complement system correlated only with ultrastructural changes upon the endothelial surface of the glomerular capillary.

It is difficult to directly extrapolate the results of the present acute study to the clinical state associated with AGBM-Ab-induced glomerulonephritis. Although large quantities of antibody can be demonstrated on the GBM of patients with this form of glomerulonephritis (Wilson and Dixon, 1973; McPhaul and Mullins, 1976), it is unlikely that such a large amount of AGBM-Ab as was utilized in this study (with respect to the weight of the animal) could be generated and released into the circulation in such a short time period in the analogous clinical condition. Therefore, it is not likely that vasoconstriction is the dominant mode of initial GFR reduction in clinical AGBM-Ab-induced nephritis but rather the decrease in L_pA. It is possible that polymorphonuclear leukocytes and other cells may contribute to further reduction in L_pA at a later time through loss of filtering capillary surface in the absence of complement activation. The present, acute studies certainly suggest that an intact complement system accelerates the process.

In the normal rat, large doses of AGBM-Ab lead to reduced nephron filtration rate due to: (1) vasoconstriction especially at higher doses, and (2) reduced glomerular permeability coefficient (L_pA). The reduction in L_pA in turn is due to ultrastructural changes on the endothelial surface of the glomerular membrane (L_p) and to the loss of capillary surface area due to adherence of polymorphs (Fig. 8).

In complement-depleted rats, vasoconstriction essentially is prevented. Complement depletion also prevents the loss of surface area by preventing the migration of polymorphs into the capillary (Fig. 8). However, there remains a reduction in L_pA which correlates with separation of the endothelial cell from the underlying membrane. These membrane alterations occur independent of the fixation of complement.

These studies have demonstrated the utility of the technique of renal micropuncture as a quantitative assay tool in the investigation of pathophysiologic states which include the definition of specific mechanisms producing immune injury to the glomerulus.

References

Allison, M. E. M., Wilson, C. B., and Gottschalk, C. W., 1974, Pathophysiology of experimental glomerulonephritis in rats, *J. Clin. Invest.* **53:**1402.

Ballow, M., and Cochrane, C. G., 1969, Two anticomplementary factors in cobra venom: Hemolysis of guinea pig erythrocytes by one of them, *J. Immunol.* **103:**944.

Baylis, C., Rennke, H. R., and Brenner, B. M., 1977, Mechanisms of gentamicin-induced defect in glomerular filtration, *Clin. Res.* **25:**426A.

Blantz, R. C., 1974, Effect of mannitol on glomerular ultrafiltration in the hydropenic rat, *J. Clin. Invest.* **54:**1135.

Blantz, R. C., 1975, The mechanism of acute renal failure after uranyl nitrite, *J. Clin. Invest.* **55:**621.

Blantz, R. C., and Wilson, C. B., 1976, Acute effects of anti-glomerular basement membrane antibody on the process of glomerular filtration in the rat, *J. Clin. Invest.* **58**:899.

Blantz, R. C., Israelit, A. H., Rector, F. C., Jr., and Seldin, D. W., 1972, Relation of distal tubular NaCl delivery and glomerular hydrostatic pressure, *Kidney Int.* **2**:22.

Blantz, R. C., Tucker, B. J., and Wilson, C. B., 1978, Acute effects of anti-glomerular basement membrane antibody on the process of glomerular filtration in the rat: Influence of dose and complement depletion, *J. Clin. Invest.* **61**:910.

Brenner, B. M., Troy, J. L., and Daugharty, T. M., 1971, The dynamics of glomerular ultrafiltration in the rat, *J. Clin. Invest.* **50**:1776.

Cochrane, C. G., Unanue, E. R., and Dixon, F. J., 1965, A role of polymorphonuclear leukocytes and complement in nephrotoxic nephritis, *J. Exp. Med.* **122**:99.

Deen, W. M., Robertson, C. R., and Brenner, B. M., 1972, A model of glomerular ultrafiltration in the rat, *Am. J. Physiol.* **223**:1178.

Gotze, O., and Müller-Eberhard, H. J., 1977, The alternative pathway of complement activation, *Adv. Immunol.* **24**:1.

McPhaul, J. J., Jr., and Mullins, J. D., 1976, Glomerulonephritis mediated by antibody to glomerular basement membrane: Immunological, clinical and histopathological characteristics, *J. Clin. Invest.* **57**:351.

Maddox, D. A., Bennett, C. M., Deen, W. M., Glassock, R. J., Knutson, D., Daugharty, T. M., and Brenner, B. M., 1975, Determinants of glomerular filtration in experimental glomerulonephritis in the rat, *J. Clin. Invest.* **55**:305.

Richards, A. N., and Walker, A. M., 1935, Urine formation in the amphibian kidney, *Am. J. Med. Sci.* **192**:727.

Rocha, A., Marcondes, M., and Malnic, G., 1973, Micropuncture study in rats with experimental glomerulonephritis, *Kidney Int.* **3**:14.

Stein, J. H., Gottschalk, J., Osgood, R. W., and Ferris, T. F., 1975, Pathophysiology of a nephrotoxic model of acute renal failure, *Kidney Int.* **8**:27.

Unanue, E. R., and Dixon, F. J., 1965, Experimental glomerulonephritis. V. Studies on the interaction of nephrotoxic antibodies with tissues of the rat, *J. Exp. Med.* **121**:697.

Wilson, C. B., and Dixon, F. J., 1973, Anti-glomerular basement membrane antibody-induced glomerulonephritis, *Kidney Int.* **3**:74.

6

Physical Interactions between Macromolecules and the Glomerular Filter

Manjeri A. Venkatachalam and Helmut G. Rennke

Recent studies have focused attention on molecular factors other than steric hindrance that determine the permeability of the glomerular filter to macromolecules (Farquhar, 1978; Brenner *et al.*, 1978; Rennke and Venkatachalam, 1977a; Rennke *et al.*, 1978, Bohrer *et al.*, 1978). Using tracer molecules of appropriate size, charge, and shape, it has been shown that glomerular permeability is markedly dependent on all of these molecular parameters. Thus, molecules of certain size, shape, and charge characteristics are excluded from the glomerular filtrate. The degree of exclusion is determined by physical interactions between molecules and the filtering membrane. Discussion of the basis for different types of filter–molecule interactions (i.e., pertaining to steric phenomena, electrostatic effects and molecular configuration) will form a large part of this review. The dynamics of glomerular blood flow and filtration also govern permeability. These considerations are treated elsewhere in this book.

1. The Nature of the Filter

The glomerular filter is comprised of both cellular and extracellular matrix elements (Fig. 1; see also Chapter 1). Both endothelial cells and visceral epithelial cells of the filter present complex, individualized features of differentiation in their overall structure and substructure. Consideration

Manjeri A. Venkatachalam and Helmut G. Rennke · Departments of Pathology, Brigham and Women's Hospital and Harvard Medical School, Boston, Massachusetts 02115.

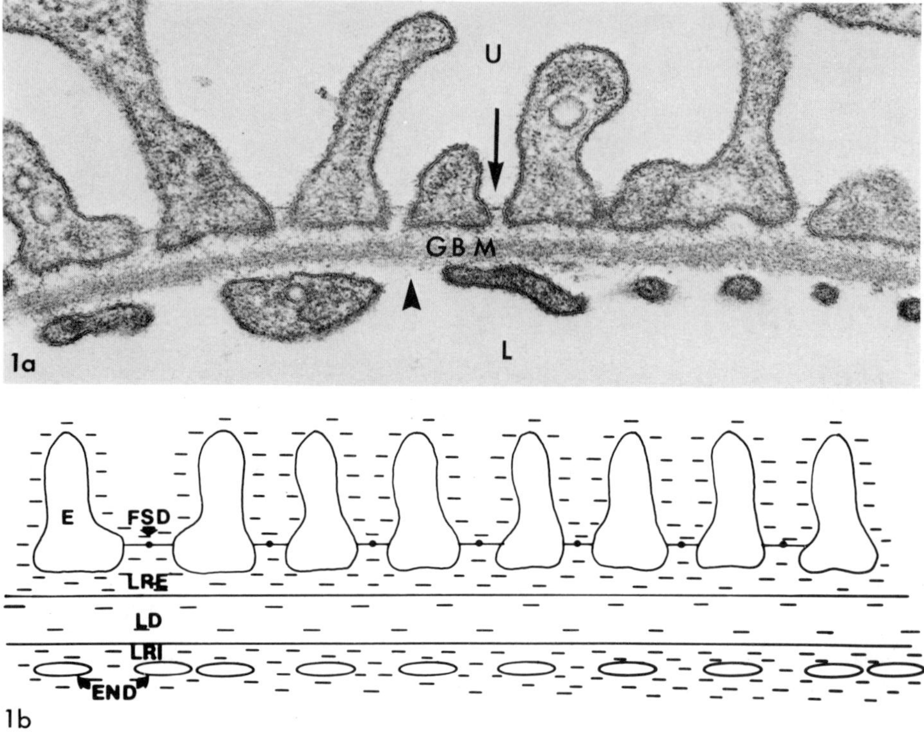

Figure 1. (a) Electron micrograph of rat glomerular capillary wall. From capillary lumen (L) outwards towards the urinary space (U), the filter is comprised of an endothelium with 500- to 1000-Å-diameter fenestrae (arrowhead), the glomerular basement membrane (GBM), and the glomerular epithelial foot processes. The latter are anchored to the outer surface of the GBM and are bridged by thin filtration slit diaphragms (arrow). The GBM has three layers, a central lamina densa and two peripheral electron-lucent layers, the lamina rara interna or the subendothelial layer, and the lamina rara externa, or the subepithelial layer. × 72,000. (b) Diagrammatic representation of the distribution of polyanionic sites (negative signs) in the filter. The concentration of the polyanion is greatest over the epithelial and endothelial cell coats and in the laminae rarae. END, endothelium; LRI, lamina rara interna; LD, lamina densa; LRE, lamina rara externa; FSD, filtration slit diaphragm.

of these features suggests that they subserve important glomerular functions. For example, the endothelial fenestrae (500–1000 Å in diameter) permit free access of plasma to the extracellular filter matrix; the number of fenestrae may partly determine the rate of filtration and thus, the high hydraulic conductivity of the filter wall. The complex interdigitating foot process architecture of the visceral epithelial cells likewise defines a large paracellular pathway (through the filtration slits) for filtered water and solutes and thus exerts control over the rate of filtration. The cellular elements of the filter provide mechanical support to the filtering membrane and appear responsible for its synthesis.

The filtering membrane is composed mainly of the extracellular matrix that occupies the entire filtration pathway from the endothelial fenestrae up to the filtration slits. This matrix is heterogeneous, but is physically continuous and is formed by the juxtaposition of the endothelial cell surface coat, the glomerular basement membrane (GBM), and the epithelial cell coat. The endothelial cell coat measures up to 120 Å in thickness, and lines the endothelial plasma membranes, including those lining the fenestrae. The latter are at least partially narrowed by cell coat material. Towards the abluminal side of the endothelium, the cell coat merges with the GBM. The GBM consists of a central electron-dense layer, the lamina densa, and two relatively electronlucent peripheral layers, the lamina rara interna and externa. The lamina rara interna is subendothelial in location. The lamina rara externa is subepithelial. The epithelial cell coat measures up to 800 Å in thickness, lines the podocyte cell bodies, and extends into the filtration slits in between the foot processes. The filtration slits measure only 240 Å in width at their narrowest points and are thus completely filled by epithelial cell coat material. Towards the base of the foot processes, the epithelial cell coat merges with the lamina rara externa of the GBM.

1.1. Physical Chemistry of the Cell Coats and GBM

Cell coats are surface extensions of the plasma membrane and consist of branching networks of sugar moieties attached to protein or phospholipid (Bretscher and Raff, 1975). In the glomerulus, abundant sialic acid residues impart a strongly polyanionic character to both endothelial and epithelial cell coats (Michael *et al.*, 1970; Mohos and Skoza, 1969; Groniowski *et al.*, 1969; Jones, 1969).

The GBM, a network of fibrillar material, consists of cross-linked chains of glycopeptides (Spiro, 1972; Kefalides, 1973; Sato and Spiro, 1976). Sialic acid, aspartic acid, and possibly other acidic moieties are present in GBM fractions (Spiro, 1972; Kefalides, 1973; Sato and Spiro, 1976) and impart a strongly polyanionic character to GBM glycoprotein (Farquhar, 1978; Rennke and Venkatachalam, 1977a). There is physical and chemical heterogeneity within the GBM. The constituent fibrils are densely packed in the lamina densa and much less so in the lamina rara interna and externa. Moreover, based on fractionation studies, GBM glycopeptide chains are of two basic types, a collagen-like nonpolar type, and a noncollagen polar type rich in sialic acid-containing heteropolysaccharides and aspartic acid (Spiro, 1972; Kefalides, 1973; Sato and Spiro, 1976). Cytochemical studies with polycationic reagents have localized the polyanionic moieties of the GBM to the lamina rara interna and externa (Farquhar, 1978; Rennke and Venkatachalam, 1977a; Groniowski *et al.*, 1969; Jones, 1969; Latta *et al.*, 1975; Behnke and Zelander, 1970; Rennke *et al.*, 1975; Seiler *et al.*, 1977: von Geyer *et al.*, 1970; Nicholes *et al.*, 1973). This suggests that there is a spatial organization of

GBM glycopeptide chains with the more polar elements being located in the laminae rarae, and the more neutral collagen-like chains in the lamina densa.

The available evidence indicates that the extracellular filter matrix is composed of branched, intertwining networks of chain polymers. Being rich in carbohydrate and polyanionic radicals, the glycopeptide network forms a hydrated gel in an aqueous environment, much like those found in artificial and in naturally occurring biological gel systems. In such gel systems, the intertwining chains of glycoproteins or polysaccharides enclose well-defined spaces within them (Laurent, 1966). These spaces in the interior of the gel are available for water and solute transport. The spatial geometry of the spaces and of their electrophysical environment will be determinants of steric as well as of electrophysical interactions between macromolecules and the filter, and thus of the limits of permeability to molecules in transit from the plasma in capillary lumina to the urinary space.

1.2. The Filtration Slit Diaphragms

Relatively little is known of these slender membranes that bridge the plasma membranes of adjacent podocyte foot processes. They occur as continuous 70-Å-thick ribbons that completely bridge the labyrinthine paracellular pathway bounded by interdigitating foot processes. Spanning the filtration slits at their narrowest points (240 Å in width), they have been thought to represent modified desmosomes that hold the cells together, but also have been considered to be mechanical barriers to the filtration of macromolecules (Rodewald and Karnovsky, 1974). With special techniques of fixation, electron microscopic images reveal them to exhibit elongated central bars with rod-like subunits connecting the bars to the outer leaflets of foot process plasma membranes. The bars, rods, and plasma membranes form the limiting boundaries of a double set of shallow repeating rectangular "pores" approximately 40 × 140 Å (Rodewald and Karnovsky, 1974). The physical and chemical nature of the slit diaphragms is unknown.

2. Filtration of Macromolecules

A convenient index of the filterability of a macromolecule is its clearance, corrected for tubular reabsorption, and expressed as a ratio relative to that of a freely filterable ideal solute such as inulin, or creatinine ("fractional clearance"). The effect of the size of macromolecules on their filtration is well known. Fractional clearances of all types of macromolecules decrease with increasing effective molecular radii (Einstein–Stokes radius or a_r), as long as other factors remain constant (Brenner *et al.*, 1978; Renkin and Gilmore, 1973). However, there are clear-cut differences in filtration behavior between various classes of macromolecules. For the same effective hydrodynamic radii, the fractional clearances of the polymers polyvinylpyrrolidone (PVP) and dextran, and globular proteins are quite different. There is extreme disparity between the fractional clearances of proteins and polymers. For some molecular radii, the differences are as much as an order of magnitude (Renkin and Gilmore, 1973). For the same effective molecular radii, fractional clearances of PVP are significantly greater than those of dextrans. These discrepancies at once suggest that molecular parameters other than size must be important determinants of filterability. As one would infer, there are important differences between diverse classes of macromolecules. Firstly, the polymers (PVP, dextran) in their native form are uncharged, with no ionizable groups. Secondly, the polymers are linear and flexible. They assume random coiled configurations in free aqueous solution, but without internal bonding or tertiary structure, unlike proteins (Renkin and Gilmore, 1973). Of interest is the fact that dextran does possess a secondary structure in that the elongated chains branch laterally. PVP is quite unbranched. Thus, dextran molecules in free solution assume more compact, albeit constantly changing globular configurations than PVP which forms coils that are relatively loose. Proteins, on the other hand, are composed of charged, amphoteric polypeptide chains that are folded upon themselves in finite, rigid, unchanging conformations held together by strong hydrophobic and disulfide bonds. Thus, unlike uncharged linear polymers, they possess a net charge, usually negative, and may be expected to be more resistant to deforming forces. That these differences between molecules may be determinants of transport across the gel matrix of the filter, in addition to well-established determinants related to glomerular hemodynamics and water flux, was suggested some years ago by Renkin and Gilmore (1973), but experimental dissection of these molecular factors has been possible only recently. That the polyanionic character of glomerular filter elements is a determinant of permeability, and indeed, of normal filter structure itself is indicated by several lines of evidence. Michael *et al.* (1970) showed that a decrease in glomerular sialoglycoprotein occurs in rat aminonucleoside nephrosis with a close temporal relationship to the proteinuria as well as the characteristic effacement of glomerular epithelial foot processes that characterizes the nephrotic disorder. At about the same time, it was suggested that the paradoxically different ultrastructural localization, within the glomerular filter, of tracer proteins such as the negatively charged ferritin and catalase, and the basic myeloperoxidase is explained if one considers that the filter, being negatively charged, may have different affinities for anionic than for cationic molecules (Venkatachalam *et al.*, 1970). In subsequent studies, it was shown that neutralization of glomerular polyanion by polycations leads to effacement of glomerular epithelial foot process architecture. This effect is rapidly reversed by heparin, a polyanion (Seiler *et al.*, 1975, 1977). The polycation-induced lesion is strikingly similar to the glomerular epithelial pathology observed in proteinuric disorders. As such, these findings lent support to the original suggestion by Michael *et al.* (1970) that decrease of glomerular polyanion may be a common pathogenetic mechanism in the causation of proteinuria and foot process abnormalities. These observations also indirectly suggested that polyanionic filter elements regulate normal glomerular barrier function and structure (Michael *et al.*, 1970; Seiler *et al.*, 1975).

In further studies, it was shown that molecules of the same size, but with different net charge, penetrate the gel matrix of the filter to different degrees. Ferritin molecules of identical size (a_c = 61 Å) but with progressively increasing isoelectric points were prepared by reacting ionized carboxyl groups with appropriate nucleophiles following carbodiimide activation (Rennke *et al.*, 1975). The results showed that there is increasing penetration of the glomerular filter by ferritin molecules of progressively higher isoelectric points. Virtually identical results were obtained in the isolated perfused kidney and *in vivo* (Rennke *et al.*, 1975; Rennke and Venkatachalam, 1977b). Preliminary tracer experiments from this laboratory suggest further that the degree of penetration of the filter by ferritin molecules correlates better with the density of charge on the molecules than with the isoelectric point (pI). Ferritin molecules of approximately similar pI were prepared using two different nucleophilic substances [glycine methyl ester (GME), hexanediamine (HMD)] to react with carboxyl groups. With GME, introduction of the nucleophile results in loss of ionized carboxyl groups only. New charged groups are not added to the molecule. When HMD is used as the nucleophile, however, a new positively charged amino group is introduced into the molecule for each reacted carboxyl (Hoare and Koshland, 1967). The results of tracer experiments using native anionic ferritin, GME ferritin, and HMD ferritin are shown in Figs. 2–4. Although both GME and HMD ferritins penetrate the glomerular filter in much greater quantities than native anionic ferritin (Figs. 2–4), these two modified ferritins of approximately similar isoelectric points differ in their behavior. The HMD ferritin (Fig. 4) can be seen to traverse the GBM in quantities appreciably greater than GME ferritin (Fig. 3). These differences may be explained by variations in the topography and in the density of ionized groups on the surface of the ferritin molecule. Further quantitative studies clearly are indicated.

Quantitative information on the effect of molecular charge on filtration

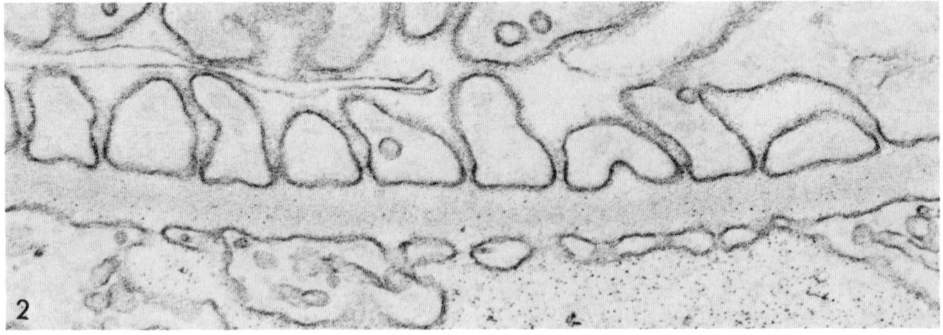

Figure 2. Electron micrograph of glomerular capillary wall from mouse intravenously injected with anionic ferritin. Kidneys were fixed by immersion in glutaraldehyde–formaldehyde fixative. There are numerous ferritin particles in the capillary lumen but few in the GBM.

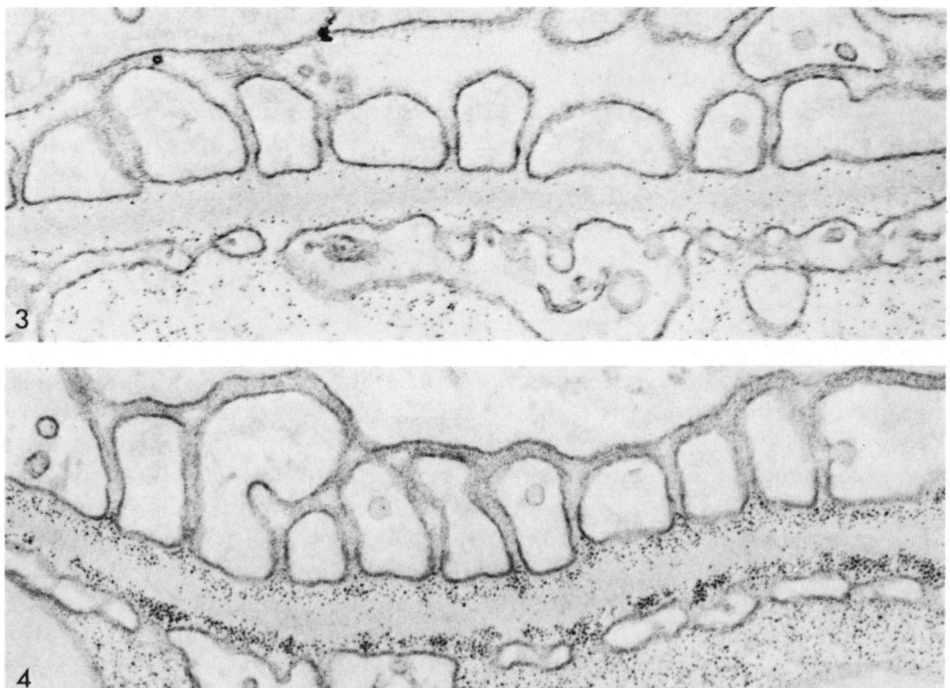

Figures 3 and 4. Electron micrographs of glomeruli from mice injected with equivalent amounts of feritins cationized with glycine methyl ester and with hexanediamine (isoelectric points between 7 and 9). Kidneys were fixed by immersion in glutaraldehyde–formaldehyde fixative. Both ferritins penetrate the GBM in amounts far greater than anionic ferritin (Fig. 2); however, ferritin modified with hexanediamine enters the filter in greater quantities (Fig. 4) than ferritin modified with glycine methyl ester (Fig. 3).

was obtained by Chang *et al.* (1975), Bohrer *et al.* (1978), and Rennke *et al.* (1978) using differently charged dextran and horseradish peroxidase molecules. These groups of workers found that fractional clearances of negatively charged macromolecules are significantly less than those of neutral or uncharged molecules. On the other hand, filtration of cationic molecules is facilitated. The impact of electrophysical effects on filtration may be gauged from the observation that for certain molecular radii, fractional clearances of cationic DEAE dextrans exceed those of anionic dextran sulfate by over two orders of magnitude (Bohrer *et al.,* 1978). The fractional clearance of cationic horseradish peroxidase (a_c = 30 Å; pI = 8.4–9.2) is 5.7 times greater than that of neutral horseradish peroxidase (pI = 7.2–7.4) of the same size, and 49 times that of negatively charged, succinylated peroxidase which is only 1.8 Å larger in radius (a_c = 32 Å; pI $<$ 4) (Rennke *et al.,* 1978). The effect of molecular configuration on glomerular permeability has been tested recently under controlled conditions (Rennke *et al.,* 1979). Clearances of uncharged dextran molecules and of neutral horseradish peroxidase were determined simultaneously. For a molecular radius of 28.45 Å, as determined by gel filtration, the fractional clearance of uncharged dextran exceeded that of the protein by a factor greater than 7. Similar results were reported for polydisperse dextrans and for Ficoll molecules (the latter possess a more compact molecular configuration than dextran) although the differences were more modest than those between proteins and dextrans (Bohrer *et al.*, 1979).

3. The Physical Basis for Glomerular Restriction

3.1. Role Played by the Cell Coats and GBM

The work of physical chemists, particularly that of Laurent and associates, has served to define the principles of steric restriction that govern the entry of permeant solutes into the interior spaces of gels. In uncharged gels, the available water volume, within the gel, for permeant nondeformable solutes, is dependent upon the equivalent hydrodynamic radii of the solute molecules (Laurent, 1966a,b). In experiments performed on a variety of gels, Laurent and associates showed that the available volume for a solute, or K_{av} of the gel, decreases progressively with increasing molecular radius, as well as with increasing concentration of the gel itself. Simply stated, the entry of a molecule into a gel is dependent upon the disparity between molecular size and the size of the spaces within the gel that are bounded by the chain-like network. The same principles should apply to the behavior of solute molecules at the plasma–glomerular filter interface.

If the gel is negatively charged, as for example in the ion-exchange gel sulfopropyl or carboxymethyl Sephadex, entry of solute molecules into the gel framework will be determined not only by molecular size, but also by molecular charge. Molecules that are too large will be excluded from the gel interior despite electrostatic interaction. Negatively charged molecules smaller than the gel spaces will tend to be excluded due to electrostatic repulsion by the ionized boundaries of the spaces. Positively charged molecules, on the other hand, will be attracted. Therefore, availability of the gel interior for solute molecules is determined by steric factors as well as by charge effects, including the density of charge on the gel and molecules. Steric and electrophysical interactions between solute molecules and the glomerular filter matrix are pictured in Figs. 5 and 6 and compared to similar interactions in artificial gel systems. The filter matrix is visualized here as one continuous flat bead of the Sephadex placed between two compartments. Molecules that appear in the filtrate in this system may be compared to those molecules in a chromatographic column that penetrate the interior of gel beads and whose appearance in the eluate is therefore delayed. Molecules that are excluded from the gel, and which therefore do not appear in the filtrate, are comparable to those molecules in the chromatographic column that quickly elute in the void volume. For analogy, the reader is referred to experiments on gelatin membranes performed by Larsen (1967). Gelatin membranes were placed

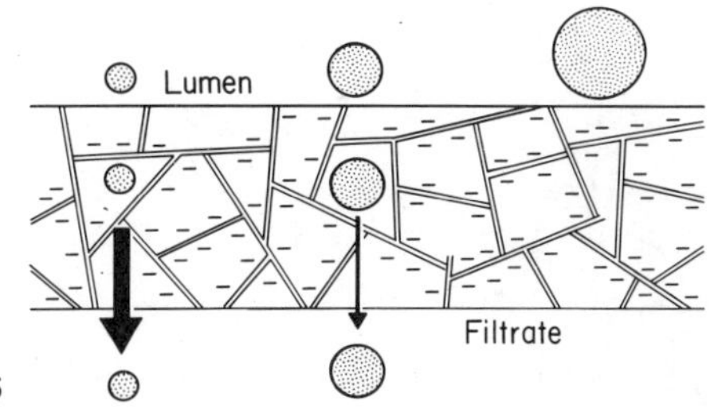

Figure 5. Effect of molecular size on the entry of uncharged molecules into a hypothetical capillary membrane and filtrate. In this and subsequent figures (6 and 7), filtering element of the capillary is represented as a gel comprised of intertwining elongated chains with fixed negatively charged radicals. Entry of molecules into the gel framework, and thus into the filtrate, is governed by steric interactions only. The available water volume, within the gel, for solute molecules, decreased with increasing molecular size.

between two aqueous compartments and the diffusion of albumin from one compartment to the other measured. If the anionic dye Congo red was bonded to the membrane, permeability to albumin decreased. Treatment of the Congo red–gelatin membranes with the polycation protamine, however, increased the permeability characteristic.

Returning to the issue of molecular configuration and flexibility, it is necessary to emphasize that estimates of the size and shape of molecules are made with reference to their physical state in free aqueous solution, that is, in a state in which they are not exposed to potential deforming forces. Ogston and Woods (1953) have shown that linear flexible chain polymers such as dextrans assume random coils in free solution, the approximate shape of the coiled configurations being globoid or ellipsoid. It is well to reiterate that these configurations are constantly changing, and that the coils are not internally bound, unlike proteins. Physical studies have shown that shearing forces tend to deform chain polymers through a process of unfolding of the random coils (Cerf and Scheraga, 1952). Solute molecules encounter such forces if they are subjected to sedimentation in gels or if they are exposed to forces of solvent drag during transport through porous matrices or gel frameworks.

For example, during such transport through a gel, the coiled configuration of a dextran or PVP molecule may be unraveled (Fig. 7). Portions of the molecule encounter obstacles in the gel. Other molecular portions which are drawn by solvent drag, uncoil. These elongated snake-like forms now behave like molecules of much smaller dimensions, then those which were measured for them in free aqueous solution. This explains the facilitation

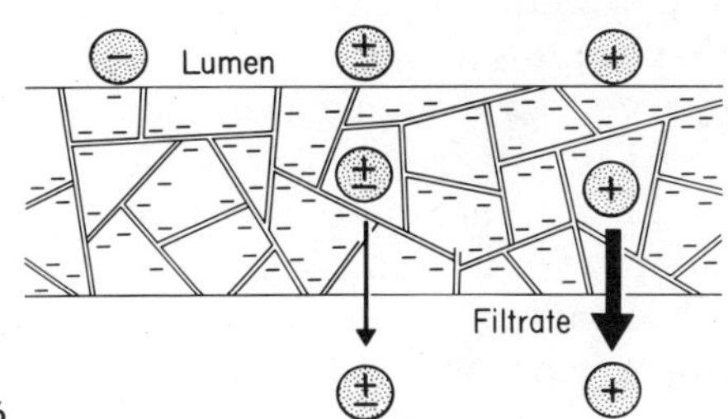

Figure 6. Effect of molecular charge on the entry of charged molecules into a hypothetical capillary membrane and filtrate. For molecules of equal size, entry of molecules into the gel is determined by electrophysical interactions. Filtration of negatively charged molecules is retarded; conversely, that of positively charged molecules is facilitated. Filtration of molecules with variable size *and* charge will be determined by steric as well as charge interactions.

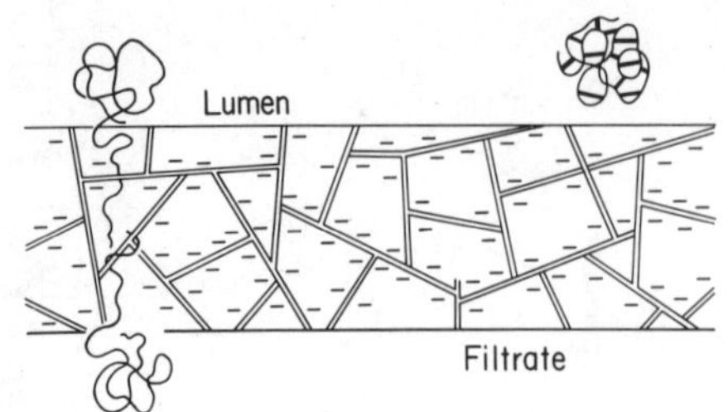

Figure 7. Effect of molecular configuration on the entry of molecules into a hypothetical capillary membrane and filtrate. Loosely coiled elongated molecules without tertiary structure, such as dextrans, pictured on the left, undergo deformation during filtration; transit of the deformed molecules through the gel is facilitated. This phenomenon is termed "reptation." On the other hand, globular proteins, pictured on the right, are not susceptible to unraveling of their polypeptide chains due to a rigid tertiary structure. Thus, for the same hydrodynamic radii measured for them in free solution, the transit of globular proteins through the gel matrix is retarded relative to that of linear chain polymers.

of transport. A theoretical treatment of such "reptilian motion" of flexible polymers through gels has been provided by de Gennes (1971). Experimental verification of this hypothesis was provided by Laurent *et al.* (1975), who measured the effective radii of a number of chain polymers during sedimentation through hyaluronate gels and compared them to their hydrodynamic radii in free solution. The true hydrodynamic radii of the molecules always greatly exceeded their effective radii (during sedimentation), for some molecules by almost 8 times. This indicates that the chain polymers behaved like much smaller molecules during transit than in free solution. Very similar results have been obtained recently by Cumming *et al.* (1977), who studied the transport of linear and globular macromolecules across thin chondroitin sulfate gels manufactured by chondrocytes in tissue culture. Linear polymers, but no globular molecules, showed marked deviations from their hydrodynamic radii during transport. The importance of these observations for glomerular transport cannot be understated. These considerations would suggest that linear polymers might be deformed to different degrees with changing hemodynamic conditions in the glomerulus, and thus affect the measured parameters of permeability.

3.2. Role Played by Slit Diaphragms and Epithelial Pinocytosis

The considerations discussed above, with respect to transport across the glomerular extracellular gel matrix, do not negate a role for other filter elements in the restrictive process. Data obtained from ultrastructural tracer experiments are consistent with a restrictive role for the filtration slit diaphragms. Thus, the GBM is not an absolute hindrance even for negatively charged large molecules like ferritin and catalase. Both anionic ferritin (a_c = 61 Å; pI = 4.5) and catalase (a_c = 52 Å; pI = 5.7) are hindered by the GBM, but incompletely (Farquhar *et al.*, 1961; Venkatachalam *et al.*, 1970; Rennke and Venkatachalam, 1977b). The molecules that do penetrate the GBM may be detected in the filtration slits proximal to the slit diaphragms, but not beyond (Venkatachalam *et al.*, 1970; Rennke and Venkatachalam, 1977b). Cationized ferritin molecules are found in the filtration slits in large numbers after intravenous injection in mice and rats, but are not found in the urinary space beyond the slit diaphragms (Rennke and Venkatachalam, 1977b). In bullfrog glomeruli, where the GBM is uneven and ill-formed, the slit diaphragms assume an important role in filtration (Schaffner and Rodewald, 1978). Rodewald and Karnovsky (1974) have postulated a role for the porous structure of the diaphragms in the filtration function. This attractive hypothesis has not been proven experimentally.

Active uptake of macromolecules by the visceral epithelial cells (podocytes) appears to be another mechanism that prevents the leakage of macromolecules into the urinary space. This "monitor" function for the epithelial cells, originally shown by Farquhar *et al.* (1961), has been confirmed repeatedly since. It seems attractive to link the retentive function of the slit diaphragms with the pinocytotic function of the epithelial cells. The bulk of plasma proteins appear to be hindered at the level of the plasma–filter interface (Ryan and Karnovsky, 1976; Ryan *et al.*, 1976). The filter, however, is not absolutely efficient, and a minority of molecules leak beyond the GBM towards the filtration slits. These molecules probably are retained by the slit diaphragms, taken up by the epithelial cells, and catabolized. The molecular limits of permeability at the level of the filtration slits remain to be determined. It seems safe to predict that these limits will be reached when molecular parameters such as size, shape, and charge approach those of serum albumin.

4. Summary

The process of ultrafiltration, whereby plasma proteins are excluded from the glomerular filtrate, is rather complex. A variety of structural and functional factors, and physical interactions between macromolecules and the main filter matrix appear to determine the limits of permeability. Imbalance at multiple levels may therefore lead to protein leakage in disease. Finally, understanding of the physical nature of the filter and its interactions with macromolecules may prove to be vital in study of the glomerular localization of humoral components of the immune response.

References

Behnke, O., and Zelander, T., 1970, Preservation of intercellular substances by the cationic dye alcian blue in preparative procedures for electron microscopy, *J. Ultrastruct. Res.* **31**:424.

Bohrer, M. P., Baylis, C., Humes, H. D., Glassock, R. J., Robertson, C. R., and Brenner, B. M., 1978, Permselectivity of the glomerular capillary wall: Facilitated filtration of circulating polycations, *J. Clin. Invest.* **61**:72.

Bohrer, M. P., Deen, W. M., Robertson, C. R., Troy, J. L., and Brenner, B. M., 1979, Influence of molecular configuration on the passage of macromolecules across the glomerular capillary wall, *J. Gen. Physiol.* **74**:583.

Brenner, B. M., Hostetter, T. H., and Humes, H. D., 1978, Molecular basis of proteinuria of glomerular origin, *N. Engl. J. Med.* **298**:826.

Bretscher, M. S., and Raff, M. C., 1975, Mammalian plasma membranes, *Nature (London)* **258**:43.

Caulfield, J. P., and Farquhar, M. G., 1976, Distribution of anionic sites in glomerular basement membranes: Their possible role in filtration and attachment, *Proc. Natl. Acad. Sci. USA* **73:**1646.

Cerf, R., and Scheraga, H. A., 1952, Flow birefringence in solutions of macromolecules, *Chem. Rev.* **51:**185.

Chang, R. L. S., Deen, W. M., Robertson, C. R., and Brenner, B. M., 1975, Permselectivity of the glomerular capillary wall. III. Restricted transport of polyanions, *Kidney Int.* **8:**212.

Cumming, G. J., Handley, C. J., and Preston, B. N., 1977, Permeability of chondrocyte cultures, *Upsala J. Med. Sci.* **81:**126 (abstract).

deGennes, P. G., 1971, Reptation of a polymer chain in the presence of fixed obstacles, *J. Chem. Phys.* **55:**572.

Farquhar, M., 1978, Structure and function in glomerular capillaries: Role of the basement membrane in glomerular filtration, in: *Biology and Chemistry of Basement Membranes* (N. A. Kefalides, ed.), pp. 43–80, Academic Press, New York.

Farquhar, M. G., Wissig, S. L., and Palade, G. E., 1961, Glomerular permeability. I. Ferritin transfer across the normal glomerular capillary wall, *J. Exp. Med.* **113:**47.

Groniowski, J., Biczyskowa, W., and Walski, M., 1969, Electron microscope studies on the surface coat of the nephron, *J. Cell Biol.* **40:**585.

Hoare, D. G., and Koshland, D. E., 1967, Method for the quantitative modification and estimation of carboxylic acid groups in proteins, *J. Biol. Chem.* **242:**2447.

Jones, D. B., 1969, Mucosubstances of the glomerulus, *Lab. Invest.* **21:**119.

Kefalides, N. A., 1973, Structure and biosynthesis of basement membranes, *Int. Rev. Connect. Tissue Res.* **6:**63.

Larsen, B., 1967, Increased permeability to albumin induced with protamine in modified gelatin membranes, *Nature (London)* **215:**641.

Latta, H., Johnston, W. H., and Stanley, T. M., 1975, Sialoglycoproteins and filtration barriers in the glomerular capillary wall, *J. Ultrastruct. Res.* **51:**354.

Laurent, T. C. 1966a, In vitro studies on the transport of macromolecules through the connective tissue, *Fed. Proc.* **25:**1128.

Laurent, T. C., 1966b, The exclusion of macromolecules from polysaccharide media, in: *The Chemical Physiology of Mucopolysaccharides* (G. Quintarelli, ed.), pp. 153–168, Little, Brown, Boston.

Laurent, T. C., Preston, B. N., Pertoft, H., Gustafsson, B., and McCabe, M., 1975, Diffusion of linear polymers in hyaluronate solutions, *Eur. J. Biochem.* **53:**129.

Michael, A. F., Blau, E., and Vernier, R. L., 1970, Glomerular polyanion alteration in aminonucleoside nephrosis, *Lab. Invest.* **23:**649.

Mohos, S. C., and Skoza, L., 1969, Glomerular sialoprotein, *Science* **164:**1519.

Nicholes, B. K., Krakower, C. A., and Greenspon, S. A., 1973, The chemically isolated lamina densa of the renal glomerulus, *Proc. Soc. Exp. Biol. Med.* **142:**1316.

Ogston, A. G., and Woods, E. F., 1953, Molecular configuration of dextrans in aqueous solution, *Nature (London)* **171:**221.

Renkin, E. M., and Gilmore, J. P., 1973, Glomerular filtration, in: *Handbook of Physiology,* Section 8, *Renal Physiology* (J. Orloff and R. W. Berliner, eds.), pp. 185–248, American Physiological Society, Washington, D.C.

Rennke, H. G., and Venkatachalam, M. A., 1977a, Structural determinants of glomerular permselectivity, *Fed. Proc.* **36:**2619.

Rennke, H. G., and Venkatachalam, M. A., 1977b, Glomerular permeability: In vivo tracer studies with polyanionic and polycationic ferritins, *Kidney Int.* **11:**44.

Rennke, H. G., Cotran, R. S., and Venkatachalam, M. A., 1975, Role of molecular charge in glomerular permeability: Tracer studies with cationized ferritins, *J. Cell Biol.* **67:**638.

Rennke, H. G., Patel, Y., and Venkatachalam, M. A., 1978, Glomerular filtration of proteins: Clearance of anionic, neutral and cationic horseradish peroxidase in the rat, *Kidney Int.* **13:**278.

Rennke, H. G., Patel, Y., and Venkatachalam, M. A., 1979, Glomerular permeability of macromolecules: Effect of molecular configuration on the fractional clearance of uncharged dextran and neutral horseradish peroxidase in the rat, *J. Clin. Invest.* **63:**713.

Rodewald, R., and Karnovsky, M. J., 1974, Porous structure of the glomerular slit diaphragm in the rat and mouse, *J. Cell Biol.* **60:**423.

Ryan, G. B., and Karnovsky, M. J., 1976, Distribution of endogenous albumin in the rat glomerulus: Role of hemodynamic factors in glomerular barrier function, *Kidney Int.* **9:**36.

Ryan, G. B., Hein, S. J., and Karnovsky, M. J., 1976, Glomerular permeability to proteins: Effect of hemodynamic factors on the distribution of endogenous immunoglobulin and exogenous catalase in the rat glomerulus, *Lab. Invest.* **34:**415.

Sato, T., and Spiro, R. G., 1976, Studies on the subunit composition of the renal glomerular basement membrane, *J. Biol. Chem.* **251:**4026.

Schaffner, A., and Rodewald, R., 1978, Glomerular permeability in the bullfrog *Rana catesbeiana, J. Cell Biol.* **79:**314.

Seiler, M. W., Venkatachalam, M. A., and Cotran, R. S., 1975, Glomerular epithelium: Structural alterations induced by polycations, *Science* **189:**390.

Seiler, M. W., Rennke, H. G., Cotran, R. S., and Venkatachalam, M. A., 1976, Distribution of glomerular anionic sites as revealed by polycationic compounds, *Am. J. Pathol.* **82:**54a (abstract).

Seiler, M. W., Rennke, H. G., Venkatachalam, M. A., and Cotran, R. S., 1977, Pathogenesis of polycation induced alterations ("fusion") of glomerular epithelium, *Lab. Invest.* **36:**48.

Spiro, R. G., 1972, Basement membranes and collagens, in: *Glycoproteins: Their Composition, Structure and Function,* 2nd ed., Part B (A Gottschalk, ed.), pp. 964–999, Elsevier, Amsterdam.

Venkatachalam, M. A., Karnovsky, M. J., Fahimi, H. D., and Cotran, R. S., 1970, An ultrastructural study of glomerular permeability using catalase and peroxidase as tracer proteins, *J. Exp. Med.* **132:**1153.

von Geyer, G., Linss, W., Schaaf, P., Moller, I., and Muller, A., 1970, Ultrahistochemische Untersuchungen and isolierten glomerularen Basalmembranen, *Acta Histochem.* **35:**67.

7

Pathologic and Functional Correlations in the Glomerulopathies

Alan M. Robson and Barbara R. Cole

1. Introduction

For many years nephrologists have looked for improved, noninvasive methods that could help in the initial evaluation of patients with renal disease and also could provide a useful tool with which to assess the response of patients to treatment. Although the measurement of protein selectivity (Joachim *et al.*, 1964; Cameron and Blandford, 1966) has gained some popularity for such purposes, there are many inherent problems in this method (Pesce *et al.*, 1970). Thus, it has not gained widespread acceptance.

An alternate approach has been taken in this laboratory. For several years the usefulness of serial measurements of glomerular permselectivity in the investigation and management of children with renal diseases has been evaluated. The results of these studies, performed in more than 100 children, as well as animal studies undertaken to supplement and to help with the interpretation of the observations in man, are summarized herein.

2. Methods

The measurement of glomerular permselectivity, using inert polyvinylpyrrolidone (PVP), is a relatively simple technique the details of which have been published previously (Robson *et al.*, 1974a). After injection of a pulse

---

Alan M. Robson and Barbara R. Cole · Edward Mallinckrodt Department of Pediatrics, Washington University School of Medicine, and Division of Nephrology, St. Louis Children's Hospital, St. Louis, Missouri 63178. This work was supported by Public Health Service Research Career Development Award 5 K04 AM 70236, Program Project Grant AM 09976, Clinical Research Center Grant RR 00036, and fellowship support from the Kidney Foundation of Greater St. Louis and Metro-East.

of polydisperse PVP and allowing approximately 20 min for equilibration throughout the PVP volume of distribution, clearance measurements of the PVP are undertaken by the usual methods. Column chromatography of the plasma and urine samples is used for separation of PVP according to molecular size, so that the clearances of individual moieties of a wide range of sizes of PVP can be calculated.

In most instances, the patient's diagnosis was established by histologic examination of a percutaneous renal biopsy. Standard methods were used to obtain and to prepare the biopsy specimen (Robson *et al.*, 1971) with recognized histologic diagnoses being made (Heptinstall, 1974). Informed consent was obtained before any studies were undertaken. Renal biopsies were performed only if they were indicated by the patient's clinical presentation and/or course.

3. Results

3.1. Normal Subjects

Figure 1 shows typical results of two studies in a normal person. The molecular radius of each fraction of PVP (depicted as the Stokes–Einstein radius or Rs) is plotted against the clearance of that PVP fraction. The clearances are expressed as a percentage of clearance of inulin determined simultaneously. Larger-molecular-weight PVP molecules were virtually excluded from the urine. Smaller molecules had higher clearances. Molecular clearance related inversely to molecular size. PVP molecules with an Rs of approximately 25 Å or less had clearances equal to that of inulin. As shown in Fig. 1, the method is quite reproducible in any individual. In addition, results from normal subjects agree closely with one another (Robson *et al.*, 1974a) and with those published by other investigators (Hulme and Hardwicke, 1968).

3.2. Minimal Change Nephrotic Syndrome (MCNS)

The results of the permselectivity studies performed in children in relapse from MCNS and who were not treated with steroids are compared to those obtained from six normal children in Fig. 2. These results are similar to those published previously (Robson *et al.*, 1974a) and were totally unexpected when first seen. Even though all of the patients in relapse from MCNS had marked proteinuria, the relative clearance of PVP molecules equivalent in size to albumin (Rs = 35 Å) was not increased as might have been expected, but rather was decreased. In fact, in patients with MCNS, all PVP molecules with an Rs of 35 Å or less had significantly decreased permselectivity (Fig. 2).

At the time these observations were first made, it was suggested that the discrepancies between the clearances of albumin and PVP could relate to the

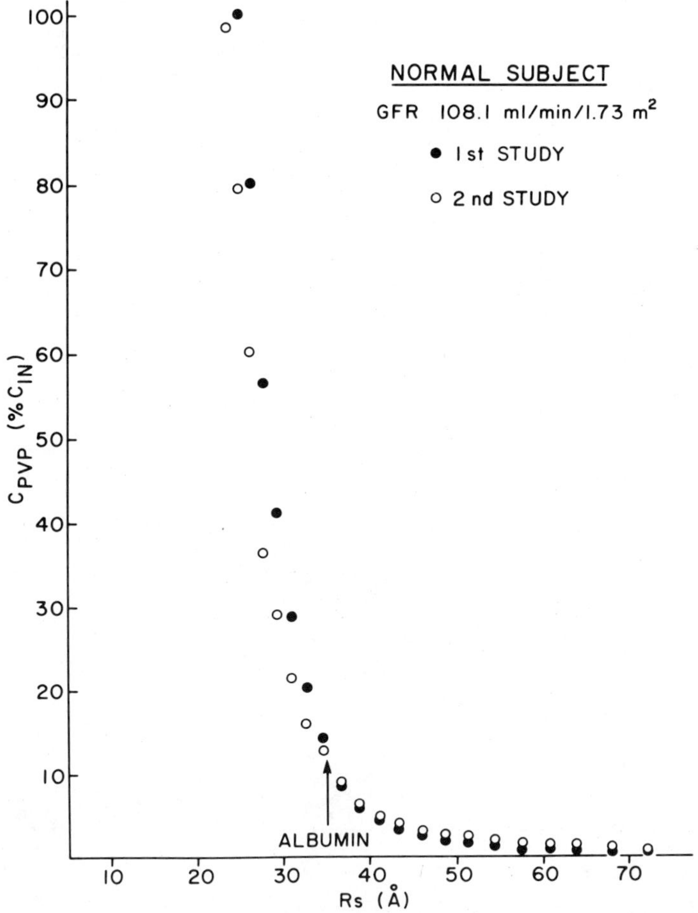

Figure 1. Clearances of different-size PVP molecules calculated from two successive clearance periods in a normal subject. The clearance of PVP molecules, expressed as a percentage of the simultaneously determined clearance of inulin, is plotted against the molecular size of that moiety of PVP. These latter values were calculated from the volumes of elution from Sephadex G-200 columns and are expressed as the Stokes–Einstein radius for a sphere of equivalent size (Rs) in angstroms. The position in which albumin is eluted from the columns (Rs 35 Å) is shown for comparison.

presence or absence of molecular charge (Robson *et al.*, 1974a). Indeed, it has now been well established that the ability of molecules to penetrate the glomerular barrier is dependent not only on molecular size and shape but also on charge (Rennke and Venkatachalam, 1977). In addition, charge has a marked effect on the clearance of molecules. Positively charged dextran molecules have a greater clearance than uncharged molecules of identical size, with the clearances of negatively charged dextran molecules being reduced markedly below the clearances of uncharged dextran molecules of equivalent size (Brenner *et al.*, 1978). These observations support the thesis

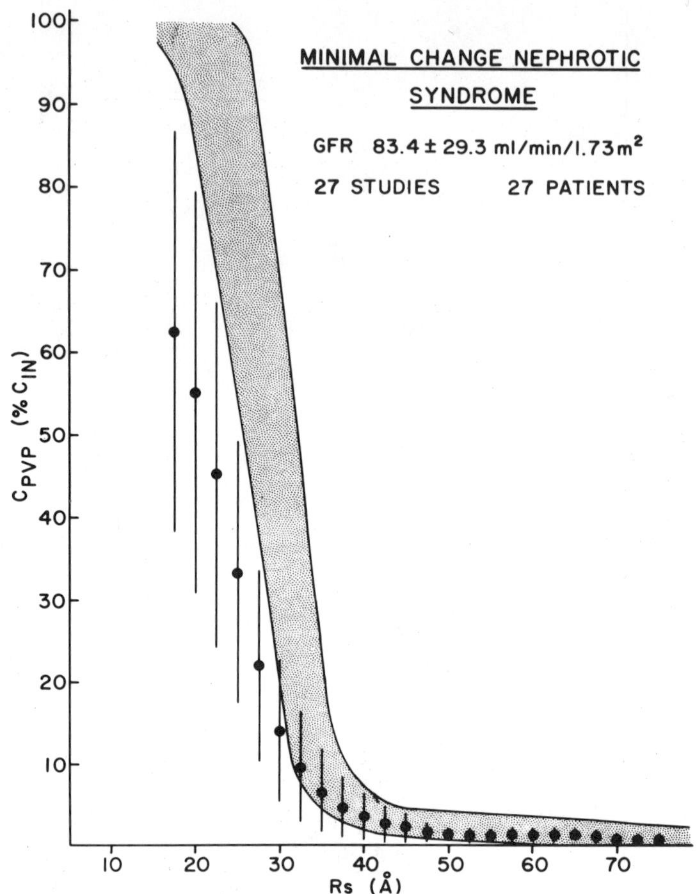

Figure 2. The pattern of permselectivity to PVP observed in 27 untreated patients in relapse from minimal change nephrotic syndrome. The shaded area represents the normal range of values observed in 6 healthy children; the values from the children with MCNS are depicted as the mean ± S.D. for each moiety of PVP shown.

(Robson *et al.*, 1974) that in MCNS the well-documented loss of glomerular polyanion (Blau and Haas, 1973) removes an electrical barrier to filtration and permits increased passage into the urine of albumin, which carries a negative charge, but does not permit concomitant increases in the clearances of the uncharged PVP molecules.

During the study of MCNS, several children were observed who were thought initially to have MCNS from their clinical presentation, but who did not respond adequately to treatment with steroids and were found subsequently to have another lesion as a cause of their nephrotic syndrome. Attempts were made to determine whether measurements of glomerular permselectivity could help to separate these children, early in the course of their disease, from those with steroid-responsive MCNS. The results are summarized in Table 1 where PVP clearances from the 6 normal subjects are compared to PVP clearances from 27 untreated patients in relapse from true MCNS, and from the 8 steroid-resistant children who were nephrotic and who were thought to have minimal change disease at the time of study. Of these 8 children, 5 were found subsequently to have mild immune complex deposition in the glomeruli, 2 had essentially normal glomeruli but responded incompletely to treatment with steroids, and 1 had focal glomerular sclerosis.

In true MCNS, the clearances of the large PVP molecules did not differ significantly from normal. The clearances of PVP molecules the size of albumin (35 Å) were reduced significantly from normal (Table 1, Fig. 2). In contrast, in the steroid-resistant children, clearance of the larger PVP molecules was increased above normal and also above the values observed in MCNS (Table 1). These increases were statistically significant for molecules with Rs values of 40 and 45 Å.

The fact that the eight steroid-resistant children studied here were thought initially to have MCNS from their clinical presentations and did not have obvious manifestations of an underlying glomerulonephritis should be emphasized. Although the data summarized in Table 1 suggest that the measurements of glomerular permselectivity may help to identify children with apparent MCNS who will not respond adequately to steroids, there is

Table 1. Comparison of PVP Clearances in Patients with Apparent and Those with True MCNS

PVP size (Rs) (Å)	C_{PVP} (% C_{IN})		
		Patients with clinical MCNS	
	Normal subjects (n = 6)	True MCNS (n = 27)	Others[a] (n = 8)
65	1.4 ± 1.7[b]	1.3 ± 1.4	1.9 ± 2.5
p vs. normal		NS	NS
p vs MCNS			NS
55	1.5 ± 0.9	1.4 ± 1.0	2.2 ± 2.5
p vs. normal		NS	NS
p vs. MCNS			NS
45	2.2 ± 0.8	2.2 ± 1.8	4.6 ± 2.6
p vs. normal		NS	< 0.05
p vs. MCNS			< 0.01
40	4.2 ± 1.5	3.5 ± 2.9	8.3 ± 4.0
p vs. normal		NS	< 0.01
p vs. MCNS			< 0.001
35	10.2 ± 3.9	6.6 ± 5.1	15.3 ± 8.9
p vs. normal		< 0.05	NS
p vs. MCNS			< 0.01

[a] Five patients with immune complex deposition in glomeruli, two with incomplete response to steroid, and one who developed focal glomerular sclerosis.
[b] Mean ± S.D.

overlap between the results obtained from the two groups of nephrotic children and more data will be required before conclusions can be reached with any degree of confidence.

3.3. Glomerulonephritis

The initial studies investigating the effects of glomerulonephritis on glomerular permselectivity concentrated on a relatively uniform lesion, poststreptococcal acute glomerulonephritis (PSAGN). This approach was taken since glomerulonephritis has many etiologies and histologic variations (Heptinstall, 1974), each of which could modify patterns of permselectivity in different ways.

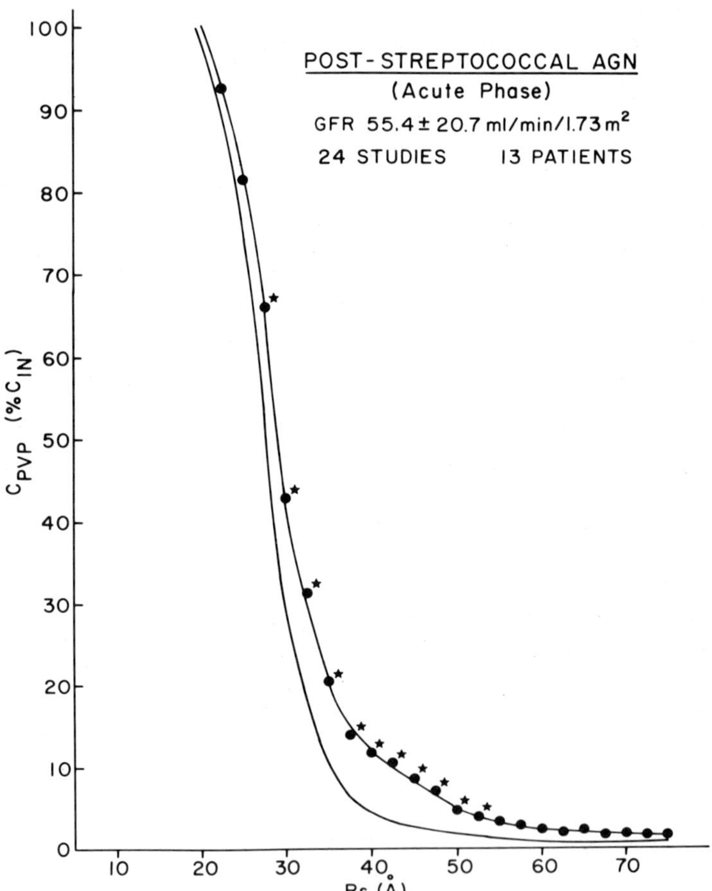

Figure 3. A summary of the 24 studies of permselectivity to PVP obtained from the 13 patients investigated during the acute phase of poststreptococcal acute glomerulonephritis (AGN). The individual points represent the mean values observed in the patients with PSAGN; the mean values from the normal subjects are shown as a solid line for comparison. Values in PSAGN which were significantly different from normal ($p < 0.05$) are marked with asterisks.

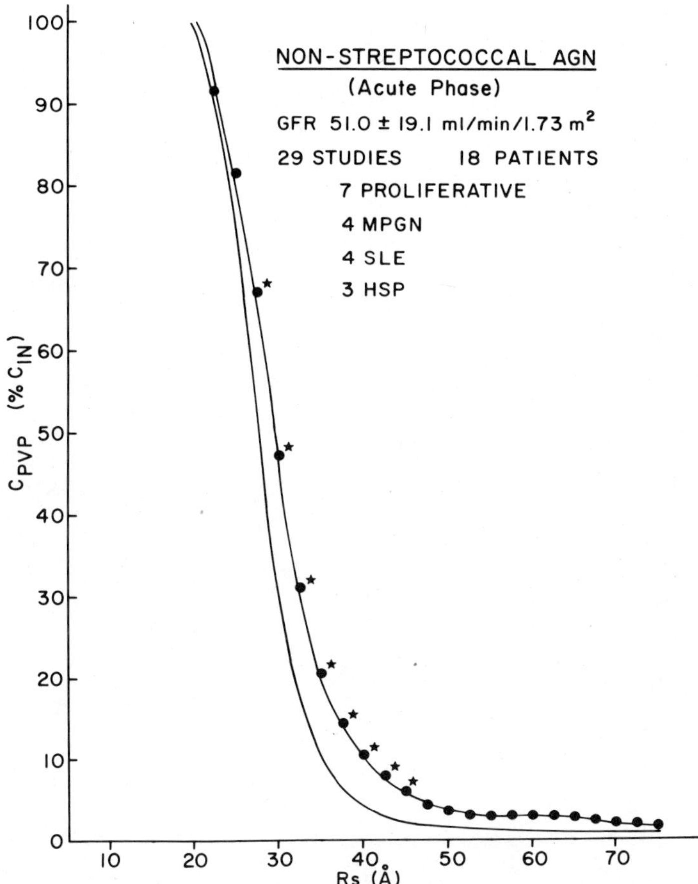

Figure 4. The influence of various forms of nonstreptococcal acute glomerulonephritis on the pattern of glomerular permselectivity. Patients with proliferative lesions and those with lesions secondary to membranoproliferative glomerulonephritis (MPGN), systemic lupus erythematosus (SLE), and Henoch–Schönlein purpura (HSP) were included in this part of the study.

The diagnosis of PSAGN was determined using criteria established previously (Alkjaersig *et al.*, 1976). Twenty-four studies were performed during the acute phase of the disease in 13 patients, each of whom had a marked reduction in GFR, the mean value being 55.4 ± 20.7 (S.D.) ml/min/1.73 m^2. The pattern of glomerular permselectivity in these patients was obviously abnormal (Fig. 3) with the curve being shifted to the right of normal as a result of statistically significant increases in the relative clearances of PVP molecules with Rs values ranging from 30 to 50 Å.

These changes in permselectivity were not unique to patients with PSAGN. Twenty-nine studies were performed in 18 children with various other forms of acute glomerulonephritis. These children also had marked reductions in GFR to a mean of 51.0 ± 19.1 ml/min/1.73 m^2. Patterns of permselectivity (Fig. 4) were modified in a manner comparable to that seen

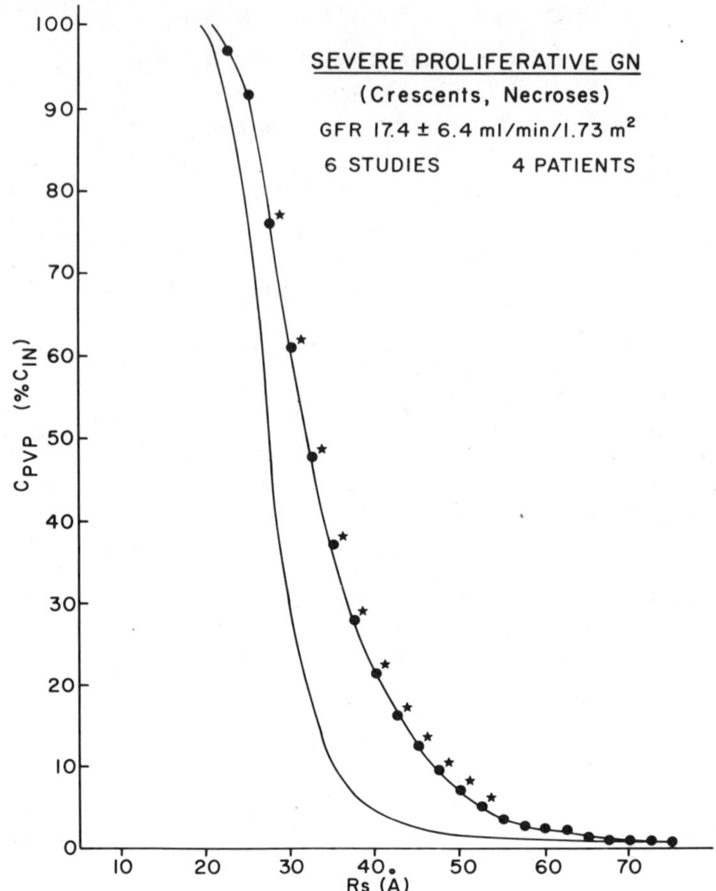

Figure 5. Pattern of glomerular permselectivity observed in four children with severe forms of glomerulonephritis. Values significantly different from normal ($p < 0.05$) are marked by asterisks. (See legends to Fig. 3 and 4 for more details.)

in PSAGN, indicating that this abnormal pattern of permselectivity was not unique to the poststreptococcal form of the disease. Indeed, when results from patients with each of the disease entities shown in Fig. 4 were analyzed separately, there were no significant differences in the results from one disease group as compared to any other.

Children with more severe glomerulonephritis had qualitatively similar but quantitatively more marked abnormalities in permselectivity. This is shown in Fig. 5 where results are summarized from four children, each of whom had glomerular crescents and glomerular necroses as well as proliferative changes on renal biopsy. The severity of the disease process in these children is illustrated by the magnitude of the reduction in GFR to a mean of only 17.4 ± 6.4 ml/min/1.73 m^2.

Even children with mild forms of glomerulonephritis had altered glomerular permselectivity (Fig. 6). Most of the 28 patients included in this part of the study presented with either hematuria and/or proteinuria. None were hypertensive or edematous, and all had glomerular filtration rates within normal limits, the mean value being 112.1 ± 15.5 ml/min/1.73 m^2. Despite the mild nature of the glomerulonephritis, permselectivity was abnormal and changes were present irrespective of the underlying renal pathology.

One further group of children that was studied comprised those who had severe glomerulonephritis complicated by a florid nephrotic syndrome. Of the seven patients in this group, five had a pathologic diagnosis of membranoproliferative glomerulonephritis and two of proliferative glomerulonephritis. Their values for GFR were reduced to only 23.4 ± 22.5 ml/min/1.73 m^2. Their pattern of permselectivity (Fig. 7) was different from that seen in any other group of children. They had greater increases in the relative clearances of the larger PVP molecules than seen in other children with glomerulonephritis. In addition, there were relative decreases in the clearances of the smaller PVP molecules. This change is similar to that seen

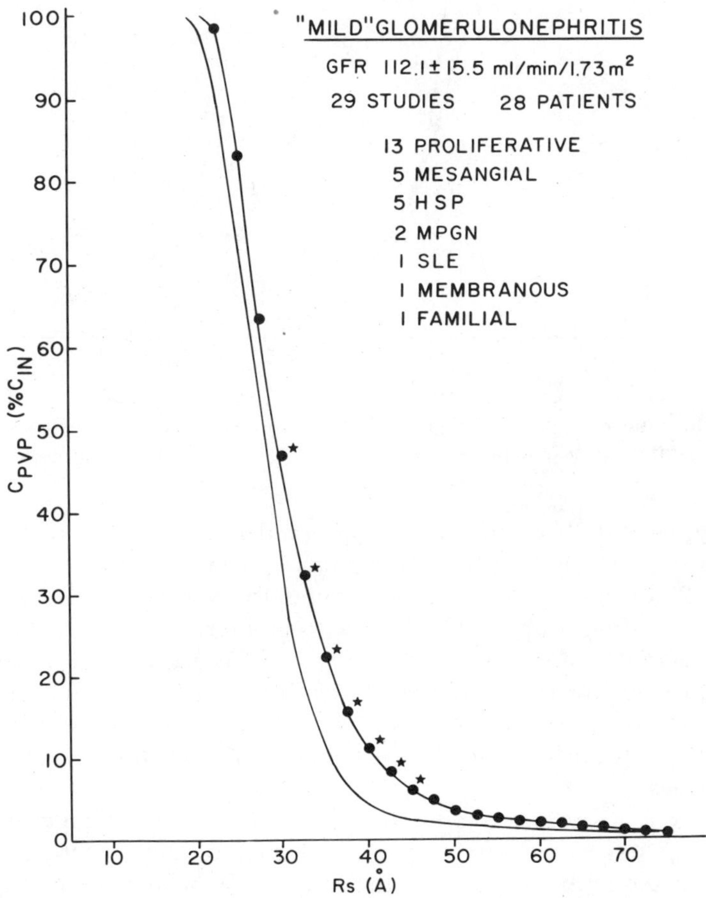

Figure 6. Influence of mild forms of glomerulonephritis on glomerular permselectivity. Values significantly different from normal ($p < 0.05$) shown by asterisks. (See legends to Fig. 3 and 4 for more details.)

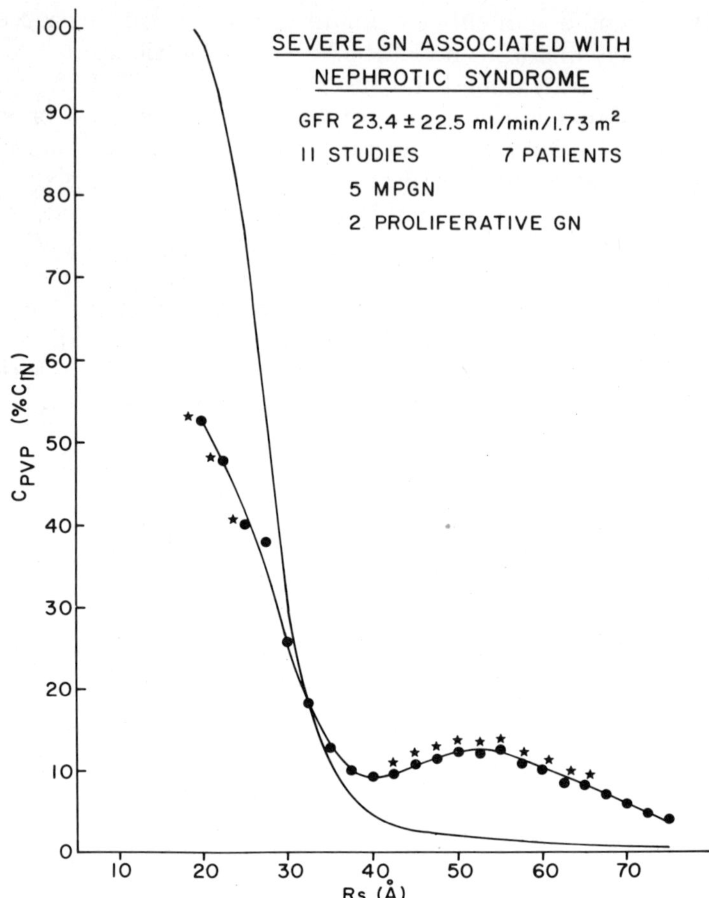

Figure 7. The pattern of glomerular permselectivity observed in patients with severe glomerulonephritis complicated by a nephrotic syndrome. (Details as summarized in Figs. 2, 3, and 4.)

in children with MCNS and was not observed in any patient with glomerulonephritis not complicated by an obvious nephrotic syndrome.

Table 2 compares the clearance values for selected molecular sizes of PVP in each of the groups of children with glomerulonephritis. It is obvious that in general the more severe the lesion and the greater the decrease in GFR, the greater are the increases in relative clearances of the larger PVP molecules. In the glomerulonephritic patients with a nephrotic syndrome, there also was a significant decrease in the relative clearance of the smaller PVP molecules.

From these observations in man, it would appear that changes in patterns of glomerular permselectivity occur irrespective of the underlying etiology of the glomerulonephritis and that the magnitude of these changes depends on the severity of the lesion. This thesis was tested by measuring glomerular permselectivity in rabbits with anti-basement membrane glomerulonephritis

(Germuth and Rodriguez, 1973). Animals with the least severe histologic lesions had well-preserved renal function and had nearly normal permselectivity (Fig. 8). Those with more severe lesions had filtration rates reduced to approximately 66% of normal and had marked increases in permselectivity. Animals with the most severe lesions had glomerular filtration rates reduced to a mean of 40% of normal, and had both increases in permselectivity to large-molecular-weight PVP and a decreased permselectivity to the smaller PVP molecules. This latter pattern is identical to that observed in patients with severe glomerulonephritis associated with the nephrotic syndrome.

Thus, the studies in animals support the concept that, in glomerulonephritis, it is the severity rather than the etiology of the renal lesion that determines the pattern of permselectivity. The one abnormal pattern of permselectivity that was not observed in the animals with anti-GBM glomerulonephritis was the one found in patients with MCNS. This pattern could be reproduced in animals by inducing a nephrotic syndrome with the aminonucleoside of puromycin (Buerkert *et al.*, 1976; Bohrer *et al.*, 1977).

3.4. Modification of Permselectivity by Treatment

As shown previously (Robson *et al.*, 1974a), the abnormal pattern of glomerular permselectivity observed in patients in relapse from MCNS will return to normal following a steroid-induced remission. Similarly, patterns of permselectivity may return to normal in many patients with glomerulonephritis even when the lesion is a severe one. This is illustrated in Fig. 9 which shows two studies obtained from a patient with severe proliferative, necrotizing glomerulonephritis. The first study, which was undertaken

Table 2. Comparison of Results from Normal Children and Those with Glomerulonephritis of Varying Severity

PVP size (Rs) (Å)	C_{PVP} (% C_{IN})				
		Patients with glomerulonephritis[a]			
	Normal subjects (n = 6)	Mild (n = 28)	Moderate (n = 31)	Severe (n = 4)	With NS[b] (n = 7)
55	1.5 ± 0.9[c]	2.5 ± 2.3	3.0 ± 2.5	3.6 ± 3.1	12.4 ± 7.8
p vs. normal		NS	NS	NS	< 0.02
45	2.2 ± 0.8	6.0 ± 5.3	7.3 ± 5.6	12.6 ± 6.8	10.7 ± 12.0
p vs. normal		< 0.05	< 0.01	< 0.001	< 0.05
35	10.2 ± 3.9	22.1 ± 17.9	20.5 ± 12.0	37.1 ± 8.7	12.8 ± 10.7
p vs. normal		< 0.02	< 0.01	< 0.001	NS
25	77.5 ± 13.9	83.1 ± 23.1	81.6 ± 18.8	91.6 ± 10.2	40.1 ± 23.9
p vs. normal		NS	NS	< 0.05	< 0.001
C_{IN} (ml/min/1.73 m^2)	121.0 ± 6.8	112.1 ± 15.5	53.0 ± 19.8	17.4 ± 6.4	23.4 ± 22.5

[a] Includes patients with poststreptococcal and other forms of acute glomerulonephritis (Heptinstall, 1974).
[b] Patients with severe glomerulonephritis and nephrotic syndrome.
[c] Mean ± S.D.

during the acute phase of the disease, showed marked abnormalities and a GFR reduced to 27.7 ml/min/1.73 m^2. The second study—performed 1 year later at a time when the patient's inulin clearance had returned to 104.0 ml/min/1.73 m^2, his urine was protein-free, and the urine sediment benign—was normal. In patients with glomerulonephritis, patterns of permselectivity usually remain abnormal until proteinuria has resolved. This was the case in the patient illustrated in Fig. 9.

3.5. *Prognostic Value of Measurements of Permselectivity*

As shown already, patterns of permselectivity may help to identify children with apparent MCNS who will not respond adequately to steroids

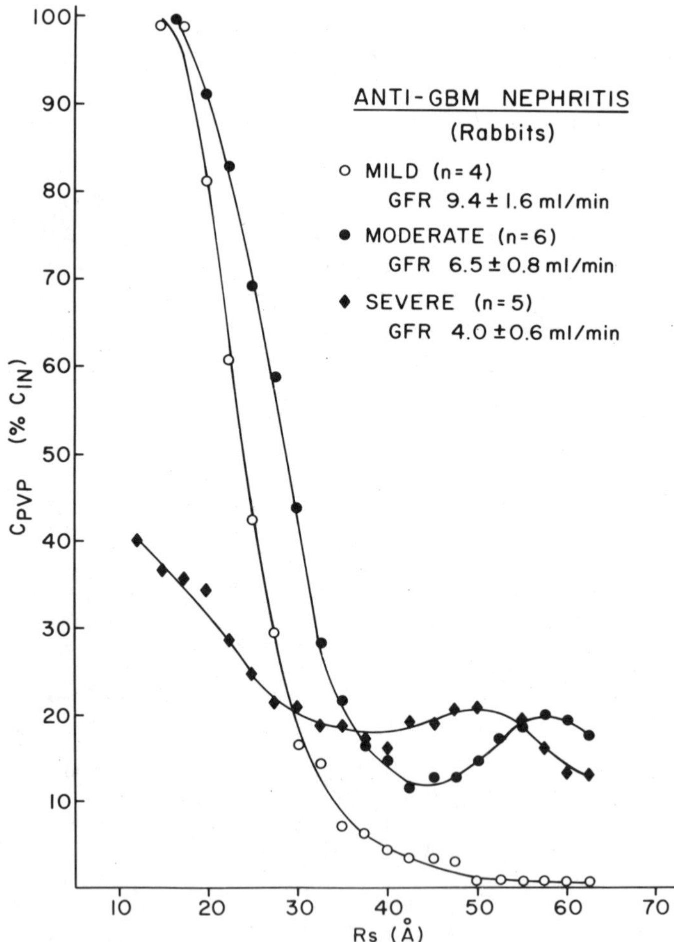

Figure 8. Glomerular permselectivity in rabbits with anti-GBM glomerulonephritis. Results are grouped according to the severity of the underlying lesion (determined from renal histology). The GFR values were determined from the clearance of inulin, and are shown as the mean ± S.D. n, number of animals studied.

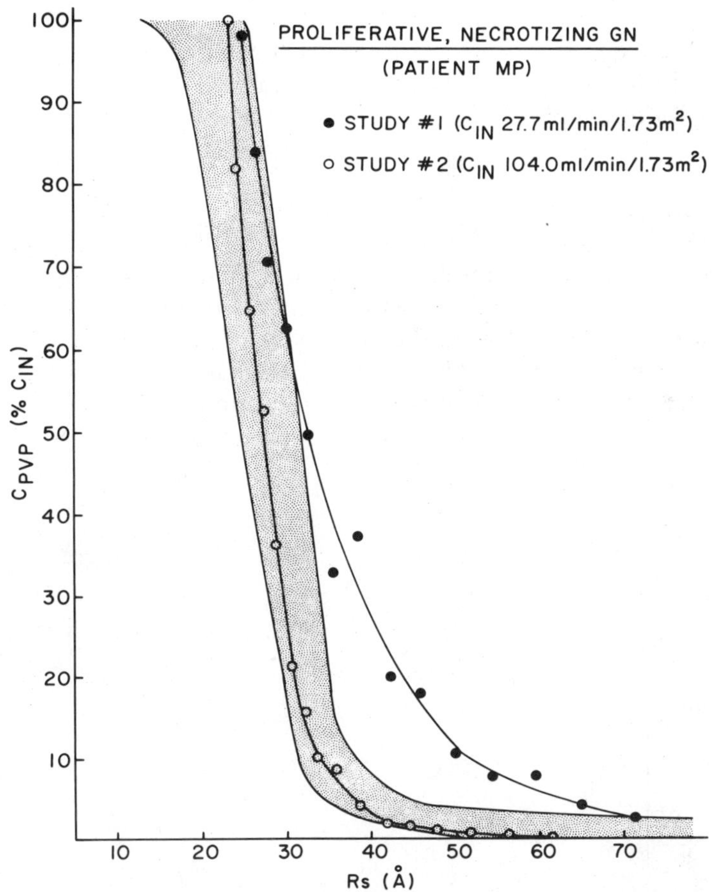

Figure 9. Two studies of glomerular permselectivity performed 1 year apart in a patient with severe glomerulonephritis characterized by glomerular proliferation and necrosis. In the first study, performed during the acute stage of the disease, the curve is abnormal, being shifted to the right of normal. With healing of the disease (second study), the curve has returned to the normal range depicted by the shaded area.

(Table 1). The prognostic value of permselectivity curves in patients with glomerulonephritis is less clear. In general, patients with the poorest prognosis are those who have both glomerulonephritis and the nephrotic syndrome with the abnormalities characteristic of this combination of clinical findings present on their permselectivity curves (Fig. 7). Improvement can occur in some of these patients and there may be concomitant improvement in the pattern of permselectivity, although the return of such a pattern to normal has not been seen. However, in animals with the most severe forms of anti-basement membrane glomerulonephritis and permselectivity characterized by increased relative clearances of larger PVP molecules and decreased clearances of the smaller molecules (Fig. 8), there may be both a return of GFR and of permselectivity to normal if the animals are treated with daily intravenous pulses of methylprednisolone (30 to 50 mg/kg body wt per pulse) for a week (Robson *et al.*, 1978). In contrast, animals treated with more conventional doses of steroids, or left untreated, rarely show comparable improvements in either renal function or in patterns of permselectivity (Robson *et al.*, 1978).

4. Discussion

Do the studies of permselectivity help gain an understanding of the pathophysiology of glomerular diseases? It has been observed that whenever there is extensive fusion of epithelial foot processes, there are decreased clearances of the smaller PVP molecules. This is illustrated in Fig. 10 which compares the patterns of permselectivity found in children with a nephrotic

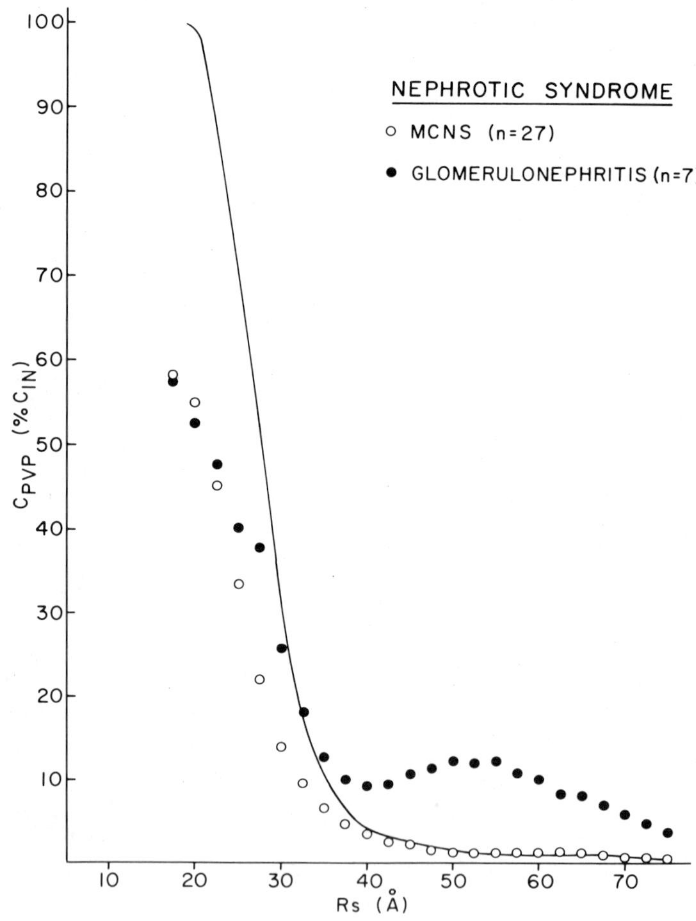

Figure 10. Comparison of the results obtained from patients with nephrotic syndrome secondary to either severe glomerulonephritis or to MCNS. The mean values observed in the normal subjects are depicted by the solid line.

syndrome secondary to either MCNS or to severe glomerulonephritis. Both groups of children had increased permselectivity to the smaller PVP molecules. In glomerulonephritis, this change was associated with increased clearances of larger PVP molecules, while in minimal change disease it was not. These observations in man are paralleled by those in animals with nephrotic syndrome secondary to either anti-basement membrane nephritis or to the administration of the aminonucleoside of puromycin.

These findings suggest that extensive fusion of epithelial foot processes per se results in significant alterations in the permeability characteristic of the glomerulus. Moreover, they provide evidence that there may be at least two mechanisms resulting in fusion of the epithelial cell foot processes. In both human and experimental forms of glomerulonephritis, it is suggested that the increased clearances of PVP molecules with Rs values of 35 Å and greater reflect a relative increase in permeability in the GBM to larger-molecular-weight compounds. This thesis is supported by previously published work which includes the observation that basement membranes from animals with experimental glomerulonephritis lose their normal ability to segregate molecules according to molecular size (Huang *et al.*, 1967). If the lesion is a severe one, resulting in major disruption of the GBM, it could cause an extensive leak of protein out of the glomerular capillary. In turn, this could result not only in proteinuria and the nephrotic syndrome, but also in loss of glomerular polyanion and fusion of epithelial foot processes. This mechanism would be similar to that of the experimental model of Vernier and his colleagues who demonstrated that such changes could be produced by the systemic infusion of protein in amounts sufficient to result in proteinuria (Vernier *et al.*, 1960; Roy *et al.*, 1972).

In human MCNS and in the animal counterpart of the disease, there is no demonstrable increase in permselectivity to PVP. If the arguments presented above are correct, then there must be an alternate mechanism for the loss of glomerular polyanion and fusion of epithelial foot processes characteristic of these disease states. Recent studies have suggested that cultured lymphocytes taken from patients with nephrotic syndrome release a protein into the culture medium and that this lymphokine modifies vascular permeability (Lagrue *et al.*, 1975). Although this observation remains to be confirmed (Trompeter *et al.*, 1978), such an agent could be toxic to the glomerular epithelial cells, causing loss of glomerular polyanion. Alternately, if this lymphokine is filtered across the glomerular barrier, it could result in the direct loss of charge on the glomerular sialoprotein. Indeed, an experimental model of this proposed mechanism is provided by the work of Seiler and colleagues who have shown that both loss of polyanion and podocyte fusion occur after perfusing the kidney with polycations such as protamine sulfate or poly-L-lysine (Seiler *et al.*, 1977). Subsequent studies from this laboratory have shown that these changes are associated with increased proteinuria (Root *et al.*, 1977).

Interpretations of these data may be too simplistic. Chang and his colleagues have demonstrated that when both convection and diffusion contribute to solute transport across the glomerulus, glomerular permselectivity is altered not only by changes in the glomerular ultrafiltration coefficient, but also by changes in any of the other primary determinants of glomerular filtration including capillary plasma flow rate, mean glomerular transcapillary hydraulic pressure, and initial glomerular capillary protein concentration (Chang *et al.*, 1975a,b). Changes in these determinants of filtration rate probably do not account for the altered patterns of permselectivity observed in our group of patients with renal disease. Changes in permselectivity cannot be correlated with alterations in the clearance of para-aminohippuric acid, with alterations in filtration fraction, with changes in arterial blood pressure, or with changes in plasma protein concentrations which were measured at the same time permselectivity was determined.

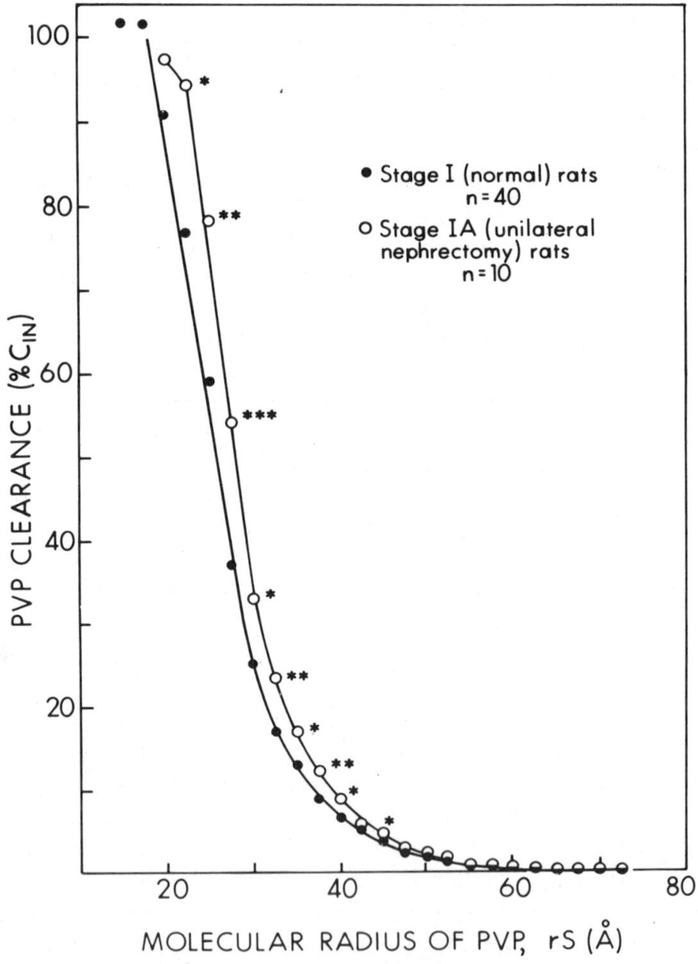

Figure 11. Glomerular permselectivity in normal rats and in those with unilateral nephrectomy. Statistically significant differences are shown as follows: $*p < 0.05$; $**p < 0.005$; $***p < 0.001$.

However, it is recognized that these are indirect measurements of the determinants of GFR and that they do not exclude entirely the possibility that such changes could play a role in the altered permselectivity seen in these patients.

Indeed, another mechanism which alters permselectivity has been observed. Figure 11 compares measurements of glomerular permselectivity in normal rats with those from unilaterally nephrectomized animals. It is obvious that the animals with reduced renal mass had significant increases in permselectivity. As detailed elsewhere (Robson *et al.*, 1974b, 1979), changes in the determinants of ultrafiltration do not explain this altered permselectivity. Another adaptive change which occurs in residual nephrons when nephron mass is reduced is probably responsible. Such a mechanism could contribute to the altered permselectivity observed in our patients with renal disease. These patients had decreases in total GFR and could well have had increases in GFR per nephron in the residual nephrons.

The present observations provide exciting new insights into how disease states modify normal glomerular permselectivity and how measurements of permselectivity could help in the management of patients with renal disease. However, more observations are required before the value of measuring glomerular permselectivity either as a clinical or as an investigational tool can be determined with certainty.

5. Summary

1. Relative increases in the clearances of PVP molecules with Rs values of 25 to 45 Å are seen both in patients and in experimental animals with glomerulonephritis or with immune complex deposition in the glomeruli. The magnitude of these changes is related to the severity of the underlying glomerulonephritis rather than to the disease process causing the glomerulonephritis.
2. Relative decreases in the clearances of PVP molecules with Rs values below 25 Å are seen whenever there is extensive fusion of glomerular epithelial cell foot processes. If this change is associated with glomerulonephritis, the clearances of the larger PVP molecules are increased.
3. From these observations it is suggested:
    a. That increases in permselectivity of larger PVP molecules indicate an increased permeability of the GBM.
    b. That extensive fusion of the epithelial foot processes results in major modification of the glomerular permeability characteristics.
    c. That extensive fusion of the epithelial foot processes probably occurs by at least two mechanisms. The first is an increased passage of proteins across a damaged GBM. The second may result from a direct effect on either the epithelial cells or on the glomerular sialoproteins causing loss of glomerular polyanion.

4. These observations do not permit a detailed assessment of the contributions of changes in the primary determinants of glomerular ultrafiltration or of loss of nephron mass, in generating the altered patterns of permselectivity.

5. Measurements of glomerular permselectivity may be of clinical value in the management of patients with renal disease. For example:

a. In patients with apparent MCNS, any relative increases in the clearances of large PVP molecules may be predictive of an incomplete response to steroids.
b. Measurements may help in determining a patient's prognosis. The association of markedly decreased clearances of smaller PVP molecules with markedly increased clearances of larger molecules often indicates a poor prognosis.
c. Abnormalities in the patterns of glomerular permselectivity do return to normal with resolution of the underlying disease process, providing a potential tool with which to assess adequacy of response to treatment.

ACKNOWLEDGMENTS. We would like to thank Drs. J. Ingelfinger, R. Kienstra, J. Giangiacomo, J. Mor, and E. Root for their help in performing some of the studies reported here; Dr. J. Kissane for his interpretations of the renal biopsies; Dr. F. Germuth, Jr., for his help with immunofluorescent and electron microscopic studies of the renal biopsies and for helping to produce rabbits with glomerulonephritis; B. Murray and L. Peterson for their technical assistance; and Wanda Shaul for her skilled assistance in preparing the manuscript.

References

Alkjaersig, N. K., Fletcher, A. P., Lewis, M. L., Cole, B. R., Ingelfinger, J. R., and Robson, A. M., 1976, Pathophysiological responses of the blood coagulation system in acute glomerulonephritis, *Kidney Int.* **10:**319.

Blau, E. B., and Haas, J. E., 1973, Glomerular sialic acid and proteinuria in human renal disease, *Lab. Invest.* **28:**477.

Bohrer, M. P., Baylis, C., Robertson, C. R., and Brenner, B. M., 1977, Mechanisms of the puromycin induced defects in the transglomerular passage of water and macromolecules, *J. Clin. Invest.* **60:**152.

Brenner, B. M., Hostetter, T. H., and Humes, H. D., 1978, Glomerular permselectivity: Barrier function based on discrimination of molecular size and charge, *Am. J. Physiol.* **234:**F455.

Buerkert, J. E., Mor, J., Murray, B. N., and Robson, A. M., 1976, Glomerular permeability in disease: A proposed role of the glomerular epithelial cell, *Abstr. Am. Soc. Nephrol.* **9:**69.

Cameron, J. S., and Blandford, G., 1966, The simple assessment of selectivity in heavy proteinuria, *Lancet* **2:**242.

Chang, R. L. S., Robertson, C. R., Deen, W. M., and Brenner, B. M., 1975a, Permselectivity of the glomerular capillary wall to macromolecules, *Biophys. J.* **15:**861.

Chang, R. L. S., Veki, I. F., Troy, J. L., Deen, W. M., Robertson, C. R., and Brenner, B. M., 1975b, Permselectivity of the glomerular capillary wall to macromolecules, *Biophys. J.* **15:**887.

Germuth, F. G., Jr., and Rodriguez, E., 1973, *Immunopathology of the Renal Glomerulus: Antibasement Membrane Glomerular Disease in Animals,* p. 181, Little, Brown, Boston.

Heptinstall, R. H., 1974, *Pathology of the Kidney,* 2nd ed., Little, Brown, Boston.

Huang, F., Hutton, L., and Kalant, N., 1967, Molecular sieving by glomerular basement membrane, *Nature (London)* **216:**87.

Hulme, B., and Hardwicke, J., 1968, Human glomerular permeability to macromolecules in health and disease, *Clin. Sci.* **34:**515.

Joachim, G. R., Cameron, J. S., Schwartz, M., and Becker, E. L., 1964, Selectivity of protein excretion in patients with the nephrotic syndrome, *J. Clin. Invest.* **43:**2332.

Lagrue, G., Xheneumont, S., Branellec, A., Hirbec, G., and Weil, B., 1975, A vascular permeability factor elaborated from lymphocytes. 1. Demonstration in patients with nephrotic syndrome, *Biomedicine* **23:**37.

Pesce, A. J., Gaizutix, M., and Pollack, V. E., 1970, Selectivity of proteinuria: An evaluation of the immunochemical and gel filtration techniques, *J. Lab. Clin. Med.* **75:**586.

Rennke, H. G., and Venkatachalam, M. A., 1977, Glomerular permeability: *In vivo* tracer studies with polyanionic and polycationic ferritins, *Kidney Int.* **11:**44.

Robson, A. M., Kissane, J. M., Manley, C. B., Jr., and Kahn, L. I., 1971, Renal biopsy: Its place in the management of renal disease, *Clin. Pediatr.* **10:**96.

Robson, A. M., Giangiacomo, J., Kienstra, R. A., Naqvi, S. T., and Ingelfinger, J. R., 1974a, Normal glomerular permeability and its modification by minimal change nephrotic syndrome, *J. Clin. Invest.* **54:**1190.

Robson, A. M., Jaeger, B. V., Ingelfinger, J. R., Kienstra, R. A., Mor, J., Shankel, S., and Bricker, N. S., 1974b, Modification of glomerular permeability characteristics following reduction in renal mass, *Abstr. Am. Soc. Nephrol.* **7:**75.

Robson, A. M., Giangiacomo, J., and Germuth, F. G., Jr., 1978, Efficacy of methylprednisolone pulses in the treatment of experimental glomerulonephritis, *Abstr. Am. Soc. Nephrol.* **11:**26A.

Robson, A. M., Mor, J., Root, E. R., Jager, B. V., Shankel, S. W., Ingelfinger, J. R., Kienstra, R. A., and Bricker, N. S., 1979, On the mechanism of proteinuria in non-glomerular renal disease, *Kidney Int.* **16:**416.

Root, E. R., Conley, S. B., and Robson, A. M., 1977, Effect of glomerular polyanion removal on proteinuria, *Pediatr. Res.* **11:**555 (abstract).

Roy, L. P., Vernier, R. L., and Michael, A., 1972, Effect of protein-load proteinuria on glomerular polyanion, *Proc. Soc. Exp. Biol. Med.* **141:**870.

Seiler, M. W., Rennke, H. G., and Venkatachalam, M. A., 1977, Pathogenesis of polycation-induced alterations ("fusion") of glomerular epithelium, *Lab. Invest.* **36:**48.

Trompeter, R. S., Barratt, T. M., and Layward, L., 1978, Vascular permeability factor and nephrotic syndrome, *Lancet* **2:**900.

Vernier, R. L., Papermaster, B. W., Olness, K., Binet, E., and Good, R. A., 1960, Morphologic studies of the mechanism of proteinuria, *Am. J. Dis. Child.* **100:**476.

8

Glomerular Mesangium: Introductory Remarks

Alfred F. Michael and Yigal Shvil

1. *Introduction*

The movement of macromolecules in the glomerulus has attracted great interest in recent years. The transport across the glomerular capillary is dependent upon the size of the molecule, electrostatic charge, and the hemodynamic determinants of glomerular filtration. Morphologic studies suggest that the glomerular basement membrane (GBM) and its epithelial coat act as a barrier which is partially dependent on fixed anionic sites as well as on the structure of the GBM. Macromolecular substances including immune complexes, aggregated proteins, and other materials also may move into and out of the glomerular mesangium. The demonstration of significant abnormalities in this site, in human renal disease indicates crucial involvement in pathologic states. These abnormalities include mesangial expansion and nodule formation in diabetic nephropathy; deposition of immunoproteins in a variety of forms of glomerulonephritis; and morphologic alterations of proliferation and increased matrix in many other diseases. This chapter also will serve as a general introduction to other studies which are discussed elsewhere in this volume. The role of the mesangium has been the subject of two recent reviews in which readers can find a more complete discussion (Michael *et al.*, 1979, 1980).

2. *Morphologic and Antigenic Relationships*

Although first recognized over 40 years ago (Zimmerman, 1933), a considerable period of time elapsed before electron microscopic studies

---

Alfred F. Michael · Department of Pediatrics, University of Minnesota Medical School, Minneapolis, Minnesota 55455. ***Yigal Shvil*** · Department of Pediatrics, Hadassah Hospital, Jerusalem, Israel.

demonstrated unequivocally that the mesangial region was separate and distinct from other parts of the glomerulus (Suzuki *et al.,* 1963; Latta *et al.,* 1960; Farquhar and Palade, 1962; Latta, 1973). The mesangial region is limited by the overlying endothelium which separates it from the capillary lumen and by the mesangial reflections of the basement membrane which separate it from the epithelium (Fig. 1). In a sense it is an intercellular space which is directly contiguous with the capillary lumen but without an interposed basement membrane. This is a rather unique site and differs from other interstitial regions of the body. The cells contain numerous organelles

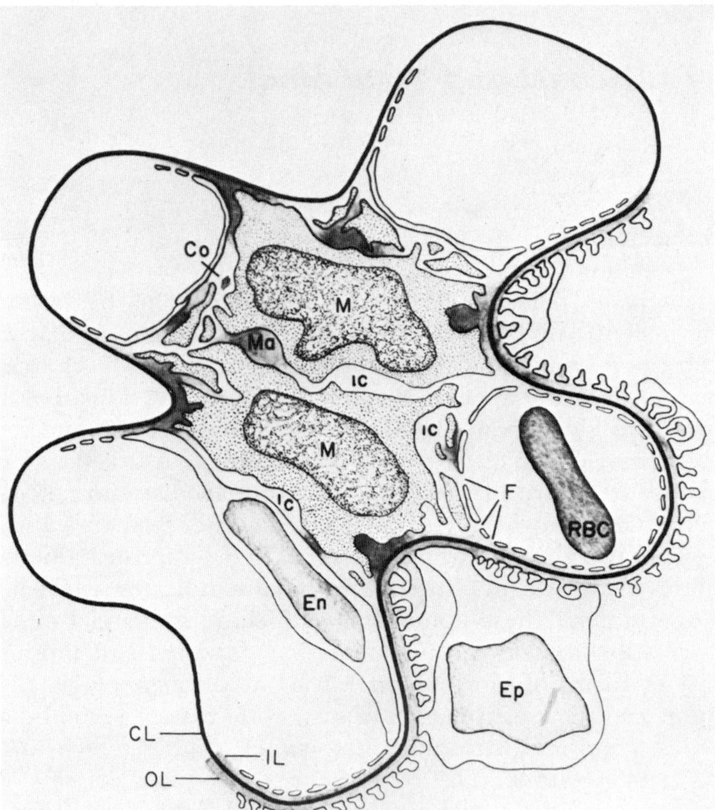

Figure 1. Diagram of a rat mesangial region surrounded by capillaries. The central layer (CL) of the basement membrane invests the capillaries like a sheet and also passes over the mesangial region. The capillary boundary of the mesangium is formed by the axial portions of endothelial cells (En). Mesangial cells (M) are partially surrounded by mesangial matrix (Ma), in which bundles of collagen (Co) can sometimes be found. Fenestrations (F) of the endothelium allow passage of particles and plasma into intercapillary and intercellular channels (IC). The thickness of the outer layer (OL) and inner layer (IL) of the basement membrane have been drawn thicker than they are to show their relationships to the adjacent cells. The central layer (lamina densa) is thin in the rabbit, mouse, and rat (as shown here) but much thicker in the monkey and human. Epithelial cell bodies (Ep) extend primary processes which branch to form the foot processes. The capillary diameter is usually somewhat greater than the diameter of a red blood cell (RBC). (Reprinted from Latta, 1973.)

including coarse microfilaments that are suggestive of smooth muscle cells. Immunohistochemical studies have clearly demonstrated the presence of myosin in this region (Becker, 1972; Scheinman *et al.*, 1974). A number of morphologic studies carried out by Latta and Maunsbach (1962a,b), Barajas and Latta (1963), and Barajas (1970) have demonstrated an intimate relationship between mesangial cells and components of the juxtaglomerular (JG) apparatus, the lacis cells and the epithelioid granulated cells of the afferent arteriole. The demonstration of gap junctions in mesangial and lacis cells indicates that an integrated contractile function may be one of the major functions of the mesangial cell although this has not been proven (Pricam *et al.*, 1974). This relationship to the JG zone, the presence of myosin, and prior evidence for contractility *in vitro* (Bernik, 1969) supports this hypothesis. It also suggests that the mesangium may be important in regulation of glomerular blood flow. The proximity to the JG zone may provide an exit for macromolecules from mesangial sites.

The mesangial matrix, located between mesangial cells, is of unknown composition and has an antigenic structure. While morphologic studies suggest that the matrix is some form of collagen, the precise type has not been defined. Although mesangial matrix has been called "basement membrane-like," and it may have some similarities to the basement membrane, there is no evidence that these two structures are identical. Antibody eluted from kidneys of patients with anti-GBM nephritis, reacts avidly with the endothelial part of the GBM but does not react with mesangial matrix. Fibronectin, which is a noncollagenous glycoprotein, also is identified in the mesangial zone by immunofluorescent techniques and is known to be a significant component of other connective tissue components (Scheinman *et al.*, 1978). Because of fibronectin's ability to bind to collagen, it has been proposed that this protein may play a role in the attachment of certain cells to connective tissue matrix (Stenman and Vaheri, 1978; Engvall *et al.*, 1978). Cyclic nucleotide (cyclic GMP) has been demonstrated in mesangial cells (Dousa *et al.*, 1977). Angiotensin II administered to animals has been shown to localize in the mesangium (Osborne *et al.*, 1975).

3. *Morphologic Tracer Studies*

A number of probes have been used to evaluate the mesangium (Michael *et al.*, 1979, 1980) (Table 1). Early classical studies by Farquhar and Palade (1962) and Latta *et al.* (1960) demonstrated mesangial localization of colloidal gold, thorotrast, and ferritin following their administration to animals. The probes which have been used are summarized in Table 1. Some of these macromolecules are present within mesangial channels and cells shortly after being administered to animals. Thereafter they are cleared gradually by mechanisms not well-defined yet. Since uptake by mesangial cells could be demonstrated, it was proposed that phagocytosis might be one mechanism by which the mesangium terminates these substances. Entry into the mes-

Table 1. Substances Taken Up by the Mesangium following Administration to Animals[a]

Probe	Molecular weight (radius or S)
Inorganic particles	
Colloidal carbon	(200–300 Å)
Thorium dioxide	(50–200 Å)
Colloidal gold	(20–100 Å)
Polysaccharides	
Iron-dextran	200,000 (37 × 220 Å)
Dextran	125,000 (78 Å); 250,000 (100 Å)
Polyvinyl alcohol polymer	35,000–240,000
Proteins	
Horseradish peroxidase	40,000 (30 Å)
Myeloperoxidase	160,000 (44 Å)
Catalase	240,000 (52 Å)
Ferritin	480,000 (61 Å)
Aggregated protein and complexes	
Aggregated globin	(250–1000 Å)
Aggregated human IgG	(18–600 S)
Aggregated human albumin	—
Antigen–antibody complexes	473,000 (11 S); > 473,000 (> 11 S)

[a] For references see Michael (1980).

angium was through endothelial fenestrae and the junctions between mesangial cells and endothelial cells, with movement into mesangial channels. The transport of carbon by way of the mesangial channels was much slower than that observed for other materials. Immune complexes in both human and experimental renal disease have been described extensively in a number of situations. Hence, it was reasonable to approach this study by use of preformed antigen–antibody complexes or aggregated proteins, such as aggregated IgG (AHIgG) and albumin (Michael *et al.*, 1979, 1980, AHIgG, which is a polydisperse population of macromolecules with sedimentation coefficients greater than 18 S, localizes in the mesangium. AHIgG achieves a peak within 2–4 hr following administration, following which is a gradual decrease in the amount present over the course of the succeeding 48 hr.

4. *Kinetic Studies of Mesangial Function*

Utilizing isotopic techniques (Michael *et al.*, 1967; Mauer *et al.*, 1972, 1974), it has been possible to carry out kinetic studies for evaluation of the uptake and disappearance of macromolecules from the mesangial zone. These studies used the administration of radiolabeled (^{125}I) AHIgG to rats. At varying periods of time, thereafter, the amount of ^{125}I present in isolated preparations of glomeruli was determined. These studies are based upon morphologic observations which demonstrate that aggregated proteins are present almost exclusively in the mesangial zone of glomeruli within 2–4 hr. Further, a prompt increase in the amount of aggregate present within the mesangial zone was demonstrated. The quantity is maximal within 2–4 hr following its administration to animals, and thereafter there is a gradual decrease in concentration over the subsequent 48 hr.

This uptake and egress of macromolecules into and out of the mesangium may be separated conveniently into afferent and efferent phases (Michael *et al.*, 1979, 1980), although it is apparent that no time line strictly separates one phase from the other. The highest concentrations of macromolecules are present within the mesangium in the initial period of time, a time when the blood level is relatively high. This time is called arbitrarily the afferent limb. During the subsequent period of time (efferent limb), there is a progressive decrease in the concentration within the glomerulus associated with relatively low blood levels.

5. Modulating Factors Affecting Afferent and Efferent Limb

5.1. Afferent Limb

There are a number of factors that are known to play an important role in the uptake of macromolecules by the mesangium (Michael *et al.*, 1979, 1980).

5.1.1. *Blood Level of the Macromolecule*

There is compelling evidence which shows that the level of the macromolecule in the blood is a major determinant of the amount that migrates into the mesangium. Evidence for this is derived from data demonstrating a dose relationship in mice and rats given aggregated proteins (Michael *et al.*, 1967, 1980; Mauer *et al.*, 1974) and a relationship to systemic mononuclear phagocytic function. The latter was demonstrated in studies in which antigen–antibody complexes (greater than 11 S) made with reduced and alkylated antibody persisted for longer periods of time in the circulation and at higher blood levels than immune complexes made with intact antibody. As a consequence, these showed greater localization in the mesangium (Haakenstad *et al.*, 1976) because of decreased hepatic uptake. Similar changes have been seen following the administration of antigen–antibody complexes or of aggregated proteins to cortisone-treated animals which have relatively higher blood levels secondary to impaired nonhepatic phagocytosis and to decreased extravascular loss of the protein.

5.1.2. *Characteristic of the Macromolecule*

As mentioned above, ultrastructural tracer studies using a variety of macromolecules of varying molecular weights have shown that these materials may be found in the mesangium following administration to animals. These findings suggest that plasma normally percolates through this zone probably under the influence of the hemodynamic factors that control glomerular filtration. Thus, the movement into and out of the mesangium does not appear to be an all-or-none phenomenon, although it is apparent on the basis of the morphologic studies described above, that certain molecules tend to become lodged in and persist in this site more than in others. For example, there is a striking difference in mesangial sequestration of monomeric IgG (7 S) as compared with AHIgG (greater than 18 S). This is apparent in the heightened uptake of AHIgG in animals with glomerular capillary injury (see below) as compared to the lack of an increase using 7 S. IgG. In addition, the time course for movement of certain molecules such as carbon is exceedingly slow with a maximal uptake at 32–36 hr, and with a persistence for weeks within the mesangium as compared to aggregated proteins in which maximal uptake is seen within 4 hr and complete disappearance by 48 hr. These findings suggest that large molecules become trapped within the mesangial channels whereas small molecules move through this zone with minimal impedance.

Studies relating the type of immune complex to localization within the glomerulus support the concept that the characteristics of the macromolecule are important determinants of its localization. In immune complex disease in animals, it has been demonstrated that poorly soluble complexes of intermediate size tend to localize within the mesangium in contrast to small or more soluble complexes which tend to become deposited in the peripheral capillary loop. Other studies have shown that passive administration of immune complexes made with antibody of high avidity or affinity localize in the mesangium in contrast to the peripheral capillary loop distribution of complexes made with low-affinity antibody (Germuth and Rodriquez, 1973; Germuth *et al.,* 1972; Cochrane and Koffler, 1973; Koyama *et al.,* 1978)

5.1.3. *Hemodynamic Factors*

It is probable that the hemodynamic factors that play a role in glomerular filtration also influence the uptake of macromolecules by the mesangium although relevant information is minimal. Studies in immune complex trapping by vascular structures have demonstrated a role for variables such as delivery rate, hydrostatic pressure, and ultrafiltration rate although, as mentioned previously, the blood level of the macromolecule appears to be a major determinant (Herbert *et al.,* 1978). The delivery of macromolecules to the glomerular capillary which is a function of concentration and of blood flow probably also plays an important role in the afferent mechanism. The precise role of other factors such as glomerular capillary pressure, tubular pressure, or oncotic pressure has not been explored. The movement of materials into the mesangial zone from the glomerular capillary suggests that pressure differences may exist between these sites.

5.1.4. *Characteristics of the Glomerular Capillary*

There is compelling evidence that damage to the integrity of the glomerular capillary has a very direct effect on mesangial kinetics. For example, the administration of aminonucleoside of puromycin or anti-GBM antibody to rats results in a striking increase to over 10-fold that of normal in the uptake of AHIgG by the mesangium. That efferent mechanisms appear to be intact in both of these models is suggested by the fact that the removal rate from the mesagnium is similar to that seen in normal animals. Changes occur very early after the administration of aminonucleoside or after relatively low doses of anti-GBM antibody, prior to the development of overt proteinuria. This suggests that gross nephrotic syndrome is not an essential feature of the altered kinetics. That these changes are not related to alterations in the systemic milieu has been demonstrated by the ability to alter the kinetics by perfusion of anti-GBM antibody or aminonucleoside into one kidney while the contralateral kidney remains perfectly normal (Hoyer *et al.,* 1975, 1976).

The mechanism of this heightened afferent limb is unknown. It may be a consequence of an alteration in glomerular capillary permeability or of the abrogation of the electronegative charge of the epithelium. Support for this concept is derived from studies carried out in autologous immune complex disease in rats in which loss of polyanion staining and increased mesangial uptake are not observed (Couser *et al.,* 1976; Schneeberger *et al.,* 1977). Thus, there may be a relationship between charge and mesangial traffic.

5.2. *Efferent Limb*

What is the route of macromolecules that have entered the mesangium?

5.2.1. *Stalk JG Traffic*

On the basis of morphologic studies, there is good evidence that a proportion of macromolecules entering the mesangium move down the stalk to the JG zone. This conclusion is drawn from studies which demonstrate the presence of aggregated proteins in the stalk and hilar region of the glomerulus at late times following administration to animals (Michael *et al.,* 1967); from studies using carbon in which over a period of weeks a gradual migration from peripheral mesangial zones via the stalk to the JG zone is demonstrated (Elema *et al.,* 1976); and from studies using iron dextran in which movement occurs down the stalk to the JG zone and along the inner aspect of the distal tubular basement membrane of cells opposite the lamina densa (Leiper *et al.,* 1977). The route that these molecules take thereafter is not known although it is possible that movement into the interstitium, lymphatics, and distal tubular cells occurs. There is no evidence for excretion in the urine at the site, although this has not been definitively excluded.

5.2.2. *Phagocytosis*

Early studies carried out with tracers such as ferritin demonstrated active uptake of the label by mesangial cells (Farquhar and Palade, 1962). Experiments have demonstrated little evidence for uptake of aggregated proteins or antigen–antibody complexes (Michael *et al.*, 1967; Striker *et al.*, 1979). The relative amount of the macromolecule taken up by the cell compared to that moving through the mesangial channels is unknown. Methodologic problems could be responsible for the failure to demonstrate uptake of aggregated proteins and of antigen–antibody complexes by mesangial cells. Therefore, this issue must remain open.

A number of studies have demonstrated clearly that monocytes may infiltrate the glomerulus, invade the mesangium, and contribute to the hypercellularity seen in pathologic states. There is no evidence at all that the mesangial cell is derived from a monocyte precursor. (1) Morphologic studies demonstrating monocytes within the glomerulus have demonstrated clearly that these are distinct from mesangial cells. (2) Studies in female human kidneys transplanted into male recipients demonstrate no cells within the mesangial zone containing Y-bodies although such cells may be seen in interstitial inflammatory infiltrates and crescents (Schiffer and Michael, 1978). (3) Studies in which kidneys from animals treated with *Habu* snake venom were transplanted into thymidine-injected recipients failed to demonstrate labeled proliferating glomerular cells. This suggested that these cells were a relatively stable population and that local proliferation was occurring (Bradfield *et al.*, 1977). It is apparent that inflammatory cells may infiltrate the glomerulus and in this site contribute actively to the phagocytosis of immune complexes that had been localized therein.

5.2.3. *Other Routes*

Although not proven by morphologic tracer studies, it is likely that regurgitation from the mesangial zone into the glomerular capillary may occur. Some evidence for this is deduced from studies carried out in animals with ureteral obstruction (see Chapter 9).

6. *Modulation of Mesangial Afferent and Efferent Limb*

As mentioned previously, modulation of uptake has been possible by raising the blood level of the circulating macromolecule by increasing the dose, or by interfering with uptake by the systemic mononuclear phagocytic system. In addition, a striking increase in uptake is observed in animals with anti-GBM nephritis and with aminonucleoside nephrosis. The mechanism of this has not been established clearly although it may be related to changes in glomerular capillary permeability secondary to alteration in the negative charge of the glomerular capillary.

Alteration in efferent kinetics has been demonstrated in animal models with unilateral or with bilateral ureteral occlusion which is described in greater detail elsewhere in this volume. Blockade, which is demonstrable at high circulating levels of AHIgG, is manifested by a plateau in the glomerular concentrations from 4 to 16 hr following administration to animals. This may be a consequence of interference with traffic through the mesangial stalk region although this remains to be proven. The fact that egress occurs even in the persistence of ureteral obstruction when the blood level becomes relatively low, suggests at least two mechanisms for loss of materials from the mesangium. One mechanism is evident at high blood levels of the circulating macromolecule and is impeded by ureteral occlusion. The other, which comes into play as the circulating level decreases, may be that of mesangial–capillary reflux. Alterations in the efferent limb also have been observed in animals with long-standing aminonucleoside nephrosis in which segmental and goobal sclerosis develops as a consequence of irreversible epithelial injury, polyanion loss, and glomerular capillary collapse. The normal mechanism for loss of AHIgG from the glomeruli of these animals is inhibited severely and may be a consequence of interference with the capillary–mesangial pathway for disposal of macromolecular substances (Glasser *et al.,* 1977; Velosa *et al.,* 1977). In this model as well as in humans with segmental sclerosis, subendothelial deposits are often present in the glomerulus and represent sequestration of immunoprotein and complement components in part. The demonstration of these materials in many different forms of glomerular hyalinization suggests that sclerosis leads to a disturbance in macromolecular traffic and accumulation of endogenous complex material (Velosa *et al.,* 1976).

7. *Conclusion*

The glomerular mesangium is a unique region containing cells and matrix material. It is located adjacent to the juxtaglomerular apparatus with which it probably has a close functional relationship. Morphologic and immunohistologic studies of the kidney in human disease have demonstrated prominent involvement of this region of the glomerulus in diseases such as diabetic nephropathy and in most forms of immune complex glomerulonephritis. Macromolecular substances enter the interstitial mesangial space without requiring to cross the capillary basement membrane. This uptake or afferent limb is dependent upon the level and characteristics of the circulating macromolecule, hemodynamic effects, and intrinsic characteristics of the glomerular capillary. The route for egress (efferent limb) from the mesangium includes JG–stalk migration, phagocytosis by resident mesangial cells and infiltrating inflammatory cells, and possibly regurgitation into the circulation. Modulation of uptake or disposal has been demonstrated in experimental models of renal disease—a striking increase in uptake after administration of anti-GBM antibody or aminonucleoside of puromycin and efferent blockade following ureteral obstruction.

References

Barajas, L., 1970, The ultrastructure of the juxtaglomerular apparatus as disclosed by three-dimensional reconstruction from serial sections, *J. Ultrastruct. Res.* **33:**116.

Barajas, L., and Latta, H., 1963, A three dimensional study of the juxtaglomerular apparatus in the rat, *Lab. Invest.* **12:**257.

Becker, C. G., 1972, Demonstration of actomyosin in mesangial cells of the renal glomerulus, *Am. J. Pathol.* **66:**97.

Bernik, M. B., 1969, Contractile activity of human glomeruli in culture, *Nephron* **6:**1.

Bradfield, J. W. B., Cattell, V., and Smith, J., 1977, The mesangial cell in glomerulonephritis. II. Mesangial proliferation caused by Habu snake venom in the rat, *Lab. Invest.* **36:**478.

Cochrane, C. G., and Koffler, D., 1974, Immune complex disease in experimental animals, in: *Advances in Immunology* (F. J. Dixon and H. G. Kunkel, eds.), pp. 185–264, Academic Press, New York.

Couser, W. G., Stilmant, M. M., and Darby, C., 1976, Autologous immune complex nephropathy. I. Sequential study of immune complex deposition ultrastructural changes, proteinuria and alterations in glomerular sialoprotein, *Lab. Invest.* **34:**23.

Dousa, T. P., Barnes, L. D., Ong, S. H., and Steiner, A. L., 1977, Immunohistochemical localization of 3′:5′-cyclic AMP and 3′:5′-cyclic GMP in rat renal cortex: Effect of parathyroid hormone, *Proc. Natl. Acad. Sci. USA* **74:**3569.

Elema, J. D., Hoyer, J., and Vernier, R. L., 1976, The glomerular mesangium: Uptake and transport of intravenously injected colloidal carbon in the rat, *Kidney Int.* **9:**395.

Engvall, E., Ruoslahti, E., and Miller, E., 1978, Affinity of fibronectin to collagens of different genetic types and to fibrinogen, *J. Exp. Med.* **147:**1584.

Farquhar, M. G., and Palade, G. E., 1962, Functional evidence for the existence of a third cell type in the renal glomerulus, *J. Cell Biol.* **13:**55.

Germuth, F. G. and Rodriguez, E., 1973, *Immunopathology of the Renal Glomerulus,* Little, Brown & Co., Boston, pp. 15–43.

Germuth, F. G., Jr., Senterfit, L. B., and Dreesman, G. R., 1972, Immune complex disease. V. The nature of the circulating complexes associated with glomerular alterations in the chronic BSA-rabbit system, *Johns Hopkins Med. J,* **130:**344.

Glasser, R. J., Velosa, J. A., and Michael, A. F., 1977, Experimental model of focal sclerosis. I. Relationship to protein excretion in aminonucleoside nephrosis, *Lab. Invest.* **36:**519.

Haakenstad, A. O., Striker, G. E., and Mannik, M., 1976, The glomerular deposition of soluble immune complexes prepared with reduced and alkylated antibodies and with intact antibodies in mice, *Lab. Invest.* **35:**293.

Hebert, L. A., Allhuser, C., and Koethe, S., 1978, Some hemodynamic determinants of immune complex trapping by the kidney, *Kidney Int.* **14:**452.

Hoyer, J. R., Mauer, S. M., and Michael, A. F., 1975, Unilateral renal disease in the rat. I. Clinical, morphologic and glomerular mesangial functional features of the experimental model produced by renal perfusion with aminonucleoside, *J. Lab. Clin. Med.* **85:**756.

Hoyer, J. R., Elema, J. D., and Vernier, R. L., 1976, Unilateral renal disease in the rat. II. Glomerular mesangial uptake of colloidal carbon in unilateral aminonucleoside nephrosis and nephrotoxic serum nephritis, *Lab. Invest.* **34:**250.

Koyama, A., Niwa, Y., Shigematsu, H., Taniguchi, M., and Tada, T., 1978, Studies on passive serum sickness. II. Factors determining the localization of antigen–antibody complexes in the murine renal glomerulus, *Lab. Invest.* **38:**253.

Latta, H., 1973, Ultrastructure of the glomerulus and juxtaglomerular apparatus, in: *Handbook of Physiology,* Section 8, *Renal Physiology* (S. R. Geiger, ed.), pp. 1–29, American Physiological Society, Washington, D.C.

Latta, H., and Maunsbach, A. B., 1962a, The juxtaglomerular apparatus as studied electron microscopically, *J. Ultrastruct. Res.* **6:**547.

Latta, H., and Maunsbach, A. B., 1962b, Relations of the centrolobular region of the glomerulus to the juxtaglomerular apparatus, *J. Ultrastruct. Res.* **6:**562.

Latta, H., Maunsbach, A. B., and Madden, S. C., 1960, The centrolobular region of the renal glomerulus studied by electron microscopy, *J. Ultrastruct. Res.* **4:**455.

Leiper, J. M., Thomson, D., and MacDonald, M. K., 1977, Uptake and transport of imposil by the glomerular mesangium in the mouse, *Lab. Invest.* **37:**526.

Mauer, S. M., Fish, A. J., Blau, E. B., and Michael, A. F., 1972, The glomerular mesangium. I. Kinetic studies of macromolecular uptake in normal and nephrotic rats, *J. Clin. Invest.* **51:**1092.

Mauer, M., Fish, A., Day, N., and Michael, A. F., 1974, The glomerular mesangium: II. Studies of macromolecular uptake in nephrotoxic nephritis in rats, *J. Clin. Invest.* **53:**431.

Michael, A. F., Fish, A. J., and Good, R. A., 1967, Glomerular localization and transport of aggregated protein in mice, *Lab Invest.* **17:**14.

Michael, A. F., Nevins, T. E., Raij, L., and Scheinman, J. I., Macromolecular transport in the glomerulus: Studies of the mesangium and epithelium *in vivo* and *in vitro,* in: *Contemporary Issues in Nephrology* (B. M. Brenner and J. H. Stein, eds.), Churchill Livingstone, Edinburgh.

Michael, A. F., Keane, W., Raij, L., Vernier, R. L., and Mauer, S. M., 1980, Editorial review of the glomerular mesangium, *Kidney Int.* **17:**141.

Osborne, M. J., Droz, B., Mayer, P., and Morel, F., 1975, Angiotensin II: Renal localization in glomerular mesangial cells by autoradiography, *Kidney Int.* **8:**245.

Pricam, C., Humbert, F., Perrelet, A., and Orci, L., 1974, Gap junctions in mesangial and lacis cells, *J. Cell Biol.* **63:**349.

Scheinman, J. I., Fish, A. J., and Michael, A. F., 1974, The immunohistopathology of glomerular antigens: The glomerular basement membrane, collagen and actomyosin antigens in normal and diseased kidneys, *J. Clin. Invest.* **54:**1144.

Scheinman, J. I., Fish, A. J., Matas, A. J., and Michael, A. F., 1978, The immunohistopathology of glomerular antigens. II. The glomerular basement membrane, actomyosin, and fibroblast surface antigens in normal, diseased and transplanted human kidneys, *Am. J. Pathol.* **90:**71.

Schiffer, M. S., and Michael, A. F., 1978, Renal cell turnover by Y-chromosome (Y-body) staining of the transplanted human kidney, *J. Lab. Clin. Med.* **92:**841.

Schneeberger, E, E., Collins, A. B., Latta, H., and McCluskey, R. T., 1977, Diminished glomerular accumulation of colloidal carbon in autologous immune complex nephritis, *Lab. Invest.* **37:**9.

Stenman, S., and Vaheri, A., 1978, Distribution of a major connective tissue protein, fibronectin, in normal human tissue, *J. Exp. Med.* **147:**1054.

Striker, G. E., Mannik, M., and Tung, M., 1979, Role of marrow-derived monocytes and mesangial cells in removal of immune complexes from renal glomeruli, *J. Exp. Med.* **149:**127.

Suzuki, Y., Churg, J., Grishman, E., Mautner, W., and Dachs, S., 1963, The mesangium of the renal glomerulus: Electron microscopic studies of pathologic alterations, *Am. J. Pathol.* **43:**555.

Velosa, J., Miller, K., and Michael, A. F., 1976, Immunopathology of the end-stage kidney: Immunoglobulin and complement component deposition in non-immune disease, *Am. J. Pathol.* **84:**149.

Velosa, J., Glasser, R. J., Nevins, T. E., and Michael, A. F., 1977, Experimental model of focal sclerosis. II. Correlation with immunopathologic changes, macromolecular kinetics and polyanion loss, *Lab. Invest.* **36:**527.

Zimmerman, K. W., 1933, Uber den bau des glomerulus der saugerniere: Weitare Mitteilunger, *Z. Mikrosk. Anat. Forsch.* **32:**176.

9

The Influence of Hemodynamic Factors upon Mesangial Kinetics of Macromolecules

L. Raij and W. Keane

1. Introduction

The mesangium is an important route for macromolecular traffic through the glomerulus (Farquhar and Palade, 1962; Michael *et al.*, 1979). In addition, the contiguity of the mesangium with the lacis cells of the juxtaglomerular zone and the presence of actomyocin (Becker, 1972; Scheinman *et al.*, 1974) suggest that this structure may play a role in the regulation of the glomerular microcirculation. By analogy, dynamic changes in the glomerular microcirculation may influence the macromolecular traffic through the mesangium.

The transglomerular passage of macromolecular proteins to the urinary space is dependent upon size, the hemodynamic determinants of glomerular filtration rate (GFR), and the electrostatic properties of the glomerular capillary wall (Fig. 1) (Brenner *et al.*, 1978). Whether these factors also have an influence upon the mesangial uptake (afferent limb) and egress (efferent limb) of macromolecular proteins is unknown. In particular, it is not known if hemodynamic factors have an influence in modulating mesangial uptake and release of macromolecules.

Previous studies demonstrated that following the intravenous administration of radiolabeled aggregated human IgG (AHIgG^{125}I), a polydispersed macromolecular protein with properties similar to antigen–antibody complexes, mesangial kinetics can be studied (Mauer *et al.*, 1972). With this technique, the concentration of AHIgG^{125}I is determined in preparations of isolated glomeruli obtained from rats sacrificed at different time intervals

L. Raij and W. Keane · Department of Medicine, University of Minnesota Medical School, Minneapolis, Minnesota 55455.

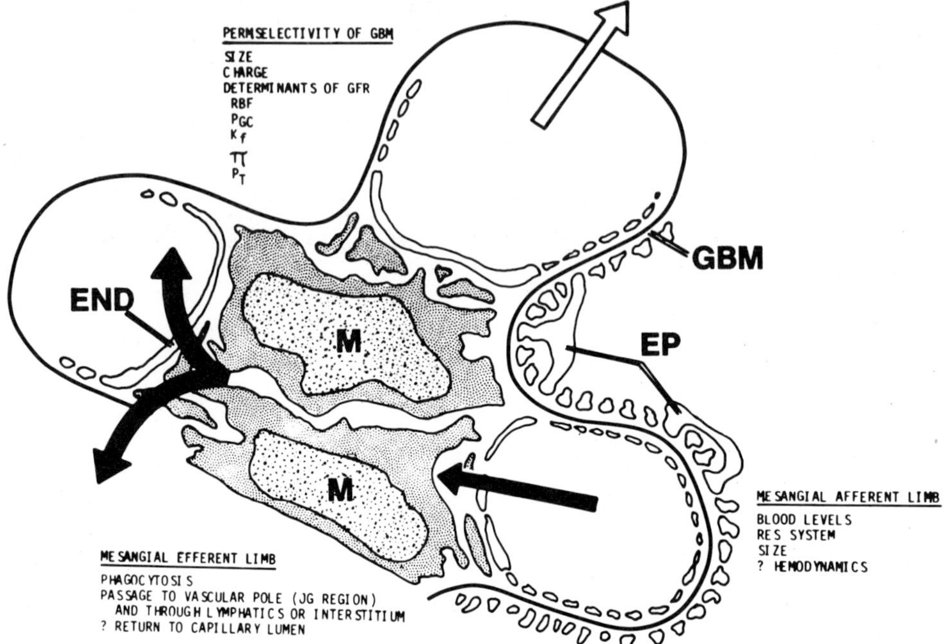

Chapter 9

Figure 1. Schematic representation of the factors that control the passage of macromolecules through the glomerular basement membrane and the mesangium.

after AHIgG^{125}I administration. This experimental design is based upon morphologic studies that demonstrated the presence of IgG exclusively in the mesangium within 2–4 hr (Michael *et al.*, 1967). In normal rats, after the administration of AHIgG^{125}I, there is prompt mesangial uptake followed by a linear fall in concentration that parallels that observed in blood, liver, and spleen (Mauer *et al.*, 1972).

These techniques were applied to the study of mesangial kinetics in normal animals and in animals with selective alterations in renal hemodynamic factors (Fig. 2).

2. Methods

Rats, 200 g, were injected with AHIgG^{125}I, 45 mg/100 g body wt. Radiolabeled aggregated IgG was prepared as described previously (Mauer *et al.*, 1972). The animals were killed at 4, 8, 16, and 24 hr following the administration of AHIgG^{125}I. Blood samples were obtained when the animals were killed and the amount of circulating aggregated IgG $>$ 7 S was determined by sucrose gradients. AHIgG^{125}I was then quantitated in preparations of isolated glomeruli as well as in spleen and liver. In some experiments, semiquantitative immunofluorescence studies were performed on tissue obtained at the time the animals were killed in order to correlate these with the uptake of AHIgG^{125}I in preparations of isolated glomeruli.

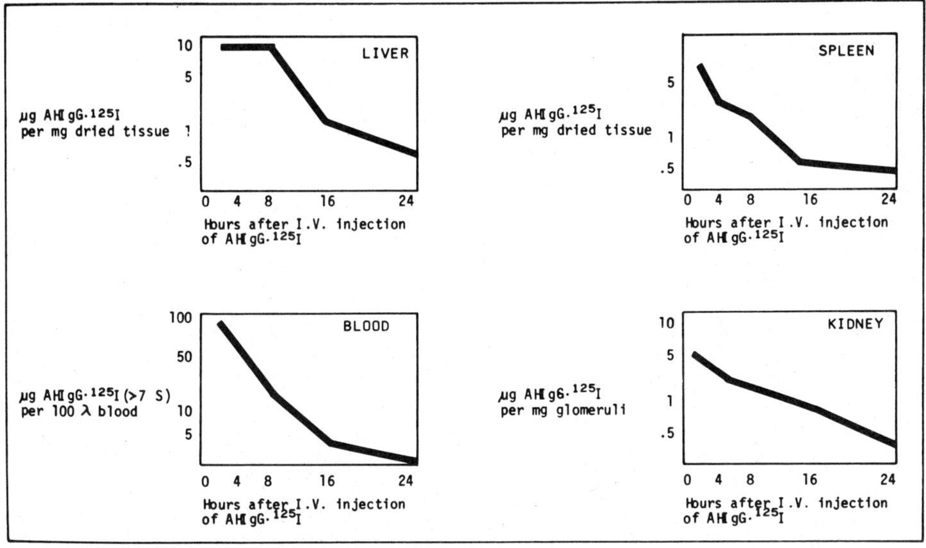

Figure 2. The concentration of AHIgG^{125}I in blood, liver, spleen, and glomeruli of normal rats sacrificed at 4, 8, 16, and 24 hr following intravenous injection of 45 mg AHIgG^{125}I/100 g body wt.

In addition, immunofluorescence microscopy was used to establish the uniformity of mesangial uptake in cortical and in juxtamedullary glomeruli.

To study the effect of blood flow alterations, the aorta was constricted with a ligature placed between the origins of the right and left renal arteries (Fig. 3). The technique utilized was such that the renal blood flow (RBF) to

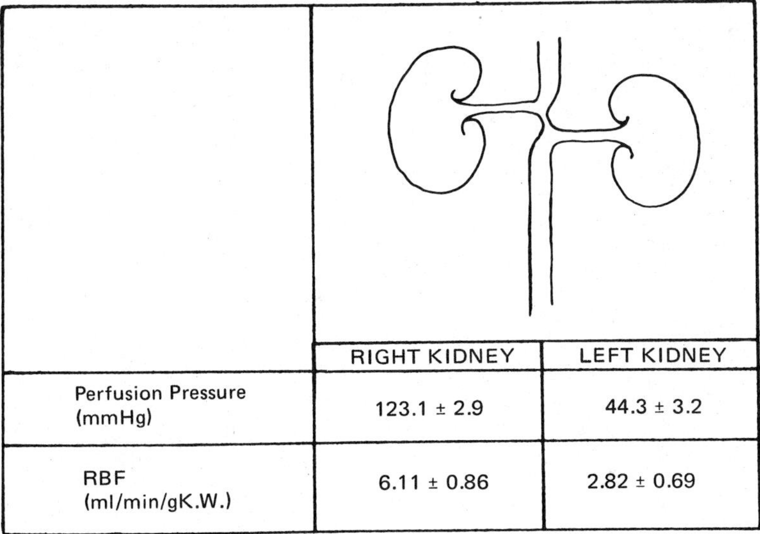

	RIGHT KIDNEY	LEFT KIDNEY
Perfusion Pressure (mmHg)	123.1 ± 2.9	44.3 ± 3.2
RBF (ml/min/gK.W.)	6.11 ± 0.86	2.82 ± 0.69

Figure 3. Renal hemodynamic changes induced by the placement of an aortic ligature between the origin of the right and left renal arteries.

the left kidney was reduced to approximately 50% of control while the mean aortic pressure below the constriction was 45 mm Hg. RBF and perfusion pressure to the right kidney were normal. The animals were injected with AHIgG^{125}I according to the general protocol described above. The animals were sacrificed at the different time intervals and blood, spleen, liver, and glomerular concentration of AHIgG^{125}I determined.

3. Results

3.1. Influence of Reduced Renal Blood Flow and Perfusion Pressure on Mesangial Uptake and Release of Macromolecules

Blood levels of AHIgG^{125}I > 7 S in animals with aortic constriction were not different from those of sham-operated animals (Fig. 4). Also, there were no differences in spleen and liver uptake of AHIgG^{125}I.

Mesangial kinetics in the right, normal kidney of animals with aortic constriction was the same as that observed in kidneys of sham-operated animals (Fig. 5). However, mesangial uptake in the left kidneys of animals with aortic constriction was decreased by 50%, which corresponded with the reduction (50%) in RBF. The AHIgG^{125}I disappearance rate from the mesangium of the left kidneys of rats with aortic constriction was not different from control and contralateral kidneys since they had similar negative slopes (Fig. 5). Hence, in the normal kidney, a reduction in RBF and perfusion pressure induces a decrease in mesangial uptake (afferent limb), but has no effect on the efferent limb.

3.2. Effects of Ureteral Obstruction upon Mesangial Kinetics of Macromolecules

The influence of hemodynamic factors upon mesangial function was also studied in animals with unilateral ureteral ligation (UUL) and in animals

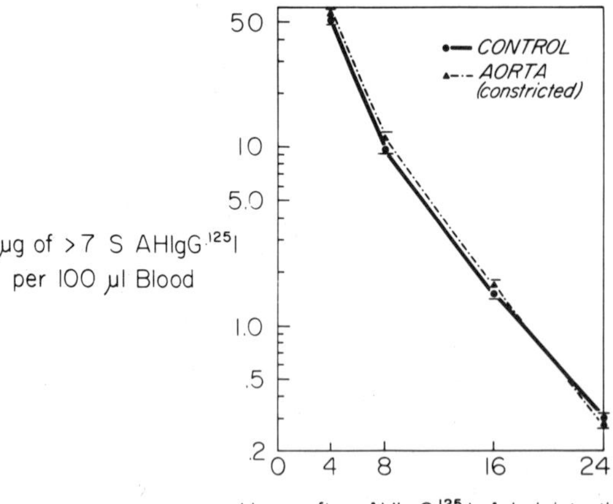

Figure 4. The blood concentration of AHIgG^{125}I > 7 S in control animals and animals with aortic constriction. Each point represents the mean ± S.E.M. obtained from five animals in each group at the time intervals noted.

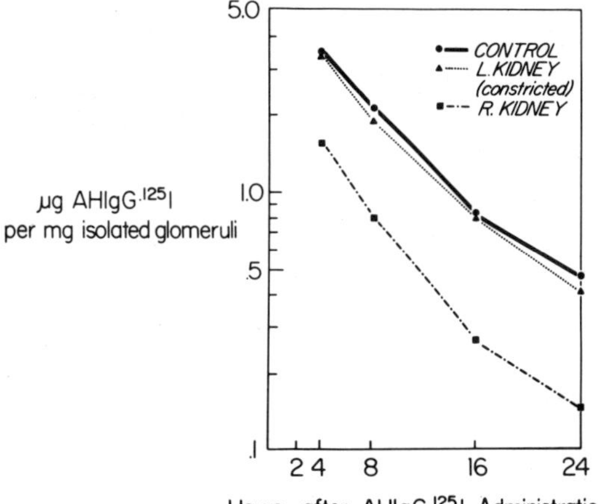

Figure 5. The concentration of AHIgG^{125}I in preparations of isolated glomeruli from control animals and animals with aortic constriction. Each point represents the concentration of AHIgG^{125}I in glomeruli from five kidneys in each group at the time intervals noted.

with bilateral ureteral ligation (BUL) followed by unilateral release (Raij *et al.*, 1972). After 24 hr of ureteral obstruction, important alterations in RBF and in GFR occur (Fig. 6). RBF is within normal limits in the contralateral kidney (control) of UUL animals; reduced 50% in the unreleased BUL and UUL kidneys; and reduced 20% in the released BUL kidney. The GFR is within control values in the contralateral kidney of UUL animals, but it is reduced by 80% in the released BUL kidney. Further, the unreleased UUL and BUL kidneys are nonfiltering.

After ureteral obstruction, AHIgG^{125}I was given to rats with either unilateral or bilateral ureteral obstruction, according to the experimental protocol described above.

	CONTROL (n=6)	BUL (n=6)		UU L (n=6)	
RBF (ml/min/100g BW)	2.84 ± 0.03	1.73 ± 0.11	2.44 ± 0.11	3.02 ± 0.04	1.47 ± 0.66
Cl_{IN} (ml/min/100g BW) per kidney	0.48 ± 0.02	-	0.11 ± 0.02	0.48 ± 0.05	-
BUN (mg/dl)	23.71 ± 0.21	184 ± 10.6		27.46 ± 0.05	

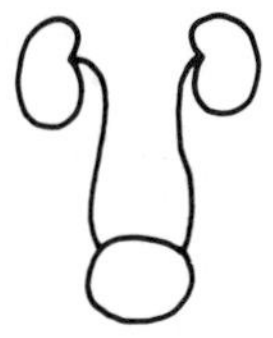

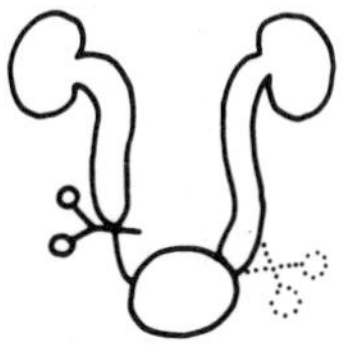

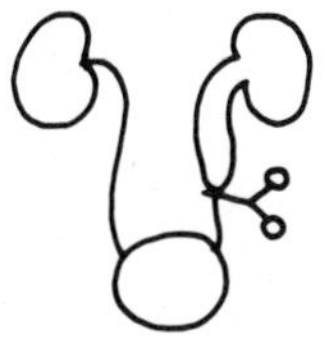

Figure 6. Renal hemodynamic changes in animals with unilateral and bilateral ureteral ligation of 24-hr duration.

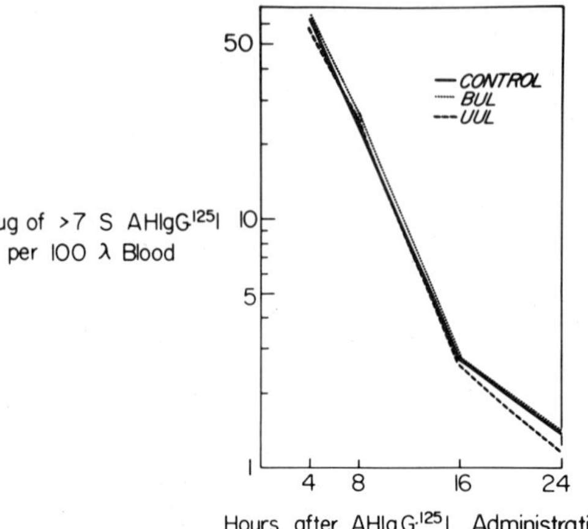

Figure 7. Blood concentration of AHIgG^{125}I > 7 S in control animals and animals with unilateral and bilateral ureteral ligation. Each point represents the mean ± S.E.M. obtained from five animals in each group at the time intervals noted.

There were no differences in the maximum levels nor the falloff curves of AHIgG^{125}I in the blood of either the control animals or the animals with unilateral or bilateral ureteral ligation (Fig. 7). Uptake of AHIgG^{125}I in glomeruli of control animals and in the normal nonobstructed kidneys of UUL animals was the same (Fig. 8). A linear logarithmic decrease in concentration of AHIgG^{125}I over a period of 24 hr was observed. However, the kinetics of AHIgG^{125}I in the mesangium of obstructed kidneys was different from that of the normal and also between themselves. (1) In BUL kidneys (released or unreleased) mesangial concentration of AHIgG^{125}I from 4 to 16 hr was approximately 10-fold the concentration found in UUL kidneys. (2) The significant decrease in concentration between 4 and 16 hr observed in control and in nonobstructed kidneys was not observed in UUL and BUL kidneys (released or unreleased). In all obstructed kidneys, a

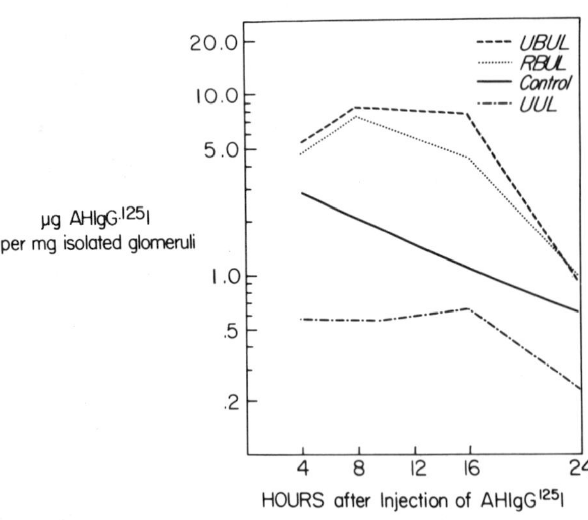

Figure 8. The concentration of AHIgG^{125}I in glomeruli from control kidneys and kidneys with ureteral obstruction. Each point represents the concentration in glomeruli from five kidneys in each group at the time intervals noted. The control values of AHIgG^{125}I were obtained from sham-operated animals and did not differ from the concentrations in the nonobstructed (normal) kidneys of the UUL. UBUL, unreleased kidney of animals with bilateral ureteral ligation; RBUL, released kidney of animals with bilateral ureteral ligation; UUL, unreleased kidneys of animals with unilateral ureteral ligation. (Modified from Raij *et al.*, 1979.)

plateau in glomerular concentration of AHIgG^{125}I was observed between 4 and 16 hr. (3) After 16 hr, a time when the blood level of AHIgG^{125}I had decreased to 3% of initial values, there was a decrease in glomerular AHIgG^{125}I. These studies showed that ureteral occlusion induced a blockade in the transport of AHIgG^{125}I out of the mesangium (efferent limb) that was primarily demonstrable at high blood levels of AHIgG^{125}I. However, during the period 16–24 hr, a significant decrease in mesangial concentration occurred in association with blood levels that were less than 3% of initial values. These observations suggest at least two mechanisms for disposal of macromolecules from the mesangium: one which is nullified by ureteral obstruction and is detectable at high levels of circulating AHIgG^{125}I, and another which is not affected by ureteral occlusion and is evident at low blood AHIgG^{125}I concentration. One possible mechanism to explain these observations is that ureteral obstruction impairs the passage of macromolecules through the glomerular stalk into the interstitium. When blood levels of AHIgG^{125}I are high, mesangial concentration does not change, probably because of a dynamic equilibrium between the circulating and the mesangial pools of AHIgG. When blood AHIgG^{125}I decreased to the low 16- to 24-hr levels, this equilibrium is offset and, in spite of ureteral obstruction, mesangial egress occurs. The disappearance of aggregates in the 16–24 hr period may be a consequence of their regurgitation into the circulation by way of the mesangial area of the glomerular capillaries. In addition, it appears that the mesangial capacity to accommodate and to retain macromolecules is different in these two models of ureteral obstruction. As compared to the controls, it is increased in BUL and is decreased in UUL kidneys.

These studies conclusively show that intrarenal dynamic factors can influence mesangial uptake (afferent limb) and egress (efferent limb) of macromolecules. The possibility that these changes may be mediated by the retention or increased production of vasoactive materials cannot be excluded. In that respect, increased production of prostaglandin E_2 and thromboxane A_2 have been shown experimentally in hydronephrotic kidneys (Morrison *et al.*, 1978; Nishikawa *et al.*, 1977).

3.3. Mesangial Kinetics of Macromolecules in Mercury Chloride Acute Renal Failure

The pathophysiology of acute renal failure (ARF) continues to be unclear. In most experimental models, as well as in human ARF, the relative contribution of glomerular and/or tubular factors to the reduction in renal function has remained controversial (Stein *et al.*, 1978). A functional assessment of the mesangium, an intraglomerular structure that may play a role in the glomerular microcirculation, can contribute to the understanding of the factors that participate in the pathogenesis of ARF. Following the administration of $HgCl_2$, 4.7 mg/kg body wt, rats develop a consistent pattern of ARF (Flamenbaum *et al.*, 1974). Physiologically, ARF is characterized by a marked reduction in whole kidney glomerular filtration rate (WKGFR) as

Table 1. Physiologic Data in $HgCl_2$ ARF

	Control	ARF	*p* value
BUN (mg/dl)	22.4	139.6	< 0.001
RBF (ml/min/g kidney wt)	6.3 ± 0.7	6.0 ± 0.2	NS
GFR (ml/min/100 g body wt)	1.14 ± 0.11	0.046 ± 0.06	< 0.001
SNGFR (ml/min)	39.7 ± 2.2	43.9 ± 3.5	NS
P_t[a] (mm Hg)	13.3 ± 0.7	17.6 ± 1.1	< 0.01

[a] P_t, pressures in the early part of proximal tubules.

determined by inulin clearance, normal RBF and a normal single nephron glomerular filtration rate (SNGFR), as determined by micropuncture techniques (Table 1). Morphologically, the glomerular architecture is normal but there is uniform necrosis of the proximal tubular epithelial cells.

In the light of these morphologic changes, investigators have proposed various hypotheses to explain the discrepancies between WKGFR, SNGFR, and RBF, and their respective contribution to renal insufficiency (Stein *et al.,* 1978). These explanations include: (1) marked nephron heterogeneity with a few nephrons functioning normally and the majority of nephrons showing minimal or absent function; (2) normal formation of glomerular filtrate with backdiffusion through damaged tubules; (3) marked tubular obstruction secondary to presence of cellular debris in the tubular lumen. This obstruction could coexist with backdiffusion of glomerular filtrate. However, the functional importance of tubular obstruction has been difficult to evaluate because of the possibility of venting the obstructed tubules during insertion of the micropuncture pipet. The study of mesangial kinetics in $HgCl_2$ ARF would be important in order to resolve the following issues: (1) if the mesangium, usually inaccessible to micropuncture, is functionally affected in this model of ARF; (2) if there is heterogeneity in mesangial AHIgG uptake and release as determined by semiquantitative immunofluorescence microscopy; (3) if tubular obstruction is the main mechanism

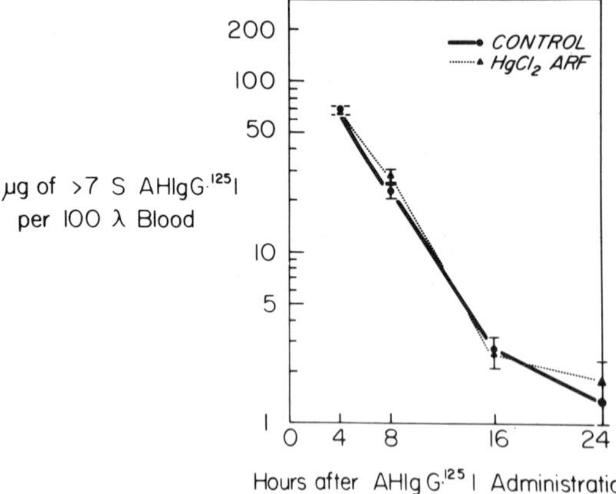

Figure 9. The blood concentration of AHIgG125I > 7 S in control animals and animals with $HgCl_2$ acute renal failure (ARF). Each point represents the mean ± S.E.M. from five animals in each group at the time intervals noted.

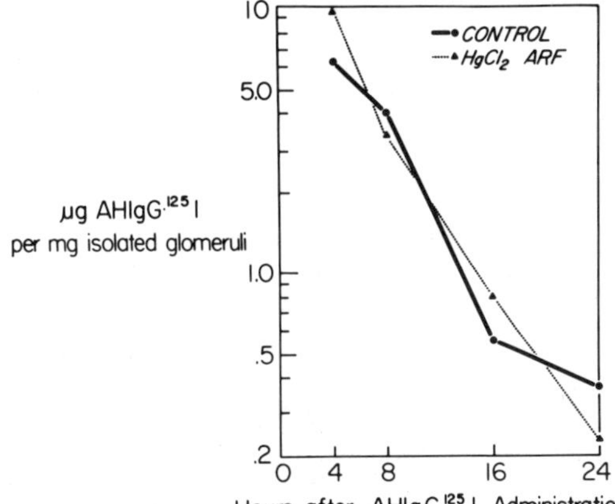

Figure 10. The concentration of AHIgG125I in preparations of isolated glomeruli from control animals and animals with $HgCl_2$ acute renal failure (ARF). Each point represents the concentration in glomeruli from 10 kidneys in each group at the time intervals noted.

operative in this model of ARF, a blockade of the mesangial efferent limb should become evident (see Section 3.2). On the other hand, if the main mechanisms of the reduced WKGFR is significant backdiffusion of glomerular filtrate, mesangial kinetics should be normal.

Following the intravenous administration of $AHIgG^{125}I$ to animals with $HgCl_2$ ARF, blood levels of > 7 S were not different from control animals (Fig. 9). Also, liver and spleen uptake of $AHIgG^{125}I$ were similar in control and in ARF animals. Mesangial uptake and release of macromolecules were similar in ARF animals and in control animals (Fig. 10). Thus, the mesangium functions normally in this model of ARF. Semiquantitative immunofluorescence microscopy did not reveal glomerular mesangial heterogeneity. Hence, in this model of nephrotoxic ARF, the studies of mesangial kinetics are supportive of the estimates of glomerular function determined by micropuncture techniques and would indicate that tubular obstruction is not an important component of this model.

4. *Conclusions*

In summary, based on the studies herein described, the following conclusions can be drawn. (1) In normal kidneys, reduction in RBF and in perfusion pressure leads to a decrease in mesangial uptake (afferent limb) but does not interfere with the mesangial disappearance of aggregates (efferent limb). (2) In $HgCl_2$ ARF, WKGFR rate is markedly decreased but SNGFR is normal. The mesangium functions normally in this model. Studies of mesangial kinetics in this model of ARF are in agreement with estimates of glomerular function obtained using micropuncture techniques. (3) Impaired disposal of aggregates through the mesangial efferent limb is the hallmark of altered mesangial kinetics in ureteral obstruction. (4) The observed changes in mesangial $AHIgG^{125}I$ kinetics in BUL and UUL are not related directly to changes in RBF (delivery rate of $AHIgG^{125}I$) or to

GFR. (5) The marked increase in mesangial AHIgG^{125}I observed in BUL may reflect changes in mesangial afferent limb and/or mesangial capacity. (6) Alteration in mesangial kinetics in ureteral obstruction appears to be related to intraglomerular or to interstitial factors.

References

Becker, C. G., 1972, Demonstration of actomyocin in mesangial cells of the renal glomerulus, *Am. J. Pathol.* **66:**97.

Brenner, B., Hostetter, T., and Humes, H. D., 1978, Molecular basis of proteinuria of glomerular origin, *N. Engl. J. Med.* **298:**826.

Farquhar, M. G., and Palade, G. E., 1962, Functional evidence for the existence of a third cell type in the renal glomerulus, *J. Cell. Biol.* **13:**55.

Flamenbaum, W., McDonald, F. D., Di Bona, G. F., and Oken, D. E., 1974, Micropuncture study of renal tubular factors in low dose mercury poisoning, *Nephron* **8:**221.

Mauer, S. M., Fish, A. J., Blau, E. B., and Michael, A. F., 1972, The glomerular mesangium. I. Kinetics studies of macromolecular uptake in normal and nephrotic rats, *J. Clin. Invest.* **51:**1092.

Michael, A. F., Fish, A. J., and Good, R. A., 1967, Glomerular localization and transport of aggregated protein in mice, *Lab. Invest.* **17:**14.

Michael, A. F., Nevins, T. E., Raij, L., and Scheinman, J., 1979, Macromolecular transport in the glomerulus: Studies of the mesangium and epithelium *in vivo* and *in vitro,* in: *Contemporary Issues in Nephrology* (B. M. Brenner and J. H. Stein, eds.), Vol. 3, p. 167, Churchill Livingstone, Edinburgh.

Morrison, A. R., Nishikawa, K., and Needleman, P., 1977, Thromboxane A_2 biosynthesis in the ureter obstructed isolated perfused kidney of the rabbit, *J. Pharmacol. Exp. Ther.* **205:**1.

Nishikawa, K., Morrison, A., and Needleman, P., 1977, Exaggerated prostaglandin biosynthesis and its influence on renal resistance in the isolated hydronephrotic rabbit kidney, *J. Clin. Invest.* **205:**1.

Raij, L., Keane, W. F., Osswald, H., Michael, A., 1979, Mesangial Function in Ureteral Obstruction in the Rat—Blockade of the Efferent Limb, *J. Clin. Invest.* **64:**1204–1212.

Scheinman, J. I., Fish, A. J., and Michael, A. F., 1974, The immunohistopathology of glomerular antigens: The glomerular basement membrane, collagen and actomyosin antigens in normal and diseased kidneys, *J. Clin. Invest.* **54:**1144.

Stein, J. H., Lifschitz, M. D., and Barnes, L. D., 1978, Current concepts on the pathophysiology of acute renal failure, *Am. J. Physiol. Renal Fluid Electrolyte Physiol.* **3:**F171.

10

Deposition and Removal of Glomerular Immune Complexes: Relationships to the Mononuclear Phagocyte System

Mart Mannik and Gary E. Striker

1. Introduction

The deposition of circulating immune complexes in renal glomeruli is well established experimentally. Their presence in glomeruli in human diseases is well documented also. The estimate has been made that over 90% of acute glomerulonephritis is caused by immune complexes. The reasons for the variations in the course and prognosis of glomerulonephritis are not known adequately at this time.

The purpose of this article is to consider the relationships between the mononuclear phagocyte system (MPS) and the deposition and removal of glomerular immune complexes. The MPS was called the reticuloendothelial system, but the term mononuclear phagocyte system was adopted when it was shown that all of the mononuclear phagocytes (monocytes) are derived from the bone marrow precursors. The tissue mononuclear phagocytes (macrophages) enter tissue sites via the circulation, particularly when augmented locally by inflammatory stimuli. Even Kupffer cells turn over slowly by being replenished with marrow-derived cells (Crofton *et al.*, 1978).

The MPS, in particular the Kupffer cells in liver, plays a major role in clearing the circulation of immune complexes, thereby decreasing the possibility of deposition of these marterials in renal glomeruli and other vascular

---

Mart Mannik · Department of Medicine, University of Washington, Seattle, Washington 98195. ***Gary E. Striker*** · Department of Pathology, University of Washington, Seattle, Washington 98195. The work reported herein was supported by Research Grants AM 11476 from the National Institute of Arthritis, Metabolism and Digestive Diseases, HL 03175 from the National Heart and Lung Institute, and GM 24990 from the National Institute of General Medical Sciences.

beds. A diminished capacity of the Kupffer cells to remove circulating immune complexes prolongs their circulation and enhances their tissue deposition. Furthermore, when immune complexes are deposited in certain areas of renal glomeruli, the influx of marrow-derived mononuclear cells contributes to the removal of these substances.

2. *Removal of Circulating Complexes by the MPS*

A large number of methods have been developed to measure the concentration of immune complexes in serum or in other body fluids (Zubler and Lambert, 1978). The concentration of immune complexes in serum at any given time depends on the rate of immune complex formation and on the rate of immune complex removal from the circulation. The former is a function of the availability of specific antigens and antibodies. Quantitative information on the rates of immune complex formation is available neither in experimental models of spontaneous immune complex diseases nor in diseases induced by single or repeated antigen injection. The removal of immune complexes from the circulation depends on uptake by the MPS and on the rate of tissue deposition. Quantitatively, as will be discussed below, the major route of removal for circulating pathogenic immune complexes is the uptake of these materials by the Kupffer cells in the liver. Only relatively small amounts of immune complexes from the circulation are deposited in tissues during acute and chronic experimental models (Wilson and Dixon, 1970, 1971). These small amounts of deposited complexes suffice to cause tissue damage.

The lattice of immune complexes, the status of the MPS, the nature of antigens in immune complexes, and the nature of antibodies in immune complexes are variables that alter the uptake of immune complexes by the MPS. The lattice structure of immune complexes is defined by the number of antigen and antibody molecules in a given immune complex. Experiments with preformed soluble immune complexes, prepared with monomeric antigens and purified antibodies of the IgG class, showed that large-latticed immune complexes, containing more than two antibody molecules (greater than Ag_2Ab_2), were removed from the circulation relatively rapidly. The disappearance of these complexes was described by a single exponential function in rabbits, monkeys, and mice (Mannik *et al.*, 1971; Mannik and Arend, 1971; Haakenstad and Mannik, 1974, 1976). The half-life of these large-latticed complexes was a function of the concentration of circulating immune complexes, demonstrated by the fact that with increasing doses of injected complexes the half-life increased. When clearance velocity of these complexes was calculated, the velocity reached a plateau, an indication that the system is saturated (Haakenstad and Mannik, 1974). Immediately after injection of complement-fixing immune complexes, a phase of increased vascular permeability occurred, which led to extravasation of plasma, large-latticed and small-latticed immune complexes, and a concomitant rise of hematocrit (Haakenstad *et al.*, 1975; Haakenstad and Mannik, 1976). This phenomenon lasted about 15 min. This initial phase of removal of circulating immune complexes by increased vascular permeability was not observed with immune complexes that were rendered ineffective in complement fixation by reduction and alkylation of the antibodies used to prepare the complexes (Haakenstad and Mannik, 1976).

The small-latticed immune complexes, defined as containing one or two antibody molecules (i.e., Ag_2Ab_2, Ag_2Ab_1, or Ag_1Ab_1), were removed more slowly than were large-latticed complexes, but faster than antibodies alone. The fate of these materials in circulation was described best by exponential curves composed of two components (Mannik *et al.*, 1971; Haakenstad and Mannik, 1976). The first exponential component was attributed to equilibration between the intra- and extravascular compartments, and the second and slower component represented catabolism. The site for catabolism of these complexes is unknown, but it probably occurs in the Kupffer cells of the liver.

Quantitative studies on the specific hepatic uptake of immune complexes indicated that the bulk of large-latticed immune complexes (90%) removed from the circulation were taken up by the Kupffer cells in the liver (Arend and Mannik, 1971). The splenic uptake accounted for less than 1% of complexes removed by the liver when small doses of complexes were injected. With large doses, the specific splenic uptake increased to 10% of the amount taken up by the liver (Haakenstad and Mannik, 1976).

With increasing doses of immune complexes, the specific hepatic uptake of immune complexes, as examined at 1 hr after the administration of complexes, also reaches a plateau, indicating saturation of the Kupffer cells (Haakenstad and Mannik, 1974). This plateau was observed at the same dose as the saturation noted in clearance kinetics and is thought to be a function of saturation of the Fc receptors on Kupffer cells. It is analogous to the saturation of the MPS demonstrated and extensively studied with carbon particles and other substances (Biozzi *et al.*, 1953; Norman, 1974) that do not rely on the presence of Fc receptors on Kupffer cells. Thus, the saturation of the Kupffer cells with large-latticed immune complexes prolongs the circulation of these materials and enhances their deposition in other organs, including in the renal glomeruli.

The nature of antigens in immune complexes may alter the fate of these complexes in circulation. For example, heavily dinitrophenylated bovine serum albumin (BSA) was rapidly removed from the circulation of unimmunized animals (Klaus and Mitchell, 1974). Similarly, human serum albumin (HSA) was removed from the circulation of unimmunized mice as a function of the number of 4-fluoro-3-nitrophenyl azide groups conjugated to the lysine residues of this protein (Mannik and Haakenstad, 1977; Mannik *et al.*, 1981). Such antigens, independent of the lattice of immune complexes, contributed to the removal of complexes from circulation (Mannik and Jimenez, 1979). DNA injected into unimmunized animals also was removed rapidly from the circulation (Natali and Tan, 1971; Chused *et al.*, 1972;

Emlen and Mannik, 1978) and over 90% of the removed DNA was found in the liver (Emlen and Mannik, 1978). Immune complexes composed of DNA and antibodies to DNA were removed from mouse circulation at a rapid rate comparable to DNA alone (Emlen and Mannik, 1982). Furthermore, galactose receptors on hepatocytes can contribute to the removal of circulating immune complexes containing asialoproteins with exposed galactose (Finbloom *et al.*, 1981).

Finally, the fate of immune complexes in circulation is influenced by the nature of antibodies in the immune complexes. IgG_2 and IgG_4 subclasses of antibodies are ineffective in reacting with phagocyte receptors *in vitro* (Spiegelberg, 1974). These observations suggest that large-latticed immune complexes, composed of such antibodies, circulate longer than immune complexes containing antibodies that bind effectively with phagocyte receptors. This question was examined with a model system, using IgG antibodies with reduced and alkylated interchain disulfide bonds. Immune complexes made with such antibodies formed lattices comparable to those obtained with intact molecules (Mannik *et al.*, 1971). The antigen–antibody complexes made with reduced and alkylated antibodies reacted ineffectively with monocyte receptors *in vitro* (Arend and Mannik, 1972). Upon injection of these complexes into unimmunized mice, rabbits, or monkeys (Mannik *et al.*, 1971; Mannik and Arend, 1971; Haakenstad and Mannik, 1976), the large-latticed immune complexes persisted longer in circulation due to decreased hepatic uptake and were removed from the circulation of mice at rates comparable to small-latticed immune complexes (Haakenstad and Mannik, 1976). As a result of prolonged circulation of these complexes, increased glomerular deposition occurred (Haakenstad *et al.*, 1976).

3. Glomerular Deposition of Circulating Immune Complexes

In human diseases and in experimental models, immune complexes have been recognized in subendothelial, mesangial, and subepithelial areas of glomerular capillary loops. In a given patient with glomerulonephritis, complexes may exist in all areas to varying degrees. In the chronic serum sickness model of glomerulonephritis in rabbits, induced by repeated bovine serum albumin injection, complexes have been found in all three areas (Germuth *et al.*, 1972). The presence of these complexes was related to the size of immune complexes after the injection of antigen. The conclusion was reached that the large-latticed complexes deposited in mesangial and subendothelial areas and relatively small-latticed complexes localized in the subepithelial area of the glomerular capillary loops. These investigations did not provide direct proof for the deposition of circulating immune complexes in the subepithelial area.

The intravenous injection of preformed soluble immune complexes into unimmunized mice has established that in this species, only large-latticed complexes are deposited in renal glomeruli. These studies also indicated the sequence of subendothelial and mesangial deposition of immune complexes (Haakenstad *et al.*, 1976).

Several observations indicate that only large-latticed immune complexes (greater than Ag_2Ab_2) are deposited in glomeruli. When a mixture of large-latticed and small-latticed immune complexes, prepared from HSA and anti-HSA, was injected intravenously into mice in a single dose, the glomerular deposition progressed as long as the large-latticed complexes persisted in circulation (Haakenstad *et al.*, 1976). During continued presence of circulating small-latticed complexes, the glomerular deposits declined (see Table 1). This disappearance of complexes already deposited was not due to the high degree of antigen excess, achieved by relatively rapid removal and destruction of the complexes. This conclusion was supported by experiments in which immune complexes freed from excess antigen by gel filtration were administered to mice and examined by methods previously published. The glomerular deposition and removal of these partially purified complexes had the same sequence as that in studies published previously (Haakenstad *et al.*, 1976) and illustrated in Table 1. The deposition of large-latticed complexes only was supported further by the finding of enhanced glomerular deposition when the large-latticed immune complexes prepared with reduced and alkylated antibodies persisted longer in circulation. Further support for this was obtained by finding minimal or no glomerular deposition upon the administration of immune complexes consisting essentially only of small-latticed complexes, prepared with 50-fold antigen excess (Mannik and Haakenstad, 1977). Finally, the role of the lattice of immune complexes in deposition of these materials in renal glomeruli is illustrated by the effective disappearance of the deposits from the subendothelial and mesangial areas upon rendering the entire mouse in antigen excess by the administration of large doses of excess antigen, as described below.

The sequential transmission electron microscopic examination of renal tissues of mice after administration of preformed immune complexes indi-

Table 1. Intensity of Glomerular Localization of Rabbit IgG following the Administration of HSA–Anti-HSA Complexes, Prepared with Intact or with Reduced and Alkylated Rabbit Anti-HSA[a]

	Intensity of rabbit IgG in glomeruli at indicated hours after administration of immune complexes[b]				
Injected complexes	1	4	12	24	96
HSA–anti-HSA (5 mg Ab)	tr–1+	2–3+	2–3+	1–2+	tr+
HSA–anti-HSA, RA[c] (5 mg Ab)	1+	3–4+	4+	4+	3+
HSA–anti-HSA, RA (1 mg Ab)	nd	nd	2–3+	2–3+	2+

[a] Modified from Haakenstad *et al.* (1976).
[b] The intensity of fluorescence was graded from 0 to 4+; tr indicates trace amounts; nd indicates experiments not done. Two mice were sacrificed at each time period.
[c] RA indicates reduced and alkylated antibodies were used to prepare the immune complexes.

cated a sequence of events in subendothelial and mesangial localization of complexes (Haakenstad *et al.*, 1976). One hour after administration of complexes, the deposits were seen in the fenestrae of endothelial cells adjacent to the mesangium. At the same time, small amounts of deposits were noted in the subendothelial area and in the mesangial matrix (see Table 2). Later, increasing electron-dense material was found in the subendothelial area and in the mesangial matrix. When most of the large-latticed complexes were removed from the circulation (12 hr), the endothelial fenestrae contained decreased deposits. Within a few hours, the subendothelial areas cleared, leaving only deposits in the mesangial matrix. By 24 hr, even these deposits were decreasing and at later times only trace amounts of deposits were recognized. Similar observations were noted after the administration of immune complexes with reduced and alkylated antibodies. However, in these experiments, the deposits were much more extensive and persisted much longer in the glomeruli. Collectively, these studies suggested that the circulating, large-latticed immune complexes were lodged initially in endothelial fenestrae and then accumulated in the subendothelial area adjacent to the mesangium. Thereafter, the subendothelial deposits appeared to be translocated into the mesangial matrix by yet undefined mechanisms. In experiments with intact IgG-class antibodies, 24 to 48 hr after the single dose of complexes even the mesangial deposits were removed. Thus, the glomerular deposition from a single shower of circulating immune complexes was a relatively transient phenomenon in the otherwise healthy glomerulus.

During these experiments the circulating immune complexes were not deposited in the subepithelial area. The same findings have been reported by others (Okumura *et al.*, 1971; Koyama *et al.*, 1978). These experiments were of short duration (96 hr) to avoid variables induced by the endogenous immune response to the injected immune complexes (HSA and rabbit IgG). The immune clearance of residual circulating complexes usually occurred 105 hr after the injection (Mannik, 1979). Longer experiments and experiments with repeated injections of preformed immune complexes could be

Table 2. Glomerular Localization of Electron-Dense Material Following the Administration of HSA–anti-HSA Complexes Prepared with Intact Antibodies[a]

	Intensity of deposits at indicated hours after administration of immune complexes[b]				
Localization of deposits	1	4	12	24	96
Endothelial cell fenestrae	+	+	±	−	−
Subendothelial area	±	+ +	+ +	−	−
Mesangial matrix	±	+	+ +	±	±
Mesangial cells	−	−	−	−	−
Subepithelial area	−	−	−	−	−

[a] Modified from Haakenstad *et al.* (1976).
[b] The amount of electron-dense material was graded: none, −; trace, ±; moderate, +; or large, + +. Two mice were sacrificed at each time period and at least six glomeruli were examined from each specimen.

carried out in mice rendered tolerant to the constituent antigens and antibodies.

4. *Removal of Immune Complexes from Glomeruli by Bone Marrow-Derived Macrophages*

During the electron microscopic studies of kidneys from mice after injection of immune complexes, the impression was gained that macrophages and not mesangial cells were engaged in phagocytosis of immune complexes in the mesangial matrix (Haakenstad *et al.*, 1976). The same observation was made by other investigators (Okumura *et al.*, 1971). The detailed study of kidneys from NZB mice did not reveal phagolysosomes in mesangial cells (Comerford *et al.*, 1968). Furthermore, the persistence of glomerular deposits of immune complexes with reduced and alkylated antibodies in contrast to the prompt removal of complexes with intact antibodies (see Table 1, the 5- and 1-mg dose with reduced and alkylated antibodies), implied that an Fc-receptor-mediated mechanism contributed to the removal of immune complexes from glomeruli. In addition, morphological studies have suggested the accumulation of macrophages in glomeruli as a cause for increased mesangial cellularity in glomerulonephritis (Schreiner *et al.*, 1978). To establish the participation of marrow-derived mononuclear phagocytes in the removal of deposited immune complexes from glomeruli, a distinctive marker was needed for marrow-derived cells. In Chediak–Higashi mice, monocytes, macrophages, neutrophils, and Kupffer cells have easily recognizable giant lysosomes. On the other hand, these mice at various ages did not have the same structures in the resident mesangial cells.

Marrow transplantation was carried out between the syngeneic normal C57BL/6J and Chediak–Higashi (beige C57BL/6 [*bg/bg*]) mice after total body irradiation (Striker *et al.*, 1979). Two to three weeks after successful marrow transplantation, the normal mice with Chediak–Higashi marrow and the Chediak–Higashi mice with normal marrow were given a single dose of soluble immune complexes, prepared with either intact antibodies or with reduced and alkylated antibodies. The clearance kinetics and the glomerular deposition of immune complexes were examined by methods previously described (Haakenstad and Mannik, 1976; Haakenstad *et al.*, 1976). Upon the administration of immune complexes to both groups of transplanted mice, the clearance kinetics of the soluble immune complexes were not significantly different from those of normal control mice. The glomerular deposition and persistence of immune complexes, prepared with intact antibodies or with reduced and alkylated antibodies, were comparable to those of normal C57BL/6J mice as determined by immunofluorescence microscopy, examined at 24 and 96 hr after injection of the complexes. At least six glomeruli from each sacrificed mouse were examined by electron microscopy. The observations indicated that phagocytosis of the immune complexes in the glomerular mesangium is accomplished primarily by marrow-derived cells. First, all glomeruli contained a number of marrow-derived cells with giant lysosomes in the normal mice with Chediak–Higashi marrow, whereas these cells were absent in the Chediak–Higashi mice with normal marrow. Thus, in the Chediak–Higashi mice with normal marrow, the administration of immune complexes did not induce the formation of giant lysosomes in the resident mesangial cells. Therefore, the cells with giant lysosomes in the normal mice with Chediak–Higashi marrow must have been derived from bone marrow. Second, careful attention was given to the presence of deposits of immune complexes in the extracellular areas, within the marrow-derived and within the resident mesangial cells. The electron-dense deposits of immune complexes and the giant lysosomes were

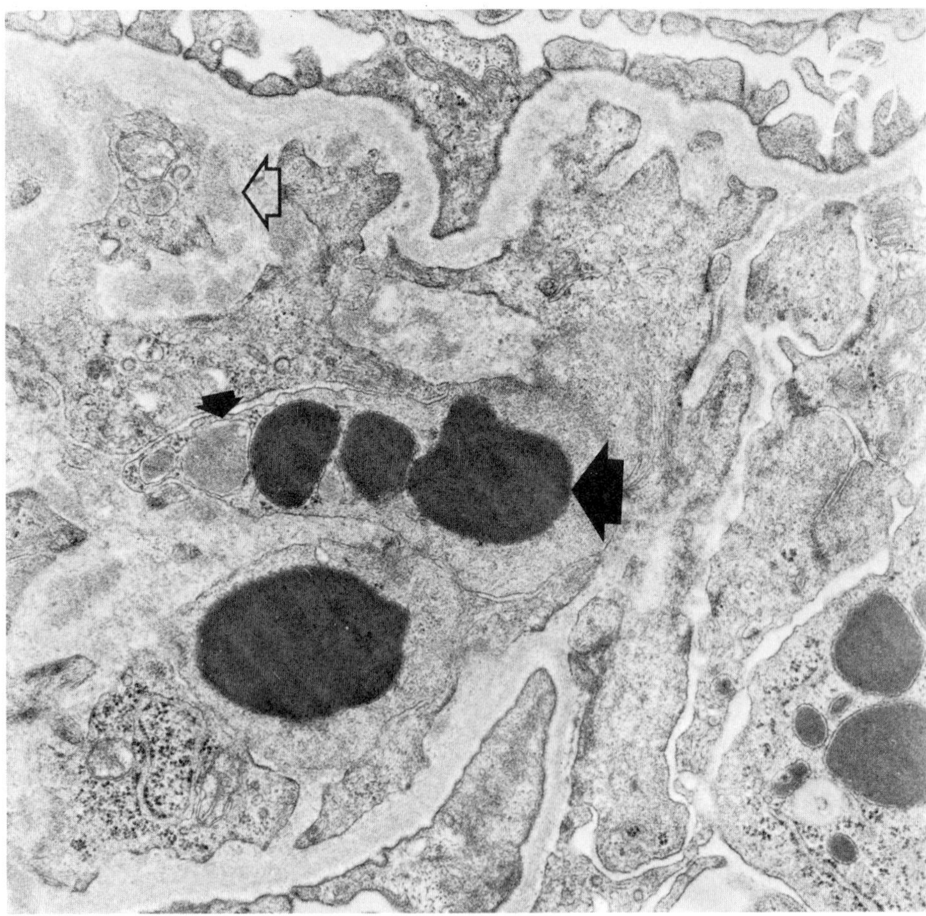

Figure 1. Electron micrograph of a glomerulus from a normal mouse with Chediak–Higashi marrow 24 hr after the administration of immune complexes prepared with reduced and alkylated antibodies. Giant lysosomes (large arrow) are evident in the cytoplasm of two marrow-derived cells. Immune complex deposits are noted within the phagolysosomes (small arrow) of one of these cells as well as in the mesangial matrix (open arrow).

Table 3. Summary of Electron Microscopic Findings in Marrow Cross-Transplanted Normal and Chediak–Higashi Mice after Administration of Immune Complexes[a]

	Mononuclear cells		Mesangial cells	
	Giant lysosomes	Immune complex deposits	Giant lysosomes	Immune complex deposits
CH (N marrow)[b]	0[c]	+	0	0
N (CH marrow)[b]	+	+	0	0

[a] Data summarized from Striker *et al.* (1979).
[b] CH (N marrow) indicates Chediak–Higashi mice that received normal marrow; N (CH marrow) indicates normal C57BL/6J mice that received Chediak–Higashi marrow.
[c] 0 indicates the absence and + indicates the presence of either giant lysosomes or immune complex deposits.

distinguished easily. In the normal mice with Chediak–Higashi marrow, the immune complex deposits were present in the mesangial matrix, in the marrow-derived cells with giant lysosomes (see Fig. 1), and not in the resident mesangial cells that possessed the characteristic peripheral cytoplasmic dense bodies. Similarly, in the Chediak–Higashi mice with normal marrow, the cells with characteristics of resident mesangial cells contained no deposits of immune complexes, whereas deposits were present in the mesangial matrix and within the phagolysosomes of the presumed marrow-derived macrophages (see Table 3). These experiments indicate that the marrow-derived macrophages contribute to the removal of immune complexes from the mesangial matrix. These experiments do not exclude other removal mechanisms. If the resident mesangial cells participate in removal of deposited immune complexes, they do not do so by the usual phagocytic process identifiable by morphologic criteria.

Of interest is that Schreiner *et al.* (1978) provided evidence that marrow-derived macrophages contributed to proteinuria and structural damage in the secondary phase (endogenous immune phase) of nephrotoxic serum nephritis in rats. In experiments described above, the contribution of macrophages to glomerular damage was not studied but the influx of these cells is likely to contribute to structural damage in glomeruli.

5. Removal of Immune Complexes from Glomeruli by Antigen Excess

As already discussed above, only large-latticed circulating immune complexes were deposited in the glomeruli following injection of preformed immune complexes, composed of HSA and rabbit anti-HSA. An increasing degree of antigen excess converted the large-latticed immune complexes to small-latticed immune complexes in this antigen–antibody system (Arend *et al.*, 1972; Arend and Mannik, 1974).

It is postulated that the injection of antigen following the administration of immune complexes with varying lattice sizes should convert all immune complexes accessible to the antigen to small-latticed complexes. The influence of large doses of antigen on the chronic serum sickness model of glomerulonephritis was examined by Valdes *et al.* (1969). The chronic disease was induced with daily injections of a constant dose of BSA. The antigen injections were discontinued in some rabbits, but some of the animals had a progression of their disease and died while others improved. In another group of rabbits, an initial dose of 500 mg BSA followed by daily doses of 100 mg BSA were given in place of the previously administered smaller daily dose. With the experimental protocol, the excess antigen administration resulted in a decrease of proteinuria and a conversion of the pattern of glomerular deposits from a coarsely granular pattern along glomerular loops to a finely beaded or mesangial pattern of immune complex deposition. The authors suggested that the mesangial area may not have been accessible to the excess antigen. In a subsequent publication, it was reported that the immune complexes in late membranous glomerulonephritis were surrounded by basement membrane and appeared to dissolve very slowly when large doses of antigen were given (Germuth *et al.*, 1977). Wilson and Dixon (1971) reported the half-life of renal-bound antigen in rabbits with BSA-induced chronic serum sickness. When the antigen administration was discontinued, the half-life of renal-bound antigen was 5.6 ± 1.1 days, but with excess antigen (1.2–3.0 g BSA/day) the half-life decreased to 0.9 ± 0.1 day. Concurrent with these quantitative studies, immunofluorescence and electron microscopy showed the deposits of immune complexes to be decreased. These studies clearly showed the accessibility of glomerular immune complexes to the excess antigen, including that in the subepithelial area of glomeruli.

In order to examine the influence of excess antigen on the fate of immune complexes deposited in the subendothelial area and in the mesangial matrix, immune complexes prepared with reduced and alkylated antibodies were injected into unimmunized mice and then at various times intravenously excess antigen was administered. In these experiments, the injected HSA–anti-HSA complexes were prepared at five fold antigen excess. The standard time chosen to administer the antigen excess was 12 hr after the intravenous injection of immune complexes, since at that time abundant deposits of immune complexes were observed by immunofluorescence microscopy and subendothelial and mesangial deposits were seen by electron microscopy (Haakenstad *et al.*, 1976). The degree of antigen excess to be administered was calculated on the basis of the same precipitin curves as those used to determine the antigen excess for preparation of the administered soluble complexes. The degree of antigen excess achieved *in vivo* exceeded the calculated values. During the 12 hr after the injection of immune complexes, these materials were catabolized and equilibrated between the intra- and extravascular spaces, so that at 12 hr, 47% of the injected material remained in circulation (Haakenstad and Mannik, 1976). In addition, the free antigen already administered with the immune complexes was catabolized with a half-life of 18.65 hr (Haakenstad and Mannik, 1974). Therefore, the administered excess antigen would create in the mouse an estimated excess twice that of the dose calculated on the basis of precipitin curves.

Provided that sufficient excess antigen was administered, the immune complexes already deposited were removed completely from the glomeruli by 12 hr after the injection of excess antigen. The results are summarized in Table 4. The calculated 40-fold excess antigen created about an 80-fold antigen excess *in vivo*. Three hours after the dose of excess antigen, the deposits in glomeruli decreased significantly and by 12 hr no deposits were seen by immunofluorescence microscopy (see Fig. 2). The antigen (HSA) similarly was removed during these experiments (see Fig. 3). Smaller doses of antigen excess decreased the glomerular deposits, but to a lesser degree (see Table 4). This might have been expected since the large-latticed immune

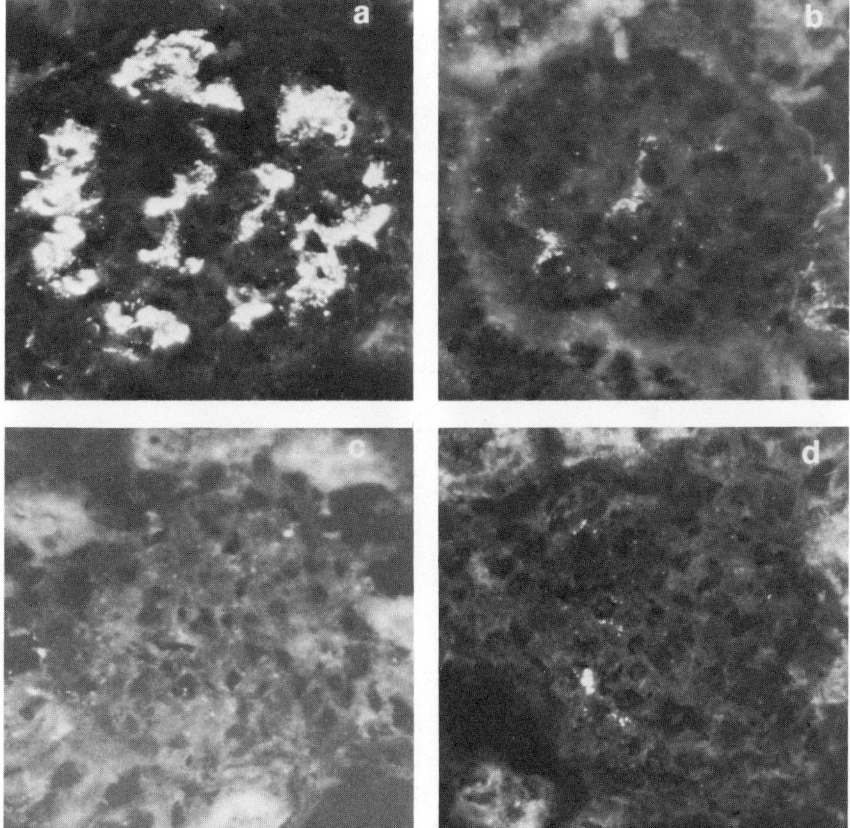

Figure 2. Resolution of immune complexes by administration of excess antigen, demonstrated by immunofluorescence microscopy. Mice initially received HSA–anti-HSA complexes prepared with reduced and alkylated rabbit antibodies. Twelve hours later, a calculated dose of 40-fold excess antigen was administered and the mice were sacrificed at varying times after that. The sections were stained with sheep antibodies to rabbit IgG, conjugated with fluorescein isothiocyanate. In (a), 4+ staining is illustrated in a control mouse at 12 hr without excess antigen administration; in (b), (c), and (d), 1+, 0, and trace staining are illustrated in mice that received the excess antigen 6, 12, and 84 hr respectively prior to sacrifice. Some staining of the tubules surrounding the glomeruli is evident; this is due to the orange autofluorescence attributed to lipofuchsin.

Table 4. Intensity of Glomerular Localization of Rabbit IgG following Administration of Excess HSA 12 hr after the Injection of HSA–Anti-HSA Complexes Prepared with Reduced and Alkylated Antibodies.

	Intensity of rabbit IgG in glomeruli at indicated hours after administration of excess antigen[a]					
Calculated dose of antigen excess	1.5	3	6	12	36	84
40-fold	3–4+	2+	1+[b]	0[b]	0	tr–1+[b]
20-fold	—	3+	3+	tr–1+	—	—
10-fold	—	—	4+	2+	—	—
None	4+[b]	4+	4+	4+	4+	3–4+

[a] The intensity of fluorescence was graded 0 to 4+; tr indicates trace amounts; — indicates time intervals where experiments were not done. At least two mice were examined for each experimental observation.
[b] Examples of these observations are illustrated in Fig. 2.

complexes decrease with increasing doses of excess HSA in this antigen–antibody system and at 50-fold antigen excess only small-latticed immune complexes were formed. By electron microscopy, the mesangial and subendothelial electron-dense deposits were no longer visible 12 hr after the administration of a calculated 40-fold antigen excess. The mesangial matrix possessed decreased density and was expanded in comparison to normal mice. When the excess antigen was administered at longer intervals after injection of immune complexes, not all the glomerular deposits were removed. By electron microscopy, the extracellular deposits were released, but the

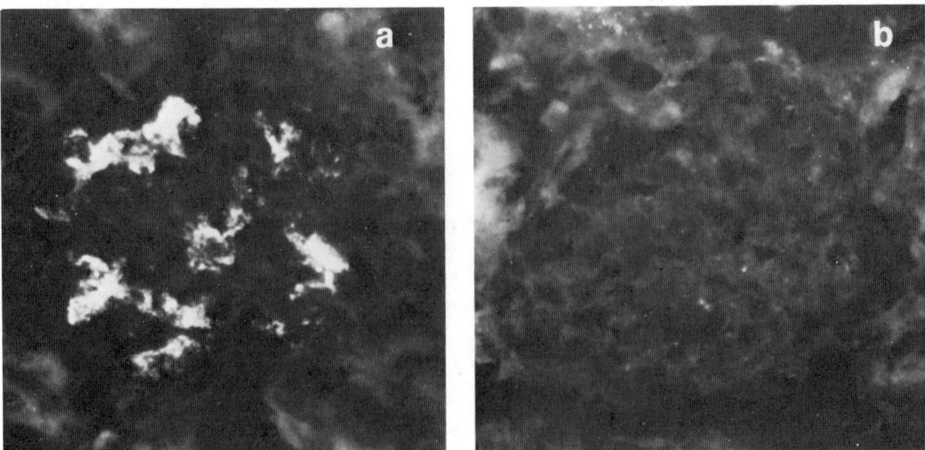

Figure 3. Resolution of glomerular immune complexes after administration of excess antigen, demonstrated by disappearance of antigen by immunofluorescence microscopy. The tissues from the same mice as in Figs. 2a and c were examined, but stained with rabbit antibodies to HSA, conjugated with fluorescein isothiocyanate. In (a), 3+ staining is illustrated in a control mouse; in (b), 0 staining is illustrated in a mouse that received excess antigen 12 hr previously. See Fig. 2 legend regarding tubular staining.

deposits phagocytized by monocytes were not altered by excess antigen (Mannik and Striker, 1980).

The experiments presented and previously published observations indicate that the subendothelial, mesangial (in mesangial matrix), and subepithelial immune complexes are readily accessible to antigens like HSA and BSA. In the preceding sections, the evidence was reviewed that only large-latticed (greater than Ag_2Ab_2) immune complexes are deposited in the subendothelial and mesangial areas. The rapid removal of immune complexes from these areas when they are converted to small-latticed (Ag_2Ab_2 or Ag_1Ab_1) immune complexes further supports this conclusion. The mechanisms responsible for the entrapment of large-latticed immune complexes in the subendothelial and mesangial areas have not been elucidated. The absolute size of immune complexes and actual precipitate formation may be important. Alternately, physicochemical characteristics of large-latticed immune complexes as multivalent ligands may contribute to binding of complexes to structural components of glomeruli. These questions are experimentally approachable with appropriate chemical alterations of antigens and antibodies. The prompt removal of immune complexes converted to small lattices indicates a fluid flow other than the formation of glomerular filtrate in the subendothelial and mesangial areas, but the direction of this "washout" is not known.

The effective removal of immune complexes deposited in glomeruli by the administration of excess antigen raises interesting possibilities. For example, the involved antigen could be degraded into small fragments that retain their antigenicity but are no longer immunogenic. Such materials, if administered in large doses, would form only small-latticed immune complexes with circulating antibodies, would not cause an anaphylactic reaction, and would not result in further glomerular deposition of complexes. The small antigenic fragments of molecules are also likely to be excreted effectively by the kidneys and should dissolve the immune complexes deposited in glomeruli. These speculations are testable in experimental models.

6. Summary

The mononuclear phagocyte system, in particular the Kupffer cells of the liver, removes circulating large-latticed immune complexes. Thereby, the glomerular deposition of these materials is decreased. Saturation of the Kupffer cells with immune complexes prolongs their circulation and enhances their deposition in glomeruli. Once immune complexes are deposited in glomeruli, phagocytosis by marrow-derived mononuclear phagocytes contributes to their removal from the mesangial matrix. The resident mesangial cells are not involved in the removal of deposited complexes by ultrastructurally recognizable phagocytic mechanisms.

Large-latticed immune complexes (greater than Ag_2Ab_2) are deposited from the circulation into the subendothelial and mesangial areas. Complexes already deposited in the endothelial or mesangial areas can be dispersed from these areas when converted to small-latticed (Ag_2Ab_2 or Ag_1Ab_1) immune complexes by exposure to high degrees of antigen excess.

During the administration of preformed immune complexes, subepithelial localization of immune complexes was not observed. As reviewed by Couser and Salant (1980), several investigations indicate that subepithelial immune complexes are formed locally by prior access of antigen to this area.

References

Arend, W. P., and Mannik, M., 1971, Studies on antigen–antibody complexes. II. Quantification of tissue uptake of soluble complexes in normal and complement-depleted rabbits, *J. Immunol.* **107:**63.

Arend, W. P., and Mannik, M., 1972, *In vitro* adherence of soluble immune complexes to macrophages, *J. Exp. Med.* **136:**514.

Arend, W. P., and Mannik, M., 1974, Determination of soluble immune complex molar composition and antibody association constants by ammonium sulfate precipitation, *J. Immunol.* **112:**451.

Arend, W. P., Teller, D. C., and Mannik, M., 1972, Molecular composition and sedimentation characteristics of soluble antigen–antibody complexes, *Biochemistry* **11:**4063.

Biozzi, G., Benacerraf, B., and Halpern, B. N., 1953, Quantitative study of the granulopectic activity of the reticuloendothelial system. II. A study of the kinetics of the granulopectic activity of the R.E.S. in relation to the dose of carbon injected. Relationship between the weight of the organs and their activity, *Br. J. Pathol.* **34:**441.

Chused, T. M., Steinberg, A. D., and Talal, N., 1972, The clearance and localization of nucleic acids by New Zealand and normal mice, *Clin. Exp. Immunol.* **12:**465.

Comerford, F. R., Cohen, A. S., and Desai, R. G., 1968, The evolution of the glomerular lesion in NZB mice: A light and electron microscopic study, *Lab. Invest.* **19:**643.

Couser, W. G., and Salant, D. J., 1980, In situ immune complex formation and glomerular injury, *Kidney Int.* **17:**1.

Crofton, R. W., Diesselhoff-den Dulk, M. M. C., and van Furth, R., 1978, The origin, kinetics, and characteristics of the Kupffer cells in the normal steady state, *J. Exp. Med.* **148:**1.

Emlen, W., and Mannik, M., 1978, Kinetics and mechanisms for removal of circulating single-stranded DNA in mice, *J. Exp. Med.* **147:**684.

Emlen, W. and Mannik, M., 1982, Clearance of circulating DNA-antiDNA immune complexes in mice, *J. Exp. Med.*, in press.

Finbloom, D. S., Magilavy, D. B., Hartford, J. B., Rifai, A., and Plotz, P. H., 1981, The influence of antigen on immune complex behavior in mice, *J. Clin. Invest.* **68:**214.

Germuth, F. G., Jr., Senterfit, L. B., and Dreesman, G. R., 1972, Immune complex disease. V. The nature of the circulating complexes associated with glomerular alterations in the chronic BSA-rabbit system, *Johns Hopkins Med. J.* **130:**344.

Germuth, F. G., Jr., Taylor, J. J., Siddiqui, S. Y., and Rodriquez, E., 1977, Immune complex disease, VI. Some determinants of the varieties of glomerular lesions in the chronic bovine serum albumin-rabbit system, *Lab. Invest.* **37:**162.

Haakenstad, A. O., and Mannik, M., 1974, Saturation of the reticuloendothelial system with soluble immune complexes, *J. Immunol.* **112:**1939.

Haakenstad, A. O., and Mannik, M., 1976, The disappearance kinetics of soluble immune complexes prepared with reduced and alkylated antibodies and with intact antibodies in mice, *Lab. Invest.* 283.

Haakenstad, A. O., Case, J. B., and Mannik, M., 1975, Effect of cortisone on the disappearance kinetics and tissue localization of soluble immune complexes, *J. Immunol.* **114:**1153.

Haakenstad, A. O., Striker, G. E., and Mannik, M., 1976, The glomerular deposition of soluble immune complexes prepared with reduced and alkylated antibodies and with intact antibodies in mice, *Lab. Invest.* **35:**293.

Klaus, G. G. B., and Mitchell, G. F., 1974, The influence of epitope density on the immunological properties of hapten–protein conjugates. II. The *in vivo* and *in vitro* metabolism of heavily and lightly conjugated protein, *Immunology* **27:**699.

Koyama, A., Niwa, Y., Shigematsu, H., Taniguchi, M., and Tada, T., 1978, Studies on passive serum sickness. II. Factors determining the localization of antigen–antibody complexes in the murine renal glomerulus, *Lab. Invest.* **38:**253.

Mannik, M., 1979, Clearance and glomerular deposition of circulating immune complexes, in: *Protides of the Biological Fluids*, 26th colloquium (H. Peters, ed.), Pergamon Press, Elmsford, N. Y.

Mannik, M., and Arend, W. P., 1971, Fate of preformed immune complexes in rabbits and rhesus monkeys, *J. Exp. Med.* **134:**19s.

Mannik, M., and Haakenstad, A. O., 1977, Circulation and glomerular deposition of immune complexes, *Arthritis Rheum.* **20:**S148.

Mannik, M., and Jimenez, R. A. H., 1979, The mononuclear phagocyte system (MPS) and immune complex diseases, in: *Immunopathology: Proceedings of the 6th International Convocation on Immunology* (F. Milgrom and B. Albini, eds.), Karger, Basel, p. 212.

Mannik, M., and Striker, G. E., 1980, Removal of glomerular deposits of immune complexes in mice by administration of excess antigen, *Lab. Invest.* **42:**483.

Mannik, M., and David, K. A., 1981, Covalently cross-linked immune complexes prepared with multivalent cross-linking antigen. *J. Immunol.* **127:**1999.

Mannik, M., Arend, W. P., Hall, A. P., and Gilliland, B. C., 1971, Studies on antigen–antibody complexes. I. Elimination of soluble complexes from rabbit circulation, *J. Exp. Med.* **133:**713.

Mannik, M., David, K. A., and Gauthier, V. J., 1981, Preparation and characterization of 4-azido-2-nitrophenyl human serum albumin as an antigen for covalent cross-linking of immune complexes, *J. Immunol.* **127:**1993.

Natali, P. G., and Tan, E. M., 1972, Experimental renal disease induced by DNA–antiDNA immune complexes, *J. Clin. Invest.* **51:**345.

Norman, S. J., 1974, Kinetics of phagocytosis. II. Analysis of *in vivo* clearance with demonstration of competitive inhibition between similar and dissimilar foreign particles, *Lab. Invest.* **31:**161.

Okumura, K., Kondo, Y., and Tada, T., 1971, Studies on passive serum sickness. I. The glomerular fine structure of serum sickness nephritis induced by preformed antigen–antibody complexes in the mouse, *Lab. Invest.* **24:**383.

Schreiner, G. F., Cotran, R. S., Pardo, V., and Unanue, E. R., 1978, A mononuclear cell component in experimental immunological glomerulonephritis, *J. Exp. Med.* **147:**369.

Spiegelberg, H. L., 1974, Biological activities of immunoglobulins of different classes and subclasses, *Adv. Immunol.* **19:**259.

Striker, G. E., Mannik, M., and Tung, M. Y., 1979, Role of marrow-derived and mesangial cells in removal of immune complexes from renal glomeruli, *J. Exp. Med.* **149:**127.

Valdes, A. J., Senterfit, L. B., Pollack, A. D., and Germuth, F. G., Jr., 1969, The effect of antigen excess on chronic immune complex glomerulonephritis, *Johns Hopkins Med. J.* **124:**9.

Wilson, C. B., and Dixon, F. J., 1970, Antigen quantitation in experimental immune complex glomerulonephritis. I. Acute serum sickness, *J. Immunol.* **105:**279.

Wilson, C. B., and Dixon, F. J., 1971, Quantitation of acute and chronic serum sickness in the rabbit, *J. Exp. Med.* **134:**7s.

Zubler, R. H., and Lambert, P. H., 1978, Detection of immune complexes in human diseases, *Prog. Allergy* **24:**1.

11

LCM Virus Infection and Nephritis

Phillip E. Hoffsten

1. Description of Chronic LCM Virus Infection in Mice

Lymphocytic choriomeningitis (LCM) virus was first described in the mid-1930s by Traub (1939) who noted that serum from certain mice was lethal when injected intracerebrally into other strains of mice. He demonstrated that the lethal agent was a vertically transmitted virus. Based on Traub's early work, chronic LCM virus infection was felt to be the result of host immunological tolerance to the virus (Burnet and Fenner, 1949). In the mid-1950s, Rowe (1954) demonstrated that LCM virus was not intrinsically cytopathic, i.e., the lethal acute meningitis following intracerebral injection of adult immunocompetent mice resulted from the animal's immune reaction to the virus. While chronic LCM virus infection was long thought to result in no disease, Hotchin and Collins (1964) noted the occurrence of "late onset disease" with glomerulonephritis in persistently infected mice. Oldstone and Dixon (1967) demonstrated that the glomerulonephritis in mice with chronic LCM virus infection had an immune complex pathogenesis, They performed studies of the immunoglobulin eluted from the kidneys of chronically infected mice and reported that the eluted antibody had binding specificity for LCM antigens. This latter observation implied that mice chronically infected with LCM virus were not immunologically tolerant to the virus as had been previously thought (Burnet and Fenner, 1949). Controversy over this observation has continued and will be addressed later in this chapter.

Studies of LCM virus-induced nephritis in SWR/J mice have been performed in mice infected neonatally (Hotchin *et al.*, 1962). The LCM virus carrier state induced is a lifelong infection which can be quantified by the intracerebral injection of serial dilutions of infectious serum into previously unexposed adult mice. Serum from the chronic LCM carrier may be diluted

Phillip E. Hoffsten · Department of Internal Medicine, Washington University School of Medicine, St. Louis, Missouri 63110.

1:500 and still be lethal for half the adult immunocompetent mice receiving a unit volume (0.03 ml) of the diluted serum. Early studies in Hoffsten's laboratory quantified parameters of renal disease occurring in chronic carrier mice. Using radial immunodiffusion techniques to quantify albuminuria, half of the carrier mice were found to have abnormal albuminuria by 6 months of age. Males and females were equally affected (Hoffsten *et al.*, 1975a). Remarkably, many chronic carrier mice are not albuminuric even after 1½ years of observation as compared to the 2-year life span of a normal SWR/J mouse. Uninfected SWR/J mice and nonalbuminuric LCM virus carrier mice have similar values for serum albumin, serum immunoglobulin, serum third component of complement, hematocrit, and blood urea nitrogen. In contrast, albuminuric LCM carrier mice have a significant reduction in serum albumin, serum third component of complement, and hematocrit. The serum concen-

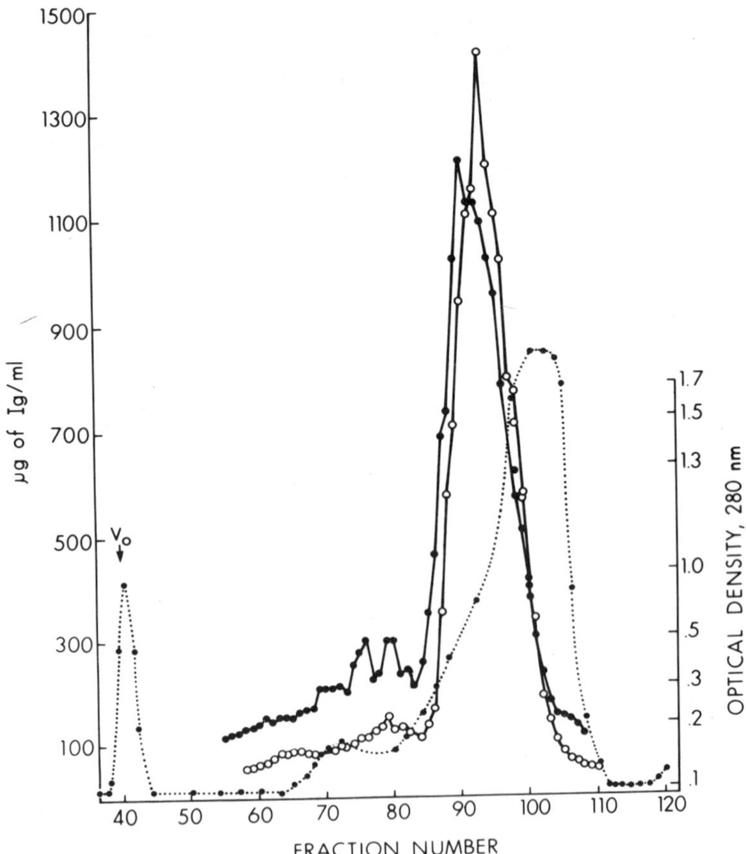

Figure 1. Bio-Gel A5 column chromatography of normal and LCM virus carrier mouse serum. The dotted line represents the optical density of the column effluent. The presence of immunoglobulin antigen (μg Ig/ml) in normal serum (○) is compared to the values in LCM virus carrier serum (●).

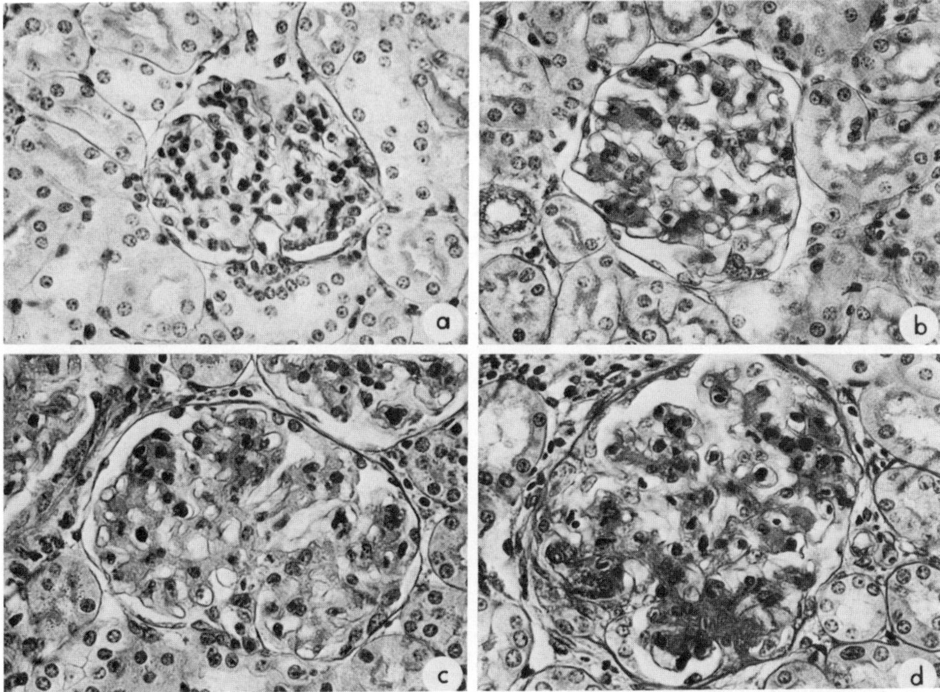

Figure 2. Light photomicrographs of glomeruli from normal and LCM virus-infected mice. (a) Glomerulus from a normal mouse; (b) glomerulus from an LCM-infected nonalbuminuric mouse; (c, d) glomeruli from LCM virus-infected albuminuric mice. PAS stain. Original magnification for all photomicrographs: × 200.

tration of immunoglobulin is elevated in albuminuric LCM virus carrier mice (Hoffsten *et al.*, 1979).

Using the Raji cell technique, Theofilopoulos has demonstrated circulating immune complexes in 9 of 10 sera from LCM carrier mice (personal communication). Nine of ten sera from normal SWR/J mice were negative using the same technique. Using Bio-Gel A5 (Bio-Rad Laboratories, Richmond, Calif.) column chromatography, an increased concentration of immunoglobulin antigen with 300,000 to 3,000,000 molecular weight in the serum of LCM virus carrier mice (Fig. 1) has been demonstrated. Concentration of the column fractions containing the high-molecular-weight immunoglobulin antigen and subsequent pH 3.2 buffer elution of the presumed immune complexes has yielded measurable amounts of 7 S immunoglobulin. This eluted immunoglobulin had no binding specificity for LCM viral antigens (complement fixation) or mouse tissue (immunofluorescence microscopy).

The severity of renal pathology in LCM virus carrier mice correlates with albuminuria (Hoffsten *et al.*, 1975b) rather than with the age of the mouse. By light microscopy, albuminuric LCM virus carrier mice have more extensive mesangial deposits of PAS-positive material and the glomeruli are larger (Fig. 2). Increased thickness of glomerular capillary walls cannot be

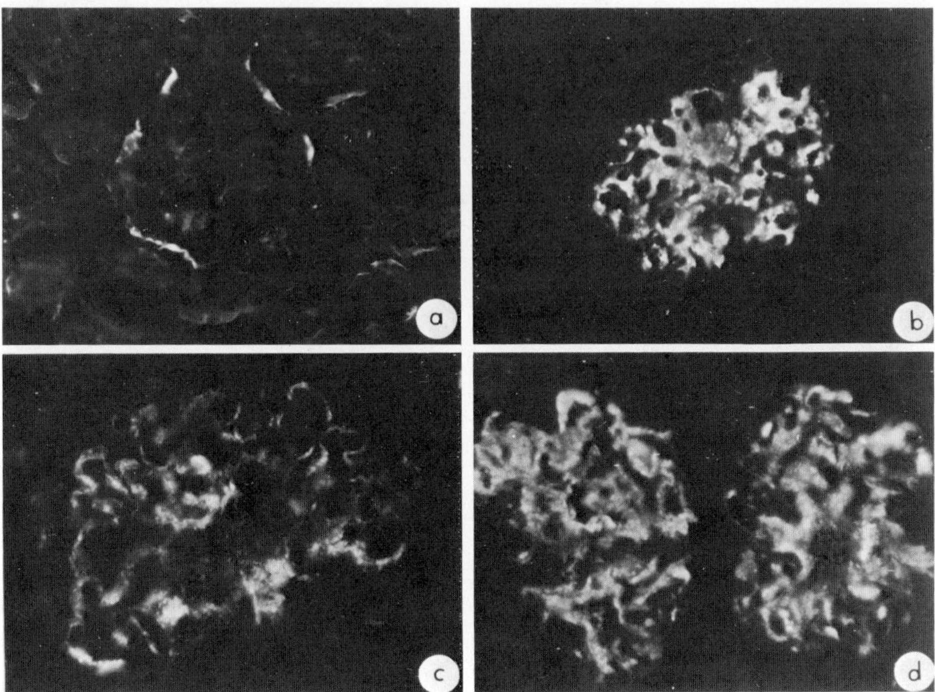

Figure 3. Immunofluorescent photomicrographs of glomeruli from normal and LCM virus-infected mice. The sections were stained with fluorescein-labeled rabbit anti-mouse immunoglobulin antiserum. (a) Glomerulus from a normal mouse; (b) glomerulus from an LCM virus-infected nonalbuminuric mouse; (c, d) glomeruli from LCM virus-infected albuminuric animals. Original magnification: × 200.

discerned consistently in the albuminuric animals. Lymphocytic perivascular cuffing commonly seen in kidneys of LCM virus carriers is no more frequent in albuminuric animals. By immunofluorescence microscopy, nonalbuminuric animals have predominantly mesangial deposits of immunoglobulin and complement while albuminuric LCM virus carriers have larger confluent mesangial deposits of immune proteins and also glomerular capillary loop deposition (Fig. 3). Glomerular deposition of LCM viral protein as observed by immunofluorescence microscopy is most frequently negative regardless of the age, sex, or quantitative proteinuria of the animal. By electron microscopy, electron-dense deposits are seen only in the mesangium of the nonalbuminuric animals (Hoffsten *et al.*, 1975b). Albuminuric mice have both mesangial and capillary loop electron-dense deposits (Hoffsten *et al.*, 1975b).

2. *Adoptive Immunization of LCM Mice*

Volkert (1963, 1971) performed a series of studies in which syngeneic LCM immune spleen cells were transferred to chronic LCM carrier mice, a procedure termed "adoptive immunization." Seven to ten days after the transfer of syngeneic LCM immune spleen cells, the titer of infectious LCM virus in the circulation decreased in association with the appearance of complement-fixing anti-LCM antibody in the serum of the adoptively immunized mouse. Cells containing LCM viral antigen disappeared from the liver although not from the brain or the kidney where many cells containing the characteristic cytoplasmic LCM viral antigen (Hoffsten *et al.*, 1977a) were seen. During the first month after adoptive immunization, a marked diminution in the glomerular deposits of immunoglobulin and complement (Hoffsten *et al.*, 1977a) occurred. Volkert *et al.* (1975) demonstrated that the effector cell for adoptive immunization is a T cell and that anti-LCM antibody is not required for adoptive immunization to occur.

Volkert's techniques of adoptive immunization have been utilized in this laboratory as a therapeutic modality for the glomerulonephritis occurring in mice chronically infected with LCM virus. Studying a series of littermate pairs of LCM carrier mice, one of which was adoptively immunized at 2–4 months of age, it was noted that only 2 of 55 adoptively immunized animals became albuminuric during the ensuing year of observation. In contrast, 15 of 28 control animals developed abnormal albuminuria. By pathological examination, glomeruli from the adoptively immunized animals had fewer immune deposits and smaller glomerular diameter than their littermate controls (Hoffsten *et al.*, 1977b).

Studies of the mechanism of adoptive immunization have been published by Volkert *et al.* (1975) and confirmed in Hoffsten's laboratory. Using either a nylon wool column or a column of glass beads coated with antibody to mouse immunoglobulin, it has been possible to fractionate mouse spleen cells and obtain a population of purified T cells. It was found that adoptive immunization of LCM carrier mice using a population of LCM immune T cells (< 1% B cells) resulted in no detectable production of anti-LCM antibody. The removal of LCM virus from the serum and of LCM antigen from liver tissue was as effective as if whole spleen cell populations had been used. Cells isolated from the thymus gland or from the bone marrow of nonimmune mice or mice immune to LCM virus did not result in adoptive immunization of LCM virus carriers (Hoffsten *et al.*, 1977b). This leads to the conclusion that adoptive immunization is mediated by peripheral T cells acting as killer T cells. This population of cells is not present in the chronic LCM virus carrier, and indicates that its T cell population is immunologically tolerant to LCM viral antigen.

As previously mentioned, Oldstone and Dixon (1967) reported that immunoglobulin eluted from the glomeruli of LCM carrier mice had binding specificity for LCM viral antigen. They stated that this demonstrated the lack of classical immunological tolerance for LCM virus in the carrier mouse. Since anti-LCM antibody is not demonstrable in the serum of chronically infected mice, the assertion of Oldstone and Dixon requires that the LCM carrier be in a state of "pseudotolerance" (Howard *et al.*, 1971) in which antigen appears in the serum in quantity sufficient to immediately neutralize circulating anti-LCM antibody. If LCM carrier mice were pseudotolerant to the virus, it could be predicted that removal of LCM antigen from the circulation by adoptive immunization would result in the appearance of large amounts of anti-LCM antibody. This is not seen as shown by experiments using purified LCM immune T cells of adoptively immunized carrier mice (Volkert *et al.*, 1975; Hoffsten *et al.*, 1977b). Similarly, if LCM carrier mice were in antigen excess, it would be predicted that the injection of large amounts of anti-LCM antibody would result in an acute glomerulonephritis in these mice. The converse has been observed in that glomerulonephritis in these animals resolves following adoptive immunization with no residual evidence of an acute glomerulonephritis. If the animals were pseudotolerent, administration of additional anti-LCM antiserum to the carrier mouse would be expected to result in a worsening of the glomerular disease. This was not observed (Hoffsten *et al.*, 1977a). Finally, immune complex glomerulonephritis with subendothelial deposits occurring in antigen excess is characterist-

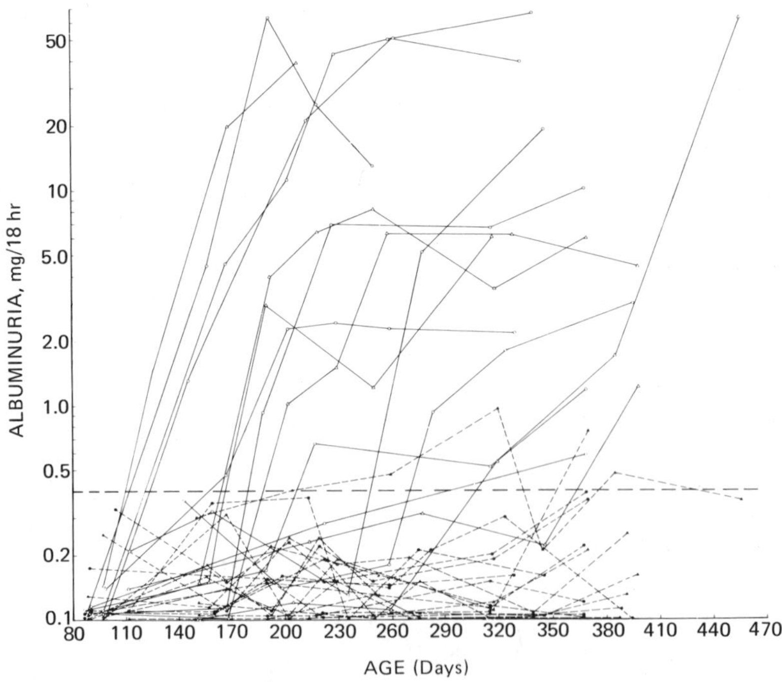

Figure 4. Albuminuria measurements in LCM virus carrier mice and adoptively immunized littermates. The horizontal heavy dashed line represents the upper limits of normal for albuminuria in SWR/J mice. Each solid line represents a single LCM virus carrier mouse which developed abnormal proteinuria during the period of observation. Each dashed line represents a single adoptively immunized littermate. Multiple albuminuria determinations were made for each individual mouse and are represented by points on the various lines.

ically a proliferative glomerulonephritis. The glomerulonephritis occurring in LCM carrier mice is not proliferative (Hoffsten *et al.*, 1975a). While none of these observations provide compelling evidence leading to a choice between the tolerant and pseudotolerant state of LCM carrier mice, a reexamination of the immunoglobulin eluted from the kidneys of LCM carrier mice seemed warranted.

Using the same technique described in the previous report by Oldstone and Dixon (1967), antibody with LCM binding specificity was not demonstrable in this laboratory (Klein *et al.*, 1977). The controls employed included the addition of anti-LCM antibody during the elution procedure and subsequent detection of anti-LCM antibody activity in the final product. The findings were consistent with the original impression of Burnet and Fenner (1949) that LCM virus carrier mice are classically immunologically tolerant to LCM virus. Since these results were published, Buckmeier and Oldstone (1978) have reasserted the previous position that LCM virus carrier mice produce anti-LCM antibody demonstrable by radioimmunoassay technique. Resolution of the controversy regarding the presence or absence of anti-LCM antibody in glomerular eluates from LCM carrier mice must await reports from additional laboratories where this critical point is examined.

3. Mesangial and Reticuloendothelial Function in LCM Virus Carrier Mice

The studies of Mauer *et al.* (1972) provided the foundation for examination of mesangial function in mice chronically infected with LCM virus. It was hypothesized that LCM virus might affect the mesangial system and thereby prevent normal clearance of material deposited in glomeruli. Quantitative isolation of glomeruli from a single mouse kidney has not been achieved. Therefore, this laboratory adapted Mauer's method and took advantage of certain histopathological observations to quantify glomerular accumulation of injected heat-aggregated human gamma globulin (AIgG). Test mice were injected intraperitoneally with 25 mg of AIgG labeled with both ^{125}I and fluorescein. Autopsies were performed at various time intervals. Protein-bound radioactive iodine adherent to renal tissue was quantified in individual kidneys from normal and LCM virus-infected mice. By immunofluorescence microscopy, AIgG deposits were found exclusively within glomeruli 24 hr after intraperitoneal injection. Using autoradiography, radioactive iodine adherent to renal tissue was seen to be doposited predominantly, although not exclusively, within the glomeruli. These two observations provided the basis for the impression that renal tissue-bound radioactive iodine represented predominantly glomerular deposits of AIgG. It was found that albuminuric LCM virus carrier mice invariably had larger glomerular accumulations of injected aggregates, although the rate of clearance of these aggregates from renal tissue was similar to the rate in normal mice (Fig. 5) (Hoffsten *et al.*, 1979). Thus, an intrinsic glomerular mesangial lesion in the

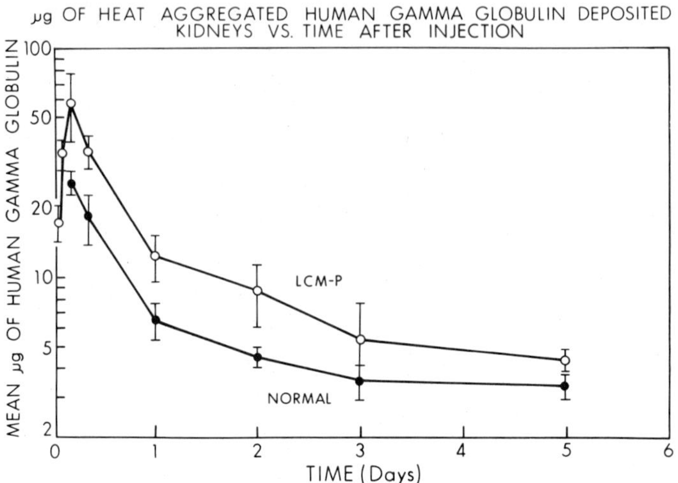

Figure 5. Rate of removal of AIgG from the glomeruli of LCM virus-infected albuminuric mice compared to normal mice. Each point represents an average value ± S.E.M. for five mice.

LCM virus carrier mouse was not seen. While mesangial clearance of accumulated AIgG was similar in LCM-infected and normal mice, the greater accumulation noted in LCM-infected proteinuric animals was associated with higher blood concentrations of AIgG.

This led to the hypothesis that LCM virus carrier mice might have a reduced rate of clearance of blood-borne immune complex-like material. This hypothesis was tested using intravenous injections of 4 mg AIgG with subsequent measurement of the rate of disappearance of AIgG from the blood. It was found that the LCM virus carriers had a significantly longer half-time for the removal of circulating aggregated gamma globulin than did normals (Fig. 6) (Hoffsten *et al.*, 1979). This observation is compatible with the hypothesis that glomerulonephritis occurring in chronic LCM virus carrier mice results from an increased rate of glomerular deposition of immune complexes as opposed to a decreased rate of glomerular immune deposit clearance.

A proposal for the pathogenesis of immune complex glomerulonephritis occurring in mice chronically infected with LCM virus integrating the observations described is presented in Fig. 7. The proposal includes consideration that the disease is associated with demonstrable circulating immune complexes. While antigen-binding specificity of the immunoglobulin contained in the circulating immune complexes or in glomerular immune deposits remains controversial based on these findings quantitatively the amount of anti-LCM antibody present must be small if any is present. The proposal considers the mesangial system to be functionally intact with glomerular accumulation of immune proteins resulting from an abnormal increased rate of glomerular deposition.

In the hypothesis presented in Fig. 7, it is suggested that the absence of

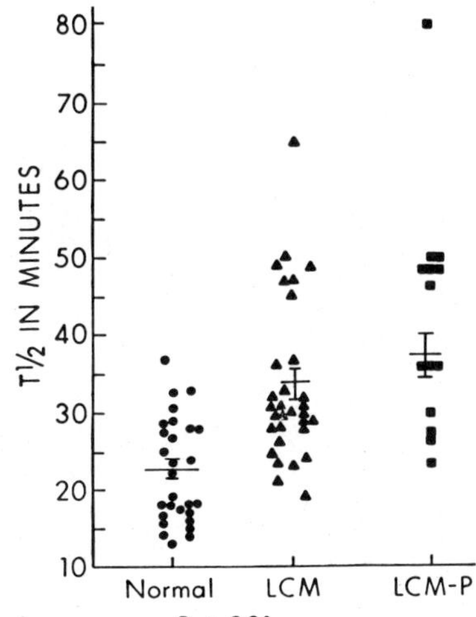

Figure 6. Half-time for the disappearance of 4 mg heat-aggregated human gamma globulin from the circulation of normal, LCM virus-infected, and LCM virus-infected albuminuric (LCM-P) mice. The mean $t^{1/2}$ value is significantly prolonged in both LCM virus-infected groups as compared to normals.

a population of LCM-specific T cells allows the persistence of LCM virions in the circulation and in the tissues of the LCM virus carrier. It is suggested that the removal of LCM virions from the circulation competitively inhibits the animal's reticuloendothelial system. Thus, the quantity of circulating immune complexes normally encountered would increase in blood and be

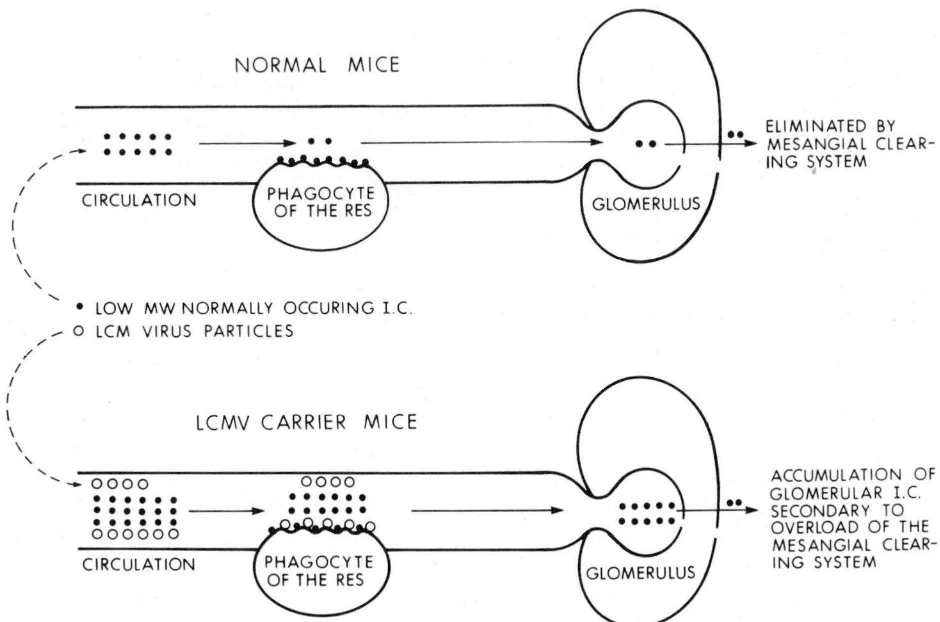

Figure 7. Proposed pathogenesis of the glomerulonephritis occurring in mice chronically infected with LCM virus.

presented to the glomeruli in increased concentrations with subsequent glomerular accumulation. This hypothesis implies that no major fraction of the immunoglobulin in glomerular deposits will have binding specificity for a single antigen.

To test the feasibility of this hypothesis, experiments were performed to determine if material as large as an LCM virion (estimated molecular weight > 150,000,000) could inhibit competitively the phagocytosis of small-molecular-weight immune complexes such as were demonstrated and are known to be associated with glomerular deposition (Germuth and Rodriguez, 1973). Using differential ultracentrifugation, a low-molecular-weight fraction (50,000–5,000,000) of ^{131}I-labeled AIgG (Fig. 8) was prepared. Using Bio-Gel A5 gel chromatography, a high-molecular-weight fraction (>50,000,000) of ^{125}I-labeled AIgG was prepared. Test animals were normal male 2- to 4-month-old SWR/J mice and each received 0.4 ml of aggregate suspension via tail vein injection. Blood samples to quantify the rate of clearance of the two populations of labeled AIgG were obtained at 2, 5, 8, and 11 min after injection. The $t_{1/2}$ for clearance of the aggregates was calculated by standard methods.

The results of these experiments are shown in Table 1. When 1 mg of a low-molecular-weight aggregate was injected intravenously into test mice, the average $t_{1/2}$ for clearance of the material was 13.7 min. If the 1 mg of low-molecular-weight aggregate was combined with 3 mg of high-molecular-weight aggregate, the removal of the low-molecular-weight material from the blood was slowed significantly with a $t_{1/2}$ of 21.3 min, a result statistically

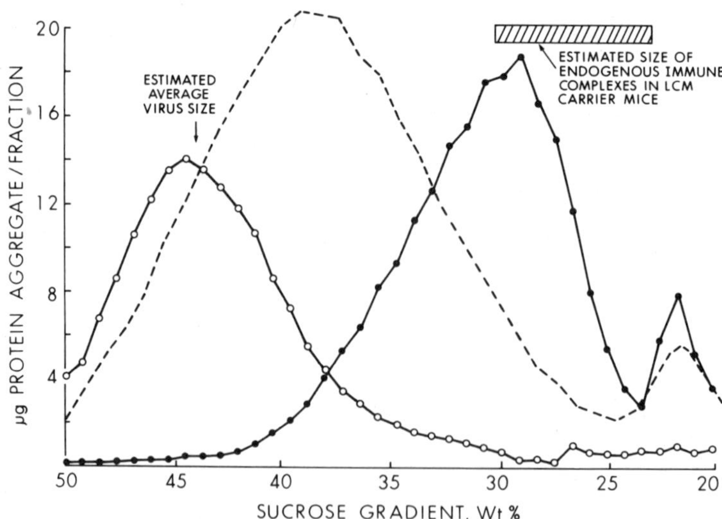

Figure 8. Sucrose density gradients of heat-aggregated human gamma globulin fractions. High-molecular-weight material (○) was labeled with 127I, and low-molecular-weight aggregates (●) were labeled with 131I. Both high- and low-molecular-weight fractions were prepared from material having a distribution of molecular sizes illustrated by the dashed line.

Table 1. $t_{1/2}$ (min) for the Clearance of Low-Molecular-Weight (500,000–5,000,000) Heat-Aggregated Human Gamma Globulin (AIgG) [Alone and in the Presence of High-Molecular-Weight (50,000,000) Aggregates]

1 mg low-MW AIgG	1 mg low-MW AIgG + 3 mg high-MW AIgG	4 mg low-MW AIgG	4 mg low-MW AIgG + 4 mg high-MW AIgG
11.1	30.1	21.0	36.1
12.6	23.0	15.4	68.3
14.0	20.5	13.2	56.8
12.1	20.3	14.7	39.4
13.8	17.1	17.1	46.5
21.8	18.0		
15.0	20.1		
8.3	19.4		
	22.9		
	21.9		

Mean ± S.E.M. 13.7 ± 1.4 ← $p < 0.001$ → 21.3 ± 1.1 ← $p < 0.01$ → 16.2 ± 1.3 ← $p < 0.001$ → 49.9 ± 6.1

different than for the injection of 4 mg of low-molecular-weight aggregate alone. A very marked slowing of the blood clearance of low-molecular-weight aggregate was produced when 4 mg of low-molecular-weight aggregate was combined with 4 mg of high-molecular-weight aggregate. With this combination, the $t_{1/2}$ for removal of the low-molecular-weight aggregate was 59.9 min.

These results provide support for the concept illustrated in Fig. 7. To establish the proposed pathogenesis, more extensive quantitative studies of the reticuloendothelial system will be required. The proposal is offered as an alternative to those pathogenetic hypotheses in which immune complex glomerulonephritis is a hypersensitivity state with predominance of a single antigenic agent in the glomerular deposits.

References

Buckmeier, J. J., and Oldstone, M. B. A., 1978, Virus induced immune complex disease: Identification of specific viral antigens and antibodies deposited in complexes during chronic lymphocytic choriomeningitis virus infection, *J. Immunol.* **120:**1297.

Burnet, F. M., and Fenner, F., 1949, *The Production of Antibodies,* 2nd ed., Macmillan, New York.

Germuth, F. G., Jr., and Rodriguez, E., 1973, *Immunopathology of the Renal Glomerulus: Immune Complex Deposit and Antibasement Membrane Disease*, Little, Brown, Boston.

Hoffsten P. E., Hill, C., and Klahr, S., 1975a, Studies of albuminuria and proteinuria in normal mice and mice with immune complex glomerulonephritis, *J. Lab. Clin. Med.* **86:**920.

Hoffsten, P. E., Hill, C., Klahr, S., Koh, S. J., Taylor, J., and Germuth, F. G., Jr., 1975b, Morphologic determinants of albuminuria in immune complex nephritis, *Kidney Int.* **8:**449 (abstract).

Hoffsten, P. E., Oldstone, M. B. A., and Dixon, F. J., 1977a, Immunopathology of adoptive immunization of mice chronically infected with lymphocytic choriomeningitis virus, *Clin. Immunol. Immunopathol.* **7:**44.

Hoffsten, P. E., Villalobos, R., Hill, C., and Klahr, S., 1977b, T-Cell deficiency in immune complex glomerulonephritis, *Kidney Int.* **11:**318.

Hoffsten, P. E., Swerdlin, A., Bartell, M., Hill, C., Brotherson, K., and Klahr, S., 1979, Reticuloendothelial and mesangial function in murine immune complex glomerulonephritis, *Kidney Int.* **15:**144.

Hotchin, J., and Collins, D., 1964, Glomerulonephritis and late onset disease of mice following neonatal virus infection, *Nature (London)* **203:**1357.

Hotchin, J., Benson, L. M., and Seamer, J., 1962, Factors affecting the induction of persistent tolerant infection of newborn mice with LCM, *Virology* **18:**71.

Howard, J. G., Christie, G. H., and Courtenay, B. M., 1971, Studies on immunological paralysis IC: The relative contributions of continuous antibody neutralization and central inhibition to paralysis with type III pneumococcal polysaccharide, *Proc. F. Soc. London B Ser.* **178:**417.

Klein, B., Hill, C., and Hoffsten, P. E., 1977, Studies of the immunoglobulin eluted from the glomeruli of mice chronically infected with lymphocytic choriomeningitis virus, *J. Immunol.* **119:**707.

Mauer, S. M., Fish, D. J., Blau, E. B., and Michael, A. F., 1972, The glomerular mesangium. I. Kinetic studies of macromolecular uptake in normal and nephrotic rats, *J. Clin. Invest.* **51:**1092.

Oldstone, M. B. A., and Dixon, F. J., 1967, Lymphocytic choriomeningitis: Production of antibody by tolerant infected mice, *Science* **158:**1193.

Rowe, W., 1954, Studies on pathogenesis and immunity in lymphocytic choriomeningitis infection of the mouse, *Naval Med. Res. Inst. Rep.* **12:**167.

Traub, E., 1939, Epidemiology of LCM in a mouse stock observed for four years, *J. Exp. Med.* **69:**801.

Volkert, M., 1963, Studies on immunological tolerance of LCM virus. 2. Treatment of virus carriers by adoptive immunization, *Acta Pathol. Microbiol. Scand.* **57:**465.

Volkert, M., and Lundstedt, C., 1971, Tolerance and immunity to the lymphocytic choriomeningitis virus, *Ann. N.Y. Acad. Sci.* **181:**183.

Volkert, M., Bro-Jorgenson, K., Marker, O., Rubin, A., and Trier, L., 1975, The activity of T and B lymphocytes in immunity and tolerance to the lymphocytic choriomeningitis virus in mice, *Immunology* **29:**455.

12

Diabetic Nephropathy: Relevance of Animal Models to the Understanding of Pathological Processes in Immune Renal Disease

S. Michael Mauer, David M. Brown, and Michael W. Steffes

Diabetic glomerulopathy represents the end result of a variety of pathogenetic processes which are dependent upon a long-standing diabetic state for their expression. Since it is reasonable to assume that the glomerulus has a limited repertoire of responses to pathologic stimuli, it is hoped that these studies of glomerular structural and functional changes in rodents with diabetes may provide insights into events occurring in immune glomerular injury.

1. The Pathology of Diabetic Nephropathy

In man, diabetic nephropathy is characterized by thickening of the glomerular basement membrane (GBM) (Østerby, 1972), tubular basement membrane (TBM), and Bowman's capsule (Warren *et al.*, 1966). Increased concentrations of plasma proteins, most strikingly IgG and albumin, can be detected immunohistochemically in all of these membranes (Miller and Michael, 1976). As with GBM thickening (Østerby, 1972), mesangial thickening, primarily due to increased mesangial matrix material, occurs early in

---

S. Michael Mauer · Department of Pediatrics, University of Minnesota Medical School, Minneapolis, Minnesota 55455. ***David M. Brown*** · Department of Laboratory Medicine and Pathology and Department of Pediatrics, University of Minnesota Medical Schools, Minneapolis, Minnesota 55455. ***Michael W. Steffes*** · Department of Laboratory Medicine and Pathology, University of Minnesota Medical School, Minneapolis, Minnesota 55455.

the disease (Østerby, 1972). This mesangial thickening is associated with markedly increased mesangial staining for smooth muscle proteins (Scheinman *et al.*, 1974).

The final pathological picture is expressed as diffuse and nodular (Kimmelstiel–Wilson) glomerulosclerosis (Heptinstall, 1974; Kimmelstiel, 1968). Hyalin (exudative) glomerular deposits (Heptinstall, 1974; Kimmelstiel, 1968) characteristically occur in the subendothelial space, and hyalin arteriolar degenerative changes are virtually diagnostic of diabetes when occurring in both afferent and efferent arterioles of the same glomerulus (Heptinstall, 1974; Bell, 1952). These hyalin lesions contain a wide variety of plasma proteins with biological activity as evidenced by their capacity to fix heterologous complement (Burkholder, 1965).

Diabetic glomerulopathy in animals is remarkably similar to that seen in man. Dogs (Bloodworth, 1965; Bloodworth *et al.*, 1969) and rats (Hägg, 1974a) with experimentally induced diabetes develop progressive GBM thickening. Although not as carefully documented, similar GBM changes occur in experimental diabetes in monkeys (Bloodworth *et al.*, 1973) and in genetic diabetes in mice (Mauer, Brown, and Steffes, unpublished observations). All of these species, when diabetic, manifest progressive mesangial thickening and, in the dog, this results in the development of Kimmelstiel–Wilson nodules (Bloodworth, 1965) similar to those in man. In rats where careful immunohistochemical studies have been performed (Mauer *et al.*, 1972b; Hägg, 1974b), hyalin glomerular nodules contain a variety of plasma proteins which are capable of heterologous complement fixation. However, in rats (Mauer *et al.*, 1972b) and mice (Wehner *et al.*, 1972), deposition of IgG, IgM, and C3 occurs in the mesangium, a finding quite unlike the characteristic linear extracellular membrane immunofluorescence pattern seen in human diabetic nephropathy. Finally, rats with long-standing diabetes develop increased mesangial staining for smooth muscle antigens (Scheinman *et al.*, 1978).

2. *The Glomerular Mesangium in Diabetic Nephropathy*

Thickening of the mesangium, as emphasized above, is characteristic of diabetic nephropathy in animals and in man. This is primarily due to an increase in mesangial matrix material (Kimmelstiel, 1968) with a lesser contribution from mesangial cell proliferation. The mesangium appears to have the important function of taking up and of processing macromolecules which circulate through the endothelial cells lining the glomerular capillary lumen. Since diabetic glomerulopathy in rodents is characterized by increased mesangial localization of immunogobulins and complement, the question may be raised as to whether or not this phenomenon represents an alteration in mesangial function. It should be emphasized that, in the early stages of diabetic nephropathy in rats, thickening of the mesangium is focal and segmental while the increased staining for IgG, IgM, and C3 is diffuse and generalized. Since nonimmunological proteins such as albumin are not present in the mesangium of diabetic rats, this suggests that the presence of increased quantities of immune reactants in the mesangium of these animals represents mesangial trapping of circulating immune complexes. However, the failure of these immune proteins to fix heterologous complement and the absence of cellular proliferation in this area (Mauer *et al.*, 1972b) may be taken as evidence against aggressive biological activity of the immunoglobulins and complement in the mesangium. It is known that normal rodents develop mesangial immunoglobulin and complement deposition with aging (Mauer *et al.*, 1972b; Guttman *et al.*, 1967; Steblay and Rudofsky, 1971). Further, it is known that certain proteinuric states are associated with increased mesangial uptake of injected and endogenous macromolecules (Mauer *et al.*, 1972a, Mauer *et al.* 1974a, Hoyer *et al.*, 1975). Since diabetic rats are known to have albuminuria at an early stage of their disease (Mauer *et al.*, 1978b), it is possible that the increased mesangial IgG, IgM, and C3 in these animals is related to their proteinuric state. The relationship of mesangial macromolecular uptake and processing to alterations in glomerular pressure–flow characteristics is incompletely understood (see Chapter 2). However, it is possible that alterations in these characteristics, known to occur in diabetic rats, may be important in the genesis of the immunohistochemical abnormalities. Whether the alterations in glomerular microcirculatory hemodynamics could explain both the proteinuria and the immunofluorescent findings in diabetic rats require further study.

In order to examine mesangial function in diabetic rats, these animals and appropriate controls were injected with colloidal carbon and studied, using the methods of Elema *et al.* (1976). The uptake and processing of this macromolecule with sequential renal biopsies were performed over an 8-week period. These studies allowed assessment of mesangial uptake of carbon and of mesangial transit of this macromolecule through the glomerular hilum to the extraglomerular portion of the mesangium (the lasis area). These studies, performed according to the methods of Elema *et al.* (1976), detected no overall quantitative differences in the mesangial uptake and processing of colloidal carbon in diabetic as compared to control rats. However, striking qualitative differences were noted in those animals with early diabetic glomerulopathy. There was a marked accumulation of colloidal carbon precisely in those areas of the mesangium thickened by the diabetic process. Further, the carbon in these thickened areas persisted in high concentrations for the 8-week duration of the study. In contrast, areas of the mesangium of these diabetic animals not yet thickened by the diabetic state, processed the carbon normally. These results suggest that mesangial dysfunction in macromolecular processing in diabetic rats is the consequence of pathological changes in the mesangium rather than the converse. This is the first demonstration in animals of a pathological process which is capable of interfering with mesangial molecular clearance mechanisms. These observations could have relevance to other forms of mesangial injury in that mesangial damage may lead to alterations in mesangial function which may predispose to further mesangial injury, and ultimately leading to destruction of this area of the glomerulus.

Present technology does not allow precise quantitation of the relative contribution of mesangial cell phagocytosis as compared with "regurgitation" into the circulation or traffic via the stalk of the glomerulus in the ultimate processing of macromolecules which have entered the mesangium from the circulation. Of these three possibilities, only the first and last have been documented. Recently, Imposil, an iron-dextran complex, has been demonstrated in mice to course rapidly through intercellular mesangial channels to the area of the juxtaglomerular apparatus and thence into the distal tubule at the level of the macula densa (Leiper *et al.*, 1977). This phenomenon to date has not been documented in other species including man and thus its importance remains open to question. The immunohistochemical studies of genetically diabetic mice support the concept that the distal tubular route plays a role in the egress of macromolecules from the mesangium. These animals, within 2 to 4 months of onset of diabetes, developed markedly increased mesangial IgG, IgM, and C3 localization which extended into the axial region of the glomerulus and into the distal tubule. This finding, uniform in all glomeruli sectioned through the juxtaglomerular apparatus, probably represents the first demonstration of endogenous proteins processed via the mesangium by this route. One could speculate that the failure to demonstrate this mechanism in species other than the mouse suggests that in the mouse, the degradation of protein macromolecules by distal tubular cells represents the rate-limiting step in the mesangial transport system.

3. *Reversibility of Mesangial Lesions of Diabetes in Animals*

As noted above, there are striking similarities in the glomerulopathy of diabetes in the rat, mouse, dog, monkey, and man. Therefore, it is postulated that diabetic glomerulopathy results from the metabolic perturbations of the diabetic state and from their physical and chemical consequences. It is theorized that species differences in the pathological expression of diabetic glomerulopathy probably result from differences in tissue responses to these abnormalities rather than to differences in the fundamental pathogenetic mechanisms. The strongest evidence to date that diabetic nephropathy in man is secondary to the disturbed diabetic environment is the development of all the typical and diagnostic pathological changes of diabetes in normal kidneys transplanted into diabetic humans (Mauer *et al.*, 1976a,b). Similar observations have been made in normal kidneys transplanted into diabetic rats (Lee *et al.*, 1974). Further, it has been shown that kidneys from diabetic rats transplanted into normal animals show striking improvement in mesangial lesions (Lee *et al.*, 1974). These studies have been extended in observations of rats cured of their diabetic state by islet tissue transplantation (Mauer *et al.*, 1974b; McMillan, 1975). As seen in Fig. 1, islet transplantation results in normoglycemia and normal nonfasting insulin levels within 2

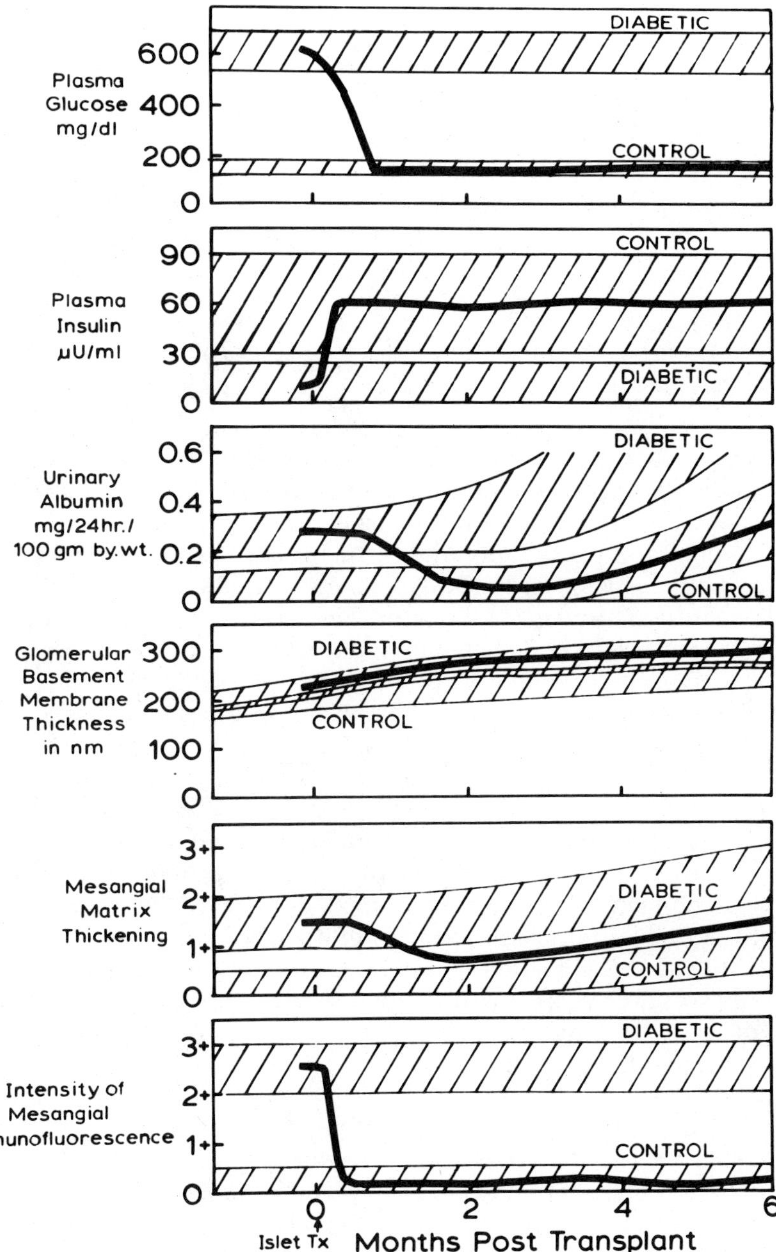

Figure 1. Effects of pancreatic islet transplantation on various parameters of glomerular structure and function in diabetic rats.

weeks. Mesangial matrix thickening returns rapidly towards normal but minimal residual thickening remains. The increased mesangial immunoglobulin and complement localization completely normalizes following islet transplantation. Thus, abnormalities in mesangial structure secondary to the disordered metabolic environment of the diabetic animal are, in large measure, reversible when diabetes is cured at a relatively early stage of the pathologic process. Whether the advanced lesions of the mesangium seen in rats with more long-term diabetes are reversible is unknown but, intuitively, one would not expect mesangial sclerosis to be amenable to therapeutic manipulation.

4. Glomerular Capillary Permeability and GBM Thickening in Diabetic Rats

Rats diabetic for 7 and 12 months have GBM thickness which is respectively about 10 and 20% greater than that in age-matched controls (Mauer, Brown, and Steffes, unpublished observations). Rats receiving successful islet tissue transplants after 7 months of diabetes and evaluated 5 months posttransplant had GBM thickness virtually identical to that of rats with 12 months of untreated diabetes (Fig. 1). These results suggest that the GBM abnormalities of diabetes are uninfluenced by islet transplantation. However, this interpretation must be tempered by the preliminary findings that diabetic rats have increased glomerular volumes which are normalized by islet transplantation (Mauer, Brown, and Steffes, unpublished observations). Thus, only when GBM mass in glomeruli of treated and of untreated diabetic rats is compared can the influence of treatment on diabetic GBM thickening be precisely established. Finally, it is important to consider that GBM turnover in the rat may be slow. Thus, the failure to find that islet transplantation has a significant influence upon GBM thickness during the 5-month period of these studies may reflect GBM turnover rate.

GBM biochemistry in diabetes remains a confused. The relevant controversy is beyond the scope of this paper. The reader is referred to studies in which differing findings and conclusions are reached (Spiro, 1976; Westberg and Michael, 1973; Kefalides, 1974; R. G. Spiro and Spiro, 1971; M. J. Spiro and Spiro, 1971; Risteli *et al.*, 1976; Cohen and Voght, 1971; Khalifa and Cohen, 1975; Wahl *et al.*, 1973; Beisswenger, 1976). For the present review it is sufficient to note that evidence that the machinery for basement membrane synthesis is increased in diabetic rats (Spiro, 1976) must be reevaluated in terms of the information referred to above. The diabetic rat glomerulus is increasing in size at a rate exceeding that of normal animals. Until increased rates of glomerular enlargement due to conditions other than diabetes such as compensatory hypertrophy are examined, data regarding levels of enzymes involved in GBM synthesis in diabetic animals must be considered uncontrolled and nonspecific.

5. *Glomerular Hemodynamics and the Development of Diabetic Nephropathy*

Ditzel (1976) has argued that alterations in microvascular flow–pressure relationships play a role in the development of the secondary complications of diabetes. He has demonstrated reduced P50 values in diabetic patients, based presumably upon increased levels of hemoglobin A_1C and disordered phosphate metabolism. He reasoned that this results in autoregulatory local tissue vasodilatation and increased tissue perfusion. Further, increased plasma viscosity (McMillan, 1976) and decreased red blood cell deformability both in diabetic animals (McMillan *et al.*, 1978) and in man (Schmid-Schönbein and Vogler, 1976; McMillan *et al.*, 1978) could contribute to the need for increased capillary pressures to achieve adequate microcirculatory flow. Mogensen (1976) has documented increased kidney size, glomerular filtration rate (GFR), and filtration fraction in juvenile diabetics and has interpreted this to represent increased glomerular filtration pressures. Gärtner (1978) has shown increased total kidney GFR without increased renal plasma flow in genetically diabetic mice. Hostetter *et al.* (1978) and Azar (personal communication) have found increased transcapillary hydraulic pressures in direct measurements in the capillaries of superficial glomeruli in diabetic Munich-Wistar rats. Evidence is accumulating to support the concept that alterations in glomerular hemodynamics exist in diabetic animals and in man. Experiments were performed to test the hypothesis that these hemodynamic forces could influence the rate at which the glomerular lesions of diabetes develop in animals.

Unilateral nephrectomy, which causes increased glomerular capillary blood flows and pressures (Azar *et al.*, 1977), accelerated the development of glomerulopathy in diabetic rats while it produced no significant pathologic changes in nondiabetic uninephrectomized animals studied over the same time period (Scheinman *et al.*, 1978; Steffes *et al.*, 1978). Hypertensive diabetic rats with two-kidney Goldblatt hypertension developed accelerated diabetic glomerulopathy in the unclipped kidney while the clipped kidney, protected from hypertension, was relatively protected from diabetic glomerulopathy as compared with the normotensive diabetic animals (Mauer *et al.*, 1978a). How hemodynamic changes in glomeruli of diabetic animals and of man combine with the diabetic state to influence the rate of development of diabetic glomerulopathy remains unknown. The finding that hypertension increases and contralateral renal artery narrowing diminishes the mesangial localization of IgG, IgM, and C3 indicates that the localization of these immune reactants in diabetic rats is hemodynamically dependent, at least in part. It is known that renal artery narrowing decreases (Germuth *et al.*, 1967) and elevation of blood pressure increases (Wilens and Henderson, 1965) immune complex localization within the glomerulus. Thus, pressure–flow relationships within glomerular capillaries appear to have marked influences upon the transport of circulating macromolecules from the lumen of the glomerular capillary into the glomerular filter system and the mesangium.

References

Azar, S., Johnson, M. A., Hertel, B., and Tobian, L., 1977, Single-nephron pressures, flow and resistances in hypertensive kidneys with nephrosclerosis, *Kidney Int.* **12:**28.

Beisswenger, P. J., 1976, Glomerular basement membrane: Biosynthesis and chemical composition in the streptozotocin diabetic rat, *J. Clin. Invest.* **58:**844.

Bell, E. T., 1952, A postmortem study of vascular disease in diabetes, *Arch. Pathol.* **53:**444.

Bloodworth, J. M. B., Jr., 1965, Experimental diabetic glomerulosclerosis. II. The dog, *Arch. Pathol.* **79:**113.

Bloodworth, J. M. B., Jr., Engerman, R. L., and Powers, K. L., 1969, Experimental diabetic microangiopathy. 1. Basement membrane statistics in the dog, *Diabetes* **18:**455.

Bloodworth, J. M. B., Jr., Engerman, R. L., and Anderson, P. J., 1973, Microangiopathy in the experimentally diabetic animal, in: *Vascular and Neurological Changes in Early Diabetes* (R. A. Camerini-Dávalos and H. S. Cole, eds.), pp. 245–250, Academic Press, New York.

Burkholder, P. M., 1965, Immunohistopathologic study of localized plasma proteins and fixation of guinea pig complement in renal lesions of diabetic glomerulosclerosis, *Diabetes* **14:**755.

Cohen, M. P., and Voght, C., 1971, Evidence for enhanced basement membrane synthesis and lysine hydroxylation in renal glomerulus in experimental diabetes, *Biochem. Biophys. Res. Commun.* **49:**1542.

Ditzel, J., 1976, Oxygen transport impairment in diabetes, *Diabetes* **25**(Suppl. 2)**:**832.

Elema, J. D., Hoyer, J. R., and Vernier, R. L., 1976, The glomerular mesangium: Uptake of intravenously injected colloidal carbon, *Kidney Int.* **9:**395.

Gärtner, K., 1978, Glomerular hyperfiltration during the onset of diabetes mellitus in two strains of diabetic mice (C57BL/6J *db*/*db* and C57BL/KsJ *db*/*db*), *Diabetologia* **15:**59.

Germuth, F. G., Jr., Keleman, W. A., and Pollack, A. D., 1967, Immune complex disease. II. The role of circulatory dynamics and glomerular filtration in the development of experimental glomerulonephritis, *Johns Hopkins Med. J.* **120:**252.

Guttman, P. H., Wuepper, K. D., and Fudenberg, H. H., 1967, On the presence of gamma G and beta-1C globulins in the renal glomeruli of aging and neonatally X-irradiated mice, *Vox Sang.* **12:**329.

Hägg, E., 1974a, Glomerular basement membrane thickening in rats with long-term alloxan diabetes: A quantitative electron microscopic study, *Acta Pathol. Microbiol. Scand.* **82:**211.

Hägg, E., 1974b, Occurrence of immunoglobulin and complement in the glomeruli of rats with long-term alloxan diabetes, *Acta Pathol. Microbiol. Scand.* **82:**220.

Heptinstall, R. H., 1974, *Pathology of the Kidney*, Little, Brown, Boston.

Hostetter, T. H., Troy, J. L., and Brenner, B. M., 1978, Glomerular dynamics in rats with diabetes mellitus, *Proc. Am. Soc. Nephrol. Abstr.* 91A.

Hoyer, J. R., Mauer, S. M., and Michael, A. F., 1975, Unilateral renal disease in the rat. I. Clinical, morphologic, and glomerular mesangial functional features of the experimental model produced by renal perfusion with aminonucleoside, *J. Lab. Clin. Med.* **85:**756.

Kefalides, N. A., 1974, Biochemical properties of human glomerular basement membrane in normal and diabetic kidneys, *J. Clin. Invest.* **53:**403.

Khalifa, A., and Cohen, M. P., 1975, Glomerular protocollagen lysyl-hydroxylase activity in streptozotocin diabetes, *Biochim. Biophys. Acta* **386:**332.

Kimmelstiel, P., 1968, Diabetic nephropathy, in: *Structural Basis of Renal Disease* (E. L. Becker, ed.), pp. 468–484, Harper & Row, New York.

Lee, C. S., Mauer, S. M., Brown, D. M., Sutherland, D. E. R., Michael, A. F., and Najarian, J. S., 1974, Renal transplantation in diabetes mellitus in rats, *J. Exp. Med.* **139:**793.

Leiper, J. M., Thomson, D., and MacDonald, M. K., 1977, Uptake and transport of imposil by the glomerular mesangium in the mouse, *Lab. Invest.* **37:**526.

McMillan, D. E., 1975, Deterioration of the microcirculation in diabetes, *Diabetes* **24:**944.

McMillan, D. E., 1976, Plasma protein changes, blood viscosity and diabetic microangiopathy, *Diabetes* **25**(Suppl. 2)**:**858.

McMillan, D. E., Utterback, N. G., and LaPuma, J., 1978, Reduced erythrocyte deformability in diabetes, *Diabetes* **27:**895.

Mauer, S. M., Fish, A. J., Blau, E. B., and Michael, A. F., 1972a, The glomerular mesangium. I. Kinetic studies of macromolecular uptake in normal and nephrotic rats, *J. Clin. Invest.* **51**:1092.

Mauer, S. M., Michael, A. F., Fish, A. J., and Brown, D. M., 1972b, Spontaneous immunoglobulin and complement deposition in glomeruli of diabetic rats, *Lab. Invest.* **25**:488.

Mauer, S. M., Fish, A. J., Day, N., and Michael, A. F., 1974a, The glomerular mesangium. II. Studies of macromolecular uptake in nephrotoxic nephritis in rats, *J. Clin. Invest.* **53**:431.

Mauer, S. M., Sutherland, D. E. R., Steffes, M. W., Leonard, R. J., Najarian, J. S., Michael, A. F., and Brown, D. M., 1974b, Pancreatic islet transplantation: Effects on the glomerular lesions of experimental diabetes in the rat, *Diabetes* **23**:748.

Mauer, S. M., Barbosa, J., Vernier, R. L., Kjellstrand, C. M., Buselmeier, T. J., Simmons, R. L., Najarian, J. S., and Goetz, F. C., 1976a, Development of diabetic vascular lesions in normal kidneys transplanted into patients with diabetes mellitus, *N. Engl. J. Med.* **295**:916.

Mauer, S. M., Miller, K., Goetz, F. C., Barbosa, J., Simmons, R. L., Najarian, J. S., and Michael, A. F., 1976b, Immunopathology of renal extracellular membranes in kidneys transplanted into patients with diabetes mellitus, *Diabetes* **25**:709.

Mauer, S. M., Steffes, M. W., Azar, S., Kupcho-Sandberg, S., and Brown, D. M., 1978a, The effects of Goldblatt hypertension on the development of glomerular lesions of diabetes mellitus in the rat, *Diabetes* **27**:738.

Mauer, S. M., Brown, D. M., Matas, A. J., and Steffes, M. W., 1978b, Effects of pancreatic islet transplantation on the increased urinary albumin excretion rates in intact and uninephrectomized rats with diabetes mellitus, *Diabetes* **27**:959.

Miller, K., and Michael, A. F., 1976, Immunopathology of renal extracellular membranes in diabetes mellitus: Specificity of tubular basement membrane immunofluorescence, *Diabetes* **25**:701.

Mogensen, C. E., 1976, Renal function changes in diabetes, *Diabetes* **25**(Suppl. 2)**:**872.

Østerby, R., 1972, Morphometric studies of the peripheral glomerular basement membrane in early juvenile onset diabetes. 1. Development of initial basement membrane thickening, *Diabetologia* **8**:84.

Risteli, J., Koivisto, V. A., Åkerblom, H. K., and Kivirikko, K. I., 1976, Intracellular enzymes of collagen biosynthesis in rat kidney in streptozotocin diabetes, *Diabetes* **25**:1066.

Scheinman, J. I., Fish, A. J., and Michael, A. F., 1974, The immunohistopathology of glomerular antigens: The glomerular basement membrane, collagen and actomyosin antigens in normal and diseased kidneys, *J. Clin. Invest.* **54**:1144.

Scheinman, J. I., Steffes, M. W., Brown, D. M., and Mauer, S. M., 1978, The immunohistopathology of glomerular antigens. III. Increased mesangial actomyosin in experimental diabetes in the rat, *Diabetes* **27**:632.

Schmid-Schönbein, H., and Vogler, E., 1976, Red-cell aggregation and deformability in diabetes, *Diabetes* **25**(Suppl. 2)**:**897.

Spiro, M. J., and Spiro, R. G., 1971, Studies on the biosynthesis of the hydroxylysine-linked disaccharide unit of basement membrane and collagens. 1. Kidney glucosyltransferase, *J. Biol. Chem.* **246**:4899.

Spiro, R. G., 1976, Search for a biochemical basis of diabetic microangiopathy, *Diabetologia* **12**:1.

Spiro, R. G., and Spiro, M. J., 1971, Effect of diabetes on the biosynthesis of the renal glomerular basement membrane: Studies on the glucosyltransferase, *Diabetes* **20**:641.

Steblay, R. W., and Rudofsky, U., 1971, Spontaneous renal lesions and glomerular deposits of IgG and complement in the guinea pig, *J. Immunol.* **107**:1192.

Steffes, M. W., Brown, D. M., and Mauer, S. M., 1978, Diabetic glomerulopathy following unilateral nephrectomy in the rat, *Diabetes* **27**:35.

Wahl, R., Deppermann, D., Descher, W., Fuchs, E., and Rexroth, W., 1973, The metabolism of the isolated renal glomerulus and its basement membranes, in: *Vascular and Neurological Changes in Early Diabetes* (R. A. Camerini-Dávalos and H. S. Cole, eds.), pp. 147–153, Academic Press, New York.

Warren, S., Le Compte, P. M., and Legg, M. A., 1966, *The Pathology of Diabetes*, Lea & Febiger, Philadelphia.

Wehner, H., Höhn, O., Faix-Schade, U., Huber, H., and Walzer, P., 1972, Glomerular changes in mice with spontaneous hereditary diabetes, *Lab. Invest.* **27:**331.
Westberg, N. G., and Michael, A. F., 1973, Human glomerular basement membrane: Chemical composition in diabetes mellitus, *Acta Med. Scand.* **194:**39.
Wilens, S. L., and Henderson, D., 1965, Glomerulonephritis in pressor drug-enhanced serum sickness in rabbits, *Proc. Soc. Exp. Biol. Med.* **120:**866.

13

Characterization of Rat Glomerular Cells in Vitro

Jeffrey I. Kreisberg and Morris J. Karnovsky

1. Introduction

The renal glomerulus contains at least three cell types: endothelial cells, glomerular epithelial cells (GEC), and mesangial cells. The endothelial cell which lines the glomerular capillary wall is characterized by the presence of fenestrae approximately 1000 Å in diameter. The role that these cells play in glomerular function is not clear. However, studies by Ryan and Karnovsky (1976) demonstrate that under good flow conditions in the rat, plasma albumin and IgG molecules do not penetrate significantly beyond the fenestrae. This suggests that this layer may participate in the restriction of macromolecular passage across the glomerular capillary wall. GEC display multiple foot processes (podocytes) applied to the outside of the glomerular basement membrane (GBM). GEC have several functions attributed to them: (1) they participate in the synthesis of the GBM (Kurtz and Feldman, 1962; Walker, 1973); (2) they participate in the filtration process through pinocytosis of filtered proteins that may have leaked through the GBM (Farquhar, 1975); and (3) they participate in the filtration process by exerting an influence upon water flux during ultrafiltration (Ryan and Karnovsky, 1975). Since is has been demonstrated that intrinsic negatively charged glycoproteins in the filtration barrier are important in restricting the passage of anionic macromolecules across the GBM (Chang *et al.*, 1975; Rennke *et al.*, 1975), the highly charged cell coat of the podocytes may participate in this effect. The mesangial cell may have several functions: (1) the clearing of debris from the mesangial region by phagocytosis (Farquhar and Palade, 1961, 1962); (2) the regulation of glomerular size and blood flow by contractility,

---

Jeffrey I. Kreisberg and Morris J. Karnovsky · Department of Pathology, Harvard Medical School, Boston, Massachusetts 02115. This investigation was supported by NIH Grant AM 13132.

since it contains myofibrillar bundles; and (3) a source of renin, since under certain physiological conditions, mesangial cells have the ability to develop granules similar to juxtaglomerular (JG) cells (Dunihue and Boldesser, 1963). Isolation and characterization of homogeneous populations of glomerular cells would aid in the study of their normal metabolism as well as their altered metabolism in disease states.

Previously, Camazine *et al.* (1976) reported the isolation and characterization of a phagocytic cell from the mesangium of the rat glomerulus. These cells also were strongly adherent to glass, developed C3 and Fc receptors after 24 hr in culture, but could not be maintained *in vitro.*

In the present study, three additional and distinct cell types from rat glomeruli have been isolated and maintained in culture. One cell type has been characterized as the GEC (Kreisberg *et al.*, 1978a). The second cell type has not been completely characterized, although it contains many bundles of microfilaments. The third cell type contains renin (Kreisberg *et al.*, 1978b). Since only 4% of the glomeruli isolated in this study contain vascular poles, it is suggested that these renin-producing cells normally populate the glomerulus. None of these cell types are phagocytic *in vitro.*

2. Materials and Methods

2.1. Culture of Whole Glomeruli and Dissociated Glomerular Cells

Glomeruli were isolated from male CD (The Charles River Breeding Laboratories, Wilmington, Mass.) rat kidneys by using a graded sieving technique (Burlington and Cronkite, 1973). Aliquots of isolated glomeruli were examined by scanning electron microscopy (SEM). The procedure employed for isolating homogeneous populations of glomerular cells has been described in great detail in a previous report (Kreisberg *et al.*, 1978a). Briefly, glomeruli were either plated directly on Falcon Tissue Culture Dishes (Falcon Plastics, Oxnard, Calif.) for outgrowths of cells, or dissociated in 0.2% trypsin (12,700 BAEE units/mg; Sigma Chemical Co.) and 0.01% deoxyribonuclease (1115 Kientz units/mg protein, Sigma Chemical Co.) in HSS at 37°C for 30 min. Before plating, dissociated glomerular cells were filtered through 10-μm Nitex (TETKO, Elsmford, N.Y.) to remove any intact glomeruli. Primary cultures from outgrowths of whole glomeruli were filtered through 10-μm Nitex (TETKO) to remove glomeruli, and dissociated glomerular cells were plated for cloning at 4000 cells per 100 cm^2 Falcon Tissue Culture Dish (Falcon Plastics). The tissue culture medium (RIC) used in this study was RPMI 1640 medium (Microbiological Associates, Bethesda, Md.) buffered with 15 mM Hepes buffer (Sigma Chemical Co.), pH 7.4, supplemented with 20% fetal calf serum (FCS), diluted in half with conditioned medium (CM) with 0.66 unit/ml insulin (Eli Lilly, Indianapolis, Ind.). The RIC medium contained 100 units of penicillin and 100 μG of streptomycin per milliliter. CM was prepared from Swiss 3T3 cells in log-phase growth maintained in Dulbecco's modified minimum essential medium (DMEM) (Microbiological Associates) with 10% FCS for 24 hr. The CM was removed and filtered through 0.22-μm Millipore filters (Millipore Corp., Bedford, Mass.) before use. Clones were randomly isolated with pennicylinders, and passaged with 0.025% trypsin–0.5 mM EDTA in Ca^{2+}/Mg^{2+}-free buffered salt solution (trypsin–versene) into Costar multiwell plates (Costar, Cambridge, Mass.) in RIC. All cells were tested for fibroblast contamination by their ability to grow in RPMI 1640 containing 20% dialyzed FCS and D-valine substituted for L-valine (Gilbert and Migeon, 1975). Fibroblasts do not grow in D-valine-containing media.

2.2. *Morphological Studies*

Transmission electron microscopy was performed on all cloned cell types by usual techniques. SEM was performed on isolated glomerular preparations to determine the percentage of glomeruli with capsules intact and the degree of contamination with tubules. SEM also was performed on cloned cell types. Isolated glomeruli were fixed in suspension in 2% glutaraldehyde in HSS, pH 7.2, washed twice in HSS, and lightly suctioned onto silver membranes (Selas Flotronics, Spring House, Pa.) which had been coated with poly-L-lysine (1 mg/ml) (Sigma Chemical Co.). Cloned cell types were allowed to settle on coverslips which had been cleaned previously by boiling for 2 hr in detergent solution (7X) (Linbro Scientific, Hamden, Conn.) and then washed thoroughly with distilled water. Coverslips with cells attached were fixed in 2% glutaraldehyde in 0.1 M phosphate buffer, pH 7.2, for 1 hr at room temperature, and washed in buffer overnight. Both silver membranes with fixed glomeruli and coverslips with cells were postfixed in 1% osmium tetroxide for 30 min at 4°C, and prepared for SEM by routine methods.

2.3. *Immunological Studies*

2.3.1. *Immunocytochemistry*

Rabbit antiserum to rat antihemophilic factor (Factor VIII) was supplied by Drs. Roger E. Benson and W. Jean Dodds (Benson and Dodds, 1976a,b). Reactivity of this antiserum to rat glomerular and vascular endothelium was verified by indirect immunofluorescence on rat frozen sections (Booyse *et al.*, 1975). Dissociated cells were tested for the presence of Factor VIII 6 days after plating, and cloned cell types were tested also.

2.3.2. *Receptors for Immunoglobulin and Complement (Rosette Formation)*

These studies were performed on rat glomerular cells maintained in tissue culture for 2 months. To identify Fc receptors, the glomerular cells were incubated at room temperature for 30 min with a suspension of sheep red blood cells (SRBC) (Colorado Serum Co., Denver, Colo.) which had been coated with a subagglutinating amount of rabbit IgM antibody to SRBC (1:200 dilution) (Becker and Benacerraf, 1966). To identify C3 receptors, glomerular cells were incubated at room temperature for 30 min with a suspension of SRBC which had been treated first with a subagglutinating amount of rabbit IgM antibody to SRBC (Cordis Laboratories, Miami, Fla.) and second with C5-deficient mouse serum (from A/St mice) (Lay and Nussenzweig, 1968). Preparations were examined for the presence of rosettes by phase microscopy and SEM.

2.4. *Phagocytosis in Vitro*

Rat glomerular cells maintained in tissue culture were exposed to polystyrene spherules (1.1-μm diameter; Dow Chemical U.S.A., Midland, Mich.), zymosan (Nutritional Biochemicals Corp., Cleveland, Ohio), ferritin 2× crystalline, cadmium free (Nutritional Biochemicals Corp.), and carbon (Gunther Wagner, Hanover, Germany) in RIC. Dissociated cells were tested for phagocytosis 6 days after plating, and cloned cell types also were tested. Phagocytosis was assumed by phase contrast and transmission electron microscopy.

2.5. *Renin Determinations*

Angiotensin I generation from sonicated and from unsonicated cell preparations was measured by a radioimmunoassay technique (Clinical Assays, Cambridge, Mass.) (Haber *et al.*, 1969). One milliliter of 10^6 unsonicated and sonicated cells was incubated with renin substrate in maleate buffer, pH 6.0, containing phenylmethylsulfonyl fluoride, to inhibit conversion and degradation of angiotension I, at 37°C for 90 min.

2.6. *Studies with Aminonucleoside of Puromycin (AMNS)*

Confluent monolayers of the different cloned cell types were treated with 0.1, 1.0, 10, and 100 μg/ml of AMNS in RIC for 24 hr and the percentage of cells detaching from the monolayer was determined. Control monolayers were maintained in RIC alone.

2.7. *Studies with Nephrotoxic Serum*

An homogenate of rat kidney cortex was washed in phosphate-buffered saline (PBS), resuspended in distilled water, and lyophilized. Rabbits were given a total of 25 mg of this antigen in each foot pad, resuspended in 0.5 ml of PBS and mixed with 0.5 ml of Freund's complete adjuvant. Four weeks later, rabbits were given booster intraperitoneal injections of 100 mg of antigen in 2 ml of PBS, administered on 3 consecutive days. The animals were bled 7–9 days after the last injection. The serum was incubated at 56°C for 1 hr and absorbed with rat erythrocytes before use. Monolayers of the different cell types were treated with 1, 10, and 50 μl/ml nephrotoxic serum (NTS) in either RPMI 1640 (Microbiological Associates) medium containing heat (complement)-inactivated FCS or unheated FCS.

3. Results

3.1. Isolation of Glomeruli

SEM of glomerular preparations revealed that 85.0 ± 6.0% were free of capsules, 15.0 ± 5.0% contained capsules, and 3.0 ± 2.1% contained vascular poles. SEM also revealed very little contamination of the preparations with tubules. Two hundred glomeruli were evaluated in each isolation.

3.2. Culture of Cells from Whole Glomeruli and Dissociated Glomerular Cells

In a previous report, RIC was compared to other growth media. It was determined that with RIC as the tissue culture medium, glomeruli attached and cells could be seen growing out from them after 1 day in culture (Kreisberg *et al.*, 1978a). Attachment and growth of dissociated glomerular cells with RIC as the growth medium was far superior to all the other media previously tested. In addition, although encapsulated glomeruli attached to the flask, cells did not grow from them. Primary cell cultures from outgrowths of glomeruli and dissociated glomerular cells reached confluency after 1 week in culture, and clones established either from primary cultures of outgrowths of glomeruli or dissociated glomerular cells, became recognizable for cloning after 1 to 2 weeks in culture.

3.3. Characteristics of Isolated Cells

One cell type (cell type A) isolated by cloning was polygonal in shape by phase contrast microscopy and displayed a cobblestone appearance when confluency was reached. The doubling time of this cell was 15 hr. This cell has been characterized positively as the GEC (Kreisberg *et al.*, 1978a) because it has receptors for C3, but not for Fc, has cilia (Fig. 1), and forms junctions in culture. Also, AMNS and NTS at low concentrations are cytotoxic towards this cell (Table 1). NTS is cytotoxic to GEC within 1 hr at all doses tested whether in medium containing heat (complement)-inactivated FCS or unheated FCS (Table 1). Ultrastructurally, these cells bear a glycocalyx rich in sialic acid. Cell type B is a very large and flat cell by phase contrast microscopy. It has an average doubling time of 10 hr. Ultrastructurally, it contains many bundles of microfilaments (Fig. 2). This cell did not possess receptors for C3 or Fc nor did AMNS or NTS have any effect on it. The third cell type (cell C) isolated in this study was spindle-shaped and criss-crossed and underlapped each other in culture. This cell had an average doubling time of 19 hr. By transmission electron microscopy, it was found to contain numerous

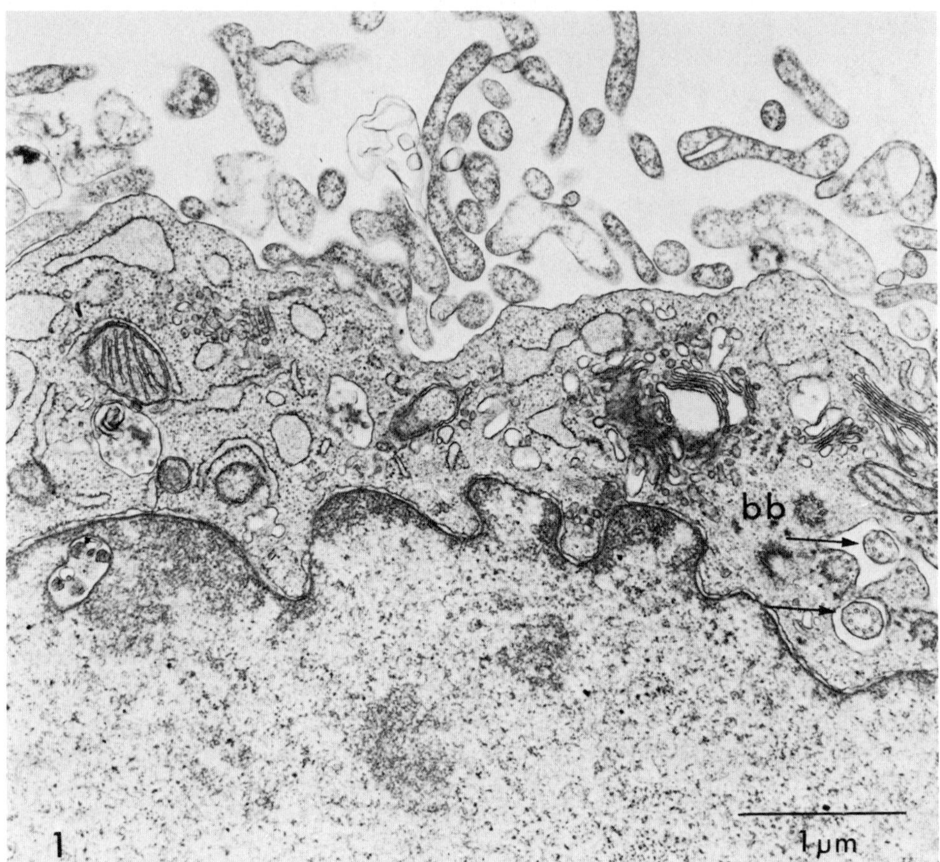

Figure 1. Transmission electron micrograph of a cultured glomerular epithelial cell. Note the two cilia in cross section (arrows). Also note the basal body (bb).

Table 1. Studies Performed on Purified Rat Glomerular Cells in Vitro

Cell type	AHF[a]	C3	Fc	Cilia	Growth in *D*-valine-substituted medium	Phagocytosis	Cytotoxicity with low doses of AMNS and NTS[b]	Renin[c]
GEC[d]	0	+	0	+	+	0	+	±
Cell with MF[e]	0	0	0	0	+	0	0	0
Renin cell	0	0	0	0	+	0	0	+

[a] AHF, antihemophilic factor.
[b] AMNS, aminonucleoside of puromycin; NTS, nephrotoxic serum.
[c] Renin cell, 2.1 ± 0.44; GEC, 0.45 ± 0.12; cell with MF, 0.09 ± 0.07 ng/10^6 cells.
[d] GEC, glomerular epithelial cell.
[e] MF, microfilaments.

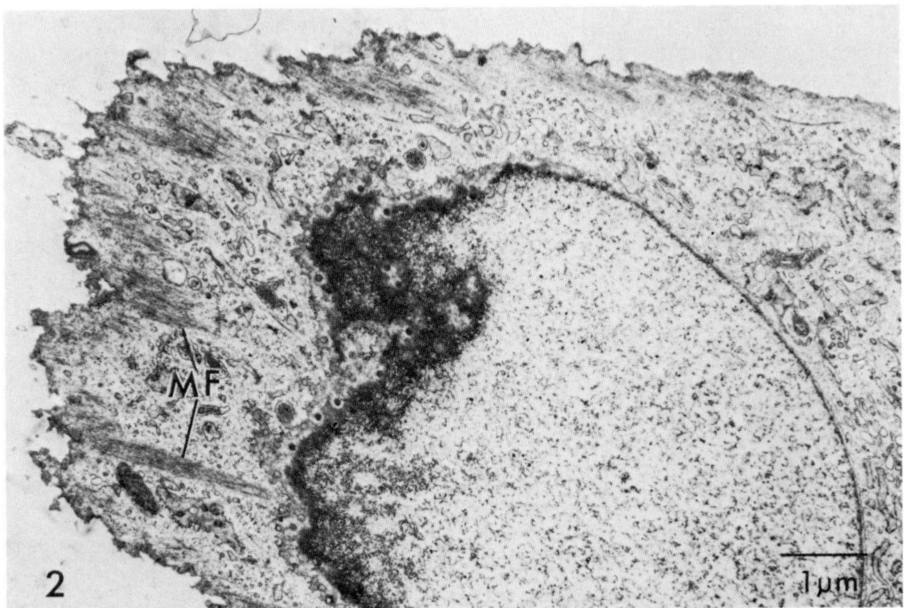

Figure 2. Transmission electron micrograph of a cultured cell that contains many bundles of microfilaments (MF).

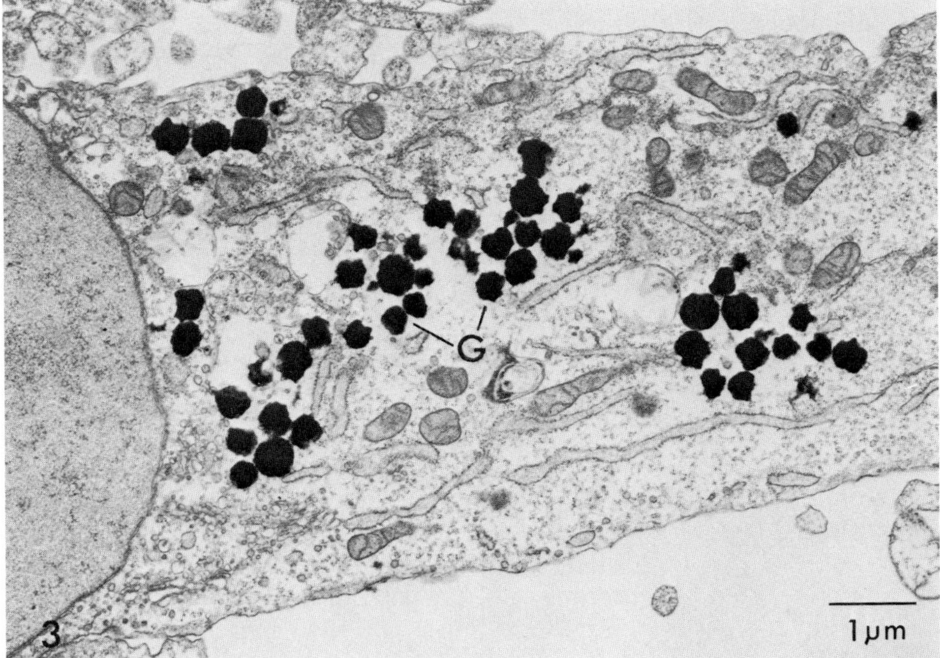

Figure 3. Transmission electron micrograph of a cultured renin cell. Note the presence of granules (G) in the cytoplasm.

electron-dense granules in its cytoplasm when fixed in 2% glutaraldehyde and stained with hafnium *en bloc* (Kreisberg and Karnovsky, unpublished data) or when fixed in a mixture of glutaraldehyde, osmium, and acrolein (Fig. 3). Cell type C did not possess C3 or Fc receptors and was not affected by AMNS or NTS in culture. However, extracts of these cells were able to convert angiotensinogen to angiotensin I, indicative of renin activity (Table I). As can also be seen in Table 1, the GEC had a small amount of renin activity. All three cell types isolated in this study grew in media containing D-valine and dialyzed FCS, indicating that they were not fibroblasts (Gilbert and Migeon, 1975). Furthermore, none of the cell types were able to phagocytose any of the particles tested, nor did any of the cells contain Factor VIII (Table 1). All three cell types have been maintained in culture for about 30 passages.

4. Discussion

In this study, three cell types were isolated from rat glomeruli. One of these cell types has been characterized as the GEC (Kreisberg *et al.*, 1978a). The presence of cilia on its surface, a characteristic of rat GEC *in situ* (Andrews and Porter, 1974; Andrews, 1975), and the cytotoxicity of the AMNS *in vitro* on GEC and not on other glomerular cells helped to identify it.

GEC injury has been observed in many human (Grisham and Ching, 1975; Cohen *et al.*, 1977) as well as in experimental glomerular disease (Andrews, 1977; Glasser *et al.*, 1977; Velosa *et al.*, 1977). AMNS administration in rats has been shown to cause GEC damage (Andrews, 1977; Glasser *et al.*, 1977; Velosa *et al.*, 1977). In this study, AMNS in low doses caused cell death to isolated GEC *in vitro*. NTS, which binds to the GBM when administered *in vivo* and causes proteinuria in two phases, injures GEC *in vitro* within 1 hr after its addition to the tissue culture medium. Mohos and Skoza (1969) observed a reduction in negative charge, demonstrated by reduced colloidal iron staining, in glomeruli that were treated with NTS *in situ*. They proposed that the nephritogenic antigen is a sialoprotein. Since GEC contain an abundant cell coat rich in sialic acid, NTS may be directed against the GEC. Binding of NTS to sialoproteins, which are also present in the GBM, may block negatively charged moieties or, alternatively, NTS or toxic substances may activate hydrolytic mechanisms of GEC. Loss of negative charge or alterations in sialic acid metabolism by GEC may lead to proteinuria.

It would be interesting to isolate glomerular endothelial cells and study their role in: (1) coagulation in glomerular disease; and (2) the renin–angiotensin system. Furthermore, it would be interesting to see whether or not isolated glomerular endothelial cells retain their fenestrae in culture. In addition, it may be possible to study the development of fenestrae *in vitro* with isolated glomerular endothelium. It is believed that none of the cell types isolated in this study are endothelium, since they did not possess Factor

VIII, a marker for endothelium *in situ* (Hoyer *et al.*, 1973; Jaffe *et al.*, 1973) and *in vitro* (Jaffe *et al.*, 1973; Booyse *et al.*, 1975). In the numerous studies that have been done on the isolation and culture of human and animal glomerular cells *in vitro* (Quadracci and Striker, 1970; Dechenne *et al.*, 1975; Camazine *et al.*, 1976; Scheinman *et al.*, 1976; Burkholder *et al.*, 1977; Scheinman and Fish, 1978), no one has been able to isolate and maintain glomerular endothelium in culture. This is probably due to the rather particular conditions (not available in this growth medium) that are required for growth by these highly differentiated fenestrated cells.

One of the cell types isolated in this study contained many bundles of microfilaments. Since mesangial cells contain microfilaments *in vivo* (Latta, 1973), one proposed function of these cells has been the control of glomerular size and blood flow by contractility. However, microfilaments have been found to exist in a variety of nonmuscle cells in culture (Lazarides and Weber, 1974; Pollack *et al.*, 1975; Fujiwara and Pollard, 1976) and therefore cannot be considered a specific marker for a particular cell type. Another proposed function of mesangial cells *in vivo* is phagocytosis of debris from the mesangium (Farquhar and Palade, 1961, 1962). None of these cell types are phagocytic *in vitro*. There are several explanations of why isolation of a phagocytic cell which could possibly be a mesangial cell has not been possible. (1) One or more of these cells may have been phagocytic *in vivo* and merely lost its ability to phagocytose in culture. (2) There may be more than one type of mesangial cell, i.e., one phagocytic and one not phagocytic *in vivo*. (3) Perhaps the function of the mesangial cell is something other than phagocytosis. The third explanation is most interesting. If the mesangial cell is not phagocytic, then perhaps cells such as the blood monocytes percolate through the mesangium to clear debris. In a previous report, a procedure was described that involved isolation of a phagocytic cell from rat glomeruli (Camazine *et al.*, 1976). These glomeruli were subjected to long enzymatic digestions. Cells that had adhered to glass overnight were examined morphologically. These cells that had adhered to glass were phagocytic, and had receptors for C3 and Fc. They had large indented nuclei, large nucleus/cytoplasm ratios, and by SEM these cells showed extensive foldings of the cell surface. Since macrophages have been shown to populate the normal human glomerulus and are able to migrate from the glomerulus (Thomson *et al.*, 1978), it is believed that the phagocytic cell isolated in this laboratory is a blood-derived monocyte that travels into and out of the mesangium to remove debris.

Direct evidence that renin was concentrated in the vascular pole of the glomerulus was provided by the studies of Bing and Kazimierczak (1960) and Cook and Pickering (1959). Edelman and Hartroft (1961) found a correlation between the degree of granulation of rabbit JG cells, immunofluorescent staining with fluorescein-labeled anti-hog renin, and renin content. However, it appears that granulated cells are not limited to the JG apparatus. Barajas (1970) found that granulated as well as agranular cells entered the glomerulus and became continuous with the glomerular mesangial cell.

Dunihue and Boldesser (1963) observed in bilaterally adrenalectomized cats that glomerular mesangial cells underwent hypertrophy and hyperplasia, and developed cytoplasmic granules similar to those of the JG cells. Since only 3% of the glomeruli isolated in this study had vascular poles attached, it is believed that the isolated renin cells described in this report are populating the glomerulus. Isolation of pure renin-producing cells, in which hemodynamic, tubular, and extrarenal influences are removed, could aid in improved understanding of the action of various stimuli on renin release.

5. Summary

Three cell types from rat glomeruli have been isolated by cloning, and growing in culture. One cell type is the GEC: it has cilia on its surface, possesses receptors for C3, and is injured when cultured in the presence of AMNS (Kreisberg *et al.*, 1978a) and NTS. The second cell type contains renin. Currently a search is under way for specific markers for the remaining unidentified cell type, which may, however, be a contractile (mesangial) cell, as judged by its morphology. In addition, a phagocytic cell has been isolated from the mesangium (Camazine *et al.*, 1976), earlier.

ACKNOWLEDGMENTS. We would like to thank Dr. Roger E. Benson and Dr. W. Jean Dodds for the preparation and gift of the anti-Factor VIII antibody. Their work was supported by NIH Grant HL 09902. We would also like to thank Dr. Walter Flamenbaum for his assistance in performing the renin radioimmunoassays. The assistance of Amy Rehfield, Robert Rubin, and Kay Cosgrove is greatly appreciated.

References

Andrews, P. M., 1975, Scanning electron microscopy of human and rheus monkey kidneys, *Lab. Invest.* **32:**610.

Andrews, P. M., 1977, A scanning and transmission electron microscopic comparison of puromycin aminonucleoside-induced nephrosis to hyperalbuminemia-induced proteinuria with emphasis on kidney podocyte pedical loss, *Lab. Invest.* **36:**183.

Andrews, P. M., and Porter, R., 1974, A scanning electron microscopic study of the nephron, *Am. J. Anat.* **140:**81.

Barajas, L., 1970, The ultrastructure of the juxtaglomerular apparatus as disclosed by three dimensional reconstructions from serial sections: The anatomical relationship between the tubular and vascular components, *J. Ultrastruct. Res.* **33:**116.

Becker, A., and Benacerraf, B., 1966, Properties of antibodies cytophilic for macrophages, *J. Exp. Med.* **123:**119.

Benson, R. E., and Dodds, W. J., 1976a, Physical relationship between canine factor VIII coagulant activity and factor VIII related antigen, *Proc. Soc. Exp. Biol. Med.* **153:**339.

Benson, R. E., and Dodds, W. J., 1976b, Immunologic characterization of canine factor VIII, *Blood* **48:**521.

Bing, J., and Kazimierczak, J., 1960, Renin content of different parts of the periglomerular circumference, *Acta Pathol. Microbiol. Scand.* **50:**1.

Booyse, F. M., Sedlak, B. J., and Rafelson, M. E., 1975, Culture of arterial endothelial cells: Characterization and growth of bovine aortic cells, *Thromb. Diath. Haemorrh.* **35:**825.

Burkholder, P. M., Oberley, T. D., Barber, T. A., Beacom, A., and Koehler, C., 1977, Immune adherence in renal glomeruli: Complement receptor sites on glomerular capillary epithelial cells, *Am. J. Pathol.* **76:**635.

Burlington, H., and Cronkite, E. P., 1973, Characteristics of cell cultures derived from renal glomeruli, *Proc. Soc. Exp. Biol. Med.* **142:**143.

Camazine, S. M., Ryan, G. B., Unanue, E. R., and Karnovsky, M. J., 1976, Isolation of phagocytic cells from the rat renal glomerulus, *Lab. Invest.* **35:**315.

Chang, R. L. S., Robertson, C. R., Deen, W. M., and Brenner, B. M., 1975, Permselectivity of the glomerular capillary wall. III. Restricted transport of polyanions, *Kidney Int.* **8:**212.

Cohen, A. H., Mampaso, F., and Zamboni, L., 1977, Glomerular podocyte degeneration in human renal disease: An ultrastructural study, *Lab. Invest.* **37:**30.

Cook, W. F., and Pickering, G. W., 1959, The localization of renin in the rabbit kidney, *J. Physiol. (London)* **149:**526.

Dechenne, C., Foidart-Willems, J., and Mahieu, P. M., 1975, Ultrastructural studies on dog renal glomerular and tubular cells in culture, *J. Submicrosc. Cytol.* **7:**165.

Dunihue, F. W., and Boldesser, W. G., 1963, Observations on the similarity of mesangial to juxtaglomerular cells, *Lab. Invest.* **12:**1228.

Edelman, R., and Hartroft, P. M., 1961, Localization of renin in juxtaglomerular cells of rabbit and dog through the use of the fluorescent antibody technique, *Circ. Res.* **9:**1065.

Farquhar, M. G., 1975, The primary glomerular filtration barrier—basement membrane or epithelial cells?, *Kidney Int.* **8:**197.

Farquhar, M. G., and Palade, G. E., 1961, Glomerular permeability. II. Ferritin transfer across the glomerular capillary wall in nephrotic rats, *J. Exp. Med.* **114:**699.

Farquhar, M. G., and Palade, G. E., 1962, Functional evidence for the existence of a third cell type in the renal glomerulus: Phagocytosis of filtration residue by a "distinct" third cell, *J. Cell Biol.* **13:**55.

Fujiwara, K., and Pollard, T. D., 1976, Fluorescent antibody localization of myosin in the cytoplasm, cleavage furrow, and mitotic spindle of human cells, *J. Cell Biol.* **71:**848.

Gilbert, S. F., and Migeon, B. R., 1975, D-Valine as a selective agent for normal human and rodent epithelial cells in culture, *Cell* **5:**11.

Glasser, R. S., Velosa, J. A., and Michael, A. F., 1977, Experimental model of focal sclerosis. I. Relationship to protein excretion in aminonucleoside nephrosis, *Lab. Invest.* **36:**519.

Grisham, E., and Ching, J., 1975, Focal glomerular sclerosis in nephrotic patients: An electron microscopic study of glomerular podocytes, *Kidney Int.* **7:**111.

Haber, E., Koerner, T., Page, L. B., Kliman, B., and Purnode, A., 1969, Application of a radioimmunoassay for angiotensin I to the physiological measurements of plasma renin activity in normal human subjects, *J. Clin. Endocrinol. Metab.* **29:**1349.

Hoyer, L. W., De Los Santos, R. P., and Hoyer, J. R., 1973, Antihemophilic factor antigen: Localization in endothelial cells by immunofluorescent microscopy, *J. Clin. Invest.* **52:**2737.

Jaffe, E. A., Hoyer, L. W., and Nachman, R. L., 1973, Synthesis of antihemophilic factor antigen by cultured human endothelial cells, *J. Clin. Invest.* **52:**2757.

Kreisberg, J. I., Hoover, R. L., and Karnovsky, M. J., 1978a, Isolation and characterization of rat glomerular epithelial cells *in vitro, Kidney Int.* **14:**21.

Kreisberg, J. I., Karnovsky, M. J., Emmett, N. L., and Barger, A. C., 1978b, Isolation and culture of a "renin" containing cell from rat glomeruli, Abstracts, 7th International Congress of Nephrology, Montreal.

Kurtz, S. M., and Feldman, I. D., 1962, Experimental studies on the formation of the glomerular basement membrane, *J. Ultrastruct. Res.* **6:**19.

Latta, H., 1973, Ultrastructure of the glomerulus and juxtaglomerular apparatus, in: *Handbook of Physiology,* Section 8, *Renal Physiology* (J. Orloff and R. W. Berliner, eds.), pp. 1–29, American Physiological Society, Washington, D.C.

Lay, W. H., and Nussenzweig, V., 1968, Receptors for complement on leukocytes, *J. Exp. Med.* **128:**991.

Lazarides, E., and Weber, K., 1974, Actin antibody: The specific visualization of actin filaments in non-muscle cells, *Proc. Natl. Acad. Sci. USA* **71:**2268.

Mohos, S. C., and Skoza, L., 1969, Glomerular sialoprotein, *Science* **164:**1519.

Pollack, R., Osborn, M., and Weber, K., 1975, Patterns of organization of actin and myosin in normal and transformed cultured cells, *Proc. Natl. Acad. Sci. USA* **72:**994.

Quadracci, L. J., and Striker, G. E., 1970, Growth and maintenance of glomerular cells *in vitro, Proc. Soc. Exp. Biol. Med.* **135:**947.

Rennke, H. G., Cotran, R. S., and Venkatachalam, M. A., 1975, Role of molecular charge in glomerular permeability: Tracer studies with cationized ferritins. *J. Cell Biol.* **67:**638.

Ryan, G. B., and Karnovsky, M. J., 1975, An ultrastructural study of the mechanisms of proteinuria in aminonucleoside nephrosis, *Kidney Int.* **8:**219.

Ryan, G. B., and Karnovsky, M. J., 1976, Distribution of endogenous albumin in the rat glomerulus: Role of hemodynamic factors in glomerular barrier function, *Kidney Int.* **9:**36.

Scheinman, J. I., and Fish, A. J., 1978, Human glomerular cells in culture: Three subcultured cell types bearing glomerular antigens, *Am. J. Pathol.* **92:**125.

Scheinman, J. I., Fish, A. S., Brown, D. M., and Michael, A. F., 1976, Human glomerular smooth muscle (mesangial) cells in culture, *Lab. Invest.* **34:**150.

Thomson, N. M., Holdsworth, S. R., Glasgow, E. F., and Atkins, R. C., 1978, The macrophage in crescentic glomerulonephritis, Abstracts, 7th International Congress of Nephrology, Montreal.

Velosa, J. A., Glasser, R. J., Nevins, T. E., and Michael, A. F., 1977, Experimental model of focal sclerosis. II. Correlation with immunopathologic changes, macromolecular kinetics, and polyanion loss, *Lab. Invest.* **36:**527.

Walker, F., 1973, The origin, turnover and removal of glomerular basement membrane, *J. Pathol.* **110:**233.

14

Culture of Human Glomerular Cells

Terry D. Oberley and Peter M. Burkholder

1. Introduction

Despite extensive knowledge about the etiology of glomerular disease, it is still not possible to prevent the excess accumulation of macromolecules (basement membrane, mesangial matrix, collagen, etc.) which results in glomerular sclerosis. In the intact animal it is difficult to study at a cellular and at a molecular level the progression of events that begins with glomerular cell injury and ends with glomerular sclerosis. It is for this reason that several investigators have begun to develop methods for the *in vitro* culture of glomerular cells. For such systems to be meaningful they must be reproducible, and various laboratories throughout the country must agree on the best model. Unfortunately, there is a great deal of controversy concerning whether adult glomeruli can be cultured successfully (Fish *et al.*, 1975), and if so, which cells are present in the resultant outgrowths (epithelial, mesangial, or endothelial) (Foidart-Willems *et al.*, 1975; Holdsworth *et al.*, 1978). The present study presents a reliable way to culture adult human glomeruli and presents preliminary morphologic and cytochemical characterization of the cultured cells.

2. Materials and Methods

2.1. Tissue Procurement

Fresh kidneys were obtained from surgical resections used for treatment of various conditions including renal hypoplasia or hypernephroma.

Terry D. Oberley and Peter M. Burkholder · Department of Pathology, University of Wisconsin Medical School, Madison, Wisconsin 53706.

2.2. Isolation and Culture of Glomeruli

The renal cortex was dissected from the renal medulla and minced into a fine paste which then successively was pestled through nylon sieves whose pore size depended on the age of the patient (adult: 450, 277, and 130 μm; fetal: 450, 130, and 73 μm). Intact glomeruli were retained on the final screen. Isolated glomeruli were pipetted directly into Tissue-Tek slide culture chambers (Miles Laboratories). Media consisted of Waymouth's medium supplemented with sodium pyruvate and nonessential amino acids (GIBCO), 20% fetal bovine serum, 10^{-5} M insulin, penicillin (100 units/ml), streptomycin (100 μg/ml), and one-half volume of conditioned medium. Conditioned medium was obtained by filtration of media harvested from confluent guinea pig glomerular cells. Media were replaced daily. After confluency of cell growth was reached, the cells were detached by exposure to 0.01% EDTA (5 sec) in PBS and 0.25% trypsin for 5 min and were subcultured in plastic flasks.

In some instances whole glomeruli were incubated in 0.25% trypsin for 30 min at 37°C in an effort to free endothelial and mesangial cells from the glomerulus by loosening the mesangial and basement membrane matrices. The products of this proteolytic digestion were cultured in tissue culture media as described for use with intact glomeruli. Cell outgrowths were monitored by phase microscopy.

2.3. Isolation of Tubular Cells and Fibroblasts

Renal cortical, nonglomerular cells were prepared from human cortex by a modification of the methods of Dechenne *et al.* (1975) and Cade-Trayer and Tsuji (1975). Human cortex was treated with 0.25% trypsin for 60 min at 37°C and the cell suspension derived was centrifuged at low speed. The supernatant was saved. The pellet was resuspended and centrifuged again. The two supernatants were combined and passed through a series of nylon screens designed to entrap glomeruli. Single cells which passed through the screens were plated in Tissue-Tek chambers. Both transmission and scanning electron microscopy have shown cells prepared in this way to consist almost entirely of tubular cells (unpublished observations). The initial cells have prominent mitochondria, dense bodies, and microvilli along one pole of the cell. After culture, these cells form confluent sheets which are easily distinguishable from glomerular cells. Although we are convinced that this technique yields tubular cells, we shall designate them nonglomerular renal cortical cells.

Human WI 38 fibroblasts were purchased from GIBCO.

2.4. Cytochemical Techniques for Light Microscopy

Limulin (Sigma) or wheat germ agglutinin (Miles) was conjugated to horseradish peroxidase (HRP) using the periodate procedure of Nakane and

Kawasi (1974). The immunoglobulin fraction of serum containing anti-basement membrane antibody from a patient with Goodpasture's syndrome was isolated by precipitation of whole serum with 50% saturated ammonium sulfate followed by chromatography on DEAE cellulose. This fraction also was conjugated to HRP.

Six-micrometer sections of human kidney, quick-frozen in isopentane, were cut on a cryostat microtome. The sections were fixed in the periodate–lysine–paraformaldehyde (PLP) fixation of McLean and Nakane (1974). The fixed sections were washed and then treated with HRP–limulin, HRP–wheat germ agglutinin, or HRP–Goodpasture's antibody for 120 min at 37°C. The diaminobenzidine (DAB)–H_2O_2 reaction then was performed. The slides were mounted in Permount. Controls included preincubation of limulin with 0.2 M sialic acid, preincubation of wheat germ agglutinin with 0.2 M *N*-acetyl-D-glucosamine, or the substitution of HRP-labeled nonimmune human immunoglobulins for HRP–anti-GBM antibody from the patient with Goodpasture's syndrome.

Cells grown in tissue culture were fixed with PLP, washed, and then stained with HRP–lectin or antibody for 120 min at 37°C. The DAB–H_2O_2 reaction then was performed and the slides mounted with Permount.

Concanavalin A (Sigma) staining of tissues and cells for light microscopy was performed as outlined by Bernhard and Avrameas (1971), in which Con A and HRP are incubated in successive steps rather than being conjugated and incubated in a single step. Con A staining of tissue for electron microscopy was performed as described by Bretton *et al.* (1976), a technique identical to that for light microscopy except that it requires prolonged incubation with lectin and constant agitation to ensure penetration of the lectin into the tissue.

2.5. D-Amino Acid Oxidase Histochemistry

Wohlrab's method (Wohlrab, 1965) was used to stain for D-amino acid oxidase.

2.6. Transmission Electron Microscopy

Suspended cells were preembedded by centrifugation in a 2% glutaraldehyde–6% bovine serum albumin gel (BSA; Cohn's fraction V) to avoid the possibility of loss during the preparative procedure. Blocks of the gel pellet containing cells were trimmed under a dissecting microscope and then processed for transmission electron microscopy by initial fixation for 4 hr at 4°C in 4% cacodylate-buffered glutaraldehyde at a total osmolal concentration of 880 mOsm followed by secondary fixation in 1% osmium tetroxide in S-collidine buffer. Then the cells were dehydrated in a graded ethanol series and embedded in an Epon 812–Araldite epoxy resin mixture. Ultrathin sections were doubly stained with lead hydroxide and uranyl acetate and examined at 50 kV on a Hitachi HS-8F electron microscope.

3. Results

3.1. Culture of Adult Human Glomeruli

The techniques outlined above resulted in nearly 100% success in culture of human glomerular cells. The following conditions were found necessary to culture adult human glomeruli. First, the tissue must be fresh. Tissue removed from autopsies several hours after death usually did not grow, whereas fresh surgical specimens of any age grew. Second, the use of nylon screens for glomerular isolation avoided the damage to epithelial cells that is frequently seen with sieving techniques (Norgaard, 1976). Finally, the culture medium used was critical. This laboratory used Waymouth's medium supplemented with nonessential amino acids, sodium pyruvate, 20% fetal bovine serum, 10^{-5} M insulin, and conditioned medium. If large quantities of glomeruli were available, conditioned medium was not necessary.

Three types of cells were seen growing around adult glomeruli. The cell type which predominated in cultures of intact glomeruli had long cytoplasmic extensions (Fig. 1). These cells with cytoplasmic extensions may have several different shapes, but they always have at least one long cell process. Furthermore, this cell seemed to change with subculture. It became extremely flattened, the number of cytoplasmic extensions decreased, and the amount of microfilament bundles increased. Also present in prominent numbers in primary cultures of intact glomeruli was a very large circular cell (Fig. 1). On the other hand, the cell which was predominant in cultures of trypsinized glomeruli was a rectangular-shaped cell (Fig. 1).

3.2. Culture of Infant Human Glomeruli

It was found much easier to culture fetal glomeruli, since these cells grew much faster and did not require conditioned medium. The morphology of infant glomerular cells in culture was much less differentiated than in the adult kidney. Furthermore, it was not necessary to trypsinize infant glomeruli in order to obtain outgrowths of three types of cells: a large circular cell, a small circular cell, and a rhomboid cell. Figures 2a and b show the difference in morphology between adult and fetal cells cultured from untrypsinized normal fetal human glomeruli following staining with HRP–wheat germ agglutinin.

3.3. Ultrastructural Characterization of Cellular Outgrowths

The predominant cell (cell with cytoplasmic extensions) which evolved in subculture of glomerular cells from intact adult glomeruli had prominent rough endoplasmic reticulum (Fig. 3) and intracellular microfilaments (Fig. 4). The predominant cell evolving from subcultured infant glomerular cells (rhomboid cell) showed prominent, branched, rough endoplasmic reticulum

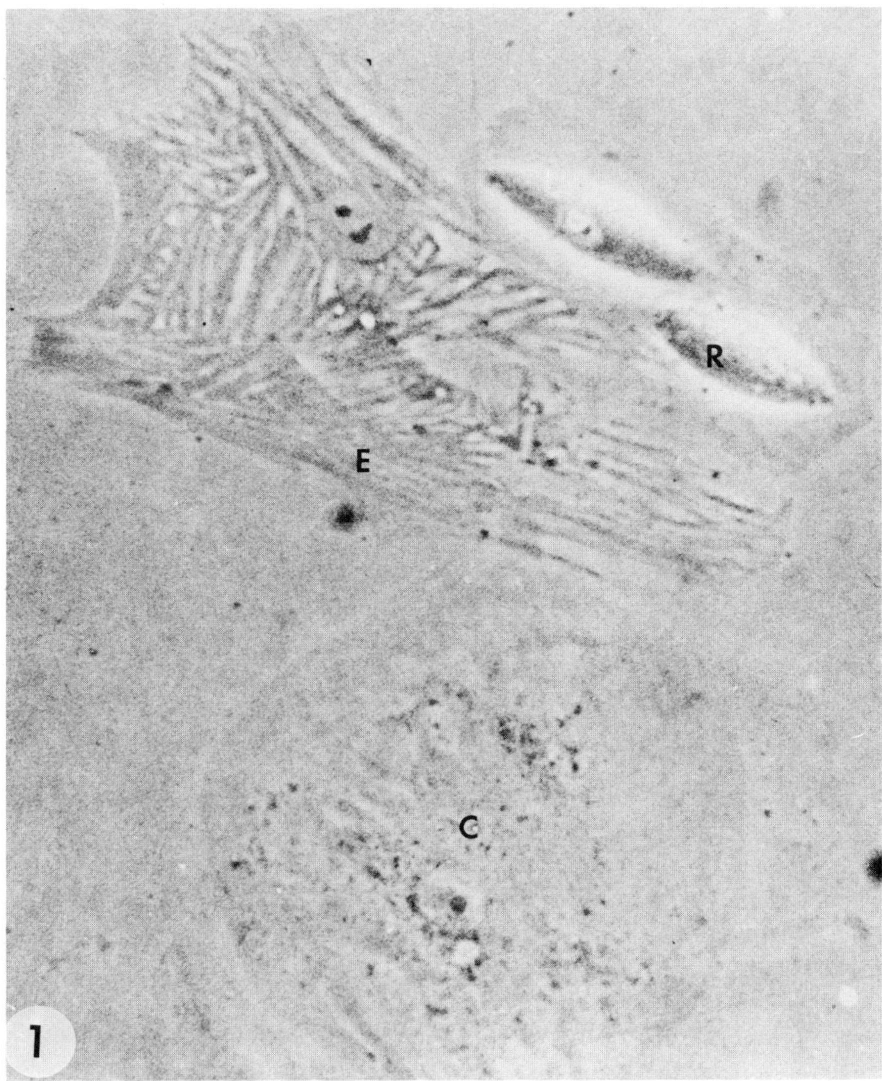

Figure 1. Mixture of cells cultured from both normal and trypsinized glomeruli, illustrating comparative cell sizes. Present are a circular cell (C) and a rectangular-shaped cell (R), and a cell with prominent intracellular bundles of microfilaments (E). The latter cell was in culture for a prolonged period of time and originally had long cytoplasmic extensions. We believe these cells to be the *in vitro* equivalents of the Bowman's capsule, mesangial, and capillary epithelial cells, respectively. × 500.

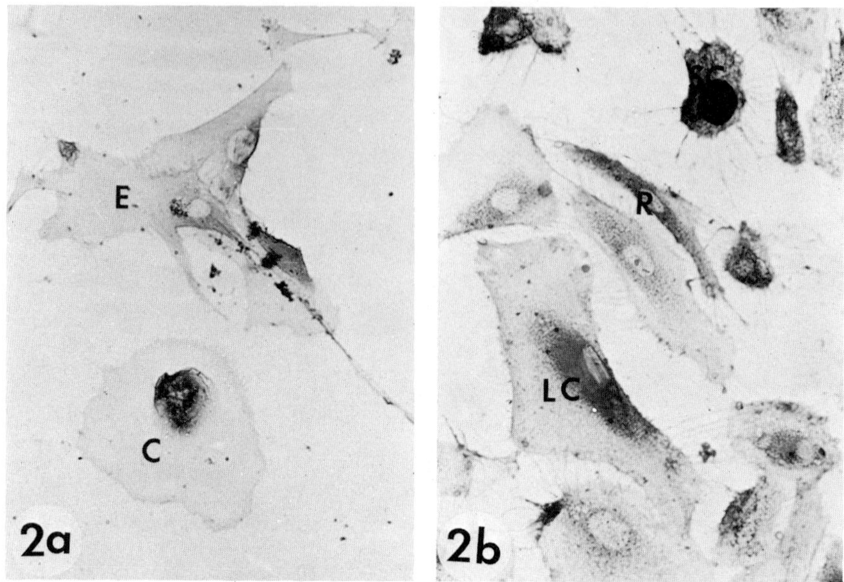

Figure 2. Adult and infant glomerular cells stained with peroxidase-labeled wheat germ agglutinin. (a) Cultures from normal adult glomeruli showed large numbers of circular cells (C) and cells with cytoplasmic extensions (E). (b) Cultures from infant glomeruli showed a large circular cell (LC), a small circular cell (SC), and a rhomboid cell (R). Both × 500.

(Fig. 5). The cells also had prominent microfilaments, but these usually were present just beneath the cell membrane.

3.4. *Cytochemical Characterization of Human Glomerular Cells*

Light microscopic examination of HRP–limulin-treated sections of normal adult kidney revealed prominent staining of glomeruli with almost no tubular staining. Similarly, both adult and fetal glomerular cells in culture showed prominent staining with HRP–limulin, while renal cortical, nonglomerular cells in culture did not stain at all.

Enzyme histochemical staining for D-amino acid oxidase showed *in vitro*-grown tubular cells to stain strongly positive (4+) while cultured fibroblasts did not stain at all. Adult glomerular cells (cell with cytoplasmic extensions) stained lightly (1+) while fetal cells (rhomboid cell) stained more strongly (2+), but clearly less than tubular cells.

3.5. *Biochemical Characterization of Extracellular Matrix Produced by Human Glomerular Cells in Culture*

If confluent adult or fetal glomerular cells in primary or secondary culture were stained by the two-step Con A–HRP reaction, an extended matrix of stained extracellular material was readily discernible.

Experiments were initiated to investigate the nature of this extracellular material. First, the nature of the Con A binding site was investigated using electron microscopy. Using the technique outlined by Bretton *et al.* (1976) for ultrastructural localization of Con A within tissue, it was found that Con A binds heavily to GBM and epithelial cell membranes. Second, reactivity of

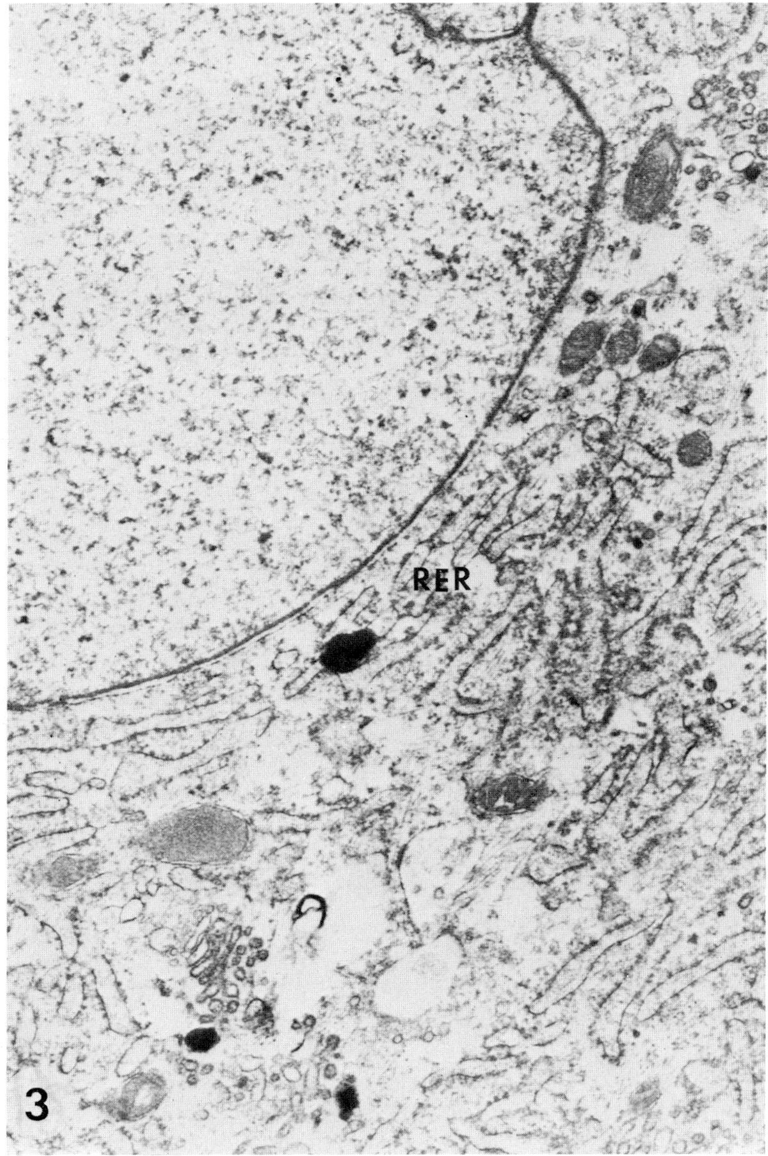

Figure 3. Transmission electron microscopy of subcultured adult glomerular cell. Note prominent rough endoplasmic reticulum (RER). × 6482.

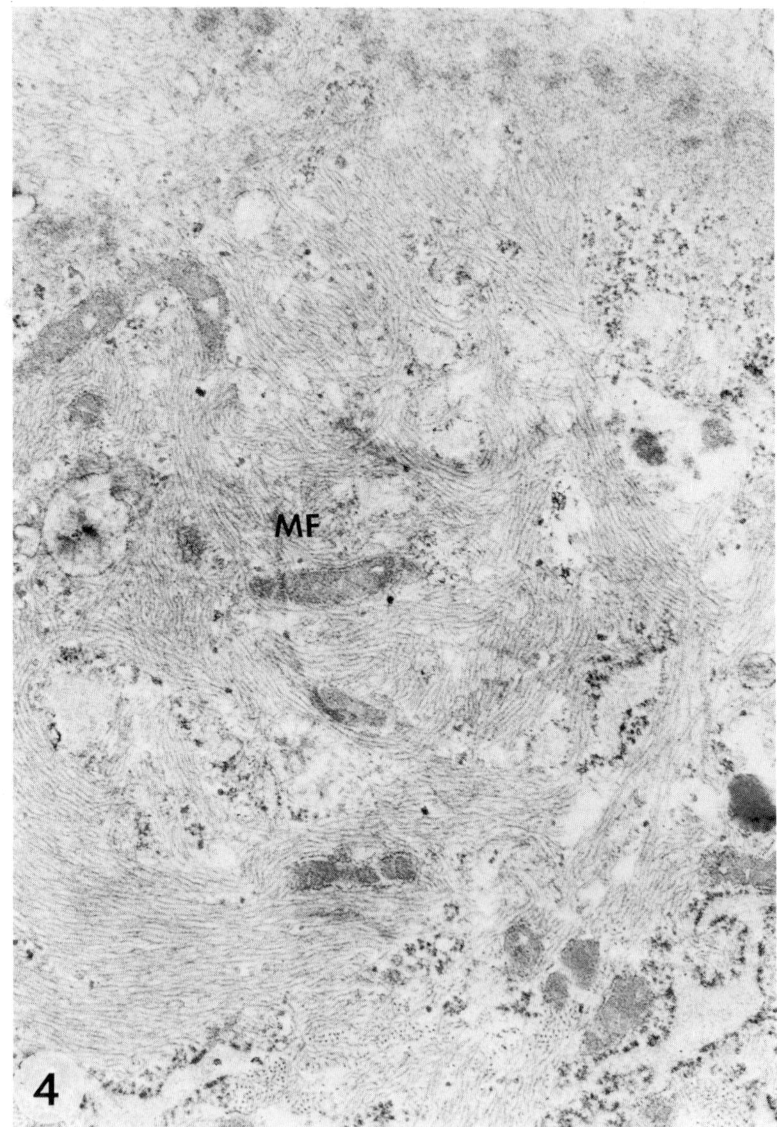

Figure 4. Transmission electron microscopy of subcultured adult glomerular cell. Note prominent intracellular microfilaments (MF). × 23,800.

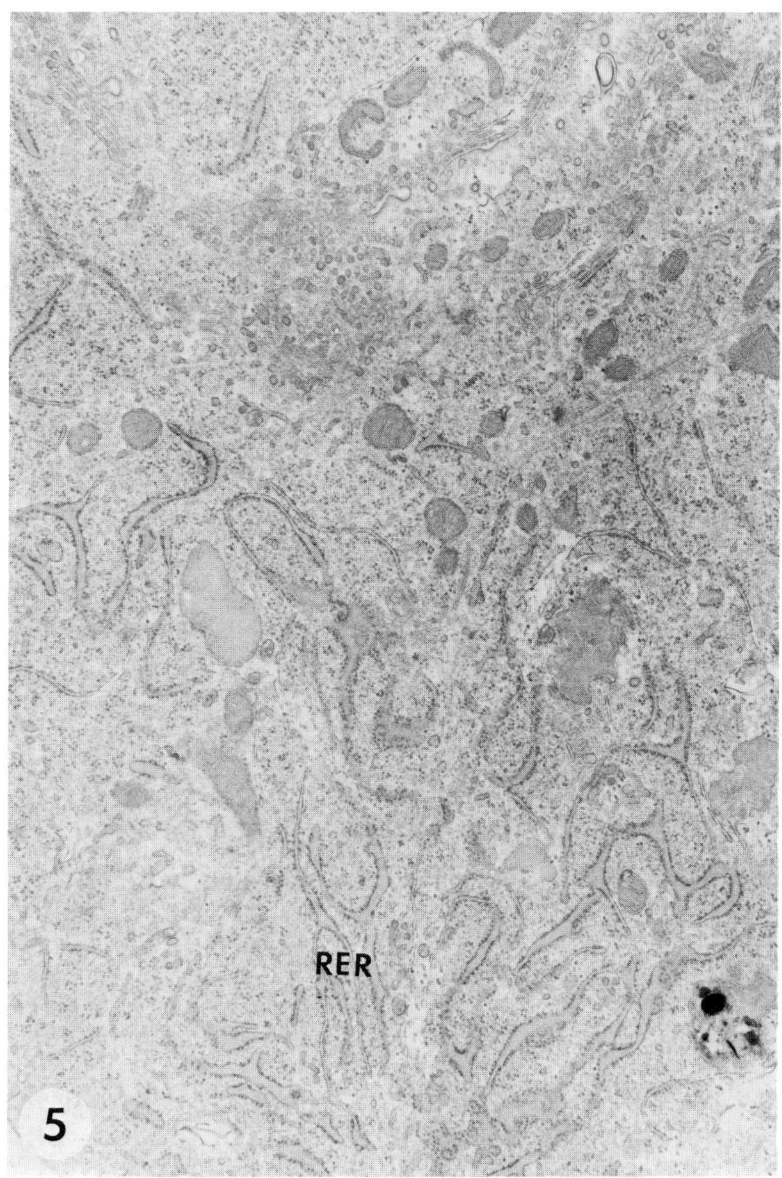

Figure 5. Transmission electron microscopy of subcultured infant glomerular cells. Note prominent branching rough endoplasmic reticulum (RER). × 15,400.

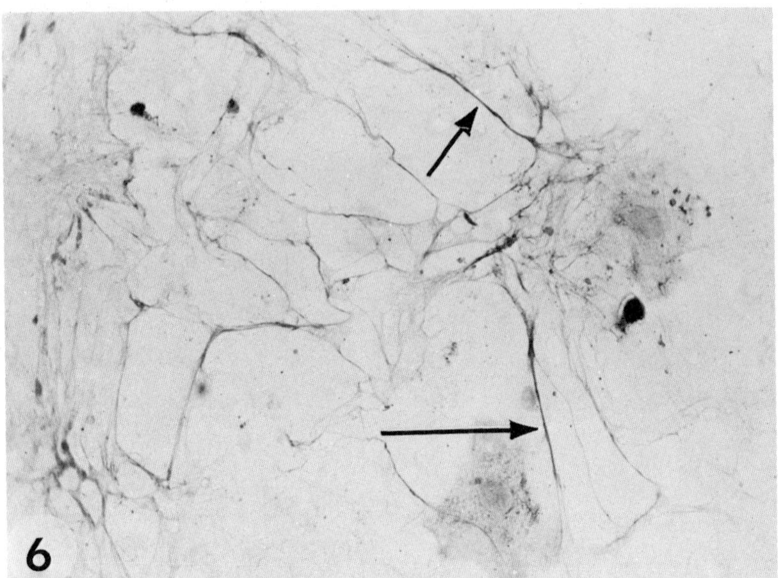

Figure 6. Reactivity with peroxidase-labeled antibody from patient with Goodpasture's syndrome of extracellular matrix produced by infant glomerular cells. Note extracellular matrix staining (arrows). × 500.

the extracellular matrix with HRP-labeled Goodpasture's serum (anti-GBM antibody) was demonstrated by staining infant glomerular cells at confluency (Fig. 6).

4. Discussion

This report presents methods for reproducible culture of adult and infant human glomerular cells. A previous study suggested that culture of adult glomeruli was not possible (Fish *et al.*, 1975), but results in other laboratories have disproved this (Foidart-Willems *et al.*, 1975; Holdsworth *et al.*, 1978). Foidart-Willems *et al.* (1975) stressed the importance of using fresh tissue to obtain cellular outgrowths from adult kidney. The use of insulin and of conditioned medium in this study definitely increased the rate of growth of human adult glomerular cells, and it is believed that these are crucial for culturing of cells from small numbers of glomeruli.

Cytochemical studies suggested that the glomerular cells were not comprised of contaminating tubular cells or fibroblasts. First, limulin, which reacts with glomerular cells, does not stain tubular cells. Second, Gilbert and Migeon (1975) demonstrated that tubular cells had high levels of D-amino acid oxidase, while fibroblasts did not contain this enzyme. These results have been confirmed and by enzyme histochemistry it was found that glomerular cells have enzyme levels intermediate between these two. Therefore, the glomerular cells grown in this fashion are not tubular cells or fibroblasts.

It is evident from this work that human glomerular cells are morphologically different from infant glomerular cells in culture. These results certainly make it easier to understand why separate laboratories have reported different morphologies for cultured glomerular cells. Fish *et al.* (1975) have stated that the predominant cell in culture of infant kidneys is the mesangial cell, while Foidart-Willems *et al.* (1975) have stated that the predominant cell in the culture of adult kidney is the epithelial cell. Holdsworth *et al.* (1978) believe that both cell types immediately grow from adult glomeruli. Although the present work did not resolve this controversy, it did show that the morphology of the glomerular cells obtained depended on several factors, including age of the cultured kidney and length of time that the cells have been in culture. The present study demonstrated that the predominant cell in cultured infant glomeruli was different morphologically from the cells cultured from adult glomeruli. While the identity of the predominant cell growing from infant glomeruli is not certain, it is reasonably definite that the predominant cell growing from adult glomeruli is the epithelial cell since the long cytoplasmic extensions are the *in vitro* equivalent of the glomerular capillary epithelial cell arbor. Future biochemical work will be directed at resolving the controversy of the origin of glomerular cells observed in culture.

The extracellular matrix produced by glomerular cells is most probably a form of basement membrane, since it binds Con A and anti-GBM antibody from a patient with Goodpasture's syndrome. These results suggest that *in vitro* culture of glomeruli provides a useful system for study of the regulation of basement membrane synthesis by glomerular cells.

References

Bernhard, W., and Avrameas, S., 1971, Ultrastructural visualization of cellular carbohydrate components by means of concanavalin A, *Exp. Cell Res.* **64**:232.

Bretton, R., Bariety, J., and Grossetete, J., 1976, Localization of concanavalin A, wheat germ, and ricinis communis on glomeruli of normal rat kidney, in: *First International Symposium on Immunoenzymatic Techniques* (G. Feldmann ed.), pp. 501–505, North-Holland, Amsterdam.

Cade-Trayer, D., and Tsuji, S., 1975, *In vitro* culture of the proximal tubule of the bovine nephron, *Cell Tissue Res.* **163**:15.

Dechenne, C., Foidart-Willems, J., and Mahieu, P. M., 1975, Ultrastructural studies on dog renal glomerular and tubular cells in culture, *J. Submicrosc. Cytol.* **7**:165.

Fish, A. J., Michael, A. F., Vernier, R. L., and Brown, D. M., 1975, Human glomerular cells in tissue culture, *Lab. Invest.* **33**:330.

Foidart-Willems, J., Dechenne, C., and Mahieu, P., 1975, Biosynthesis of basement membrane collagen in cultures of renal glomerular and tubular epithelial cells, *Diabete Metab.* **1**:227.

Gilbert, S. F., and Migeon, B. R., D-Valine as a selective agent for normal human and rodent epithelial cells in culture, *Cell* **5**:11.

Holdsworth, S. R., Thomson, N. M., Glasgow, E. F., Dowling, J. P., and Atkins, R. C., 1978, Tissue culture of isolated glomeruli in experimental crescentic glomerulonephritis, *J. Exp. Med.* **147**:98.

McLean, I. W., and Nakane, P. K., 1974, Periodate-lysine-paraformaldehyde fixative: A new fixative for immunoelectron microscopy, *J. Histochem. Cytochem.* **22**:1077.

Nakane, P. K., and Kawasi, A., 1974, Peroxidase-labeled antibody: A new method of conjugation, *J. Histochem. Cytochem.* **22:**1894.

Norgaard, J. O. R., 1976, A new method for the isolation of ultrastructurally preserved glomeruli, *Kidney Int.* **9:**278.

Wohlrab, F., 1965, Uber die Histochemische Erfass barkeit der Aminosaure-Dehydrogenasen in Saugetierogan, *Histochemie* **5:**311.

15

Immunochemical and Biochemical Studies of Human Glomerular Cells in Culture

Jon I. Scheinman

1. Introduction

Glomerular culture makes it possible to determine the contributions of the different cells of the glomerulus to normal and abnormal *in situ* glomerular structure and function. The confident identification of glomerular cells *in vitro* with the differentiated cells of the glomerulus requires more certain cell markers than are currently available.

However, with the field of study not yet a decade old (Bernik, 1969), certain areas of agreement are emerging from the various pieces of "soft" evidence used to identify presumptively the surviving cells of the explanted glomerulus. First, there is no evidence yet of the survival of the glomerular endothelial cell *in vitro*. Second, enzymatic methods of tissue disociation (Scheinman *et al.*, 1976; Schienman and Fish, 1978; Killen and Striker, 1979: Oberley and Burkholder, this volume; Kreisberg and Karnovsky, this volume) allow the vigorous early outgrowth and proliferation of "epithelioid" cell types. Finally, areas of striking agreement are noted when characterization studies have been comparable: Oberley *et al.*'s preliminary observations (1979) on the morphology of three types of human neonatal glomerular cells fit quite well with published observations (Scheinman *et al.*, 1976; Scheinman and Fish, 1978). The immunochemical and biochemical studies of rat glomerular cells, whose morphology differs from human cells (Foidart *et al.*,

Jon I. Scheinman · Department of Pediatrics, University of Minnesota Medical School, Minneapolis, Minnesota 55455. This work was supported by grants from the American Diabetes Association, the American Heart Association, the Juvenile Diabetes Foundation, the Minnesota Medical Foundation, and the Graduate School of the University of Minnesota. The author is a recipient of a Research Career Development Award (K04 AM 00126) from the NIAMDD.

1980, 1981), corroborate entirely studies of the immunochemical and biochemical characteristics of the epithelioid and smooth muscle-like human cells from this laboratory (Scheinman *et al.*, 1976, 1978c; Scheinman and Fish, 1978),and with the biochemical studies of Striker *et al.* (1978) and Killen and Striker (1979). The morphologic similarities between those cells from rat glomeruli reported by Foidart *et al.* (1980, 1981) and two of the cell types (epithelioid and smooth muscle-like) described by Kreisberg *et al.* (1978 and this volume) and the more recent observation of Ishikawa *et al.* (1980) make it quite likely that more comparable studies will provide even greater convergence.

This summary will review briefly the application and limitations of immunohistologic and biochemical approaches to the characterization of human glomerular cells in culture and efforts to define the optimal conditions for glomerular cell growth.

2. *The Immunochemical Approach to Glomerular Cell Specialization: Limitations*

The immunochemical dissection of the glomerulus (Fig. 1) (Scheinman *et al.*, 1974, 1978a) has shown the predominant mesangial cell localization of

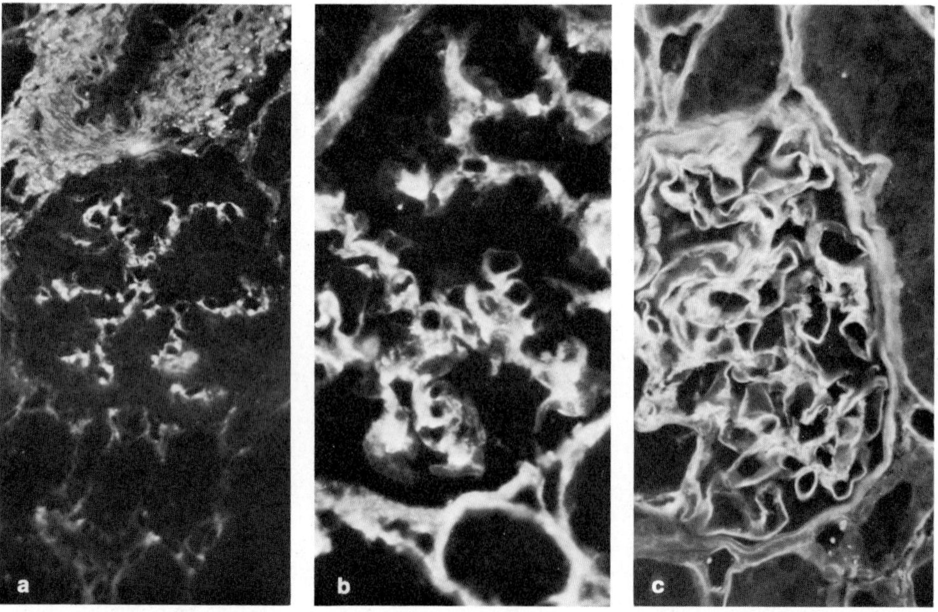

Figure 1. The immunohistology of normal glomerular antigens (Scheinman *et al.*, 1978a). (a) Anti-human smooth muscle myosin, localized in a restricted pattern (intracellular) in the mesangium. Note arterial wall stained above the glomerulus. (b) Anti-human fibronectin, localized in the mesangium (of part of a glomerulus) but more extensively (extracellular) compared to myosin. (c) Heterologous anti-GBM antibody localizing to the full thickness of the GBM by transmitted fluorescent microscopy. Mesangial staining also present.

smooth muscle myosin (Fig. 1a) and the extracellular mesangial localization of fibronectin (Fig. 1b). Fibronectin may not derive from the mesangial cell, but may localize, from the circulation to the mesangial matrix by its special affinity to collagen (Engvall and Ruoslahti, 1977). The collagen of the glomerulus has been characterized as a "type IV" (Kefalides, 1973), but both type IV and V collagens are probably present, the former perhaps in two immunochemically and anatomically distinct species (Scheinman, 1980b). Currently, there is no evidence of collagen Type I, II, and III (Nowack *et al.*, 1976) in the glomerulus. The several (noncollagen) basement membrane antigens, elicited in rabbits by immunization with whole human GBM (Fig. 1c), may derive from any or from all of the cells of the glomerulus, deposited in different zones of the GBM and mesangial matrix (Fish *et al.*, this volume). Therefore, they cannot serve as selective markers for glomerular cells. Likewise, the non-collagen glycoprotein laminin may be common to all cells of the glomerulus (Scheinman, 1980a). The autoantibodies to basement membrane eluted from the kidneys of patients with Goodpasture's disease appear to localize exclusively to epithelial aspect of the GBM (Fish, this volume). This antigen could serve as a marker of the epithelial cell if *synthesized* by glomerular cells *in vitro*, but we have not found this antigen on cells in culture. Antihemophilic Factor VIII antigen is localized on extraglomerular endothelia, and on cultured endothelial cells (Jaffe *et al.*, 1973). Factor VIII antigen synthesis by the specialized glomerular endothelium is not certain, so that its absence from glomerular cells *in vitro* (Scheinman *et al.*, 1976; Scheinman and Fish, 1978) cannot alone rule out possible endothelial origin.

3. Human Glomerular Cell Types in Vitro

Given these cautions, it is likely that, in glomerular cell cultures, the elongated overlapping rhomboid glomerular cells (Fig. 2a) containing large amounts of smooth muscle myosin in periodic fibrils and in cytoplasmic aggregates (Fig. 2b), are smooth muscle-type cells. Contact-inhibited circular cells (Fig. 2c) that excrete large amounts of GBM antigens in a cascade of granules (Fig. 2d) are epithelioid cells. These epithelioid cells excrete into the medium relatively large collagen polypeptide subunits, with approximately 15% of 3-Hyp as the 3-Hyp form, and greater lysine hydroxylation than found in the smooth muscle cells (Scheinman *et al.*, 1978c). The smooth muscle-like cells excrete collagenous polypeptides whose sulfhydryl linkage and migration on polyacrylamides resemble both Type I and III collagens, but which have greater proline 3-hydroxylation (up to 8%) than is found in dermal Types I and III collagens. Whether these are genetically distinct (mesangial) collagens or special posttranslation modifications of Types I and III collagens has not been resolved. These results were similar to those of Killen and Striker (1979) and may indicate *in vitro* dedifferentiation, in view of the absence of types I and III collagen in the intact glomerulus.

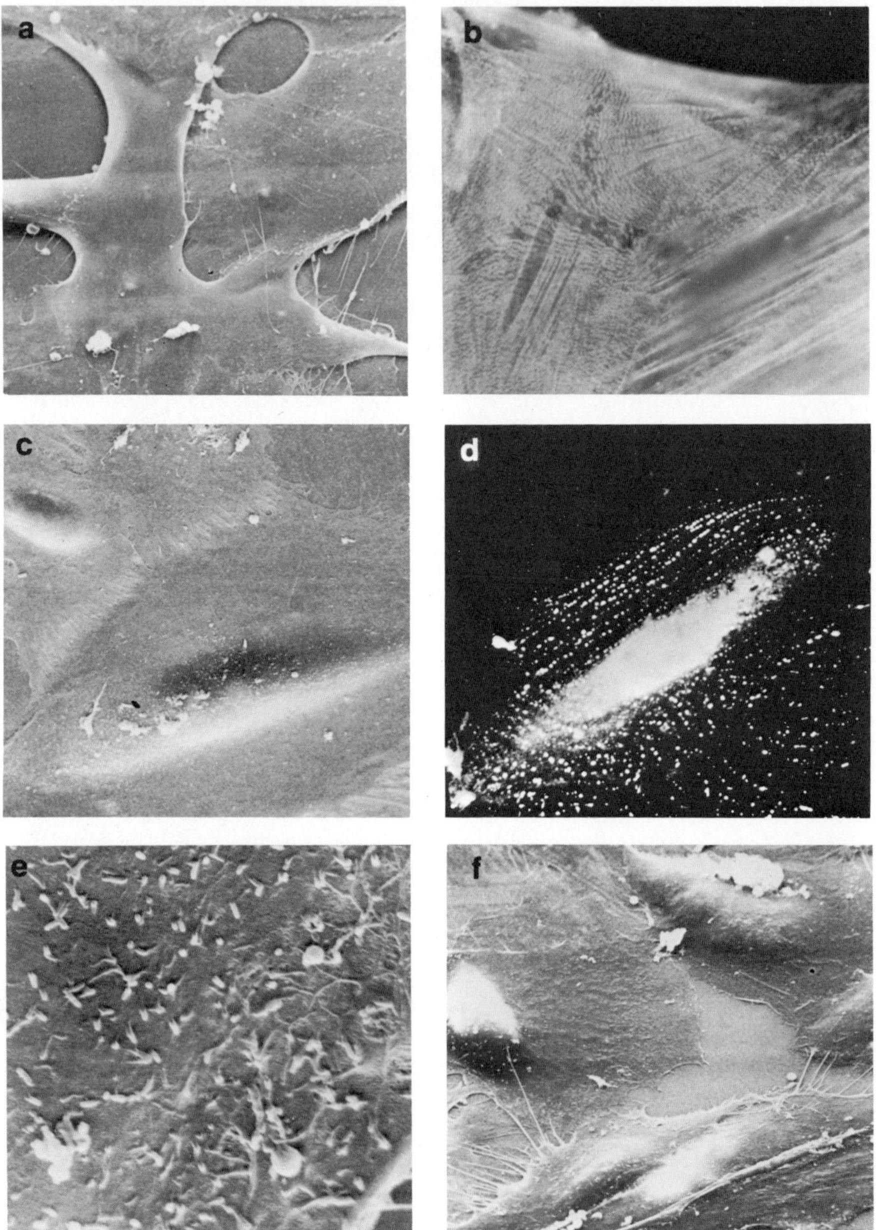

Figure 2. Human glomerular cells in culture. (a) Scanning electron microscopy of rhomboid glomerular cells, elongated, overlapping, forming syncytia with adjacent cells. (b) Antimyosin staining of central portion of rhomboid glomerular cell, showing periodic fibrils and aligned cytoplasmic myosin aggregates. (c) Two large circular glomerular cells, contact inhibited. (d) Anti-GBM staining of circular glomerular cell, showing palisade of granules excreted from the cell surface. (e) SEM of surface of large circular cell, with numerous cytoplasmic projections. (f) Small ovoid glomerular cell, derived from same explant as Fig. 2a. Magnification is the same as Fig. 2c. (SEM performed with the courtesy of Dr. J. G. White. Fluorescent pictures from Scheinman and Fish, 1978.)

4. *Early Events in Glomerular Explant Culture*

Some clues to the identification of glomerular cells in culture can be obtained from early observations of the changes in glomeruli *in vitro* under different culture conditions. Norgaard (1978) has described a retraction of epithelial cell foot processes, a decrease in colloidal iron staining, and the appearance of microvilli on the surface of the glomerular epithelium cultured *in vitro* with serum-supplemented medium. These changes resemble those seen *in situ* in proteinuric states. Surface microvilli on large circular glomerular cells *in vitro* (Fig. 2e) have been used to suggest their origin from the glomerular epithelium, but this is somewhat imaginative. Bernik (1969) observed the development of a giant arborized cell form in nonproliferating glomerular epithelial cells still attached to the mechanically isolated glomerulus *in vitro*. These observations have been confirmed more recently by Atkins *et al.* (1976). It has been noted that there is development of a similar morphology in explants of adult human glomeruli, of mechanically isolated infant glomeruli, but not of collagenase-perfused glomeruli cultured in the presence of serum, whose cells proliferate more vigorously. The small oval glomerular cells (Fig. 2f) rapidly proliferate as epithelioid types and overgrow after confluency. They may be a dedifferentiated form of the larger epithelioid cells.

5. *Glomerular Explant Conditions: Comparative Studies from Bovine Glomeruli*

In an attempt to make reproducible observations, glomeruli from 10 pairs of newborn bovine kidneys were isolated. One of each pair was perfused immediately with Lacted Ringer's solution. The other, in addition, was perfused with 0.1% collagenase and incubated at 37°C for 1 hr before the glomerular isolation that utilized a 105 μm micro-etched conical-holed stainless screen (Buckbee Mears Co., St. Paul, Minn.), followed by sieving through a 112 μm and onto a 105 μm micro-etched conical-holed stainless screen (Buckbee Mears Co.), followed by sieving through a 112 μm and onto a 105 μm (Nytex) nylon screen. Aliquots of each sample were explanted in 199, Waymouth's, RPMI 1640, and MCDB 104 (McKeehan *et al.*, 1977) media, with or without 20% fetal calf serum (Reheis), and with or without fibroblast growth factor (FGF) (Gospodarowicz *et al.*, 1976), and/or epidermoid growth factor (EGF; obtained from Collaborative Research). The use of multiple wells in HLA plates with one to three glomeruli per well, allowed repetitive observation of the same glomeruli, with no nonglomerular contaminants present. Under these conditions, the optimal cellular outgrowths occurred more slowly than those from human infant glomeruli, in spite of almost immediate glomerular attachment. The elongated (rhomboid, smooth muscle-like) cells emerged under most conditions at about 2 weeks. An exception was in medium RPMI 1640, where both with and without serum, the interior of the glomeruli became very dark within 2–3 days, and the emergence of the rhomboid cells was unusual and sparse. On the other hand, the sequence of surface outgrowth was similar under all conditions, but marked differences in the timing of this sequence occurred. Explants onto glass without serum in Eagle's basal medium (BME) showed a stream of small stellate cells with long processes that rapidly (1–5 min) migrated from the surface of glass, but that did not proliferate (Fig. 3a). Time-lapse studies to determine whether these formed giant cells were not performed. In media with serum from collagenase-perfused glomeruli, the epithelial

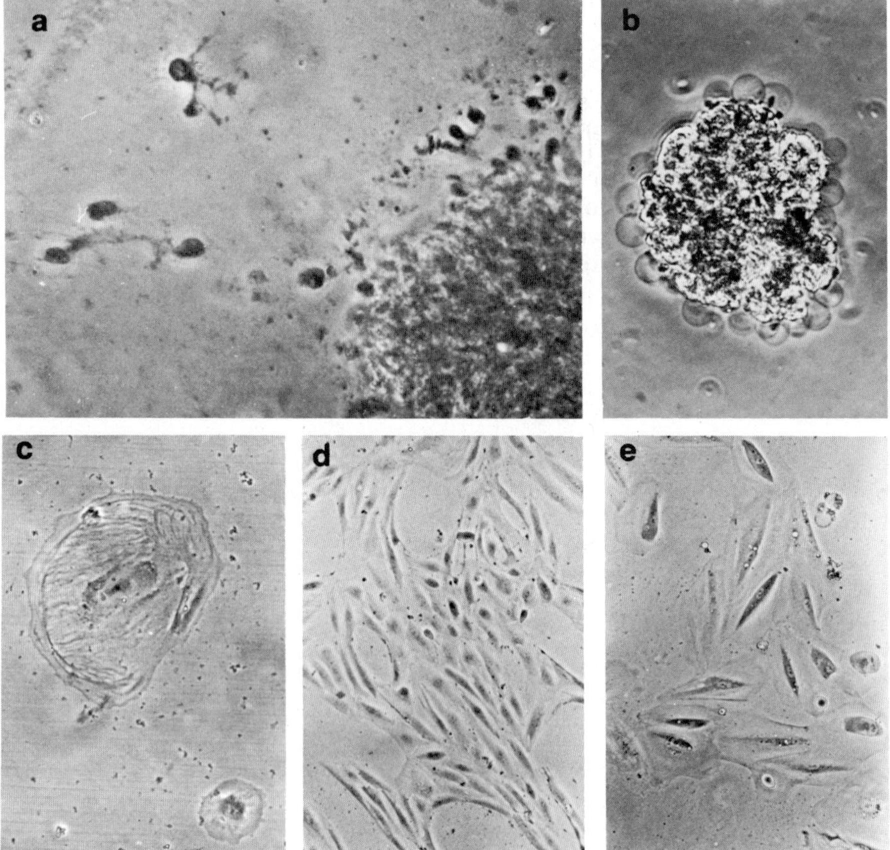

Figure 3. (a) Glomerular explant in Eagle's basal medium without serum. Small stellate cells migrate within minutes from the glomerular surface onto glass, but do not proliferate. (From Michael *et al.*, 1978.) (b) Enlarged epithelial cells on the surface of glomerulus explanted 2 days in Waymouth's medium with serum (Michael *et al.*, 1978). (c) Giant, arborized cell from third passage of cloned calf circular glomerular cells. Usual sized circular cell is in lower right, for comparison. (d) Small oval glomerular cells from explant in Waymouth's medium without serum, but with fibroblast growth factor. (e) Eighth passage of cloned human circular glomerular cells. These cells appear identical to the larger calf circular cells grown most frequently in RPMI 1640 medium.

cells first enlarged on the basement membrane (Fig. 3b), then began to form an extraglomerular confluent epithelioid monolayer at 4–5 days, except in medium 199, in which even at 7–11 days only one-half of explants grew. Frequently, several large arborized cell forms were seen, that did not proliferate in a fashion similar to that of cells in nutritionally deprived media (Fig. 3c). The epithelioid outgrowth sequence was similar without serum, as long as EGF and/or FGF were present, but the epithelial swelling was delayed to approximately 7 days, and the outgrowth appeared at 8–10 days. Even under these conditions, the more rapidly proliferating small oval glomerular cells were usual (Fig. 3d). In medium 199, without growth factors or serum, glomeruli turned totally dark within 2–3 days and outgrowth did not occur.

Glomeruli not perfused with collagenase gave slower epithelioid outgrowths at 10 or more days even in Waymouth's medium with serum. The large arborized cells were seen frequently in all of these cultures in media without serum (with FGF or EGF) when confluent outgrowths did not occur. While conditioned media may provide some help in growth at clonal density, a systematic study has not been performed.

Subcultures of these cultures using trypsin–citrate (Scheinman and Fish, 1978) did not permit quantitation of plating efficiency, but was successful for all outgrowths, even without serum, as long as EGF or FGF were present. Selective serial passage and cloning can separate the cell types. Epithelioid subcultures in RPMI 1640 with serum grew more slowly than in Waymouth's or 104, but cells were larger (Fig. 3e).

It is clear from these observations and others (Oberley *et al.*, 1979, 1980, 1981) that not only the methods of tissue isolation but the explant environment both influence the results of glomerular culture. If indeed endothelial cells do not grow *in vitro*, and if numerous cell types are observed *in vitro*, either there are more than two other cell types present in the normal glomerulus, or a single cell type can take several forms when grown *in vitro*. The latter interpretation is favored.

6. Summary of Published Reports of Human Glomerular Cells in Vitro

These results from bovine studies help to clarify some apparent discrepancies between different reports of human glomerular cells in culture and their attempted identification by morphologic criteria. Table 1 lists the published human glomerular cell types and groups them to propose a likely derivation and state of dedifferentiation. Smooth muscle-like cells are elongated cells that grow in multilayered fasciculi, have a dense extracellular matrix, and intracellular myosin fibrils. They appear late in human glomerular cultures. Epithelioid cells are more variable. Enzymatic treatment and media such as Waymouth's or RPMI 1640 with serum result in confluent outgrowths of large contact-inhibited circular cells. Smaller ovoid cells may or may not also be epithelial, but they can form multilayers after confluency.

Table 1. *Human Glomerular Cells in Vitro*[a]

Methods of isolation	Medium		Cell types[b]	Properties	Probable derivation[c]	Authors
Enzyme (Collagenase, Trypsin); Intermediate Optimal	Waymouth's	Proliferating (↑)	*Circular*, epithelioid	Large, contact inhibited. GBM antigen, "Type IV" collagen. Phagocytic. No C3b or Factor VIII	Epithelium—mild proliferation	Scheinman *et al.* (1976, 1978b,c), Scheinman and Fish (1978)
			Fusiform or *small oval*	Small, early contact inhibition, late multilayer. Mixed collagen. Phagocytic. No C3b or Factor VIII	Epithelium—rapid proliferation	Scheinman *et al.* (1976, 1978b,c), Scheinman and Fish (1978)
			Rhomboid, smooth muscle	Elongated, multilayered fasciculi. Type III and I collagen. Myosin fibrils	Mesangium	Scheinman *et al.* (1976, 1978b,c), Scheinman and Fish (1978)
	199		*Epithelial*	Monolayer, tight junctions. GBM antigen. "Type IV" collagen	Epithelium	Dechenne *et al.* (1976)
Optimal	Waymouth's		*Epithelial*	Large, irregularly shaped. Overlap. "Type IV" collagen	Epithelium—rapid proliferation	Quadracci *et al.* (1970), Striker *et al.* (1978)
			Smooth muscle	Elongate, multilayers, basal lamina. Interstitial collagen	Mesangium	Quadracci *et al.* (1970), Striker *et al.* (1978)
	Dulbecco's		*Circular* (rare)	Large, circular-oval	Epithelium—minimal proliferation	Scheinman *et al.* (1976)

Mechanical	Intermediate		Proliferating ↓	*Rhomboid*	Elongated, processes	Mesangium	Fish *et al.* (1975)
		199		*Epithelioid*	Small, tightly packed	Epithelium[d] (parietal)	Burlington and Cronkite (1973)
				Fibroblastic	Fibroblastic	Mesangium	Burlington and Cronkite (1973)
		199		*Type II* (mesangial)	Mobile, proliferating, phagocytic	Epithelium[e]	Atkins *et al.* (1976), Holdsworth *et al.* (1978)
			Nonproliferating ↑	*Type I* (epithelial)	Very large, arborized, immobile	Epithelium[e]	Atkins *et al.* (1976), Holdsworth *et al.* (1978)
(Attached)	Minimal			*Macrophage*		Macrophage	Atkins *et al.* (1976), Holdsworth *et al.* (1978)
		Eagle's basal		*Giant*	Arborized, interdigitating processes, giant, immotile	Epithelium	Bernik (1969)
				Mesangial	Large, motile	Epithelium[f]	Bernik (1969)
				Mesangial	Intercapillary. Contractile	Mesangium	Bernik (1969)
		MEM		*Epithelial*	Small, arborized (stellate). C3b receptors	Epithelium	Burkholder *et al.* (1977)

[a] Modified from Michael *et al.* (19).
[b] The author's term is in italics.
[c] Readers should understand that considerable license is used in implicating a probable derivation of any cell in culture; this has not been proven. Authors, whose cell designations have been changed, should be understanding since we may be proven wrong.
[d] The authors suggest that these cells derive from Bowman's capsule. The lack of proliferation of visceral epithelial cells is most consistent with this isolation method and medium.
[e] The authors describe type II as mesangial, but these resemble the epithelioid cells described by other authors.
[f] The author feels these polymorphic cells derive from the mesangium, as do the contractile cells. Their tentative designation here as epithelial cells better fits more recent observations.

These cells, like the larger circular cells, can be phagocytic (Schiffer *et al.*, and Scheiman, 1982). Giant, nonproliferating, arborized cells appear most often in cultures of glomeruli not exposed to enzymes and in less optimal media such as 199.

7. *Specific Markers and the Future of Glomerular Cell Culture*

Specific markers to identify human glomerular cells *in vitro* with their *in situ* counterparts have not been found yet. C3b receptors detected with fluoresceinated *E. coli*, present on explanted glomeruli, have not been preserved reliably on cellular outgrowths (Scheinman *et al.*, 1978b), although reports from other laboratories suggest their preservation (Striker *et al.*, 1978; Killen and Striker, 1979; Oberley and Burkholder, this volume). The nature of the collagen synthesized by human glomerular cells *in vitro* is suggestive of a basement membrane type of collagen derived from epithelioid cells (Foidart-Willems *et al.*, 1975; Scheinman *et al.*, 1978b). However, lack of knowledge of the origin of normal glomerular collagens and their localization (Scheinman *et al.*, 1980b) precludes their use as definitive identification of the parent cell type. Some of the features found in rat glomerular cells by Kreisberg *et al.* (1978), if applicable to human glomerular cells, may assist in their identification. However, differences in morphology, growth potential, and growth patterns between human and rat glomerular cells (Michael *et al.*, 1978) make direct translations between these systems difficult.

It is thus only an attractive working hypothesis that smooth muscle-like cells derive from the mesangium and the epithelioid forms from the glomerular visceral epithelium. Even if this hypothesis is correct, it is evident that the study of any property of a glomerular cell studied *in vitro* must first demonstrate the differentiation of that property, as compared to the glomerulus *in situ*. Thus, the field of human glomerular culture now has evolved reliable techniques for the growth of different cell types. Their confident identification requires more reliable markers, which may emerge from the many structural, biochemical, and immunochemical studies of the glomerulus discussed in this volume.

ACKNOWLEDGMENTS. I wish to thank Kathryn LaCroix, Laura Marxen, and Dan Heieren for excellent technical assistance, Marshall Hoff for illustrations, Nancy Kirschling for editorial assistance, and Drs. Alfred Fish, Alfred Michael, and David Brown for their advice and collaborative assistance in the work from which this review was derived. Dr. James G. White provided invaluable assistance in scanning electron microscopy.

References

Atkins, R. C., Holdsworth, S. R., Glasgow, E. F., and Mathews, F. E., 1976, The macrophage in human rapidly progressive glomerulonephritis, *Lancet* **1**:830.

Bernik, M. B., 1969, Contractile activity of human glomeruli in culture, *Nephron* **6:**1.

Burkholder, P. M., Oberley, T. D., Barber, T. A., Beacom, A., and Koehler, C., 1977, Immune adherence in renal glomeruli: Complement receptor sites on glomerular capillary epithelial cells, *Am. J. Pathol.* **86:**635.

Burlington, H., and Cronkite, E. P., 1973, Characteristics of cell cultures derived from renal glomeruli, *Proc. Soc. Exp. Biol. Med.* **142:**143.

Dechenne, C., Foidart-Willems, J., and Mahieu, P. M., 1976, Collagen biosynthesis in cultures of epithelial cells isolated from malignant hypertensive kidneys, *J. Submicrosc. Cytol.* **8:**101.

Engvall, C., and Ruoslahti, E., 1977, Binding of soluble form of fibroblast surface protein, fibronectin, to collagen, *Int. J. Cancer* **20:**1.

Fish, A. J., Michael, A. F., Vernier, R. L., and Brown, D. M., 1975, Human glomerular cells in tissue culture, *Lab. Invest.* **33:**330.

Foidart-Willems, J., Dechenne, C., and Mahieu, P., 1975, Biosynthesis of basement membrane collagen in cultures of renal glomerular and tubular epithelial cells, *Diabete Metab.* **1:**227.

Foidart, J. B., Dubois, C. H., Foidart, J-M, Dechenne, C. A., and Mahieu, P., 1980, Tissue culture of normal rat glomeruli. Basement membrane biosynthesis by homogeneous epithelial and mesangial cell lines, *Int. J. Biochem.* **12:**197.

Foidart, J. B., Dechenne, C. A., and Mahieu, P., 1981, Tissue culture of normal rat glomeruli: Characterization of collagenous and non-collagenous basement membrane antigens on the epithelial and mesangial cells, *Diag. Histopathol.* **4:**71.

Gospodarowicz, D., Moran, J. S., and Bialecki, H., 1976, Mitogenic factors from the brain and the pituitary: Physiological significance, *Excerpta Med. Int. Congr. Ser.* pp. 141–155.

Holdsworth, S. R., Glasgow, E. F., Thomson, N. M., and Atkins, R. C., 1978, Tissue culture of isolated human glomeruli, *Pathology* **10:**59.

Ishikawa Y., Wada, T., and Sakaguchi, H., 1980, The possibility of three types of cells in cultured glomeruli *in vitro, Am. J. Pathol.* **100:**779.

Jaffe, E. A., Nachman, R. L., Becker, C. B., and Minick, C. R., 1973, Culture of human endothelial cells derived from umbilical veins: Identification by morphologic and immunologic criteria, *J. Clin. Invest.* **52:**2734.

Kefalides, N. A., 1973, Structure and biosynthesis of basement membranes, *Int. Rev. Connect. Tissue Res.* **6:**63.

Killen, P. D., and Striker, G. E., 1979, Human glomerular visceral epithelial cells synthesize a basal lamina collagen *in vitro, Proc. Natl. Acad. Sci, USA*, **76:**3518.

Kreisberg, J. I., Hoover, R. L., and Karnovsky, M. J., 1978, Isolation and characterization of rat glomerular epithelial cells in vitro, *Kidney Int.* **14:**21.

McKeehan, W. L., McKeehan, K. A., Hammond, S. L., and Ham, R. G., 1977, Improved medium for clonal growth of human diploid fibroblasts at low concentrations of serum protein, *In Vitro* **13:**399.

Michael, A. F., Nevins, T., Raij, L., and Scheinman, J. I., 1978, Macromolecular transport in the glomerulus: Studies of the mesangium and epithelium *in vivo* and *in vitro*, in: *Contemporary Issues in Nephrology* (B. M. Brenner and J. H. Stein, eds.), Churchill Livingstone, Edinburgh.

Norgaard, J. D. R., 1978, Retraction of epithelial foot processes during culture of isolated glomeruli, *Lab. Invest.* **38:**320.

Nowack, H., Gay, S., Wick, G., Becker, U., and Timpl, R., 1976, Preparation and use in immunohistology of antibodies specific for type I and III collagen and pro-collagen, *J. Immunol. Methods* **12:**117.

Oberley, T. D., Burkholder, P. M., and Mills, M. D., 1979, Culture of human glomerular cells, *Am. J. Pathol.* **96:**101.

Oberley, T. D., VicMuth, J., and Murphy-Ulrich, J. E., 1980, Growth and maintenance of glomerular cells under defined conditions, *Am. J. Pathol.* **101.**195.

Oberley, T. D., Murphy-Ullrich, J. E., Steinert, B. W., and VicMuth, J., 1981, The growth of primary glomerular cells as a confluent monolayer in a chemically defined serum-free medium, *Am. J. Pathol.* **104:**181.

Quadracci, L. J., and Striker, G. E., 1970, Growth and maintenance of glomerular cells in vitro, *Proc. Soc. Exp. Biol. Med.* **135:**947.

Scheinman, J. I., and Fish, A. J., 1978, Human glomerular cells in culture: Three subcultured cell types bearing glomerular antigens, *Am. J. Pathol.* **92:**125.

Scheinman, J. I., Fish, A. J., and Michael, A. F., 1974, The immunohistopathology of glomerular antigens: The GBM, collagen and actomyosin antigens in normal and diseased kidneys, *J. Clin. Invest.* **54:**1144.

Scheinman, J. I., Fish, A. J., Brown, D. M., and Michael, A. F., 1976, Human glomerular smooth muscle (mesangial) cells in culture, *Lab. Invest.* **34:**150.

Scheinman, J. I., Fish, A. J., Matas, A. J., and Michael, A. F., 1978a, The immunohistopathology of glomerular antigens. II. The glomerular basement membrane, actomyosin and fibroblast surface antigens in normal, diseased and transplanted human kidneys, *Am. J. Pathol.* **90:**71.

Scheinman, J. I., Fish, A. J., Kim, Y., and Michael, A. F., 1978b, C3b receptors on human glomeruli in vitro: Loss in culture, *Am. J. Pathol.* **92:**147.

Scheinman, J. I., Brown, D. M., and Michael, A. F., 1978c, Collagen synthesis by human glomerular cells in culture, *Biochim. Biophys. Acta* **542:**128.

Schiffer, M. S., and Scheinman, J. I., 1982, submitted.

Striker, G. E., Killen, P. D., Agodoa, L. C. Y., Savin, V., and Quadracci, L. J., 1978, *In vitro* basal lamina synthesis by human glomerular epithelial and mesangial cells, evidence for post-translational heterogeneity, in: *Biology and Chemistry of Basement Membranes* (N. A. Kefalides, ed.), Academic Press, New York.

16

Results of Immune Complex Detection in Human Glomerular Diseases

Wayne A. Border

1. Introduction

Techniques for detection of soluble immune complexes (IC) in serum have become a subject of considerable scientific interest and potential clinical importance. The bulk of human glomerulonephritis probably is due to IC deposition (Wilson and Dixon, 1974, 1976). There is hope that IC detection might serve as a tool for diagnosis, prognosis, and management. This chapter will summarize the results of IC detection in patients with glomerular diseases and will indicate what the future holds for such investigations.

Despite the demonstration by Dixon *et al.* (1958) of the IC pathogenesis of acute serum sickness, detection of IC in man necessarily has awaited development of methods which do not depend upon specific recognition of an antigen. In the past 5 years, such techniques have been perfected, in large part, as a by-product of the rapid progress both in cellular immunology and in the biochemistry of the complement system. Such advances have been so productive that over 30 separate methods for IC detection have been described in the literature (Wager and Mannik, 1977; Maini and Holborow, 1977).

2. Detection of IC in Patients with Glomerulonephritis

In 1975 this laboratory set out to determine the prevalence of IC in patients presenting with glomerulonephritis. A strictly prospective study was

Wayne A. Border · Division of Nephrology and Hypertension, Los Angeles County Harbor/UCLA Medical Center, Torrance, California 90502. This work was supported in part by a grant from the Kidney Foundation of Southern California.

conducted in which serum samples from 107 patients undergoing diagnostic renal biopsy at UCLA-Harbor General Hospital were carefully collected, aliquoted, and frozen at −70°C before being tested within 1 month in parallel by C1q binding assay (C1q-BA), Raji cell assay (Raji), and microcomplement consumption assay (Woodroffe *et al.*, 1977). The findings were that IC were most prevalent in systemic lupus erythematosus (SLE) and glomerulonephritis associated with systemic disease, e.g., vasculitis or bacterial endocarditis, and were less frequent in patients manifesting only IC glomerulonephritis (Table 1). The three methods correlated poorly within each disease category, probably due to the heterogeneous IC present and their different reactivity with each method. If all three methods were considered, then 87, 65, and 39% respectively of patients with SLE, systemic disease, and glomerulonephritis and primary IC glomerulonephritis had positive results, and such results may indicate that a panel of assays should be used in clinical studies instead of a single method. There were no apparent clinical differences at presentation between IC positive and negative patients in the same disease category.

In order to determine if IC detection is of diagnostic or prognostic value, this laboratory undertook two long-term studies. The first was retrospective and involved 112 patients with adult idiopathic nephrotic syndrome, participating in a controlled, randomized trial of prednisone versus placebo, who were evaluated using C1q-BA, C1q solid-phase assay (C1q-SP), and Raji assays. All patients were diagnosed by renal biopsy. Serum samples were obtained prior to and following therapy and at frequent intervals thereafter. As shown in Table 2, IC were demonstrated in all disease categories. When the data were analyzed in terms of clinical outcome, the presence or absence of IC in individual patients seemed to have little importance. Results of IC testing did not predict response to prednisone or placebo or the likelihood of remission of nephrotic syndrome. Finally, the rate of decline of renal function was no different in patients with and without IC. In the second study, 48 patients with SLE were followed for 6 to 18 months (Abrass *et al.*, 1980b). During each clinic visit, disease activity and manifestations were recorded and serum obtained for C1q-BA, C1q-SP, C3 level, and DNA-binding activity. Analysis of the data revealed that a decline in C3 level, increase in DNA-binding activity, or positive C1q-BA often occurred in

Table 1. Prospective Study of Immune Complex Detection in Glomerular Diseases[a]

Glomerular disease (n)	Percent positive patients		
	Clq-BA	Raji	MCT
Systemic lupus erythematosus (23)	35	74	27
Systemic disease with GN (17)	41	29	18
GN without systemic disease (36)	17	14	14
Normal controls (31)	3	3	6

[a] Abbreviations used: GN, glomerulonephritis; Clq-BA, Clq binding assay; Raji, Raji cell assay; MCT, microcomplement consumption assay.

Table 2. Retrospective Study of Immune Complex Detection in Idiopathic Nephrotic Syndrome[a]

Glomerular disease (*n*)	Percent positive patients		
	Clq-BA	Raji	MCT
Minimal change disease (13)	38	46	18
Focal glomerular disease (31)	19	30	19
Membranous nephropathy (68)	22	37	32
Normal controls (23)	0	13	9

[a] Abbreviations used: Clq-BA, Clq binding assay; Clq-SP, Clq solid-phase assay; Raji, Raji cell assay.

association with an exacerbation of SLE activity, but that these tests did not significantly correlate with or predict SLE activity. This is in contrast to the C1q-SP which correlated with disease activity and when it converted from negative to positive, the change correctly predicted an exacerbation in SLE within 2 months in 78% of the cases. Whether or not a therapeutic intervention based on C1q-SP results will abort the predicted disease exacerbation is unknown. Other investigators also have found a correlation between disease activity, renal function, and the presence of IC in a selected group of patients with SLE, vasculitis, or IC-mediated rapidly progressive glomerulonephritis (Pussel *et al.*, 1978).

It is interesting to compare these results with those of other investigators who have employed the same or different IC assays. Recently, Lambert *et al.* (1978) compared 18 methods of IC detection. Six of the eighteen methods stood out as being superior in their ability to distinguish various concentrations of IG aggregates, detect all sizes of aggregates, not be adversely affected by interfering substances, and discriminate between pathological and normal serum samples. These six methods are: C1q-BA, C1q-SP, C1q-deviation (C1q-DV), monoclonal rheumatoid factor binding inhibition (mRF-I), conglutinin solid-phase binding (Kg-SP), and Raji. Several investigators have used one or more of these six methods to study groups of patients with glomerulonephritis (Woodroffe *et al.*, 1977; Abrass *et al.*, 1980a; Lambert *et al.*, 1978; Levinsky and Soothill, 1977; Levinsky *et al.*, 1977a,b; Casali *et al.*, 1977; Eisenberg *et al.*, 1977; Izui *et al.*, 1977; Ooi *et al.*, 1977a,b,c; Caro *et al.*, 1977; Tung *et al.*, 1978; Rossen *et al.*, 1976; Sobel *et al.*, 1976; Cohen *et al.*, 1978) and the results are summarized in Table 3 [for purposes of comparison, other rheumatoid factor (RF) methods in addition to mRF-I were included in the RF column].

The highest percent positive patients were found in acute glomerulonephritis, 58%; SLE, 50% (this group included patients with and without clinical evidence of nephritis), and polyarteritis/vasculitis, 46%. The lowest prevalence of IC was in patients with IgA nephropathy, 4%, probably reflecting the inability of most methods to detect IgA complexes. Not unexpectedly, a small number of patients, 10%, with anti-GBM nephritis were positive; IC have been demonstrated by immunofluorescence as a

Table 3. Use of Six Methods to Detect Immune Complexes in Glomerular Diseases[a,b]

Glomerular disease	No. patients studied/percent positive						
	Clq-BA	Clq-SP	Clq-DV	RF	Kg-SP	Raji	Total
Acute glomerulonephritis	33/55	4/100	U/90	U	U	18/56	55/58
Rapidly progressive GN	9/11	6/67	U	U	U	20/20	35/26
Systemic lupus erythematosus[c]	388/51	93/60	U	53/66	301/30	233/70	1058/50
Membranoproliferative GN	50/30	2/0	U/25	U	19/5	18/17	89/20
Minimal change disease	19/21	16/50	U/40	18/44	U	21/19	74/45
Focal Glomerular Disease[d]	31/23	27/33	U	U	U	37/27	95/28
Membranous GN	86/21	63/35	U/70	U	16/19	70/16	235/23
Mesangial proliferative GN	17/41	U	U	U	U	8/13	25/32
IgA nephropathy	7/14	7/0	U/10	U	7/0	7/0	28/4
Henoch–Schönlein purpura GN	13/3	1/0	U	U	9/3	3/0	26/23
Polyarteritis/vasculitis	67/58	17/41	17/47	17/53	88/33	48/52	154/46
Hemolytic-uremic syndrome	2/50	U	U	U	U	2/0	4/25
Chronic or unspecified GN	101/26	7/14	U	U	21/10	33/18	162/25
Anti-GBM GN	29/10	3/0	U	U	26/4	13/15	71/9
Transplant patients	35/40	U	U	U	U	23/26	58/34
Normal controls	197/3	129/3	U/5	U	177/3	218/6	721/4

[a] Table compiled from Woodroffe *et al.* (1977), Abrass *et al.* (1980a), Lambert *et al.* (1978), Levinsky and Soothill (1977), Levinsky *et al.* (1977a,b), Casali *et al.* (1977), Eisenberg *et al.* (1977), Izui *et al.* (1977), Ooi *et al.* (1977a,b,c), Caro *et al.* (1977), Tung *et al.* (1978), Rossen *et al.* (1976), Sobel *et al.* (1976), Cohen *et al.* (1978).

[b] Abbreviations used: U, data unavailable; GN, glomerulonephritis; GBM, glomerular basement membrane; Clq-BA, Clq binding assay; Clq-SP, Clq solid-phase assay; Clq-DV, Clq deviation; RF, all rheumatoid factor methods; Kg-SP, conglutinin solid-phase binding; Raji, Raji cell assay.

[c] With and without clinical renal disease.

[d] Predominantly focal-segmental glomerulosclerosis.

complicating mechanism of immunologic injury in a few such patients. quite unexpected, however, was the 45% of patients with minimal change disease that were positive since the usual diagnostic criteria for this entity include negative immunofluorescence (Abrass *et al.*, 1980a Cohen *et al.*, 1978). Several factors, such as the prompt response of the proteinuria to immunosuppressive drugs, have suggested an immunological pathogenesis for minimal change disease (Levinsky *et al.*, 1977a; Poston *et al.*, 1978). It is possible that IC may play a pathological role by interacting with cellular receptors causing a release of mediators or interfering with helper or suppressor functions without accumulating in glomerular deposits. The significance of IC detected in transplant patients remains unclear since IC may be part of the original disease or the rejection process. However, IC appear to be more prevalent in patients undergoing acute rejection (Ooi *et al.*, 1977a). Finally, low levels of IC were detectable in 4% of 721 healthy controls. A striking finding is the uniformity of test results within a disease category (i.e., SLE, minimal change disease, polyarteritis/vasculitis, etc.) despite the use of methods sensitive to different IC properties.

In summary, data are now available from application to the best IC methods to study hundreds of patients with glomerular diseases. Certainly immunopathologists are pleased that IC are detectable in the majority of patients with IC-mediated glomerulonephritis. Despite the enthusiasm of some investigators, the fact that IC are present in nearly all forms of glomerulonephritis means that their detection and quantitation will not serve as a diagnostic tool—a major disappointment to the clinical nephrologist. Perhaps qualitative differences between IC will be found that may prove useful in terms of diagnosis, but this remains to be proven. In terms of prognosis at least in adult idiopathic nephrotic syndrome, IC testing did not provide useful clinical information (Abrass *et al.*, 1980a) and another study in a general population of patients with chronic nephritic syndromes yielded similar results (Gluckman *et al.*, 1978).

Given the state-of-the-art, it can be concluded that a single IC measurement, regardless of the method employed, provides little information of clinical merit. On the other hand, serial determination of IC is likely to be useful in certain diseases such as SLE where remission and exacerbation are directly related to the quantity of circulating IC. When such patients are treated with immunosuppressive drugs, pulse methylprednisolone, or plasmapheresis, quantitation of IC may aid in determining duration or need to reinstitute therapy.

3. Ubiquitous Occurrence of IC in Man

In addition to glomerular diseases IC have been detected in a spectrum of patients with acute and chronic liver disease (Thomas *et al.*, 1978; Abrass *et al.*, 1980c) and with various kinds of cancer (Theofilopoulos *et al.*, 1977; Rossen and Barnes, 1978). Such data suggest that IC are prevalent in human disease regardless of etiology and their presence need not be associated with glomerulonephritis or imply an immunological pathogenesis for the disease in question. Thus, the results of IC detection must be interpreted in light of the likely ubiquitous presence of IC in chronically ill patients (Abrass *et al.*, 1980c).

4. The Future Use of IC Methods

The most important use of IC methods will be to provide a means for isolation and recovery of IC from patients with glomerulonephritis as has already been accomplished in experimental animals (Abrass *et al.*, 1980d). Research on the critical unanswered question of the nature and source of the antigen in the IC has been hampered by the lack of sufficient material for study. Current methods can be modified to allow processing of large volumes of serum for bulk recovery of IC material. Characterization of isolated IC as to molecular size, electrical charge, and immunoglobulin and complement composition may provide a new basis for categorizing patients with glomerulonephritis, as well as explaining why some IC are nephritogenic while others apparently circulate without producing glomerular injury.

ACKNOWLEDGMENTS. The author acknowledges the invaluable collaboration of Drs. A. J. Woodroffe, C. K. Abrass, and R. J. Glassock, the superior technical work of David Strong, and the excellent secretarial assistance of Kay Anderson.

References

Abrass, C. K., Hall, C. L., Border, W. A., Brown, C. A., Glassock, R. J., and Coggins, C. H., 1980a, Circulating immune complexes in adults with idiopathic nephrotic syndrome: Relationship to histologic category and clinical course, *Kidney Int.* **17:**545.

Abrass, C. K., Nies, K. M., Louie, J. S., Border, W. A., and Glassock, R. J., 1980b, Correlation and predictability of circulating immune complexes with disease activity in patients with systemic lupus erythematosus, *Arthritis Rheum.* **23:**273.

Abrass, C. K., Border, W. A., and Hepner, G., 1980c, Nonspecificity of circulating immune complexes in patients with acute and chronic liver disease, *Clin. Exp. Immunol.* **40:**292.

Abrass, C. K., Border, W. A., and Glassock, R. J., 1980d, Detection and characterization of circulating immune complexes in rats with autologous immune complex nephritis, *Lab. Invest.* **43:**18.

Caro, P. O., Jeny, L. M., Sladowski, J. P., and Osterland, C. K., 1977, Circulating immune complexes in systemic lupus erythematosus, *Clin. Exp. Immunol.* **29:**197.

Casali, P., Bossus, A., Carpentier, N. A., and Lambert, P. H., 1977, Solid phase enzyme immunoassay or radioimmunoassay for the detection of immune complexes based on their recognition by conglutinin: Conglutinin-binding test, *Clin. Exp. Immunol.* **29:**342.

Cohen, A., Border, W. A., and Glassock, R. J., 1978, Nephrotic syndrome with glomerular mesangial IgM deposits, *Lab. Invest.* **38:**610.

Dixon, F. J., Vazquez, J. J., Weigle, W. O., and Cochrane, C. G., 1958, Pathogenesis of serum sickness, *Arch. Pathol.* **65:**18.

Eisenberg, R. A., Theofilopoulos, A. N., and Dixon, F. J., 1977, Use of bovine conglutinin for the assay of immune complexes, *J. Immunol.* **118:**1428.

Gluckman, J. C., Jacob, N., Beaufils, H., Baumelou, A., Salah, H., German, A., and Legrain, M., 1978, Is immune complex detection of clinical significance in chronic glomerulonephritis?, *Kidney Int.* **14:**202.

Izui, S., Lambert, P. H., and Miescher, P. A., 1977, Failure to detect circulating DNA–anti-DNA complexes by four radioimmunological methods in patients with SLE, *Clin. Exp. Immunol.* **30:**384.

Lambert, P. H., Dixon, F. J., Zubler, R. H., Agnello, V., Cambiaso, C., Casali, P., Clarke, J., Cowdery, J. S., McDuffie, F. C., Hay, F. C., MacLennan, I. C. M., Masson, P., Müller-Eberhard, H. J., Penttinen, K., Smith, M., Tappeiner, G., Theofilopoulos, A. N., and Verroust, P., 1978, A collaborative study for the evaluation of eighteen methods for detecting immune complexes in serum, *J. Clin. Lab. Immunol.* **1:**1.

Levinsky, R. J., and Soothill, J. F., 1977, A test for antigen–antibody complexes in human sera using IgM of rabbit antisera to human immunoglobulin, *Clin. Exp. Immunol.* **29:**428.

Levinsky, R. J., Malleson, P. N., Barratt, T. M., and Soothill, J. F., 1977a, Circulating immune complexes in steroid responsive nephrotic syndrome, *N. Engl. J. Med.* **298:**126.

Levinsky, R. J., Cameron, J. S., and Soothill, J. F., 1977b, Serum immune complexes and disease activity in lupus nephritis, *Lancet* **1:**564.

Maini, R. N., and Holborow, E. J. (eds.), 1977, *Detection and Measurement of Circulating Soluble Immune Complexes, Ann. Rheum. Dis.* **36**(Suppl.)**:**1.

Ooi, Y. M., Ooi, B. S., Vallota, E. H., Furst, M. R., and Pollak, V. E., 1977a, Circulating immune complexes after renal transplantation, *J. Clin. Invest.* ***60:***611.

Ooi, Y. M., Vallota, E. H., and West, C. D., 1977b, Serum immune complexes in membranoproliferative and other glomerulonephritides, *Kidney Int.* **11:**275.

Ooi, Y. M., Ooi, B. S., and Pollak, V. E., 1977c, Relationships of levels of circulating immune complexes to histologic patterns of nephritis: A comparative study of membranous glomerulonephropathy and diffuse proliferative glomerulonephritis, *J. Lab. Clin. Med.* **90:**891.

Poston, R. N., Cerio, R., and Cameron, J. S., 1978, Circulating immune complexes in minimal change nephritis (Letter), *N. Engl. J. Med.* **298:**1089.

Pussel, B. A., Lockwood, C. M., Scott, D. M., and Pinching, A. J., 1978, Value of immune complex assays in diagnosis and management, *Lancet* **2:**359.

Rossen, R. D., and Barnes, B. C., 1978, Measuring serum immune complexes in cancer, *Ann. Intern. Med.* **88:**570.

Rossen, R. D., Reisberg, M. A., Singer, D. B., Schloeder, F. X., Suki, W. N., Hill, L. L., and Eknoyan, G., 1976, Soluble immune complexes in sera of patients with nephritis, *Kidney Int.* **10:**256.

Sobel, A., Gobay, Y., and Lagrue, G., 1976, Recherche de complexes immuns circulants par le test de déviation de la fraction C1q du complément, *Nouv. Presse Med.* **5:**1465.

Theofilopoulos, A. N., Andrews, B. S., Urist, M. M., Morton, D. L., and Dixon, F. J., 1977, The nature of immune complexes in human cancer sera, *J. Immunol.* **119:**657.

Thomas, H. C., DeVilliers, D., Potts, B. Hodgson, H., Gain, S., Jewell, P., and Sherlock, S., 1978, Immune complexes in acute and chronic liver disease, *Clin. Exp. Immunol.* **31:**150.

Tung, S. K., Woodroffe, A. J., Ahlin, T. D., Williams, R. C., and Wilson, C. B., 1978, Application of the solid phase C1q and Raji cell radioimmune assays for the detection of circulating immune complexes in glomerulonephritis, *J. Clin. Invest.* **62:**61.

Wager, O., and Mannik, M., 1977, Detection and relevance of circulating immune complexes, in: *Progress in Immunology II,* Proceedings of the Third International Congress of Immunology, pp. 776–778, Sydney, Australia.

Wilson, C. B., and Dixon, F. J., 1974, Diagnosis of immunopathologic renal disease, *Kidney Int.* **5:**389.

Wilson, C. B., and Dixon, F. J., 1976, Renal response to immunologic injury, in: *The Kidney* (B. M. Brenner and F. C. Rector, Jr., eds.), Saunders, Philadelphia.

Woodroffe, A. J., Border, W. A., Theofilopoulos, A. N., Gotze, O., Glassock, R. J., Dixon, F. J., and Wilson, C. B., 1977, Detection of circulating immune complexes in patients with glomerulonephritis, *Kidney Int.* **12:**268.

17

Nephritogenic Immune Responses Involving Basement Membrane and Other Antigens in or of the Glomerulus

Curtis B. Wilson

The immune response, normally a life-protecting device, can injure and destroy body tissue, and lead to such diseases as glomerulonephritis and tubulointerstitial nephritis. Studies in experimental animals begun over 70 years ago, and similar studies in man over the past 10 to 15 years, have identified two ways in which the humoral immune system can lead to renal injury (Wilson and Dixon, 1976). These two mechanisms can be divided for purposes of discussion into groups, dependent on the physical state of the antigens involved. The first group of reactions, involves soluble antigens that react with antibody to form immune complexes (Dixon, 1963). If the soluble antigens are present in the circulation, circulating immune complexes form and later deposit nonspecifically in vascular sites throughout the body, including the glomeruli and peritubular capillaries. If the soluble antigens are in the extravascular renal tissue, an Arthus–like immune complex formation occurs in the interstitium, leading to a localized immune complex disease at the site of reaction (Unanue *et al.*, 1967; Klassen *et al.*, 1971). It should be noted that immune complexes remain in equilibrium with antigen or antibody present in the body fluids, so that the composition of an immune complex deposit may be continually modified (Wilson and Dixon, 1978). Immune complexes actually can be dissolved and removed from the site of injury if a state of great antigen excess is achieved (Wilson, 1974).

The second group of immune reactions would be those involving antigens that are insoluble and fixed within tissue. Basement membrane antigens are

Curtis B. Wilson · Department of Immunopathology, Scripps Clinic and Research Foundation, La Jolla, California 92037.

the best example of this class, and a long history of experimental and human studies clearly demonstrate the pathogenicity of anti-basement membrane antibodies (Unanue and Dixon, 1967; Wilson and Dixon, 1976). Recent investigative work suggests that non-basement membrane glomerular capillary wall antigens or antigens from nonrenal sites, which are first trapped or "planted" within the glomerular capillary wall, may be involved in local nephritogenic immune reactions (Wilson, 1978b) As with immune complex disease, once the antigen–antibody reaction has taken place, common mediators of inflammation, including the complement system, polymorphonuclear leukocytes, mononuclear cells, possibly prostaglandins, and potentially the coagulation and Hageman factor-related kinin-forming systems can be activated, leading to inflammation and, when severe, actual destruction of tissue (Schreiber and Müller-Eberhard, 1979; Cochrane, 1979)

Some of the features of this interesting group of nephritogenic immune responses involving tissue-fixed antigens are reviewed herein. A good deal is known about the mechanisms of anti-basement membrane antibody; knowledge about nephritogenic immune reactions involving either non-basement membrane antigens of the glomerular capillary wall or antigens "planted" at that site is increasing. Work dealing with these latter antigens in experimental animals has clear potential for contributing to knowledge of immunologic renal injury in humans as well.

1. Anti-Basement Membrane Antibody Mechanisms

The best understood of the nephritogenic immune processes involving fixed antigens is that of anti-basement membrane disease. Studies at the turn of the century demonstrated the nephritogenic potential of antikidney antisera, and the glomerular basement membrane (GBM) was subsequently shown to contain the nephritogenic antigen (Krakower and Greenspon, 1951). Experimentally, heterologous anti-basement membrane antibodies cause injury in two phases following passive administration into an appropriate host. An immediate phase of injury occurs if sufficient amounts of antibody are administered (75, 15, and 5 μg/g kidney in rats, rabbits, and sheep, respectively) (Unanue and Dixon, 1967). The model has been very useful in outlining the principles of anti-basement membrane antibody damage and has been applied widely to the study of nephritis and its mediator systems, such as complement, polymorphonuclear leukocytes, and coagulation.

If insufficient amounts of antibody are given to induce immediate phase injury (as little as 2 μg/g kidney), a delayed or autologous phase of injury ensues when the host makes an antibody response directed toward the foreign or "planted" anti-GBM antibody bound in its kidney (Unanue and Dixon, 1965). This phase of injury is a classic example of the response to a "planted" or foreign antigen that now serves as a tissue-fixed antigen in a nephritogenic immune reaction. This phase of injury may be augmented by active immunization to the foreign immunoglobulin or by passive administration of preformed anti-immunoglobulin antibody. Recently, mononuclear cells also were proposed as participants in this phase of injury (Schreiner *et al.*, 1978; Bhan *et al.*, 1978; Holdsworth *et al.*, 1981).

A variety of experimental models have been described in which animals are immunized with basement membrane antigens and subsequently produce anti-basement membrane antibodies reactive with their own GMB or tubular basement membrane (TBM) (Unanue and Dixon, 1967; Wilson and Dixon, 1976). The sheep is particularly susceptible to this type of nephritogenic immune response and develops a rapidly fatal glomerulonephritis after immunization with a few hundred milligrams of human basement membrane (Steblay, 1962). Anti-GBM antibodies can be identified in the circulation or found fixed along the GBM in a linear pattern. Antibodies recovered from nephritic sheep have been used to transfer the disease to normal lambs, establishing the pathogenicity of the anti-basement membrane antibody (Lerner and Dixon, 1966).

Rats immunized with bovine renal basement membrane develop antibodies reactive with TBM and manifest acute tubulointerstitial nephritis (Lehman *et al.*, 1974a). This model is of particular interest because it points up strain-related variations in the antigenic composition of the TBM. Brown Norway rats, for example, have the nephritogenic TBM antigen although it is lacking in the Lewis rat strain. Lewis rats are capable of mounting an immune response to the antigen and do so when transplanted with a Brown Norway/Lewis F_1 hybrid kidney (Lehman *et al.*, 1974b). The antibodies formed bind to the TBM of the transplant but not to the host's own kidney. The strain-related difference in TBM antigens in rats is of particular interest in relation to human nephritis. Occasionally, one of these patients lacks the usual nephritogenic antigens in either their GBM or TBM (Wilson *et al.*, 1974a; McCoy *et al.*, 1976). Transplantation in this situation can lead to the induction of an anti-basement membrane antibody response similar to that just described in the rat.

Anti-basement membrane antibodies also can be induced in experimental animals by immunization with basement membrane-rich fractions of urine. About one-third of rabbits immunized with concentrated fractions of their own urine develop anti-basement membrane antibody-induced nephritis (Lerner and Dixon, 1968). Similar antigens have been identified in the sera of both rats and humans (McPhaul and Dixon, 1969; Willoughby and Dixon, 1970) and, although they probably serve normally as tolerogens, they might, under appropriate circumstances, act as immunogens.

2. *Anti-Basement Membrane Antibodies and the Diseases They Produce in Man*

Anti-basement membrane antibodies were shown convincingly as the cause of human nephritis in studies performed by Lerner *et al.* (1967). They evaluated a group of patients with possible anti-basement membrane antibody disease in view of the immunofluorescent localization of linear immunoglobin deposits along their GBMs. These investigators were able to isolate anti-basement membrane antibodies from the patients' circulations as well as from acid eluates of the involved kidneys. The pathogenicity of the isolated antibody was shown by experiments in which the antibody was used to transfer nephritis to subhuman primates. These workers also documented the transfer of anti-basement membrane antibody nephritis to a renal transplant inadvertently placed in a patient with residual circulating anti-GBM antibody, confirming the pathogenicity of the antibody in man. Subsequent studies have revealed several additional examples of recurrent anti-GBM nephritis in individuals transplanted while circulating antibody remained (Wilson and Dixon, 1973).

Anti-basement membrane antibodies now are known to be responsible for a spectrum of diseases varying from mild to severe and rapidly progressive glomerulonephritis, often with associated pulmonary injury and pulmonary hemorrhage, a condition referred to as Goodpasture's syndrome. Because the clinical picture of nephritis and pulmonary hemorrhage can have several causes (Wilson, 1979a) Goodpasture's syndrome should carry an etiologic qualification such as anti-basement membrane antibody induced, immune complex induced, etc. Some patients with a clinical presentation of idiopathic pulmonary hemosiderosis have anti-basement membrane antibodies bound in their lungs and present in their circulation. In one of the first individuals of this type evaluated in our laboratory, anti-basement membrane antibodies also were identified in the kidney along with histologic evidence of a mild glomerulitis. However, overt clinical renal symptomatology never developed (Wilson and Dixon, 1974). It is currently unknown how many individuals with idiopathic pulmonary hemosiderosis have anti-basement membrane antibodies as a cause. Some patients also have anti-basement membrane antibodies bound in the choroid plexus, and one such individual with Goodpasture's syndrome had an unexplained convulsive disorder, possibly related to the antibody deposit (Wilson and Dixon, 1976). Roughly 70% of patients with anti-GBM antibodies have anti-TBM antibodies as well, with some correlation between the presence of anti-TBM antibodies and the amount of tubulointerstitial damage observed (Lehman *et al.*, 1975; Andres *et al.*, 1978). Anti-TBM antibodies also have been noted to develop in the absence of anti-GBM antibodies in a few patients with immune complex-induced glomerulonephritis (Morel-Maroger *et al.*, 1974; Harner *et al.*, 1974; Tung and Black, 1975) or, occasionally, in association with drug-induced tubulointerstitial nephritis (Border *et al.*, 1974; Hayman *et al.*, 1975), and perhaps as a primary immune process (Andres and McCluskey, 1975; Bergstein and Litman, 1975; Wilson and Dixon, 1976). Anti-TBM antibodies in the absence of anti-GBM antibodies have been reported in transplant recipients, sometimes apparently related to the rejection process itself (Klassen *et al.*, 1973), and otherwise related to antigenic differences in the TBM between the host and the transplanted kidney (Wilson *et al.*, 1974a). The recognized spectrum of diseases caused by anti-basement membrane antibodies can be expected to grow. For example, studies have been performed on one individual with anti-TBM antibodies associated with immune complex nephritis and intractable diarrhea who had antibodies that, when eluted from the kidney, reacted with the basement membrane of the intestine (Wilson, C. B., unpublished observations). The possibility that these antibodies related to his intestinal problems is a reasonable speculation.

The most common presentation of anti-basement membrane antibody disease is Goodpasture's syndrome, i.e. pulmonary hemorrhage, accompanied with proliferative, crescent forming and often rapidly progressive glomerulonephritis. By immunofluorescence, linear deposits of IgG are observed along the GBM, occasionally with IgA or IgM as well. C3 deposits accompany the immunoglobulin in two-thirds to three-fourths of these individuals, although the deposit of C3 is often less striking than that of immunoglobulin (Wilson and Dixon, 1973). Circumferential linear deposits of immunoglobulin are observed on the TBM of about 70% of patients with anti-GBM antibody-induced nephritis. The TBM deposition may be confined to segments of the tubule or scattered diffusely throughout its length. Care must be taken in interpreting linear immunofluorescent deposits in the GBM and TBM. A troublesome background of nonimmunologic linear immunoglobulin deposits, usually accompanied by albumin, appears in kidney specimens obtained from patients with diabetes mellitus, from kidneys perfused prior to transplantation or obtained at autopsy and, for as yet unexplained reasons, in some relatively normal kidney specimens (Wilson and Dixon, 1974). The specificity of linear deposits of immunoglobulin should, then, be confirmed when possible by elution study or by detection of circulating anti-basement membrane antibodies.

The basement membrane is composed of collagenous and noncollagenous glycopeptides with variations in composition notable among different basement membrane sites. The GBM contains approximately 25% of noncollagenous glycoproteins that remain after collagenase digestion and extensive dialysis. This collagenase-solubilized GBM is capable of completely inhibiting the reaction of human anti-GBM antibodies detected by indirect immunofluorescence and is nephritogenic when used to immunize experimental animals. The collagenous portion of the GBM does not appear to be as nephritogenic, but definitive exclusion of the role of collagen awaits similar experiments using GBM collagen. From the results of one radioimmunoassay that utilized an autoclaved sodium dodecyl sulfate and immunoabsorbent-purified GBM antigen, some reactivity seemed to reside in the disaccharide moiety associated with the collagenous portion (Mahieu *et al.*, 1974).

Our studies suggest that most human anti-GBM antibodies react predominantly with 53,000 and 27,000 dalton noncollagenous glycoproteins remaining after collagenase digestion (Holdsworth *et al.*, 1979). These antigens were used in developing a radioimmunoassay to detect circulating and eluted anti-GBM antibodies (Wilson and Dixon, 1974; Wilson *et al.*, 1974b). The results are reproducible, with some sera binding up to 65% of the radiolabeled antigen. No binding is observed in normal serum. The assay is more sensitive than the standard indirect immunofluorescent technique but does not detect anti-TBM antibodies identifiable by immunofluorescence in the absence of anti-GBM antibodies. When comparing the results of this radioimmunoassay to the immunopathologic diagnosis of patients studied in this laboratory, an excellent correlation has been found. Seventy-six of seventy-eight patients with evidence of anti-GBM antibody-induced Goodpasture's syndrome and 43 of 52 patients with anti-GBM antibody-induced glomerulonephritis alone have had circulating antibody detectable with this technique. Of 329 patients with immune complex glomerulonephritis, only 2 had circulating antibody and both developed the antibody during an accelerated phase of chronic membranous glomerulonephritis. Of interest, 4 of 56 patients with systemic lupus erythematosus had evidence of circulating antibody according to the radioimmunoassay. Previous studies yielded occasional linear staining in patients with this disease (Koffler *et al.*, 1969a), suggesting that anti-GBM antibody might be numbered among the many autoantibodies such patients produce. To date, elution studies to assess the presence of anti-basement membrane antibodies in patients with systemic lupus erythematosus have not been available to confirm this suspicion. Only 1 of over 200 patients with negative renal immunopathologic studies had detectable anti-GBM antibody. This patient subsequently developed anti-GBM antibody-induced nephritis in a transplant; the original diagnosis was based on examination of only a small piece of tissue which must have been inadequate to detect the antibody.

The mean amounts of antibody detected by the radioimmunoassay do not differ between this group of patients with anti-GBM antibody-induced Goodpasture's syndrome and those with glomerulonephritis alone (Wilson and Dixon, 1978). Indeed, some of the highest levels of antibody have been found in patients without pulmonary symptoms. There is also little correlation between episodes of pulmonary hemorrhage and the absolute amount of antibody present in the circulation, although pulmonary hemorrhages rarely occur in the absence of detectable circulating antibody. Radioimmunoassays for anti-alveolar basement membrane antibody now are being developed to see if other reactivities may be present that are not detected using the GBM-derived antigen. Prior studies with antibodies eluted from the lungs of patients with Goodpasture's syndrome demonstrated cross-reactivity with the GBM, suggesting that absolute differences in the reactive antibody may not be the significant factor (Koffler *et al.*, 1969b; McPhaul and Dixon, 1970). It is probable that some additional event, perhaps physiologic or infectious in nature, is necessary before the pulmonary damage presumably mediated by the antibody becomes clinically overt (Rees *et al.*, 1977; Johnson *et al.*, 1978). Patients with anti-GBM antibody-induced Goodpasture's syndrome generally have linear deposits along the alveolar basement membranes when examined. It is not clear how many patients whose clinical disease is confined to the kidney also have antibodies bound in their lungs, since specimens from these patients are rarely available for study. However, one such individual has been seen by our group (Wilson, C. B., unpublished observations).

Serum samples generally are not drawn sufficiently early in the course of disease to allow correlation between the amount or level of antibody produced and the severity of the ensuing involvement. When serial samples are available, the first sample is almost always the highest in antibody content. A decline in reactivity in samplings taken over the subsequent weeks or months follows. When examined by indirect immunofluorescence, the mean disappearance time of the antibody is around 8 months, while with the more sensitive radioimmunoassay the mean disappearance increases to around 13 months. It is very unusual for antibody to persist over 2 years. Reappearance of antibody is unusual although large numbers of patients have not yet been followed for long periods. One interesting exception is an individual who had three episodes of disease, predominantly lung involvement, over an 11-year period and reasonably well-documented anti-GBM antibody during the first and last episodes (Dahlberg *et al.*, 1978).

Working with many nephrology and transplant-related nephrology groups throughout the country, our group has been fortunate to obtain sera and/or tissue samples from over 400 patients with anti-basement membrane antibody-induced diseases since the last series of over 50 patients reported in 1973 (Wilson and Dixon, 1973). The clinical and immunopathologic features of this new group are being reviewed. Preliminary analysis of the first 272 patients has shown that 64% have Goodpasture's syndrome, 34% have apparent glomerulonephritis alone, and the remaining few have clinical involvement confined to the lung. Sixty-nine percent of the Goodpasture's patients and 57% of the glomerulonephritis patients are males, and over 90% of both groups are Caucasian. The disease is most common in the second and third decades of life, except in a small grouping of patients, particularly of females with kidney involvement only, in the fifth and sixth decades. The disease can occur at any age, with some patients below 10 years old or over 70 also in the group. The presentation is generally either as rapidly progressive glomerulonephritis or as Goodpasture's syndrome, which often is preceded by a prodrome of flu-like illness, with a few patients having arthralgia or arthritis as a prominent early complaint. In patients presenting with Goodpasture's syndrome, pulmonary hemorrhage is generally episodic, varying from mild hemoptysis to severe and sometimes fatal pulmonary hemorrhage. The onset of pulmonary hemorrhage and glomerulonephritis may be simultaneous or one may precede the other separated by periods sometimes over a year. About three-fourths of the patients develop renal failure, and the mortality rate of the group has been about 20%. In spite of the general severity of the disease, increasing numbers of milder and self-remitting examples are being observed.

In most instances, nephrectomy makes little or no immediate impact on the amount of circulating anti-GBM antibodies, suggesting that the damaged kidney has little residual immunoabsorptive capacity. In the few patients whose serial blood samples have been available pre- and postnephrectomy, the rate of antibody decline seems to hasten after nephrectomy.

The events leading to the induction of an anti-basement membrane response are poorly understood. Some loose associations have been made with infectious or noxious environmental stimuli such as influenza A2 infection (Wilson and Smith, 1972; Wilson and Dixon, 1973) or hydrocarbon solvent inhalation (Beirne *et al.*, 1977). In reviewing the histories obtained from patients in our ongoing study, less than 20% mentioned significant environmental exposure; of these about half had experiences with hydrocarbons or cleaning fluids and a few worked as either plumbers or painters. Renal injury associated with drugs, immunologic insults, or ischemia also has been associated occasionally with anti-basement membrane antibodies (Hume *et al.*, 1970; Klassen *et al.*, 1974; Border *et al.*, 1974). Of interest are samples submitted to our laboratory from at least four patients with Hodgkin's disease or lymphoma who subsequently developed anti-basement membrane disease. This latter observation is noteworthy because of the previous finding that anti-basement membrane antibodies contaminate some antilymphocyte antibody preparations generated for immunosuppressive use (Wilson *et al.*, 1971). The anti-basement membrane antibodies recovered from one of the Hodgkin's patients had reactivity with the stromal elements of lymph nodes, the structure postulated as responsible for the induction of the antilymphocyte antibody activity in the antilymphocyte globulins (Ma *et al.*, 1978).

Differences in basement membrane antigens among individuals are of interest. Not all human kidneys used as targets for indirect immunofluorescent testing, for example, react equally well with anti-GBM antibodies. Some individuals with hereditary nephritis of the Alport type seem to lack the usual nephritogenic antigens in their basement membranes (McCoy *et al.*, 1976). At least one of these patients, upon transplantation, developed an anti-basement membrane antibody response to basement membrane antigens present in the transplant but not in his native kidneys. How extensive the antigenic differences between indivduals are is not yet clear. The recent observation of an unusual frequency of the DRw2 antigen in patients with Goodpasture's syndrome (Rees *et al.*, 1978) suggests a genetic factor in the disease, perhaps related in part to antigenic variation.

The clinical outcome of patients with anti-GBM antibody-induced glomerulonephritis or Goodpasture's syndrome has improved, with a current mortality rate of 20% compared to 47% in the initial series (Wilson and Dixon, 1973). Over 30% of the present large group are surviving with adequate renal function as compared to 11% of the previous series. Improvements in diagnostic techniques allowing identification of patients with milder forms of the disease, as well as more ready access to dialysis therapy and the now common use of high-dose steroids in the management of severe pulmonary hemorrhage, certainly have contributed to this improved outcome. More patients are being treated with immunosuppression, and recently with immunosuppression combined with intensive plasmapheresis (Lockwood *et al.*, 1975, 1976, 1979; Johnson *et al.*, 1978; Rosenblatt *et al.*, 1979). Since the production of anti-basement membrane antibodies is usually relatively short-lived, any maneuver to hasten the disappearance or removal of antibody theoretically should have therapeutic benefit. Accordingly, immunosuppression has been used to suppress antibody production coupled with removal of circulating antibody by plasmapheresis. The current impression is that the combined immunosuppressive and plasmapheresis therapy offers a further incremental benefit over that produced by immunosuppression alone. At least one controlled study is currently under way to assess this clinical impression, which is largely based on compilation of small series and anecdotal cases handled in a generally similar but not identical manner. It is apparent that the severity of disease at the time when therapy begins has a great bearing on the outcome, since patients with very severe renal damage usually do not recover function and patients who do not develop rapidly progressive renal failure initially may never do so, even though untreated. The best candidate for therapy, then, would be the patient with mild to moderate renal damage that appears to be advancing. As the number of patients given treatment grows and follow-up becomes available, it is seen that some patients experience an eventual decline in renal function even after initial improvement and apparent stabilization of their course with disappearance of circulating anti-GBM antibody (Finch *et al.*, 1979).

Renal transplantation during the active phase of anti-GBM antibody production generally results in the recurrence of severe anti-GBM antibody-induced nephritis in the graft (Lerner *et al.*, 1967; Wilson and Dixon, 1973, 1976). Yet, once detectable circulating anti-GBM antibody has declined or disappeared, renal transplantation is usually satisfactory and without great danger of recurrent nephritis in the immunosuppressed transplant recipient. Samples which were taken from a woman with Goodpasture's syndrome who, following nephrectomy, had been free of detectable circulating anti-basement membrane antibody for a period of 2 years prior to receipt of an identical-twin kidney transplant (Almkuist *et al.*, 1978) were studied. Within 3 months, this unimmunosuppressed recipient again developed circulating anti-GBM antibody with clinical, histologic, and immunofluorescent evidence of recurrent anti-GBM antibody-induced nephritis. Immunosuppressive and plasmapheresis therapy was instituted at that point, with a subequent decline in antibody levels and retention of function in the transplant. This patient is of particular interest because of the implication that there is a potential for redevelopment of the anti-basement membrane antibody response in the unimmunosuppressed transplant recipient. These events also strongly suggest that the antigens responsible for inducing the anti-GBM response in this particular patient were resident in the kidney.

3. Nephritogenic Immune Responses Involving Non-Basement Membrane Antigens in or of the Glomerulus

Recent studies in experimental animals have shown that non-classical GBM antigens present in the glomerular capillary walls, as well as extrarenal antigens which first become trapped or "planted" within the glomerulus, can be involved in nephritogenic immune reactions and appear to have a similar potential in causing immune glomerular injury in man.

3.1. Non-GBM Glomerular Capillary Wall Antigen in Glomerulonephritis

In 1959, Heymann and colleagues described the induction of experimental nephritis in rats by repeated immunization with rat kidney homogenate in adjuvant (Heymann *et al.*, 1959). Subsequent studies utilizing nephritogenic fractions of renal tubules (Fx1A) led to the concept that this was an immune complex-induced form of membranous glomerulonephritis in which complexes composed of renal tubular brush border antigen and antibody lodged in the GBM (Edgington *et al.*, 1967). The passive administration of sera obtained from rats immunized in this way or of heterologous antibodies raised in animals immunized with Fx1A results in an immunofluorescent pattern of immunoglobulin deposition in the recipient similar to that seen in the glomeruli of the immunized nephritic rat (Sugisaki *et al.*, 1973; Feenstra *et al.*, 1975). This observation raises the possibility of direct binding of antibody to antigens within glomeruli, and recent studies using perfused kidneys have suggested that heterologous anti-Fx1A antibodies do bind directly to non-GBM glomerular capillary wall antigens in a situation designed to prevent formation of circulating immune complexes (Couser *et al.*, 1978; Van Damme *et al.*, 1978). This recent observation has, then, reopened the question as to the pathogenesis of Heymann's nephritis in the rat, and perhaps of membranous nephritis in man. Indeed, antibodies eluted from kidneys of rats with Heymann's nephritis do react directly with normal rat glomeruli and identify antigens distributed in discrete areas at the bases of the epithelial cell foot processes (Neale and Wilson, 1979).

Another model of probable non-GBM antigen glomerulonephritis that occurs spontaneously in New Zealand White rabbits (Neale and Wilson, 1978; Woodroffe *et al.*, 1978) is being evaluated. Five percent of rabbits studied have abnormal proteinuria with 15 to as high as 30% have morphologic or immunofluorescent evidence of immunologically induced glomerulonephritis. The glomerular immune deposits are irregular and are nearly confluent as viewed with the fluorescence microscope. They have a sawtooth, almost continuous electron-dense pattern along the subepithelial aspect of the GBM when viewed by electron microscopy. The deposits, then, do not have the typical discrete granularity usually associated with deposits of circulating immune complexes. Of great interest, antibodies recovered from eluates of the involved kidneys from these rabbits contain antibodies reactive with a non-GBM glomerular capillary wall antigen when studied by indirect immunofluorescence using normal rabbit kidney sections as a target. With some eluates a variable reactivity is also notable with material in the walls of arterioles in these sections. Immunoperoxidase techniques using the sensitivity of the electron microscope yield results suggesting that reactivity of the eluate is greatest in the area of the epithelial foot process where it attaches to the GBM. This spontaneously occurring model of nephritis emphasizes the potential importance of non-GBM glomerular capillary wall antigens in nephritogenic immune reactions. It has not yet been established whether the immune deposits occur in the rabbits by primary localization of the antibody with the antigen, as in the case of anti-basement membrane antibody disease, or whether antigens are also released from the glomerular capillary wall or arterioles, then form circulating immune complexes with subsequent and perhaps specific entrapment within the glomerular capillary wall. Of great interest is the observation that certain human sera, as well as occasional eluates from nephritic kidneys, appear to react with non-GBM glomerular capillary wall antigens of the human kidney when tested in a similar system. This latter observation indicates that reactivity with non-basement membrane glomerular capillary wall antigens may be yet another form of immune renal injury in man.

3.2. Foreign Antigens Which Become Trapped or "Planted" within the Glomerulus

The classic example of a trapped or "planted" foreign antigen in experimental nephritis is that already described in the autologous phase of nephrotoxic nephritis, in which an immune response is generated against heterologous anti-GBM antibody previously bound to the GBM. Since deposited immune complexes are continuously in equilibrium with antigen or antibody from the circulation, once immune complex deposition has occurred the continued interaction with trapped or "planted" antigen or antibody continues and presumably contributes to the ongoing injury (Wilson and Dixon, 1976). Rheumatoid factor or anti-idiotypic antibodies also might contribute to glomerular immune deposits by reacting with previously deposited immune complexed antibody (Agnello *et al.*, 1973). Immunoconglutinins, antibodies reactive with certain complement components, could similarly fix to complement components trapped within glomeruli. Furthermore, nephritic factor, an immunoglobulin with reactivity for components of the activated alternative complement pathway (Schreiber and Müller-Eberhard, 1979), might interact with these deposits in certain patients with hypocomplementemic membranoproliferative glomerulonephritis. Mauer and his associates have described a model in which aggregated immunoglobulin as an antigen is taken up by the glomerular mesangium with nephritis induced by subsequent interaction with anti-immunoglobulin antibody (Mauer *et al.*, 1973). Recently, it has been suggested that DNA released by administration of bacterial lipopolysaccharide might bind to the GBM of mice for subsequent interaction with anti-DNA antibodies, leading to *in situ* immune complex formation (Izui *et al.*, 1976, 1977).

The lectin concanavalin A (Con A), an extract of *Canavalia ensiformis*, that binds to the glucose and mannose of the GBM, can be used as a "planted" antigen for subsequent interaction with passive or active antibody to induce glomerulonephritis (Golbus and Wilson, 1979). Sufficient amounts of Con A are infused into the renal artery of a rat to allow binding of about 75 μg Con A/g rat kidney. Rabbit anti-Con A antibody then is given intravenously with resulting glomerular injury related to the amount of anti-Con A antibody administered and bound to the kidney. When approximately 75 μg of antibody is bound, overt glomerulonephritis can be detected histologically. It is of interest that this is about the same amount of antibody that is required to induce heterologous phase anti-GBM antibody-induced injury (Unanue and Dixon, 1967). By immunofluorescence of the perfused kidney, an irregular but nearly continuous deposition of Con A, heterologous anti-Con A antibody, and rat C3 is observed along the GBM. Proliferative glomerulonephritis with polymorphonuclear leukocyte infiltration follows within 24 hr and persists and intensifies over the next 5 days. It is also possible to cause an autologous form of the disease by administering Con A into the renal artery of rats previously immunized with and producing anti-Con A antibody.

The potential importance to humans of this new model lies in the fact that many infectious agents pathogenic to man contain molecules with lectin-like properties. It is reasonable to speculate, then, that molecules from infectious agents might localize first in capillary walls through their lectin-like properties and subsequently interact with antibody when an immune response is established. Streptococcal antigens have been identified in glomeruli of patients early in the course of poststreptococcal glomerulonephritis, but the antigen later becomes undetectable perhaps because it is saturated with host antibody (Treser *et al.*, 1970). It may be that direct binding of antigen to the basement membrane is yet another contributor to the pathogenesis of poststreptococcal glomerulonephritis as part of a group that presumably also includes formation of circulating immune complexes, glomerular deposition of cryoglobulins, and perhaps alterations in complement activation (Wilson *et al.*, 1980).

4. Conclusions

The category of nephritogenic immune reactions involving a combination of circulating antibody with tissue-fixed antigens such as the GBM and TBM now should be expanded to include similar interactions with non-GBM glomerular capillary wall antigens and antigens unrelated to the kidney but first trapped or "planted" within the glomerular capillary wall. Although not yet a certainty, there is reasonable evidence to suspect that non-basement membrane glomerular capillary wall antigens and perhaps antigens trapped or "planted" at the same sites may be contributing to nephritogenic immune reactions in man.

References

Agnello, V., Koffler, D., and Kunkel, H. G., 1973, Immune complex systems in the nephritis of systemic lupus erythematosus, *Kidney Int.* **3**:90.

Almkuist, R. D., Buckalew, V. M., Jr., Hirszel, P., Maher, J. F., James, P. M., and Wilson, C. B., 1978, Recurrence of anti-glomerular basement membrane antibody (AGBM Ab) mediated glomerulonephritis in an isograft, National Kidney Foundation Clinical Dialysis and Transplant Forum, New Orleans (November 1978), abstract.

Andres, G. A., and McCluskey, R. T., 1975, Tubular and interstitial renal disease due to immunologic mechanisms, *Kidney Int.* **7:**271.

Andres, G., Brentjens, J., Kohli, R., Anthone, R., Anthone, S., Baliah, T., Montes, M., Mookerjee, B. K., Prezyna, A., Sepulveda, M., Venuto, R., and Elwood, C., 1978, Histology of human tubulo-interstitial nephritis associated with antibodies to renal basement membranes, *Kidney Int.* **13:**480.

Beirne, G. J., Wagnild, J. P., Zimmerman, S. W., Macken, P. D., and Burkholder, P. M., 1977, Idiopathic crescentic glomerulonephritis, *Medicine* **56:**349.

Bergstein, J., and Litman, N., 1975, Interstitial nephritis with antitubular basement membrane antibody, *N. Engl. J. Med.* **292:**875.

Bhan, A. K., Schneeberger, E. E., Collins, A. B., and McCluskey, R. T., 1978, Evidence for a pathogenic role of a cell-mediated immune mechanism in experimental glomerulonephritis, *J. Exp. Med.* **148:**246.

Border, W. A., Lehman, D. H., Egan, J. D., Sass, H. J., Glode, J. E., and Wilson, C. B., 1974, Antitubular basement membrane antibodies in methicillin-associated interstitial nephritis, *N. Engl. J. Med.* **291:**381.

Cochrane, C. G., 1979, Mediation systems in neutrophil-independent immunologic injury of the glomerulus, in: *Contemporary Issues in Nephrology* (C. B. Wilson, B. M. Brenner and J. H. Stein, eds.), pp. 106–121. Churchill Livingston, New York.

Couser, W. G., Steinmuller, D. R., Stilmant, M. M., Salant, D. J., and Lowenstein, L. M., 1978, Experimental glomerulonephritis in the isolated perfused rat kidney, *J. Clin. Invest.* **62:**1275.

Dahlberg, P. J., Kurtz, S. B., Donadio, J. V., Jr., Holley, K. E., Velosa, J. A., Williams, D. E., and Wilson, C. B., 1978, Recurrent Goodpasture's syndrome, *Mayo Clin. Proc.* **53:**533.

Dixon, F. J., 1963, The role of antigen–antibody complexes in disease, *Harvey Lect.* **58:**21.

Edgington, T. S., Glassock, R. J., and Dixon, F. J., 1967, Autologous immune complex pathogenesis of experimental allergic glomerulonephritis, *Science* **155:**1432.

Feenstra, K., Lee, R., v.d. Greben, H. A., Arends, A., and Hoedemaeker, Ph. J., 1975, Experimental glomerulonephritis in the rat induced by antibodies directed against tubular antigens. I. The natural history: A histologic and immunohistologic study at the light microscopic and the ultrastructural level, *Lab. Invest.* **32:**235.

Finch, R. A., Rutsky, E. A., McGowan, E., and Wilson, C. B., 1979, Treatment of Goodpasture's syndrome with immunosuppression and plasmapheresis, *South. Med. J.* **72:**1288.

Golbus, S. M., and Wilson, C. B., 1979, Experimental glomerulonephritis induced by the in situ formation of immune complexes in the glomerular capillary wall, *Kidney Int.* **16:**148.

Harner, M. H., Nolte, M., Wilson, C. B., Talwalker, Y. B., Musgrave, J. E., Brooks, R. E., and Campbell, R. A., 1974, Anti-TBM antibody and nephrotic syndrome associated with milk hypersensitivity, Third International Symposium on Pediatric Nephrology, Washington, D.C. (1974), p. 8, abstract.

Heymann, W., Hackel, D. B., Harwood, S., Wilson, S. G. F., and Hunter, J. L. P., 1959, Production of nephrotic syndrome in rats by Freund's adjuvants and rat kidney suspensions, *Proc. Soc. Exp. Biol. Med.* **100:**660.

Holdsworth, S. R., Golbus, S. M., and Wilson, C. B., 1979, Characterization of collagenase solubilized human glomerular basement membrane antigens reacting with human antibodies, *Kidney Int.* **16:**797 (abstract).

Holdsworth, S. R., Neale, T. J., and Wilson, C. B., 1981, Abrogation of immune glomerulonephritis (GN) in rabbits by antimacrophage (M) serum, *Kidney Int.* **19:**193 (abstract).

Hume, D. M., Sterling, W. A., Weymouth, R. J., Siebel, H. R., Madge, G. E., and Lee, H. M., 1970, Glomerulonephritis in human renal homotransplants, *Transplant. Proc.* **2:**361.

Hyman, L. R., Ballow, M., and Knieser, M. R., 1975, Diphenylhydantoin nephropathy: Evidence for an autoimmune pathogenesis, *Kidney Int.* **8:**450 (abstract).

Izui, S., Lambert, P. H., and Miescher, P. A., 1976, In vitro demonstration of a particular affinity of glomerular basement membrane and collagen for DNA: A possible basis for a local formation of DNA–anti-DNA complexes in systemic lupus erythematosus, *J. Exp. Med.* **144:**428.

Izui, S., Lambert, P. H., Fournie, G. J., Turler, H., and Miescher, P. A., 1977, Features of systemic lupus erythematosus in mice injected with bacterial lipopolysaccharides: Identification of circulating DNA and renal localization of DNA–anti-DNA complexes, *J. Exp. Med.* **145:**1115.

Johnson, J. P., Whitman, W., Briggs, W. A., and Wilson, C. B., 1978, Plasmapheresis and immunosuppressive agents in antibasement membrane antibody-induced Goodpasture's syndrome, *Am. J. Med.* **65:**354.

Klassen, J., McCluskey, R. T., and Milgrom, F., 1971, Nonglomerular renal disease produced in rabbits by immunization with homologous kidney, *Am. J. Pathol.* **63:**333.

Klassen, J., Kano, K., Milgrom, F., Menno, A. B., Anthone, S., Anthone, R., Sepulveda, M., Elwood, C. M., and Andres, G. A., 1973, Tubular lesions produced by autoantibodies to tubular basement membrane in human renal allografts, *Int. Arch. Allergy Appl. Immunol.* **45:**675.

Klassen, J., Elwood, C., Grossberg, A. L., Milgrom, F., Montes, M., Sepulveda, M., and Andres, G. A., 1974, Evolution of membranous nephropathy into anti-glomerular-basement-membrane glomerulonephritis, *N. Engl. J. Med.* **290:**1340.

Koffler, D., Agnello, V., Carr, R. I., and Kunkel, H. G., 1969a, Variable patterns of immunoglobulin and complement deposition in the kidneys of patients with systemic lupus erythematosus, *Am. J. Pathol.* **56:**305.

Koffler, D., Sandson, J., Carr, R., and Kunkel, H. G., 1969b, Immunologic studies concerning the pulmonary lesions in Goodpasture's syndrome, *Am. J. Pathol.* **54:**293.

Krakower, C. A., and Greenspon, S. A., 1951, Localization of the nephrotoxic antigen within the isolated renal glomerulus, *Arch. Pathol.* **51:**629.

Lehman, D. H., Wilson, C. B., and Dixon, F. J., 1974a, Interstitial nephritis in rats immunized with heterologous tubular basement membrane, *Kidney Int.* **5:**187.

Lehman, D. H., Lee, S., Wilson, C. B., and Dixon, F. J., 1974b, Induction of antitubular basement membrane antibodies in rats by renal transplantation, *Transplantation* **17:**429.

Lehman, D. H., Wilson, C. B., and Dixon, F. J., 1975, Extraglomerular immunoglobulin deposits in human nephritis, *Am. J. Med.* **58:**765.

Lerner, R., and Dixon, F. J., 1966, Transfer of ovine experimental allergic glomerulonephritis (EAG) with serum, *J. Exp. Med.* **124:**431.

Lerner, R., and Dixon, F. J., 1968, The induction of acute glomerulonephritis in rabbits with soluble antigens isolated from normal homologous and autologous urine, *J. Immunol.* **100:**1277.

Lerner, R., Glassock, R. J., and Dixon, F. J., 1967, The role of anti-glomerular basement membrane antibody in the pathogenesis of human glomerulonephritis, *J. Exp. Med.* **126:**989.

Lockwood, C. M., Boulton-Jones, J. M., Lowenthal, R. M., Simpson, I. J., Peters, D. K., and Wilson, C. B., 1975, Recovery from Goodpasture's syndrome after immunosuppressive treatment and plasmapheresis, *Br. Med. J.* **2:**252.

Lockwood, C. M., Rees, A. J., Pearson, T. A., Evans, D. J., Peters, D. K., and Wilson, C. B., 1976, Immunosuppression and plasma-exchange in the treatment of Goodpasture's syndrome, *Lancet* **1:**711.

Lockwood, C. M., Pussell, B., Wilson, C. B., and Peters, D. K., 1979, Plasma exchange in nephritis. *Adv. Nephrol.* **8:**383.

Ma, K. W., Golbus, S. M., Kaufman, R., Staley, N., Londer, H., and Brown, D. C., 1978, Glomerulonephritis with Hodgkin's disease and herpes zoster, *Arch. Pathol. Lab. Med.* **102:**527.

McCoy, R. C., Johnson, H. K., Stone, W. J., and Wilson, C. B., 1976, Variation in glomerular basement membrane antigens in hereditary nephritis, *Lab. Invest.* **34:**325 (abstract).

McPhaul, J. J., Jr., and Dixon, F. J., 1969, Immunoreactive basement membrane antigens in normal human urine and serum, *J. Exp. Med.* **130:**1395.

McPhaul, J. J., Jr., and Dixon, F. J., 1970, Characterization of human anti-glomerular basement membrane antibodies eluted from glomerulonephritic kidneys, *J. Clin. Invest.* **49:**308.

Mahieu, P., Lambert, P. H., and Miescher, P. A., 1974, Detection of anti-glomerular basement membrane antibodies by a radioimmunological technique: Clinical application in human nephropathies, *J. Clin. Invest.* **54:**128.

Mauer, S. M., Sutherland, D. E. R., Howard, R. J., Fish, A. J., Najarian, J. S., and Michael, A. F., 1973, The glomerular mesangium. III. Acute immune mesangial injury: A new model of glomerulonephritis, *J. Exp. Med.* **137:**553.

Morel-Maroger, L., Kourilsky, O., Mignon, F., and Richet, G., 1974, Antitubular basement membrane antibodies in rapidly progressive post-streptococcal glomerulonephritis: Report of a case, *Clin. Immunol. Immunopathol.* **2:**185.

Neale, T. J., and Wilson, C. B., 1978, Non-GBM glomerular antigen in spontaneous nephritis in rabbits, *Kidney Int.* **14:**706 (abstract).

Neale, T. J., and Wilson, C. B., 1979, Fixed glomerular antigen in Heymann's nephritis: Eluted antibody reactivity with normal rat glomeruli, *Kidney Int.* **16:**799 (abstract).

Rees, A. J., Lockwood, C. M., and Peters, D. K., 1977, Enhanced allergic tissue injury in Goodpasture's syndrome by intercurrent bacterial infection, *Br. Med. J.* **2:**723.

Rees, A. J., Peters, D. K., Compston, D. A. S., and Batchelor, J. R., 1978, Strong association between HLA-DRW2 and antibody-mediated Goodpasture's syndrome, *Lancet* **1:**966.

Rosenblatt, S., Knight, W., Bannayan, G., Wilson, C. B., and Stein, J. H., 1979, Treatment of Goodpasture's syndrome with plasmapheresis: A case report and review of the literature. *Am. J. Med.* **66:**689.

Schreiber, R. D., and Müller-Eberhard, H. J., Complement and renal disease, in: *Contemporary Issues in Nephrology*, Vol. III (C. B. Wilson, B. M. Brenner and J. H. Stein, eds.), p. 67, Churchill Livingstone, New York.

Schreiner, G. F., Cotran, R. S., Pardo, V., and Unanue, E. R., 1978, A mononuclear cell component in experimental immunological glomerulonephritis, *J. Exp. Med.* **147:**369.

Steblay, R. W., 1962, Glomerulonephritis induced in sheep by injections of heterologous glomerular basement membrane and Freund's complete adjuvant, *J. Exp. Med.* **116:**253.

Sugisaki, T., Klassen, J., Andres, G. A., Milgrom, F., and McCluskey, R. T., 1973, Passive transfer of Heymann nephritis with serum, *Kidney Int.* **3:**66.

Treser, G., Semar, M., Ty, A., Sagel, I., Franklin, M. A., and Lange, K., 1970, Partial characterization of antigenic streptococcal plasma membrane components in acute glomerulonephritis, *J. Clin. Invest.* **49:**762.

Tung, K. S. K., and Black, W. C., 1975, Association of renal glomerular and tubular immune complex disease and antitubular basement membrane antibody, *Lab. Invest.* **32:**696.

Unanue, E. R., and Dixon, F. J., 1965, Experimental glomerulonephritis. VI. The autologous phase of nephrotoxic serum nephritis, *J. Exp. Med.* **121:**715.

Unanue, E. R., and Dixon, F. J., 1967, Experimental glomerulonephritis: Immunologic events and pathogenetic mechanisms, *Adv. Immunol.* **6:**1.

Unanue, E. R., Dixon, F. J., and Feldman, J. D., 1967, Experimental allergic glomerulonephritis induced in the rabbit with homologous renal antigens, *J. Exp. Med.* **125:**163.

Van Damme, B. J. C., Fleuren, G. J., Bakker, W. W., Vernier, R. L., and Hoedemaeker, P. J., 1978, Experimental glomerulonephritis in the rat induced by antibodies directed against tubular antigens. V. Fixed glomerular antigens in the pathogenesis of heterologous immune complex glomerulonephritis, *Lab. Invest.* **38:**502.

Willoughby, W. F., and Dixon, F. J., 1970, Experimental hemorrhagic pneumonitis produced by heterologous anti-lung antibody, *J. Immunol.* **104:**28.

Wilson, C. B., 1974, Immune complex glomerulonephritis, *Proceedings of the 5th International Congress on Nephrology* (Mexico, 1972), Vol. 1, p. 68, Karger, Basel.

Wilson, C. B., 1979a, Immunologic diseases of the lung and kidney (Goodpasture's syndrome), in: *Pulmonary Diseases* (A. P. Fishman, ed.), McGraw–Hill/Blakiston, New York, pp. 699–706.

Wilson, C. B., 1979b, Immune reactions with antigens in or of the glomerulus, in: *Immunopathology*, (F. Milgrom and B. Albini, eds.), Karger, Basel, p. 127.

Wilson, C. B., and Dixon, F. J., 1973, Anti-glomerular basement membrane antibody-induced glomerulonephritis, *Kidney Int.* **3:**74.

Wilson, C. B., and Dixon, F. J., 1974, Diagnosis of immunopathologic renal disease (Editorial), *Kidney Int.* **5:**389.

Wilson, C. B., and Dixon, F. J., 1976, The renal response to immunological injury, in: *The Kidney* (B. M. Brenner and F. C. Rector, Jr., eds.), p. 838, Saunders, Philadelphia.

Wilson, C. B., and Dixon, F. J., 1978, Glomerulonephritis: Immunopathology and clinical manifestations, in: *Immunological Diseases*, 3rd ed., Vol. II (M. Samter, ed.), p. 1348, Little, Brown, Boston.

Wilson, C. B., and Smith, R. C., 1972, Goodpasture's syndrome associated with influenza A2 virus infection, *Ann. Intern. Med.* **76:**91.

Wilson, C. B., Dixon, F. J., Fortner, J. G., and Cerilli, J., 1971, Glomerular basement membrane-reactive antibodies in anti-lymphocyte globulin, *J. Clin. Invest.* **50:**1525.

Wilson, C. B., Lehman, D. H., McCoy, R. C., Gunnels, J. C., Jr., and Stickel, D. L., 1974a, Antitubular basement membrane antibodies after renal transplantation, *Transplantation* **18:**447.

Wilson, C. B., Marquardt, H., and Dixon, F. J., 1974b, Radioimmunoassay (RIA) for circulating anti-glomerular basement membrane (GBM) antibodies, *Kidney Int.* **6:**114a (abstract).

Wilson, C. B., Golbus, S. M., Neale, T. J., and Woodroffe, A. J., 1980, Nephritogenic immune responses involving antigens in or of the glomerulus, *Streptococcal Diseases and the Immune Response* (S. E. Read and J. B. Zabrinskie, eds.), Academic Press, New York, pp. 463–475.

Woodroffe, A. J., Neale, T. J., and Wilson, C. B., 1978, Spontaneous glomerulonephritis (GN) in New Zealand White (NZW) rabbits, VIIth International Congress of Nephrology, (Montreal, June 1978), abstract.

18

Autoimmune Disease Induced in Rabbits by Administration of Mercuric Chloride: Evidence Suggesting a Role for Antigens of the Connective Tissue Matrix

Boris Albini and Giuseppe Andres

1. Introduction

There is evidence that autologous antigens may have a role in the pathogenesis of various types of nephritides spontaneously developing in animals and in man. Data available suggest the involvement of antigens of glomerular basement membrane (GBM), cell nuclei, thyroid, and, possibly, brush border of proximal tubules, and tumors (Wilson and Dixon, 1976). The mechanisms of autoimmunization, however, are not well understood.

The nature of the autoimmune response *per se* is controversial. It is considered by some as a special and pathologic immune response differing from responses to heteroantigens (Burnet, 1959). Others think that autoimmunity is characterized by an immune response identical to that following sensitization with a foreign antigen (Lachmann, 1975; Levine, 1979). During the last two decades, the extensive experimental and clinical work invested in the search for autoimmunity has produced a considerable amount of new, albeit not always congruous, data which allow the formulation of some hypotheses concerning the etiology and the pathogenesis of these diseases (for review see Allison, 1977; Beutner *et al.*, 1979; Milgrom, 1969; Talal, 1978). Thus, it has been proposed that normally sequestered or hidden antigens are released into the circulation and thereby induce autoimmune

---

Boris Albini Department of Microbiology, State University of New York, Buffalo, New York 14214 ***Giuseppe Andres*** Departments of Microbiology, Pathology, and Medicine, State University of New York, Buffalo, New York 14214. This study was supported by USPHS Grant AI 10334.

responses, or that the amount of autoantigens present in the circulation increases, inducing a switch from tolerance to sensitization (Weigle, 1979). Alternatively, autoantigens may be altered and acquire new antigenic determinants (Milgrom, 1979); exogenous "non-self" and endogenous "self" epitopes are both present on such antigens.

2. *Mercuric Chloride-Induced Autoimmune Disease*

The possibility that exogenous toxic agents may initiate an autoimmune response has been proposed for several kidney diseases. Some forms of anti-GBM disease have been associated with exposure to hydrocarbon solvents (Beirne and Brennan, 1972). Administration of heavy metal is often associated with renal damage (Edwards, 1942). Large doses of cadmium, gold, or mercury salts produce toxic tubular lesions (Gritzka and Trump, 1968). Prolonged administration of smaller doses frequently induces immune complex nephritis in animals (Bariéty *et al.*, 1971) and in man (Mendema *et al.*, 1963). Administration of $HgCl_2$ to rabbits, over a prolonged period of time, first induces formation of antibody to antigens of the basement membranes and later formation of immune complexes and development of membranous glomerulonephritis (Roman-Franco *et al.*, 1976). Some of these findings have been confirmed by studies performed in rats (Sapin *et al.*, 1977). In the following discussion, a review of the immunopathological features of the disease developing in rabbits exposed to $HgCl_2$ will be presented.

2.1. *Induction and Course of the Disease*

$HgCl_2$ was injected into the thigh muscle of New Zealand White rabbits twice a week. The rabbits received 2 mg $HgCl_2$/kg body wt in 0.2 ml distilled water per injection (Roman-Franco *et al.*, 1978). Sixty-two rabbits were injected throughout the course of the experiment; 10 rabbits received $HgCl_2$ for the first 3 weeks only and were sacrificed 1 to 28 weeks after the last injection. Ten rabbits, housed in the same facilities as those of the experimental group, served as untreated, age-matched controls.

Soon after the first injections of $HgCl_2$, most rabbits developed diarrhea with concomitant weight loss. These acute toxic symptoms subsided after 7 to 14 days. At this stage, tissues examined by direct immunofluorescence showed no immune deposits. By electron microscopy and autoradiography, mercury was seen in the cytoplasm of tubular and intestinal epithelial cells and in the hepatocytes. Moreover, mercury was found in the elastic layer of medium-sized arteries.

After 2 weeks, the acute intoxication resolved spontaneously and the rabbits had no manifest signs of disease. Nevertheless, tissue sections obtained in this stage of the experiment showed linear deposits of IgG in the GBM (Fig. 1)., tubular basement membrane (TBM), the basement membrane-like substance of the media of medium-sized and large vessels, the reticulum of the spleen, and the endo- and perimysium of skeletal (Fig. 2) and heart

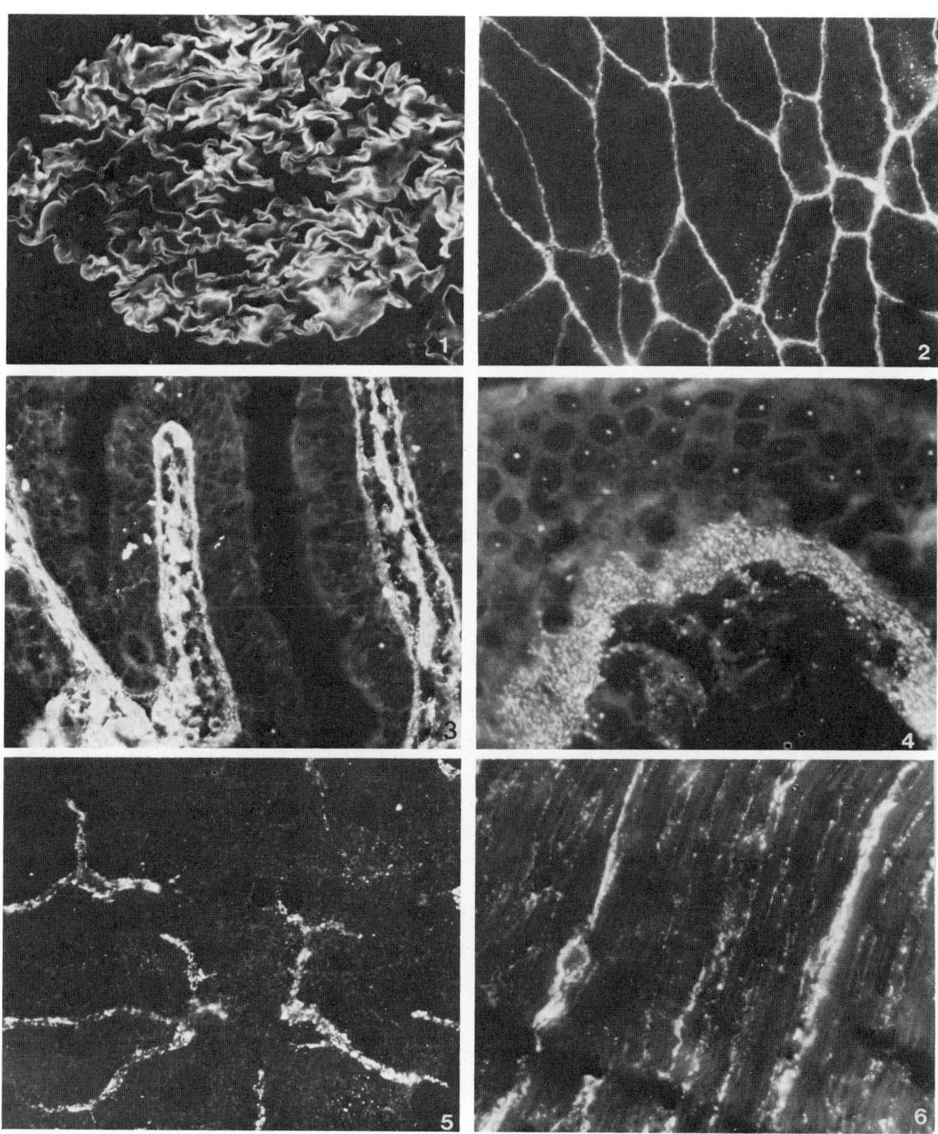

Figures 1–12 and 15. Immunopathologic aspects of tissues from rabbits injected with $HgCl_2$.
Figure 1. Renal tissue 2 weeks after injections of $HgCl_2$. Linear deposits of IgG in GBM and TBM. × 300.
Figure 2. Skeletal muscle 2 weeks after injections of $HgCl_2$. Deposits of IgG in the peri- and endomysium. × 300.
Figures 3–6. Rabbit tissues after 10–22 weeks of $HgCl_2$ injections.
Figure 3. Granular deposits of IgG in the lamina propria of intestinal villi. × 250.
Figure 4. Granular deposits of IgG in the basal lamina of an intestinal villus. × 450.
Figure 5. Granular deposits of IgG in the walls of peritoneal vessels. × 150.
Figure 6. Granular deposits of IgG in the capillaries and in the connective tissue interposed between muscle fibers in the heart. × 400.

muscles. Mild proteinuria, which was always of short duration (1–2 days), was seen in a few rabbits. Late in this stage, the rabbits developed abscesses and necrotic lesions at the sites of injection. These sometimes involved the bone and required amputation of a limb.

Four to five weeks after the first injections of $HgCl_2$, a few granular deposits of rabbit IgG and C3 were seen in the glomeruli (Fig. 7, inset). Electron microscopy revealed scattered subepithelial electron-opaque deposits (Fig. 7). The density of the deposits in glomeruli increased over the next 2–4 weeks, and after 2–3 months the rabbits developed a severe membranous glomerulonephritis (Fig. 8). At this time, granular deposits of rabbit IgG and C3 were found in the TBM (in 20% of the rabbits); in the lamina propria of intestinal villi (Fig. 3) and, more frequently, in their basement membrane (Fig. 4); in the muscularis mucosae and in the muscularis externa of the intestine; in the walls of peritoneal (Fig. 5) and cardiac vessels (Fig. 6); in the walls of hepatic arteries, veins, and sinusoids (Figs. 9 and 10); and in the walls of the sinuses, in the reticulum of Billroth's cords, and in lymphatic follicles (Fig. 11) of the spleen. In elastic arteries, linear and granular immune deposits were found in the internal and external basal laminae, and possibly in the elastica and in the elastic and collagenous fibrils of the media. By electron microscopy, foreign deposits were seen between the elastica and the internal basal lamina and between the plasma membrane of smooth muscle cells and the external basal lamina (Fig. 15). In the arterioles, linear and granular immune deposits were seen along the basal lamina and around smooth muscle cells (Fig. 15, inset a). In the peritoneal arterioles, studied in unsectioned tissue preparation (Albini *et al.*, 1977), deposits of IgG were found in a linear pattern perpendicular to the major axis of the vessel, presumably in the collagenous or basement membrane matrix interposed between smooth muscle cells; granular deposits were seen most commonly at the entrance of anastomosing branches (Fig. 15, inset b). Only five rabbits receiving continuous injections of $HgCl_2$ had preferential deposition of IgG and C3 in glomerular mesangial regions. Sixty percent of the rabbits developed proteinuria and hematuria which lasted for 1–3 weeks. Many animals had ascites, pleural or pericardial exudation, and a few had anasarca. The rabbits often contracted respiratory infections and the body weight rapidly decreased.

Rabbits given $HgCl_2$ for only 3 weeks showed, 1–28 weeks later, preferentially deposits of immunoglobulins and complement in the mesangium (Fig. 12). Some deposits, especially of C3, however, were seen in peripheral glomerular capillary walls. These rabbits, too, had a systemic pattern of immune deposits. They had mild intermittent proteinuria and sometimes hematuria. However, the progress of the disease was slower than that observed in rabbits receiving continuous injections of $HgCl_2$.

2.2 *Antibodies and Immune Complexes*

Sera from three rabbits had antibodies to basement membranes detectable in immunofluorescent staining tests; two of these rabbits were nephrec-

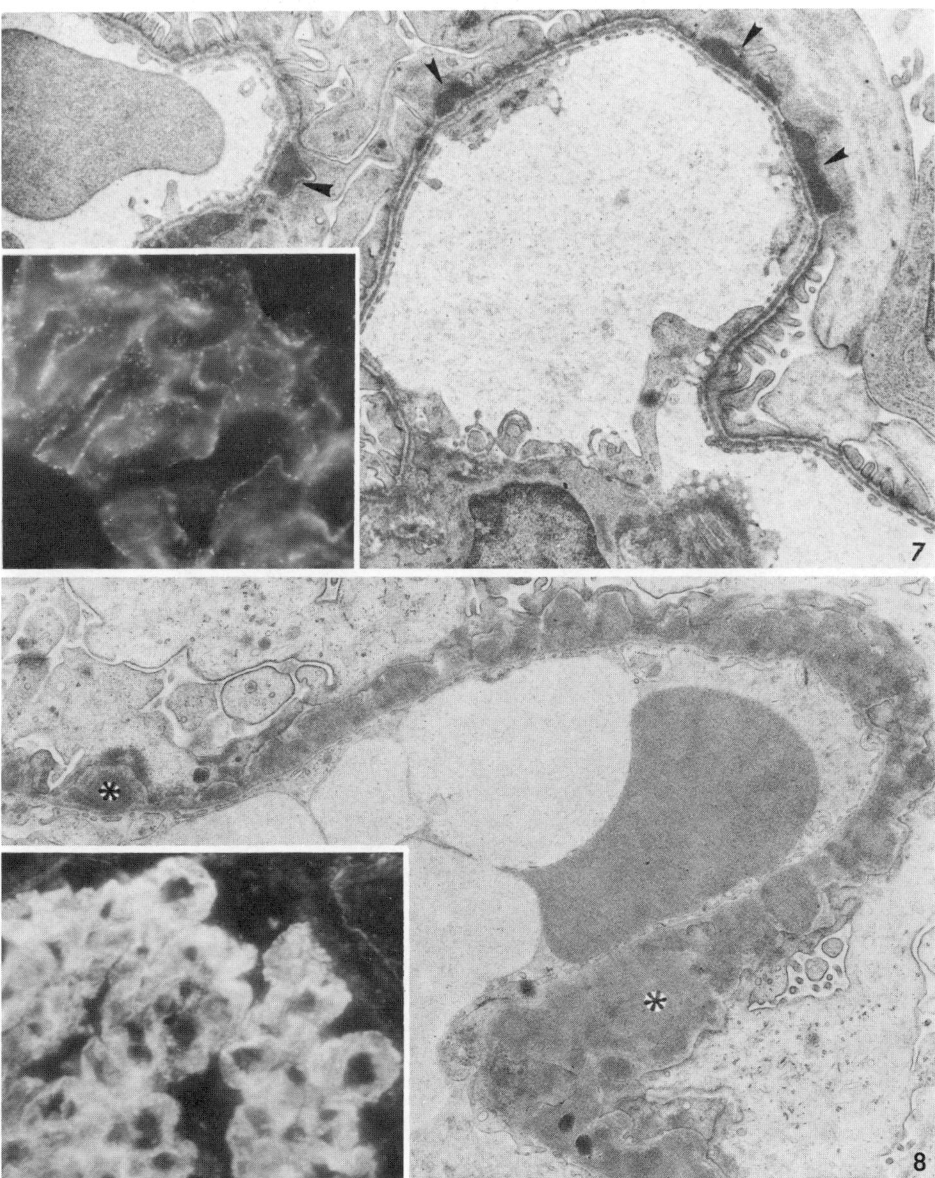

Figure 7. Electron micrograph showing part of a renal glomerulus after 4 weeks of $HgCl_2$ injections. Focal electron-opaque deposits (arrowheads) are present between the lamina densa and the epithelial cytoplasm. × 7000. The inset shows fine, granular deposits of IgG along the glomerular capillary walls in a rabbit injected for 4 weeks with $HgCl_2$. × 800.

Figure 8. Electron micrograph showing diffuse subepithelial deposits (asterisks) in a rabbit with membranous glomerulonephritis, 4 months after the beginning of $HgCl_2$ injections. × 7000. The inset shows patchy, ribbon-like deposits of IgG in the glomeruli of the same rabbit. × 400.

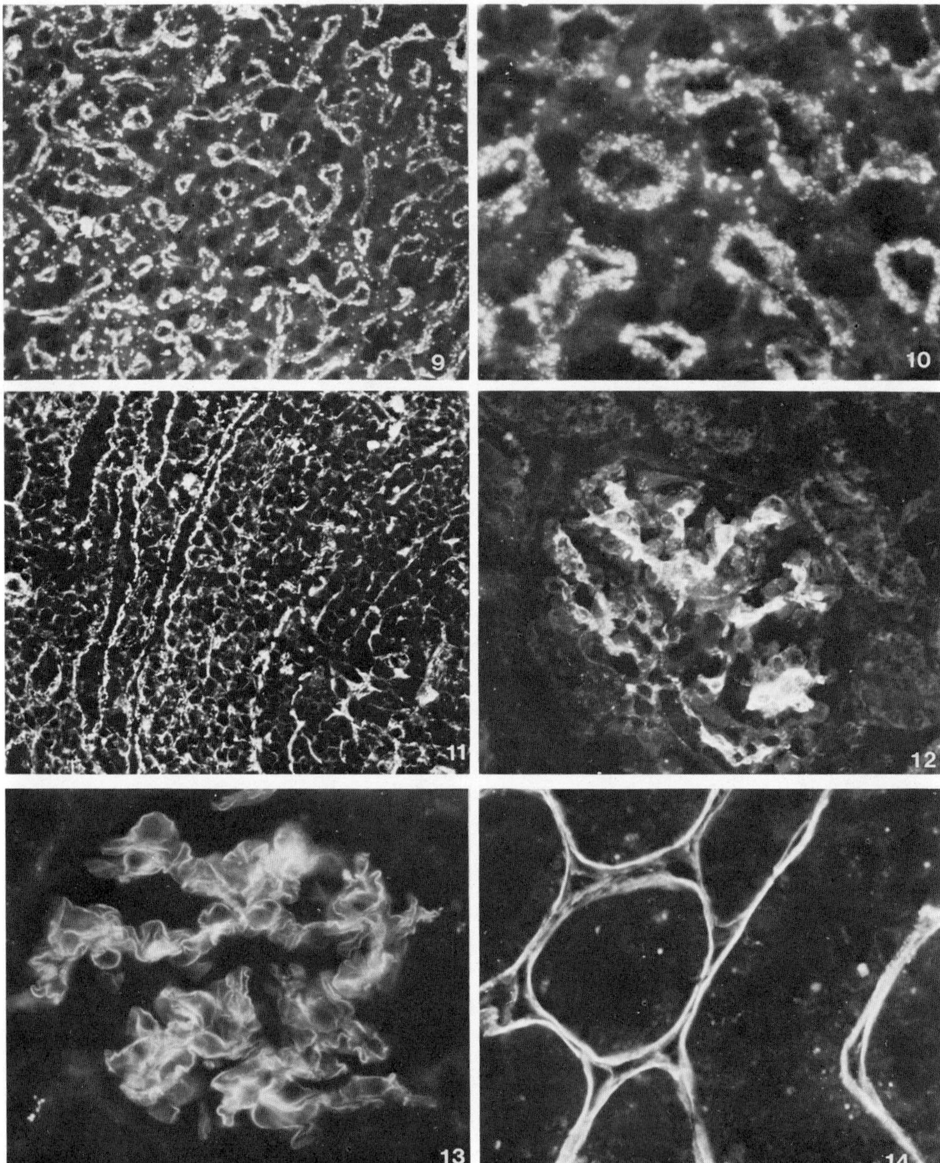

Figure 9. Granular deposits of IgG in the sinusoids of the liver in a rabbit injected for 4 months with $HgCl_2$. × 250.

Figure 10. Higher magnification of the section shown in Fig. 9. The granular deposits of IgG are localized in the walls of the sinusoids. × 400.

Figure 11. Granular deposits of IgG in the venous sinuses, in the reticulum, and in the lymphatic stroma of the spleen of a rabbit, 4 weeks after injection of $HgCl_2$. × 250.

Figure 12. Mesangial deposits of IgG in the glomerulus of a rabbit injected with $HgCl_2$ for 3 weeks only, and sacrificed 18 weeks after the last injection. × 250.

Figures 13 and 14. Sections of normal rabbit kidney incubated with the acid eluate from a nephritic kidney and stained with fluorescein-conjugated goat anti-rabbit IgG. Linear IgG deposits are present in GBM and TBM. Figure 13, × 250; Fig. 14, × 400.

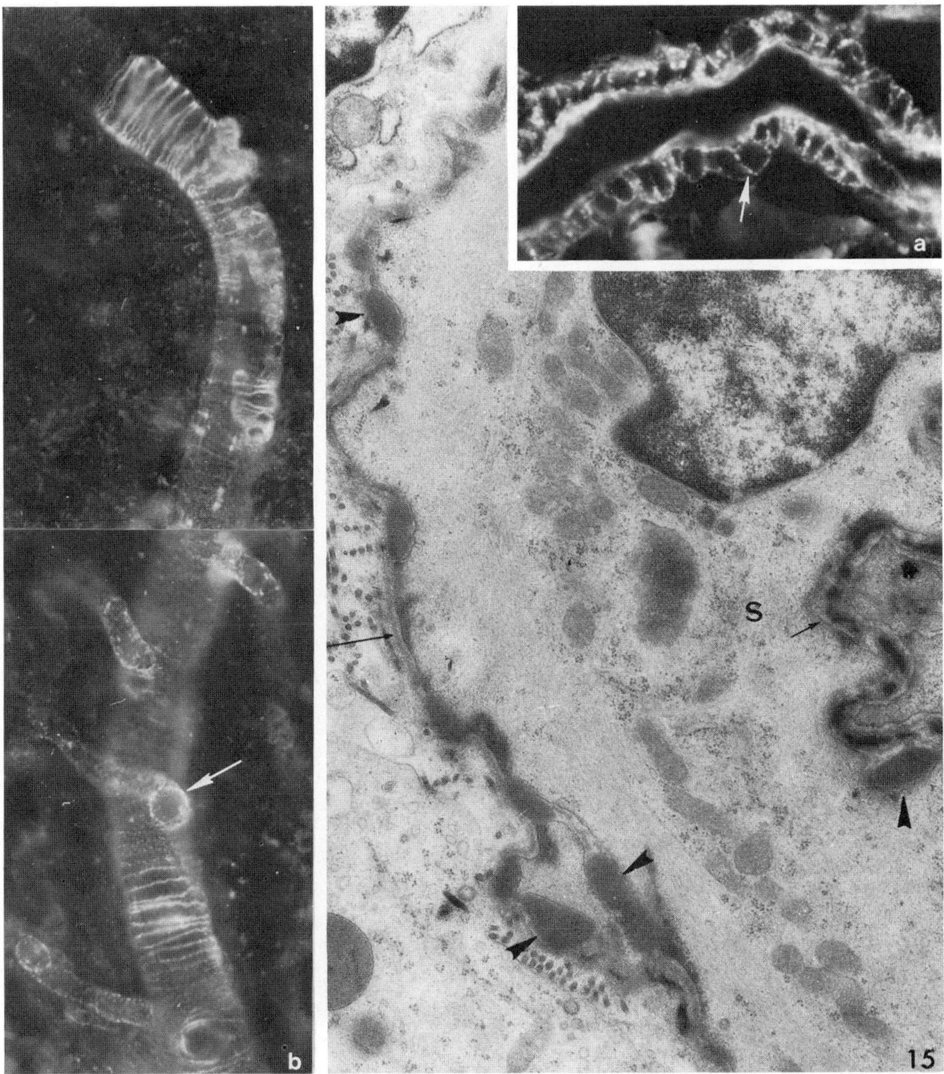

Figure 15. Electron micrograph of part of an elastic artery. Electron-opaque foreign deposits (arrowheads) are present between the elastica and the internal basal lamina (short arrow) and between the smooth muscle cell(s) and the external basal lamina (long arrow). × 15,000. (Inset a) Arteriole. Deposits of IgG along the basal lamina and around the smooth muscle cells (arrow). × 500. (Inset b) Unsectioned peritoneal arteriole. Linear deposits of IgG are seen on the surface of the vessel. The deposits are probably located in the connective tissue interposed between smooth muscle cells. Fine granular deposits are seen in the wall of anastomosing vessels (arrow). × 400.

tomized 48 hr prior to sacrifice. By indirect immunofluorescence, none of the animals had circulating antibodies reacting with nuclear or tubular brush border antigens. The sera did not react with GBM preparations or kidney homogenates in double diffusion in gel.

Eluates obtained from rabbit kidneys removed either 2–3 weeks after the beginning of the experiments or 2–3 months later reacted with the GBM (Fig. 13), the mesangial matrix, and the TBM (Fig. 14) in a linear immunofluorescent pattern. The eluates showed a similar reactivity with the peri- and endomysium of the skeletal muscles (Fig. 16), the plasma membrane of smooth muscle cells, the lamina propria of the intestine (Fig. 17), the reticulum of the spleen (Fig. 18), the walls of hepatic sinusoids (Fig. 19) and the walls of the vessels in several organs (Fig. 19). The antibody reactivity seemed to be restricted in species specificity.

In double staining immunofluorescence, the renal eluates from rabbits with mercury-induced nephropathy and a nephrotoxic serum to rabbit GBM raised in a sheep appeared to react with the same structures of the GBM. In blocking experiments, the nephrotoxic serum could block the reactivity of the GBM with the renal eluates, but the eluates could not block completely the reactivity of the nephrotoxic serum. These results indicate a partial

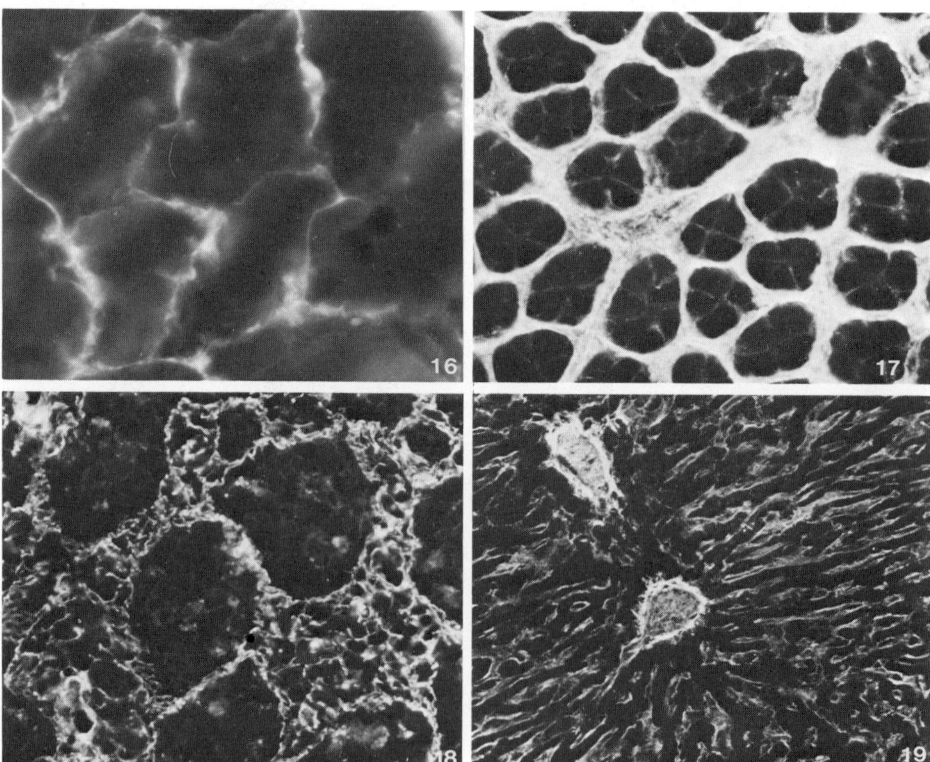

Figures 16–19. Sections of normal rabbit tissues stained as described for Figs. 13 and 14. Linear deposits of IgG are seen in the endomysium (Fig. 16; × 400), in the muscularis mucosae and in the cell coat of goblet cells of the intestine (Fig. 17; × 250), in the reticulum of Billroth's cord of the spleen (Fig. 18; × 250), in the walls of the large vessels and of the sinusoids of the liver (Fig. 19; × 150).

identity of antibody specificities of the nephrotoxic serum and the antibodies of mercury-treated rabbits. In some instances (2 out of 9), the renal eluates reacted weakly with kidney homogenate in double diffusion in gel in 0.5% agarose; no lines were seen with preparations of purified GBM or TBM. Whole kidney homogenates were able to absorb the anti-basement membrane activity of the renal eluates.

Antinuclear antibodies were found in the renal eluates of two rabbits with membranous glomerulonephritis.

Using the Raji cell assay (Albini *et al.*, 1977; Theofilopoulos *et al.*, 1974), circulating immune complexes in low titers were first demonstrable 1 to 4 weeks after the beginning of $HgCl_2$ injections. In both experimental groups, the titers of immune complexes increased with the progression of the disease. Immune complexes could also be detected in the sera of rabbits using the anti-antibody assay (Milgrom and Kano, 1978). The titers were comparable to those obtained using the Raji cell assay.

2.3. Search for the Antigen(s) Responsible for the Autoimmune Disease

The elution experiments indicate that the antibodies found early after beginning the $HgCl_2$ injections have the same reactivity as those found in late stages of disease. At present, the antibody specificity is best defined by the results of direct and indirect immunofluorescence tests. The antigen(s) responsible for the immune response apparently is localized in most basement membranes, in the reticulin fibers of lymphatic tissues, in the loose connective tissue and in the basement membrane-like material between smooth muscle cells. The antigen(s) seems to be partially related to that responsible for the induction of nephrotoxic serum (as suggested by the blocking experiments described above), and seems to be relatively species specific.

Commercially available collagenase preparations were not able to destroy the antigen(s) in kidney sections. Prolonged incubation of tissue sections in saline decreased or abolished the reactivity with kidney eluates. In immunoprecipitation tests, nephritic kidney eluates reacting with basement membranes in indirect immunofluorescence did not react with normal or with mercury-treated rabbit serum proteins. Therefore, it seems unlikely that some of the serum components to which $HgCl_2$ binds play a role in the pathogenesis of the disease. Antinuclear antibodies were never detected in the sera, but were found in the renal eluates of two rabbits with membranous glomerulonephritis. Therefore, in contrast to one of the rat models of mercury intoxication (Weening *et al.*, 1978), antinuclear antibodies do not appear to have a major role in the pathogenesis of rabbit disease.

These studies do not establish the nature of the antigen(s) responsible for the immune response developing in rabbits injected with $HgCl_2$. They indicate, however, that the antigen(s) is localized mainly in the basement membranes, in the reticulin stroma of lymphatic tissue, and in the collagen matrix.

2.4. *Systemic Localization of Immune Deposits*

As demonstrated earlier, the antigens responsible for autoimmunization in rabbits seem to be present in many organ systems throughout the body. Similarly, granular immune deposits may be found in many sites. In addition to the kidney, immune deposits are found in the spleen, liver, intestines, peritoneum, heart, muscle, adrenals, choroid plexus, and arteries of several organs. The immunofluorescence pattern varies from animal to animal, and finely granular or patchy immune deposits of IgG and C3 can be seen superimposed on the linear basement membrane deposits, which become less marked with the progression of the disease. It is conceivable that part of the immune deposits may result from local trapping of circulating antigen–antibody complexes and part from *in situ* formation of antigen–antibody complexes. The distribution of the immune deposits is comparable, in part, to that seen in BSA-treated rabbits with chronic serum sickness. Thus, in rabbits, both heterologous and autologous antigens may induce a systemic immune complex disease.

2.5. *Transformation of Anti-GBM Disease into Immune Complex Disease*

In 1967, Lerner and Dixon described that rabbits immunized with basement membrane components obtained from rabbit urine first developed antibodies to GBM. Later, these rabbits developed subepithelial immune deposits, presumably representing immune complexes. More recently, Shibata *et al.* (1972) have induced a membranous glomerulonephritis in rats immunized with a glycoprotein from the GBM. These reports, together with the experiments described here, indicate that basement membrane antigens first may induce formation of antibodies and subsequently formation of antigen–antibody complexes.

3. *Relevance for Human Diseases*

In humans, the transformation of anti-GBM nephritis into an immune complex disease seems to be a rare event. One such patient has been described by Agodoa *et al.* (1976). Some patients described by Richet *et al.* (1974) showed clinical and histopathological signs indicative of a similar transformation.

The model discussed here is relevant to problems of environmental pollution. Gold, mercury, and other metals have been associated with nephropathies in humans, and pathologic changes in various organs have been reported in intoxications with either mercury salts or organic mercury components. Further studies concerned with the identification of the antigen(s) stimulating the immune response in animals exposed to heavy metals may contribute to elucidate the etiology and the pathogenesis of some forms of human autoimmune diseases.

Table 1. Stages of Autoimmune Disease Induced in Rabbits by Mercuric Chloride[a]

Stage	Time	IX	DIF	IIF	Glomerular pathology	Proteinuria	Clinical signs
—	1 week after first $HgCl_2$ injection	0	0	0	0	0	+
I	3–5 weeks after first $HgCl_2$ injection	+	BM, 1	Bm, 1	0	±	0
II	4–10 weeks after first $HgCl_2$ injection	+ + +	BM, g	BM, 1	membranous glomerulonephritis	+	+ + +
(IIa)	1–28 weeks after last $HgCl_2$ injection	+ +	BM, g, M, g	BM, 1	mesangial glomerulonephritis	±	±

[a] Abbreviations: IX, circulating immune complexes; DIF, direct immunofluorescent staining for rabbit IgG; IIF, indirect immunofluorescent staining of normal rabbit tissue with eluates from nephritic kidneys; BM, positive immunofluorescence in basement membranes; 1, linear staining pattern; g, granular staining pattern; M, positive immunofluorescence in glomerular mesangium; 0, absent; ±, minimal; +, mild; + +, moderate; + + +, marked; IIa, rabbits injected with $HgCl_2$ for 3 weeks only, and sacrificed 1 to 28 weeks after the last injection.

4. Summary

The results reported here demonstrate that rabbits injected intramuscularly with $HgCl_2$ over prolonged periods of time develop a self-perpetuating, biphasic autoimmune disease. Immunologically, the disease is first characterized by development of antibodies to basement membranes and collagen matrix; linear deposits of rabbit IgG are present in the basement membranes. In a subsequent stage, granular deposits of IgG and C3, presumably containing immune complexes, develop in the basement membranes and in the collagen matrix of several organs. Antibodies eluted from nephritic kidneys show a tissue specificity similar to that of antibody to fibronectin, suggesting that this glycoprotein may be the antigen (or one of the antigens) stimulating the autoimmune reaction. The serological, pathological, and clinical findings are summarized in Table 1.

ACKNOWLEDGMENTS. We wish to thank Drs. A. A. Roman-Franco, M. Turiello, and E. Ossi for their contribution to these studies.

References

Agodoa, L. C. Y., Striker, G. E., George, C. R. P., Glassock, R., and Quadracci, L. J., 1976, The appearance of nonlinear deposits of immunoglobulins in Goodpasture's syndrome, *Am. J. Med.* **61**:407.

Albini, B., Ossi, E., and Andres, G., 1977, The pathogenesis of pericardial, pleural, and peritoneal effusions in rabbits with serum sickness, *Lab. Invest.* **37**:64.

Allison, A. C., 1977, Autoimmune diseases: Concepts of pathogenesis and control, in: *Autoimmunity* (N. Talal, ed.), p. 92, Academic Press, New York.

Bariéty, J., Druet, P., Laliberté, F., and Sapin, C., 1971, Glomerulonephritis with gamma and beta 1 C globulin deposits induced in rats by mercuric chloride, *Am. J. Pathol.* **65:**293.

Beirne, G. J., and Brennan, J. T., 1972, Glomerulonephritis associated with hydrocarbon solvents, *Arch. Environ. Health* **25:**365.

Beutner, E. H., Chorzelski, T., and Binder, W., 1979, Nature of autoimmunity: Pathologic versus physiologic responses and a unified concept, in: *Immunopathology of the Skin* (E. H. Beutner, T. Chorzelski, and S. Bean, eds.), p. 147, Wiley, New York.

Burnet, F. M., 1959, *The Clonal Selection Theory of Acquired Immunity*, Vanderbilt University Press, Nashville, Tenn.

Edwards, J. G., 1942, The renal tubule (nephron) as affected by mercury, *Am. J. Pathol.* **18:**1011.

Gritzka, T. L., and Trump, B. F., 1968, Renal tubular lesions caused by mercuric chloride, *Am. J. Pathol.* **52:**1225.

Lachmann, P. J., 1975, Auto-allergy, in: *Clinical Aspects of Immunology* (P. G. H. Gell, R. R. A. Colmbs, and P. J. Lachmann, eds.), p. 59, Blackwell, Oxford.

Lerner, R. A., and Dixon, F. J., 1968, The induction of acute glomerulonephritis in rabbits with soluble antigens isolated from normal homologous and autologous urine, *J. Immunol.* **100:**1277.

Levine, P., 1979, Postscript to Dr. Fudenberg's lecture, in: *Immunopathology: Proceedings of the VIth International Convocation for Immunology* (F. Milgrom and B. Albini, eds.), p. 172, Karger, Basel.

Mendema, E., Arends, A., van Zeijst, J., Vermeer, G., von der Hem, G. K., and von der Slikke, L. B., 1963, Mercury and kidney, *Lancet* **1:**1266.

Milgrom, F., 1969, Autoimmunity, *Vox Sang.* **16:**286.

Milgrom, F., 1979, Antibodies to altered autologous antigens, in: *Immunopathology: Proceedings of the VIth International Convocation for Immunology* (F., Milgrom and B. Albini, eds.), p. 56, Karger, Basel.

Milgrom, F., and Kano, K., 1978, Comparison of various procedures for the detection of antigen–antibody complexes, *Int. Arch. Allergy Appl. Immunol.* **56:**224.

Richet, G., Fillastre, J. P., Morel-Maroger, L., and Bariety, J., 1974, Change from diffuse proliferative to membranous glomerulonephritis: Serial biopsies in four cases, *Kidney Int.* **5:**57.

Roman-Franco, A. A., Turiello, M., Albini, B., Ossi, E., and Andres, G. A., 1976, Anti-basement membrane antibody (A-BM-Ab) and immune complexes (IC) in rabbits injected with mercuric chloride, *Kidney Int.* **10:**549.

Roman-Franco, A. A., Turiello, M., Albini, B., Ossi, E., Milgrom, F., and Andres, G. A., 1978, Anti-basement membrane antibodies and antigen–antibody complexes in rabbits injected with mercuric chloride, *Clin. Immunol. Immunopathol.***9:**464.

Sapin, C., Druet, E., and Druet, P., 1977, Induction of anti-glomerular basement membrane antibodies in the Brown-Norway rat by mercuric chloride, *J. Clin. Exp. Immunol.* **28:**173.

Shibata, S., Sakaguchi, H., Nagasawa, T., and Naruse, T., 1972, Nephritogenic glycoprotein. II. Experimental production of membranous glomerulonephritis in rats by a single injection of homologous renal glycopeptide, *Lab. Invest.* **27:**457.

Talal, N., 1978, Autoimmunity and the immunologic network, *Arthritis Rheum.* **21:**853.

Theofilopoulos, A. N., Dixon, F. J., and Bokisch, V. A., 1974, Binding of soluble immune complexes to human lymphoblastoid cells. I. Characterization of receptors for IgG Fc and complement and description of the binding mechanisms, *J. Exp. Med.* **140:**877.

Weening, J. J., Fleuren, J., and Hoedemaeker, P. J., 1978, Demonstration of antinuclear antibodies in mercuric chloride-induced glomerulonephritis in the rat, *Lab. Invest.* **39:**405.

Weigle, W. O., 1979, Induction of autoimmunity with inaccessible tissue antigens, in: *Immunopathology: Proceedings of the VIth International Convocation for Immunology* (F. Milgrom and B. Albini, eds.), p. 45, Karger, Basel.

Wilson, C. B., and Dixon, F. J., 1976, The renal response to immunological injury, in: *The Kidney* (B. M. Brenner and F. C. Rector, Jr., eds.), p. 838, Saunders, Philadelphia.

19

Experimental Autoimmune Renal Tubulointerstitial Disease

Ulrich H. Rudofsky and Bernard Pollara

1. *Introduction*

It is well established that many types of glomerular diseases are caused by immune complexes or by autoantibodies to glomerular basement membrane (GBM) (Wilson, this volume). In experimental models and in cases of human glomerulonephritis, there also has been immunopathologic evidence for deposition of immune reactants along the tubular basement membrane (TBM) (Andres *et al.*, 1978) although their role in the pathogenesis of tubular lesions remained largely unrecognized until about 7 years ago. As in glomerular diseases, compelling evidence for immune mechanisms in renal tubular diseases in man was obtained only after convincing animal models had been established (Andres and McCluskey, 1975) (Table 1).

This chapter describes studies on the first model of autoimmune renal tubulointerstitial disease (RTD) induced in guinea pigs by immunization with xenogeneic TBM (Steblay and Rudofsky, 1971). The morphologic and immunopathologic observations indicate that RTD in guinea pigs is a unique inflammatory reaction which involves anti-TBM autoantibodies, lymphocytes, macrophages, and the alternative complement pathway.

2. *Induction of RTD in Guinea Pigs*

2.1. *TBM Antigens*

RTD was first induced in guinea pigs by intradermal injections of rabbit TBM in Freund's complete adjuvant (Steblay and Rudofsky, 1971). Several

Ulrich H. Rudofsky and Bernard Pollara · New York State Kidney Disease Institute, Division of Laboratories and Research, New York State Department of Health, Albany, New York 12201, and Department of Pediatrics, Albany Medical College, Albany, New York, 12208.

Table 1. Models of Renal Tubulointerstitial Disease: Anti-TBM Autoantibody-Induced Disease

1. Immunization with xenogeneic TBM: guinea pigs and rats (Steblay and Rudofsky, 1971; Lehman *et al.*, 1974b)
2. Immunization with allogeneic renal antigens: Sprague–Dawley → BN or Lewis × BN rats (Sugisaki *et al.*, 1973)
3. Immunization by renal allografts: Lewis × BN → Lewis (Lehman *et al.*, 1974a)

studies indicate that there is a similar or identical cross-reacting TBM antigen in a variety of species which can be used to induce an autoimmune response to TBM in guinea pigs. Although rabbit TBM has been used most frequently (Steblay and Rudofsky, 1971; Hyman *et al.*, 1967a; Hall *et al.*, 1977), bovine (Lehman *et al.*, 1974b; Van Zwieten *et al.*, 1976), human (Franklin, 1975), ovine, and murine (U. H. Rudofsky, unpublished observations) TBM preparations induce RTD of similar severity. It should be noted that detailed immunologic comparisons of the specificity of the anti-TBM autoantibodies evoked by these various antigens have not been made.

Homologous or isologous TBM has not been used successfully in inducing the formation of anti-TBM autoantibodies in guinea pigs. Experiments in rats indicate that certain strains will respond to allogeneic TBM provided that there is a sufficient genetic difference (Table 1) (Sugisaki *et al.*, 1973; Lehman *et al.*, 1974a). Recent studies indicate that guinea pigs may make an autoimmune response to autologous, presumably altered, TBM after transferred isologous anti-TBM autoantibodies have reacted with the target tissue. This process, termed *autoimmune amplification*, shows that autoantibodies can induce loss of self tolerance (Hall *et al.*, 1977; McCluskey *et al.*, this volume).

In actively immunized animals, the severity and onset of disease is dose dependent (Table 2). By day 18, virtually all animals given approximately 0.5 mg of TBM have severe lesions. A low dose of antigen evokes a variable

Table 2. Active Immunization of Guinea Pigs with Rabbit Renal Tubular Basement Membrane: Dose Response

Dose[a] (mg)	Number of animals	Severity of lesions (day 18)	
		Mean	Range
0.1	7	1 ± 2	0–4
0.5	6	4 ± 1	3–4
1.0	7	4 ± 0	3–4
2.0	8	4 ± 1	3–4

[a] TBM in 1 ml of Freund's complete adjuvant.

response by day 18, but disease may also be severe and uniform after an additional week.

2.2. Adjuvants

Adjuvant, in particular mycobacteria or *Bordetella pertussis*, plays a crucial role in the induction of a variety of autoimmune diseases in guinea pigs, e.g., thyroiditis (McMaster *et al.*, 1967). In contrast, RTD can be readily induced by injection of TBM in several adjuvants. Although we have not observed that one adjuvant is superior to another in this model (Rudofsky, 1976), other investigators have found a difference (Lehman *et al.*, 1974b). It is possible that at a low antigen dose, there is some distinction among the adjuvants. RTD also can be induced without adjuvant by multiple injections of TBM (Rudofsky, 1976).

2.3. Strain Differences

Most guinea pigs used in these studies have been from the Albany (A) strain, a closed colony established before 1914 by the New York State Department of Health. Histocompatibility typing indicates that they are not inbred, but that all share the strain 2 MHC antigens B1., Ia 2,4 (E. M. Shevach, personal communication). These studies indicate that the relationship to strain 2 is further substantiated by the fact that all A strain guinea pigs develop strain 2-specific L_2C leukemia (U. H. Rudofsky and G. D. Hsuing, unpublished observations; Shevach and Schwartz, 1977).

Studies by Hyman *et al.* (1976a,b) showed that strain 2 may be resistant to the induction of RTD by active and passive immunization. Under the experimental conditions reported here, strain 2 develops typical progressive lesions, although the onset of lesions is somewhat delayed (Rudofsky and

Table 3. Comparison of the Effect of Antigen Competition on the Induction of Autoimmune Thyroiditis and Autoimmune RTD in Guinea Pigs

Antigens[a]	Lesions on days 18 to 21	
	Kidney (No. positive/No. tested)	Thyroid (No. positive/No. tested)
TBM	33/39	0/39
Thyroid	0/44	38/44
TBM and thyroid	43/47	7/45
TBM and lung	17/20	0/20
Lung and thyroid	0/10	2/9
Lung	0/5	0/5
TBM and BGG	10/10	0/10
Thyroid and BGG	0/10	1/10

[a] Injected on opposite flanks in Freund's adjuvant.

Pollara, 1977). The MHC-linked diminished immune response of strain 2 (Hyman *et al.*, 1976b) apparently is overcome by adequate immunization (see Section 3.2). Strain 13, A strain, and C4 deficient, as well as guinea pigs obtained from a variety of commercial sources, are highly susceptible to the induction of RTD.

2.4. *Lack of an Effect of Antigen Competition on RTD*

In collaboration with Dr. P. R. B. McMaster, the effect of antigen competition on the induction of RTD and thyroiditis was studied. These data are summarized in Table 3. As previously described by McMaster and Kyriakos (1970), antigen competition inhibited the induction of thyroiditis. RTD could not be inhibited by thyroid, lung, or bovine gamma globulin (BGG) while thyroiditis was inhibited by TBM, lung, and BGG. Dose–response data indicated that lowering the dose of TBM and keeping the dose of thyroid antigen constant merely gave a typical dose response to TBM. Doses of 2 mg and of 0.5 mg of TBM induced RTD and inhibited thyroiditis, while a dose of 0.1 mg of the preparation of TBM did not suppress thyroiditis or induce RTD. The immune response in these two autoimmune diseases appears to differ qualitatively and/or quantitatively.

3. *Passive Transfer of RTD*

Early studies (Steblay and Rudofsky, 1971) showed that the development of RTD is associated with linear deposition of IgG along the TBM (Fig. 1) and with high titers of serum anti-TBM autoantibodies. Serum transfers resulted in IgG deposition of maximal immunofluorescent intensity on the TBM, but lesions were not observed. Adoptive transfers of RTD by S. H. Stone and R. W. Steblay in 1970–1971 (personal communication) were unsuccessful when well-established methods for the transfer of autoallergic encephalomyelitis (Stone, 1961) were used.

3.1. *Transfer of RTD with Serum Antibodies*

Serum transfers of RTD from affected donors to unmanipulated recipients solely require injection of a sufficient amount of autoantibodies to TBM (Steblay and Rudofsky, 1973). Removal by specific absorption renders sera incapable of inducing RTD. The onset and severity of the lesions is dose dependent (Rudofsky *et al.*, 1975). Recipients of high doses of anti-TBM serum have focal lesions as early as days 1 to 2 while low doses can delay the onset of RTD for as long as 5 to 8 days. Serum factors other than IgG are not required for passive transfer of RTD to unmanipulated recipients. IgG_1 and IgG_2 anti-TBM autoantibodies are present in the serum and in kidney eluates (Rudofsky *et al.*, 1974; Ma *et al.*, 1974; Hall *et al.*, 1977). Both IgG isotypes transfer disease (Hall *et al.*, 1977; McCluskey *et al.*, this volume).

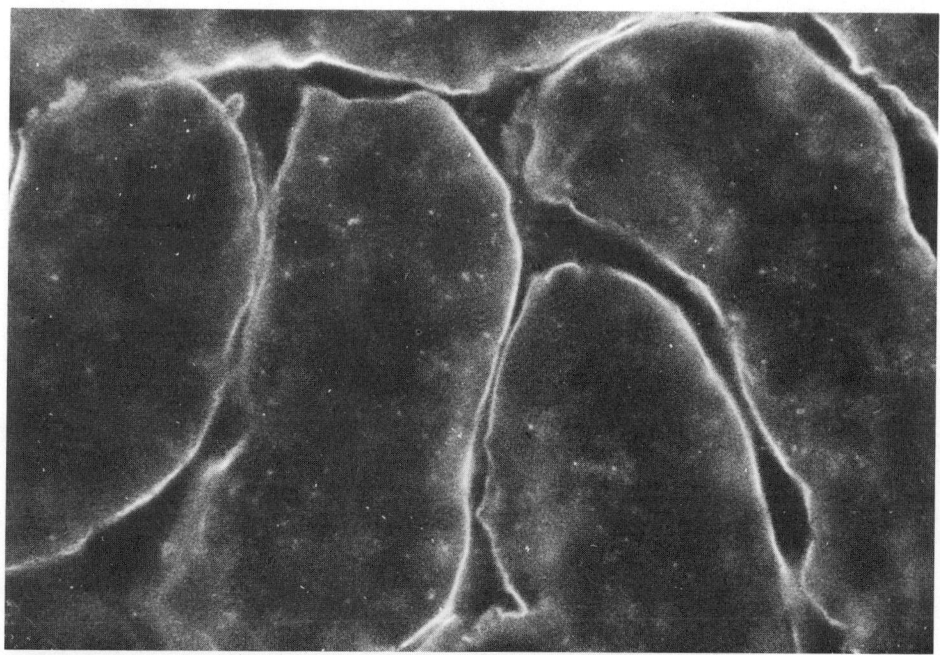

Figure 1. Immunofluorescent staining pattern in RTD. The linear deposition of IgG anti-TBM autoantibodies is characteristic for antibody-mediated renal diseases. C3 and factor B stained similarly. C4 and properdin were undetectable.

3.2. Differences in the Time Course of Passively Induced RTD in Strain 2 and A Strain Guinea Pigs

Failure to induce RTD in strain 2 guinea pigs by active immunization (Hyman *et al.*, 1976a,b) probably is related to antigen dose (see Section 2.3; Rudofsky and Pollara, 1977). The reported lack of an inflammatory response in strain 2 passive transfer recipients was reexamined. Under these experimental conditions (Steblay and Rudofsky, 1973), strain 2 developed RTD after injection of A strain anti-TBM serum. Evidently, the amount required to induce RTD in high-responder, genetically related animals (see Section 2.3) was sufficient to induce lesions in strain 2 (Fig. 2). Onset was delayed and severity diminished in this latter group.

This delay in the *inflammatory response* in strain 2 guinea pigs does not appear to be due to the diminished *immune response* as noted in actively immunized animals, i.e., lack of sufficient *autoimmune amplification* (Hall *et al.*, 1977). As shown in Fig. 2, the difference in degree of the inflammatory reactions could not be altered by passive immunization of A → 2 and 2 → A radiation chimeras (Rudofsky and Pollara, 1977). A → 2 recipients reacted like low-responder strain 2 and 2 → A like high-responder A strain guinea pigs. Thus, host factors other than those related to cells involved in the immune or inflammatory response appear to be involved in the diminished

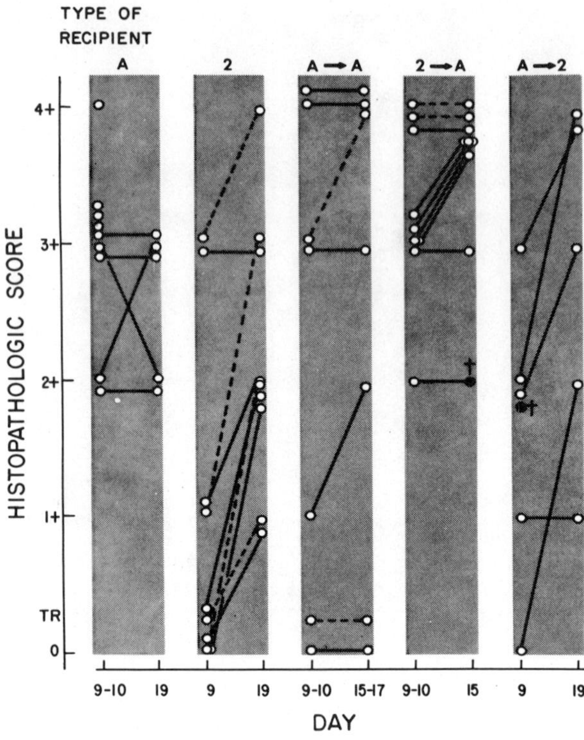

Figure 2. Comparative scores of renal histopathology of passive transfer recipients. Scores for individual guinea pigs at nephrectomy and sacrifice are connected by lines (dashed lines indicate experiments done on a different day). Two animals (+) died from causes other than renal disease.

reaction seen in strain 2 after a large dose of anti-TBM serum is injected. There may be differences in the amount of antibodies which strain 2 TBM can fix although genetic studies such as in the rat models of RTD have not been done (Sugisaki *et al.*, 1973; Lehman *et al.*, 1974a).

4. *Characteristics of Lesions in RTD*

Table 4 summarizes the morphologic characteristics of the renal lesions and the time during which these usually are observed in actively immunized

Table 4. Characteristics of Lesions of RTD of Guinea Pigs

Early Days:[a] A. 7–12 B. 1–3	Advanced 12–20 5–10	Chronic 28+ 14+
No polymorphonuclear leukocytes	Diffuse tubular and TBM destruction	Fibrosis, plasma cells
Focal intra- and intertubular small mononuclear cells (lymphoytes)	Giant cells, macrophages Hemorrhages	Few polymorphonuclear leukocytes Cyctic glomeruli

[a] A, Active immunization; B, passive transfer.

guinea pigs or in passive transfer recipients given a maximal to moderate dose of anti-TBM autoantibodies.

The most unique and fascinating morphologic feature is the absence of polymorphonuclear leukocytes (PMN) at the onset of histologic abnormalities (Rudofsky *et al.*, 1974; Van Zwieten *et al.*, 1976), in contrast to the rat (Lehman *et al.*, 1974c). As illustrated in Fig. 3, the earliest lesions involve small mononuclear cells which infiltrate the cortical interstitium. These cells appear focally around proximal tubules, and it can be seen that they can penetrate into the tubular epithelium.

Within 2–3 days, the lesions progress to involve most of the cortex but they spare the glomeruli and blood vessels (Fig. 4). At that stage, most cell infiltrates are composed of typical macrophages. Some of these appear to be intimately involved with the destruction of tubules and TBM. The most characteristic features are the multinucleated structures which resemble giant cells. Some of these seem to arise from damaged tubules while others are derived from macrophages. Both infiltrating and tubular epithelial cells may proliferate.

Those animals which survive the first 3 weeks go on to develop interstitial fibrosis. Plasma cells and neutrophils then are focally present.

5. *The Role of Complement*

After it was established that RTD can be induced in unmanipulated recipients by transfer of anti-TBM serum or of purified IgG, it became possible to study some of the cellular–humoral interactions which account for the unique lesions.

5.1. *Immunofluorescent Observations*

As shown in Table 5, IgG_1, IgG_2, C3, and factor B (Rudofsky *et al.*, 1977) are detected along the TBM of proximal tubules in actively immunized guinea pigs and in passive transfer recipients (Fig. 1). GBM is variably positive for IgG; C3 deposition is seen less frequently. C4 cannot be

Table 5. The Role of Complement in RTD

Animals	TBM deposition					RTD
	IgG[a]	C3	C4	Factor B	P	
Normal	+	+	0	+	0	+
C3-depleted	+	0	0	ND[b]	ND	0
C4-deficient	+	+	0	+	0	+

[a] IgG_1 and IgG_2.
[b] ND, not done.

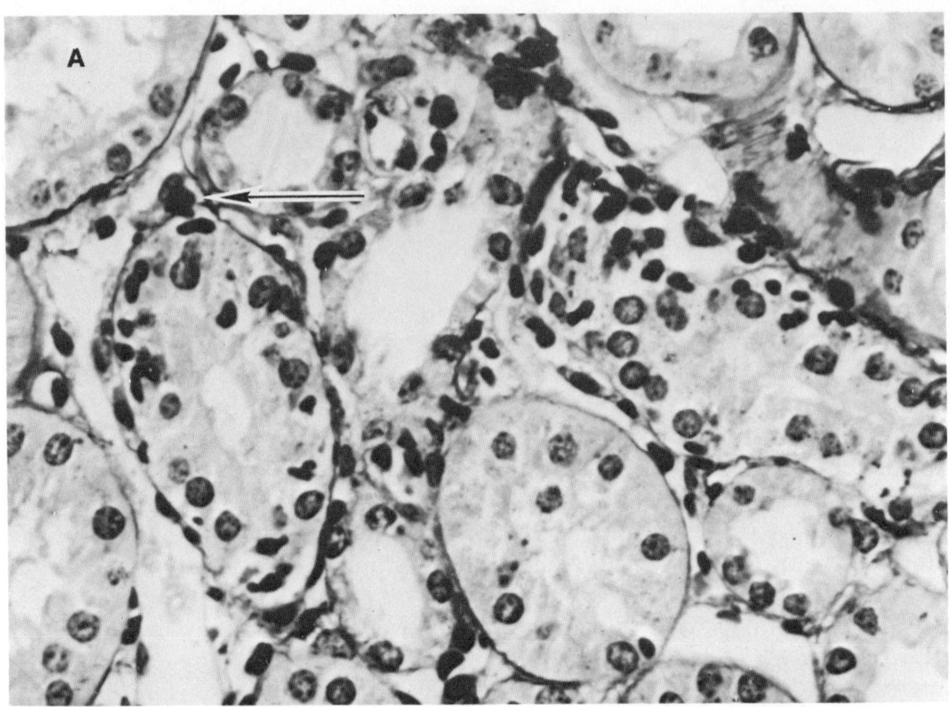
A

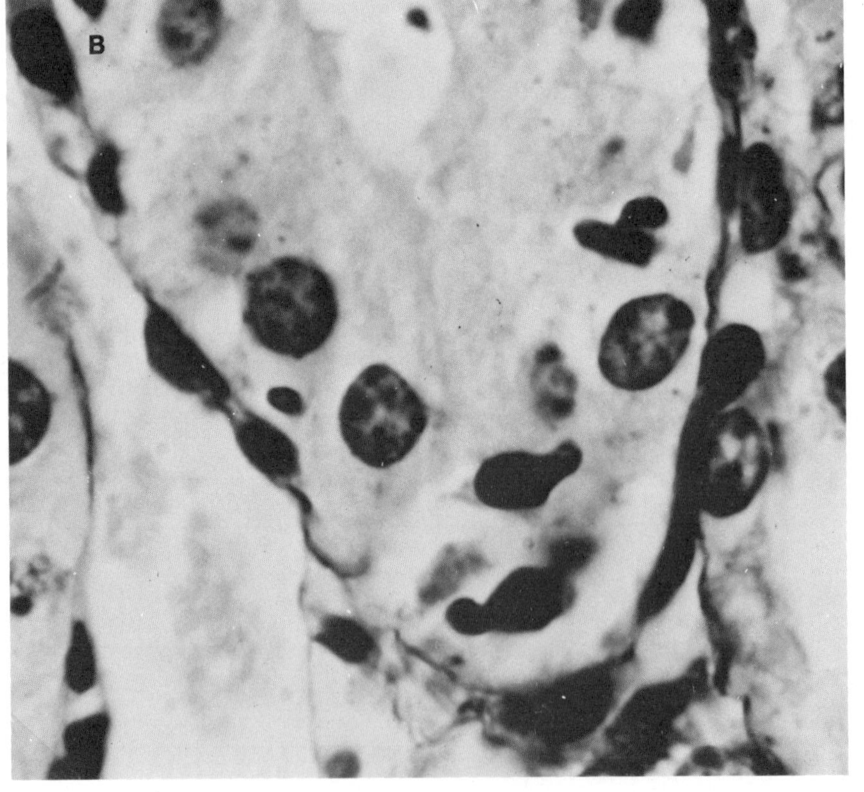
B

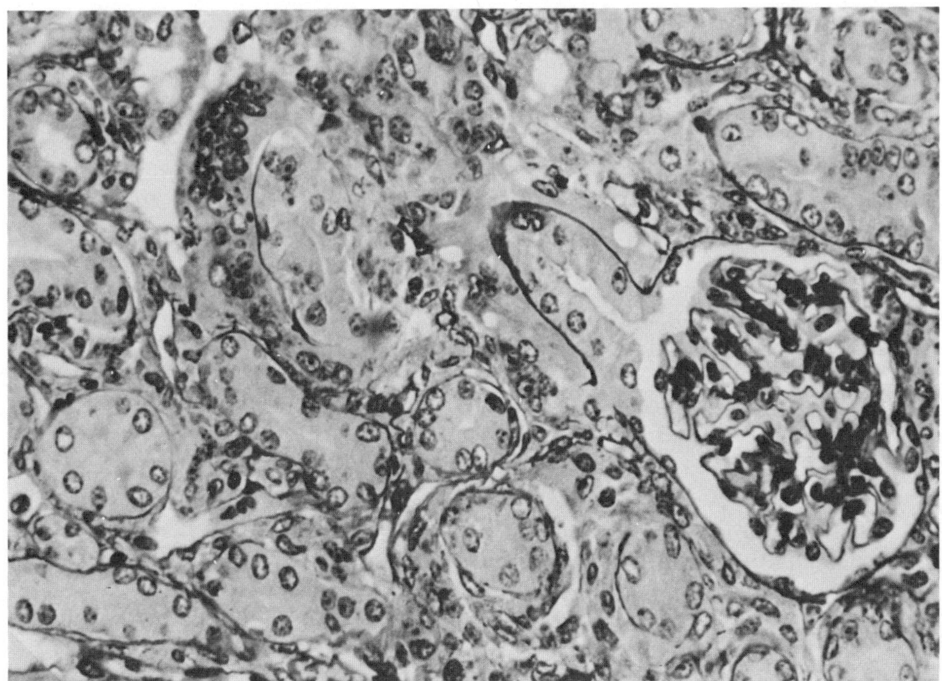

Figure 4. Advanced tubulointerstitial lesion. Rampant destruction of tubules and TBM is seen throughout the cortex. The glomerulus is not affected (silver methenamine).

demonstrated on the basement membranes. Unexpectedly, properdin is not detectable on the TBM (U. H. Rudofsky and A. Nicholson, unpublished data) with monospecific high-titered antiserum (Nicholson and Austen, 1977).

In some previous reports, detection of C3 on the TBM has been inconsistent. Lehman *et al.* (1974b) found C3 deposition in some animals only, while others (Van Zwieten *et al.*, 1976; Hyman *et al.*, 1976a; Hall *et al.*, 1977) could not demonstrate complement on the TBM. Rudofsky's observations indicate that antisera prepared to intact C3, rather than to zymosan–C3b (Mardiney and Müller-Eberhard, 1968), give consistently positive results (Rudofsky *et al.*, 1977).

5.2. Depletion of C with Cobra Venom Factor

When passive transfer recipients were pretreated with cobra venom factor (CVF), onset of renal lesions could be delayed as long as 14 days (Rudofsky *et al.*, 1975). When CVF treatment was given 4 days after passive

←

Figure 3. Early tubulointerstitial lesion. (A) Small mononuclear cells are present in the interstitium and some have invaded the tubular epithelium. One cell (arrow) appears to penetrate the TBM. (B) At higher magnification, some mononuclear cells appear to have broken through the TBM while others are in close proximity with the TBM (silver methenamine stain).

transfer, i.e., after antibodies and C3 had become fixed to the TBM, RTD could not be inhibited. Furthermore, RTD developed after C levels were reestablished. Thus, it became apparent that C3 deposition on the TBM is necessary. The presence of antibody on the TBM alone did not induce the accumulation of mononuclear cells. This suggests that either Fc is blocked or that Fc receptor cells are not part of the initial infiltrate. That CVF-treated animals had been depleted of other factors or perhaps cell types was not determined.

5.3. RTD in C4-Deficient Guinea Pigs

Although the CVF experiments and immunofluorescent data seemed to implicate C3 as a mediator of inflammation, experiments with guinea pigs with a total genetic deficiency of C4 made it clear that this component of the classic pathway is not required for the development of severe RTD (Rudofsky *et al.*, 1974).

These observations (Table 5) support the view that the alternative pathway is involved in this inflammatory reaction.

5.4. Differences in Reactivity of in Vivo and in Vitro Bound Anti-TBM Antibodies with Protein A

Protein A of *Staphylococcus aureus* Cowan strain I (SPA) reacts with the Fc portion of IgG (Biberfeld *et al.*, 1975). Fluorescein-labeled SPA was used to probe the nature of IgG deposition in RTD. As shown in Tables 6 and 7, the Fc portion of *in vivo* bound anti-TBM antibodies (IgG) is obscured either by a substance or by steric hindrance. Although IgG bound to GBM reacted well with SPA, the TBM-bound antibodies reacted only focally and faintly. By contrast, *in vitro* bound IgG was readily identified with anti-IgG or SPA on the TBM (Fig. 5).

This phenomenon is not explained simply by the greater quantity of antibody which is fixed *in vivo* and there may not be steric hindrance. However, as can be seen in the time course of IgG deposition on TBM and

Table 6. Differences in Reactivity of FITC–Anti-IgG and FITC–Staphylococcal Protein A (SPA) with in Vivo and in Vitro Bound GBM and TBM Autoantibodies

Substrate	Reagent	Intensity	
		GBM	TBM
Diseased kidney	Anti-IgG	4+	4+
	SPA	3–4+	±–1+
Normal kidney	Anti-IgG	0	4+[a]
+ anti-TBM	SPA	0	3+[b]

[a] Titer 1:320.
[b] Titer 1:40.

Table 7. Time Course of Direct Staining of Kidneys with FITC–Anti-IgG and FITC–Protein A

	Day[a]					
	7	11	13	15	18	20
Lesions						
Mean	0	1 ± 0	2 ± 1	3 ± 1	4 ± 0	4 ± 1
Range	0	0–1	1–4	2–4	4	3–4
Anti-IgG						
TBM	0	1–2	2–3	4	4	4
GBM	0	tr–1	1–2	1–2	1–4	1–4
Protein A						
TBM	0	0	tr–1	tr–1	tr–1	tr–1
GBM	0	tr–1	1	1	2–3	2–3

[a] Days after immunization; four guinea pigs per group.

GBM (Table 7), even when IgG deposition is of 1–2+ intensity, SPA does not react with anti-TBM deposits. By contrast, GBM deposits are detectable with SPA and increase in intensity parallel to IgG deposition.

The availability of the Fc portion is not required for the activation of the alternative pathway. Guinea pig $F(ab')_2$ of both IgG isotypes (Sandberg *et al.*, 1971) as well as human and rabbit F(ab) and F(ab') (Ehrnst, 1978) are efficient in activating the alternative pathway.

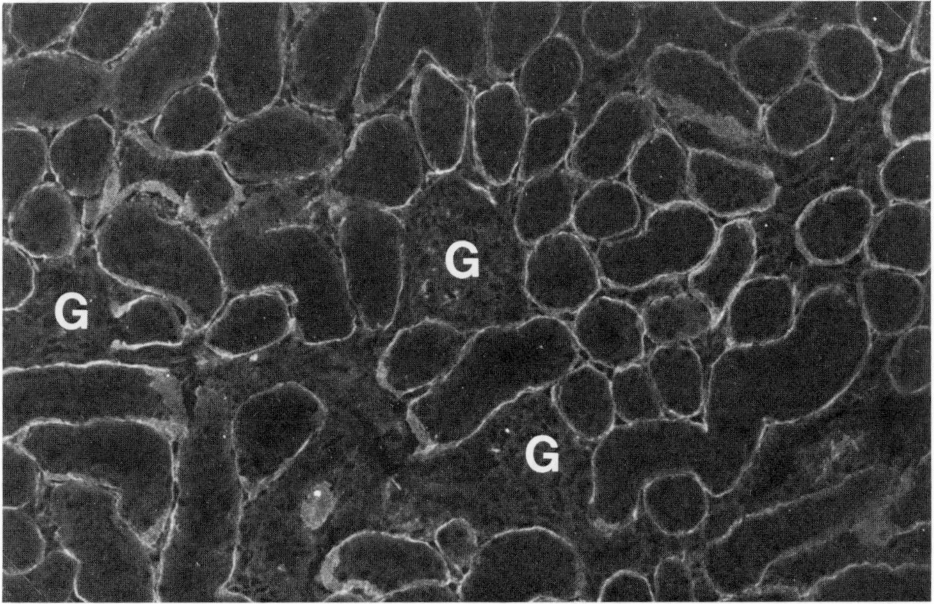

Figure 5. *In vitro* fixed anti-TBM autoantibody reaction with FITC–Protein A. Note the linear staining of TBM; glomeruli (G) are negative.

6. *The Nature and Origin of the Cellular Infiltrates*

Morphologic observations give the impression that lymphocytes and macrophages are the main cell types in RTD lesions. Lymphocytes seem to precede the influx of macrophages. A mechanism of cell-mediated immunity as the primary cause is ruled out by the passive transfer studies (Steblay and Rudofsky, 1973; Hyman *et al.*, 1976a; Van Zwieten *et al.*, 1976; Hall *et al.*, 1977) and by the failure to induce RTD by adoptive transfers with cells from sensitized donors obtained early (day 5) and late (at the time of severe disease) (S. H. Stone and R. W. Steblay, personal communication; van Zwieten *et al.*, 1976). Recently, cell-mediated lymphocytotoxicity to guinea pig kidney cells has been observed in this model (Neilson and Phillips, 1978).

The following experiments were done to examine the nature and origin of the inflammatory cells.

6.1. *Inhibition of Passive Transfer of RTD in Leukocyte-Depleted Recipients*

The purpose of the first experiments was to determine: (1) Whether the interaction of autoantibody, complement, and TBM has a direct injurious effect on the TBM, renal tubules, and interstitium, which could result in a secondary inflammatory infiltrate; or (2) whether the interaction of antibodies with complement gives rise to factors which mediate the accumulation of lymphocytes and macrophages in the target tissue.

To test these hypotheses, passive transfer experiments were performed using unmanipulated and leukocyte-depleted recipients (Rudofsky and Pollara, 1975). Guinea pigs were leukocyte-depleted with 640-rad whole body irradiation either on day 0 (shortly before injection) or on days 1 or 3 after passive immunization with a dose of anti-TBM autoantibody which would cause disease in unmanipulated recipients. Kidneys were examined by unilateral nephrectomy on days 3–4 and at sacrifice or death on days 7–9 after transfer.

Figure 6 summarizes the results. No renal lesions were observed in animals which were irradiated before or 1 day after injection of antibody. These data were confirmed in further experiments described in Section 6.2. Complete inhibition of RTD could be achieved by depletion of radiosensitive leukocytes.

In contrast, a delay in leukocyte depletion of 3 days after passive transfer of antibody had a variable effect. Those animals which did not have lesions by day 3 at nephrectomy did not develop RTD by days 7–9. In those animals which had early focal lymphocytic infiltrates on day 3, the lesions progressed despite irradiation and resembled those of nonirradiated controls. All controls developed RTD by day 7–9 regardless of whether lesions were noted on day 3.

The data were interpreted as follows: circulating, radiosensitive, nonsensitized mononuclear cells (lymphocytes?) accumulate in the target tissue first after antibody and complement have reacted with the TBM; the presence

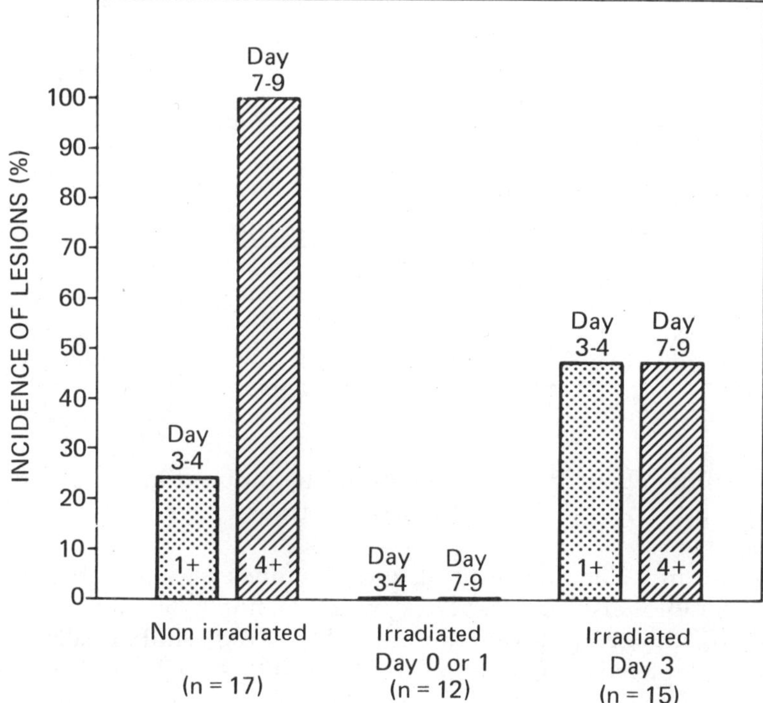

Figure 6. Effect of leukocyte depletion on passive transfer of RTD. Lesions were suppressed in animals irradiated before or 1 day after injection of autoantibodies.

of antibody and complement on TBM in the absence of these cells does not result in visible tissue destruction. Progression of RTD involves radioresistant mononuclear cells (macrophages). Neutrophils were not present in the lesions although these cells were present in the circulation after irradiation for at least 3 days. These cells were capable of infiltrating skin test sites. Macrophages persisted after irradiation and could form foreign-body granulomas on plastic implants (U. H. Rudofsky, unpublished observations).

6.2. Passive Transfer of Renal Lesions by Anti-TBM Antibody and Nonimmune Bone Marrow Cells to Leukocyte-Depleted Recipients

After it was established that there is a requirement of nonsensitized, radiosensitive mononuclear cells in the initiation of inflammation in RTD (Rudofsky and Pollara, 1975), the question about the nature and origin of these cells was pursued further in irradiated recipients given antibodies and lymphoid cells (Rudofsky and Pollara, 1976).

Preliminary experiments in the Albany strain guinea pigs indicated that lethally irradiated guinea pigs could be rescued by an allogeneic bone marrow

Table 8. Induction of Renal Lesions in Irradiated Guinea Pigs by Simultaneous Transfer of Anti-TBM Antibody and Normal Bone Marrow Cells

Group	Type of transfer	No. cells × 10^6	Incidence of lesions
1	Anti-TBM only (no irradiation)	0	36/36
2[a]	Irradiation only (no anti-TBM)	0	0/5
3	Anti-TBM	0	0/45
4	Anti-TBM + viable marrow	160–400	18/25
5	Anti-TBM + irradiated marrow	180	0/9
6	Anti-TBM + spleen cells	97	0/8
7	Anti-TBM + thymus cells	300	0/10
8	Anti-TBM + lymph node cells	60	0/4
9	Anti-TBM + leukocytes	60	0/4

[a] Groups 2–9: 750 rads 18 hr before transfer.

transplant from Albany donors. RTD could be induced in these "chimeras" (Rudofsky and Pollara, 1975) by passive transfer as well as by active immunization.

As shown in Table 8, groups of normal guinea pigs and of guinea pigs depleted of radiosensitive leukocytes by irradiation (750 rads) during the preceding 18 hr were passively immunized to TBM. Additionally, a group of leukocyte-depleted recipients received 1.6–4.0 × 10^8 allogeneic normal viable or irradiated (750 rads) marrow cells 2 to 3 hr after injection of anti-TBM serum. By days 6–8, RTD was present in all 36 unmanipulated recipients, in none of 45 depleted recipients, but in 18 of 25 animals given anti-TBM antibody and viable bone marrow from nonimmunized donors. Controls given anti-TBM antibody and irradiated marrow did not have renal lesions (Table 8).

By days 6–8, the RTD lesions were similar to those of guinea pigs given antibody only, those given anti-TBM antibody and marrow cells simultaneously, or in "chimeras," i.e., irradiated guinea pigs with marrow transplants surviving for 18–19 days before injection of antibody.

Similar experiments using cells teased from thymus, spleen, or lymph nodes of nonimmunized animals had negative results. These cells neither accumulated in the target organ in anti-TBM-injected recipients nor did they protect these animals from irradiation death. Thus, only cells which could readily proliferate, were effective. It is entirely possible that the proper number of cells from these organs was not used.

7. *Conclusions and Speculation*

The present observations on the pathogenesis of RTD in guinea pigs indicate that anti-TBM autoantibodies, complement and other factors, lymphocytes, and macrophages interact to cause severe damage to tubules and TBM. This unique inflammatory reaction differs from other types of inflammation which are known to be complement and PMN dependent (Cochrane *et al.*, 1970).

The evidence that these renal lesions are caused by autoantibodies which react with the TBM of proximal tubules is indisputable (Steblay and Rudofsky, 1973; Hyman *et al.*, 1976a; Van Zwieten *et al.*, 1976; Hall *et al.*, 1977). Less well understood are the events that take place after deposition of sufficient amounts of antibodies has occurred. The data on the participation of complement are limited by the available *in vivo* technology. The CVF experiments imply that deactivation of C3 and other components has an inhibitory effect on the influx of inflammatory cells until normal C levels are regained. Although the data are quite limited, it was observed that if CVF treatment was delayed for 4 days after passive transfer, onset of lesions was not affected. C3 and factor B are deposited on the TBM of all guinea pigs with RTD (Rudofsky *et al.*, 1977), but the reasons for the exclusively mononuclear cell infiltrates are not entirely clear.

Other antibody-induced lesions, e.g., Arthus reaction, also are mediated by complement (Cochrane *et al.*, 1970), but PMNs predominate in early infiltrates even in C4-deficient animals (Frank *et al.*, 1973). If, indeed, complement is the major mediator in RTD, it is difficult to explain the apparently exclusive participation of the alternative pathway. A clue for the lack of classic pathway activation may be in the manner in which anti-TBM antibodies are deposited *in vivo* (Section 5.4).

Morphologic and cell reconstitution studies indicate that there is a requirement for radiosensitive mononuclear cells in the initial phase of inflammation, while lesions progress when radioresistant mononuclear cells appear in the target tissue (Rudofsky and Pollara, 1975, 1976). However, it had been proposed that the irradiation experiments may have depleted the passive transfer recipients of lymphocytes which are necessary for autoantibody formation in the *autoimmune amplification* phase (Hall *et al.*, 1977). Some observations argue against the hypothesis that the immune response of passive transfer recipients must be intact. Severe lesions can be induced within 3 days and lesions progress when animals are irradiated 3 days after transfer. More work is necessary to clarify these matters.

Direct studies of the cells which infiltrate the target tissue are limited. Van Zwieten *et al.* (1976) detected Fc receptor monocytes on tissue sections of kidneys with advanced lesions, and observations also indicate the presence of Fc receptors on some of the infiltrating cells as seen by immunofluorescence (Rudofsky and Pollara, 1975). Isolation of viable mononuclear cells from kidneys with severe lesions (days 12–18) reveals a heterogeneous mixture of T and B lymphocytes and macrophages, but very few PMNs (U. H. Rudofsky, unpublished; McCluskey *et al.*, this volume). The most important identification, however, is that of the initiator cells, but recovery of cells from the early focal lesions has been difficult.

These, as yet fragmentary, observations suggest the following working hypothesis for RTD in guinea pigs: the interaction of TBM antigen and autoantibodies activates the alternative complement pathway (Müller-Eberhard, this volume) and a C3-amplifying convertase that includes C3 and factor B is assembled on the TBM. For undetermined reasons, this leads to the preferential accumulation of C3b or C3d receptor, radiosensitive, bone marrow-derived mononuclear cells (B lymphocytes?). This initial infiltrate may be activated by C3 to release factors which account for the prominent accumulation of macrophages and destruction of tubules and TBM ensues. Tubular injury may result in altered TBM antigen and leads to autoimmune amplification (Hall *et al.*, 1977) and, possibly, an as yet undefined, cell-mediated mechanism may also be present after injury and autoimmunization have occurred (Neilson and Phillips, 1978).

These speculations are supported by a number of *in vitro* observations on the interactions of C3 with B cells: (1) activation of B cells by C3b (Dukor *et al.*, 1974); (2) requirement for B cells for macrophage activation (Wilton *et al.*, 1975); (3) production of macrophage inhibition factor by C3b-activated B cells (Yoshida *et al.*, 1973; Sandberg *et al.*, 1975).

References

Andres, G. A., and McCluskey, R. T., 1975, Tubular and interstitial renal disease due to immunologic mechanisms, *Kidney Int.* **7:**271.

Andres, G., Brentjens, J., Kohli, R., Anthone, R., Anthone, S., Baliah, T., Montes, M., Mookerjee, B. K., Prezyna, A., Sepulveda, M., Venuto, R., and Elwood, C., 1978, Histology of human tubulo-interstitial nephritis associated with antibodies to renal basement membranes, *Kidney Int.* **13:**480.

Biberfeld, P., Ghetie, V., and Sjöquist, J., 1975, Demonstration and assaying of IgG antibodies in tissues and on cells by labelled staphylococcal protein A, *J. Immunol. Mehtods* **6:**249.

Cochrane, C. G., Müller-Eberhard, H. J., and Aikin, B. S., 1970, Depletion of plasma complement *in vivo* by a protein of cobra venom: Its effect on various immunologic reactions, *J. Immunol.* **105:**55.

Dukor, P., Schumann, G., Gisler, R. H., Dierich, M., König, W., Hadding, U., and Bitter-Suermann, D., 1974, Complement-dependent B-cell activation by cobra venom factor and other mitogens?, *J. Exp. Med.* **139:**337.

Ehrnst, A., 1978, Separate pathways of C activation by measles virus cytotoxic antibodies: Subclass analysis and capacity of F(ab) molecules to activate C via the alternative pathway, *J. Immunol.* **121:**1206.

Frank, M. M., Ellman, L., Green, I., and Cochrane, C. G., 1973, Site of deposition of C3 in Arthus reactions of C4 deficient guinea pigs, *J. Immunol.* **110:**1447.

Franklin, W. A., 1975, Antigenicity of renal tubular basement membranes, *Fed. Proc.* **34:**878.

Hall, C. L., Colvin, R. B., Carey, K., and McCluskey, R. T., 1977, Passive transfer of autoimmune disease with isologous IgG_1 and IgG_2 antibodies to the tubular basement membrane in strain XIII guinea pigs: Loss of self-tolerance induced by autoantibodies, *J. Exp. Med.* **146:**1246.

Hyman, L. R., Colvin, R. B., and Steinberg, A. D., 1976a, Immunopathogenesis of autoimmune tubulointerstitial nephritis. I. Demonstration of differential susceptibility in strain II and strain XIII guinea pigs, *J. Immunol.* **116:**327.

Hyman, L. R., Steinberg, A. D., Colvin, R. B., and Bernard, E. F., 1976b, Immunopathogenesis of autoimmune tubulointerstitial nephritis. II. Role of an immune response gene linked to the major histocompatibility complex, *J. Immunol.* **117:**1894.

Lehman, D. H., Lee, S., Wilson, C. B., and Dixon, F. J., 1974a, Induction of antitubular basement membrane antibodies in rats by renal transplantation, *Transplantation* **17:**429.

Lehman, D. H., Marquardt, H., Wilson, C. B., and Dixon, F. J., 1974b, Specificity of autoantibodies to tubular and glomerular basement membranes induced in guinea pigs, *J. Immunol.* **112:**241.

Lehman, D. H., Wilson, C. B., and Dixon, F. J., 1974c, Interstitial nephritis in rats immunized with heterologous tubular basement membrane, *Kidney Int.* **5:**187.

Ma, W., Rudofsky, U., Esposito, L., Dilwith, R., Pollara, B., and Steblay, R. W., 1974, A rapid method for the separation of guinea pig IgG_1 and IgG_2, *Immunol. Commun.* **3:**285.

Mardiney, M. R., and Müller-Eberhard, H. J., 1965, Mouse β_{1c}-globulin: Production of antiserum and characterization in the complement reaction, *J. Immunol.* **94:**877.

McMaster, P. R. B., and Kyriakos, M., 1970, The prevention of autoimmunity to thyroid and allergic thyroiditis by antigen competition, *J. Immunol.* **105:**1201.

McMaster, P. R. B., Lerner, E. M., II, Kyriakos, M., and Mueller, P. S., 1967, The influence of the dose of thyroid extract and mycobacteria upon experimental autoimmune thyroiditis in inbred histocompatible and random-bred guinea pigs, *J. Immunol.* **90:**201.

Neilson, E. G., and Phillips, S. M., 1978, Cell mediated lymphocytotoxicity in interstitial nephritis: *In vitro* and *in vivo* observations, *Kidney Int.* **14:**715, (abstract).

Nicholson, A., and Austen, K. F., 1977, Isolation and characterization of guinea pig properdin, *J. Immunol.* **18:**103.

Rudofsky, U. H., 1976, Studies on the pathogenesis of experimental autoimmune renal tubulointerstitial disease in guinea pigs. 3. The role of adjuvants in the induction of disease, *Clin. Exp. Immunol.* **25:**455.

Rudofsky, U. H., and Pollara, B., 1975, Studies on the pathogenesis of experimental autoimmune renal tubulointerstitial disease in guinea pigs. 1. Inhibition of tissue injury in leukocyte-depleted passive transfer recipients, *Clin. Immunol. Immunopathol.* **4:**425.

Rudofsky, U. H., and Pollara, B., 1976, Studies on the pathogenesis of experimental autoimmune renal tubulointerstitial disease in guinea pigs. 2. Passive transfer of renal lesions to leukocyte-depleted recipients by anti-tubular basement membrane autoantibodies and non-immune bone marrow cells, *Clin. Immunol. Immunopathol.* **6:**107.

Rudofsky, U. H., and Pollara, B., 1977, Autoimmune renal tubulointerstitial disease (RTD) in strain 2 guinea pigs, *Fed. Proc.* **36:**1059.

Rudofsky, U. H., McMaster, P. R. B., Ma, W., Steblay, R. W., and Pollara, B., 1974, Experimental autoimmune renal cortical tubulointerstitial disease in guinea pigs lacking the fourth component of complement (C4), *J. Immunol.* **112:**1387.

Rudofsky, U. H., Steblay, R. W., and Pollara, B., 1975, Inhibition of experimental autoimmune renal tubulointerstitial disease in guinea pigs by depletion of complement with cobra venom factor, *Clin. Immunol. Immunopathol.* **3:**396.

Rudofsky, U. H., Esposito, L. L., Dilwith, R. L., and Pollara, B., 1977, Studies on the pathogenesis of experimental autoimmune renal tubulointerstitial disease in guinea pigs. 5. Deposition of C3PA on the tubular basement membranes, *Clin. Immunol. Immunopathol.* **8:**467.

Sandberg, A. L., Oliviera, B., and Osler, A. G., 1971, Two complement interaction sites in guinea pig immunoglobulins, *J. Immunol.* **106:**282.

Sandberg, A. L., Wahl, S. M., and Mergenhagen, S. E., 1975, Lymphokine production by C3b-stimulated B cells, *J. Immunol.* **115:**139.

Shevach, E. M., and Schwartz, B. D., 1977, Overview of the structure and function of the major histocompatibility complex of the guinea pig, *Fed. Proc.* **36:**2260.

Steblay, R. W., and Rudofsky, U. H., 1971, Renal tubular disease and autoantibodies of tubular basement membrane induced in guinea pigs, *J. Immunol.* **107:**589.

Steblay, R. W., and Rudofsky, U., 1973, Transfer of experimental autoimmune renal cortical tubular and interstitial disease in guinea pigs by serum, *Science* **180:**966.

Stone, S. H., 1961, Transfer of allergic encephalomyelitis by lymph node cells in inbred guinea pigs, *Science* **134:**619.

Sugisaki, T., Klassen, J., Milgrom, F., Andres, G. A., and McCluskey, R. T., 1973, Immunopathologic study of an autoimmune tubular and interstitial renal disease in Brown Norway rats, *Lab. Invest.* **28:**658.

Van Zwieten, M. J., Bhan, A. K., McCluskey, R. T., and Collins, A. B., 1976, Studies on the pathogenesis of experimental antitubular basement membrane nephritis in the guinea pig, *Am. J. Pathol.* **83:**531.

Wilton, J. M., Rosenstreich, D. L., and Oppenheim, J. J., 1975, Activation of guinea pig macrophages by bacterial lipopolysaccharide requires bone marrow-derived lymphocytes, *J. Immunol.* **114:**388.

Yoshida, T., Sonozaki, H., and Cohen, S., 1973, The production of migration inhibition factor by B and T cells of guinea pigs, *J. Exp. Med.* **138:**784.

Addendum

Since the preparation of this manuscript several major findings have been published on the pathogenesis of RTD. Cell-mediated immune mechanisms have been elucidated by Neilson and Phillips (1979, *J. Immunol.* **123:**2373; 1979, *J. Immunol.* **123:**2381; 1980, *J. Immunol.* **125:**1708; 1981, *J. Immunol.* **126:**1980). Brown *et al.* (1979, *J. Immunol.* **123:**2102) have described inhibition of RTD with anti-idiotype serum. We have extended this model of RTD to mice and demonstrated the spontaneous occurrence of anti-TBM autoantibodies in murine lupus nephritis (Rudofsky, U. H., 1980, *Clin. Immunol. Immunopathol.* **15:**200). The experimental induction of RTD in mice is associated with an *H-2K*-restricted cellular mechanism (Rudofsky, U. H., Dilwith, R. L., and Tung, K. S. K., 1980, *Lab. Invest.* **43:**463).

20

Experimental and Human Anti-Tubular Basement Membrane Nephritis

Robert T. McCluskey, Atul K. Bhan, and Robert B. Colvin

1. Introduction

In Chapter 19, a review of the salient features of the model of anti-tubular basement membrane (TBM) nephritis in guinea pigs was given. This discussion will focus upon certain additional aspects of this model and also comment briefly on experimental anti-TBM disease in rats. Finally, current knowledge of the role of anti-TBM antibodies in human renal disease will be reviewed.

2. Experimental Anti-TBM Nephritis

2.1. Guinea Pigs

2.1.1. Passive Transfer with Serum

The transfer of appropriate amounts of serum or IgG fractions from guinea pigs with anti-TBM disease to normal guinea pigs results in the development of the characteristic features of the disease in the recipient, namely linear accumulation of IgG along the TBM and severe tubulointerstitial nephritis, with accumulation of mononuclear and multinuclear cells, as well as tubular cell damage (Steblay and Rudofsky, 1973; Hyman *et al.*, 1976a; Van Zwieten *et al.*, 1976). These observations provide the most direct evidence that the disease is mediated by antibodies. Nevertheless, a puzzling

Robert T. McCluskey, Atul K. Bhan, and Robert B. Colvin · Departments of Pathology, Massachusetts General Hospital and Harvard Medical School, Boston, Massachusetts 02115. Supported in part by NIH Grants 1 R01 AM 18729 and CA 19393.

aspect of the disease seen in some serum recipients is the length of time required for the development of severe lesions. Although small mononuclear cell infiltrates can be seen as early as 2 days, the lesions in some animals continue to progress in severity for 2 weeks or more.

One possible explanation for this protracted development of lesions was provided by the observation of Van Zwieten *et al.* (1976) that the transferred antibodies accumulate only slowly in the TBM. At four hours after transfer of anti-TBM serum to normal guinea pigs, bright staining for IgG was seen along the GBM, but there was only faint irregular staining along the TBM. On day three, both the TBM and GBM stained brightly; on day five only the TBM exhibited bright staining. Studies of guinea pig anti-TBM serum by indirect immunofluorescence indicate that most of the antibodies are directed against constituents of the TBM, and relatively little against the GBM. The early accumulation of IgG along the GBM following transfer probably results from the greater access of antibodies to the GBM, possibly reflecting the filtration function of the glomerulus.

Although the slow binding of antibodies to the TBM is probably a factor in the delayed development of lesions in serum recipients, it does not appear to provide the entire explanation, since progression is seen in some animals for more than two weeks. Another explanation emerged from the study of Hall *et al.* (1977), in which it was shown that recipients of anti-TBM antibodies were stimulated to produce their own anti-TBM antibodies (a process we call autoimmune amplification). The study was undertaken to determine whether antibodies of the IgG_1 or IgG_2 isotype (or both) mediate anti TBM disease. Serum was collected from a large number of strain 13 guinea pigs that had been immunized 14–18 days earlier with a rabbit TBM preparation in adjuvant. To this pool of serum was added guinea pig antiserum against bovine gamma globulin (BGG), 10% by volume; this provided a means for monitoring the effectiveness of the separation of the IgG_1 and IgG_2 fractions, through assays of passive cutaneous anaphylaxis (PCA) activity (a property of IgG_1) or hemolytic activity (a property of IgG_2). The pooled serum was separated into IgG_1 and IgG_2 components by DEAE chromatography. The IgG_2 fraction employed for transfer had no measurable PCA activity against BGG and the IgG_1 fraction no hemolytic activity. On the basis of these results it was estimated that there could not have been more than 0.1% reciprocal contamination of the IgG_1 and IgG_2 fractions.

Purified IgG_1 or IgG_2 fractions with approximately equal anti-TBM antibody titers and protein content were transferred to normal strain 13 guinea pigs. The animals were sacrificed 14 days later when it was anticipated that there would be severe renal lesions if transfer was effective. Recipients of either isotype were found to have developed renal lesions. Severe abnormalities were seen more frequently in guinea pigs given IgG_2 antibodies. The histological findings in the kidney were qualitatively the same in the two groups of recipients and were indistinguishable from those seen in actively immunized guinea pigs. Both groups of recipients exhibited the typical linear accumulation of IgG along the TBM. The production of the same type of tissue damage by IgG_1 and IgG_2 antibodies was surprising, in view of the distinctive biological properties of the two isotypes (Bloch *et al.*, 1963; Vuagnat, 1974).

Another puzzling finding in the study of Hall *et al.* (1977) was the wide range of anti-TBM antibody titers in the sera of the recipients, which were determined at the time of sacrifice (14 days). This was unexpected since each guinea pig received approximately the same amount of anti-TBM antibodies. These observations led to the suspicion that the recipients had been stimulated to produce their own anti-TBM antibodies to a variable extent. Compelling evidence for this conclusion was obtained by analysis of the isotypes of anti-TBM antibodies in the recipients at 14 days. As shown in Table 1, anti-TBM antibodies of both isotypes were found in recipients of either IgG_1 or IgG_2 fractions. In contrast, anti-BGG antibodies were found exclusively in the isotype that had been transferred.

Analysis of the titers of anti-TBM antibodies in the recipients showed a good correlation between the levels of antibodies and the severity of the renal lesions, which indicated that the autoantibodies produced by the host participated in the production of renal damage. However, the question raised—whether IgG_1 or IgG_2 antibodies mediate the renal damage—could not be answered, since both isotypes were produced by the recipients and presumably were present along the TBM. (The goat anti-guinea pig IgG antiserum used to detect TBM-bound antibodies by immunofluoresence is reactive with either isotype.)

The mechanism of autoimmune amplification was not elucidated. It is not clear whether or not TBM damage is required to initiate the autoimmune response, although it seems probable that this is the case. It is of interest that, in 1957, Milgrom and Dubiski predicted the phenomenon of autoimmune amplification on theoretical grounds. It is unclear whether or not the stimulation of autoantibodies by autoantibodies is an unusual event, or whether, in many situations where this phenomenon occurs, it goes unnoticed because its detection is difficult or impossible. At least one well-documented example of an analogous process has been reported. Autoantibody produc-

Table 1. IgG_1 and IgG_2 Antibodies in Recipients of IgG_1 or IgG_2 Anti-TBM Fractions: Evidence for an Active Autoimmune Response

Anti-TBM fraction transferred[a]	Extent of disease[b]	Anti-TBM titers[c]			Anti-BBG titers		
		Serum	IgG_1	IgG_2	Serum	IgG_1	IgG_2
IgG_1, 10 ml	1.7	1/40	1/20	< 1	1/267	1/80	< 1
IgG_1, 20 ml	18.7	1/132	1/320	1/40	1/400	1/160	< 1
IgG_1, 30 ml	62.2	1/704	1/640	1/640	1/896	1/160	< 1
IgG_2, 20 ml	88.0	1/960	1/1280	1/320	1/896	< 1	1/160
IgG_1, 5 ml + IgG_2, 5 ml	9.2	1/98	1/20	1/10	1/187	1/80	1/80
NGPS + anti-BGG serum	0.3	< 1	< 1	< 1	1/960	1/640	1/640

[a] One milliliter of serum from each animal in a group was pooled and separated into IgG_1 and IgG_2 antibodies by DEAE chromatography. The peaks containing IgG_1 and IgG_2 were reconcentrated to the original serum volume and assayed for anti-TBM and anti-BGG antibodies.

[b] The extent of the anti-TBM disease is the percent of cortex affected as determined morphometrically.

[c] Indirect immunofluorescence, 14 days after transfer.

tion has been demonstrated during experimental isoimmune hemolytic anemia in human volunteers (Mohn *et al.,* 1965). Seventy days after the infusion of serum containing anti-CD antibodies into a normal subject of the cDE/cE rhesus genotype, anti-E antibodies developed in the recipient. It was concluded that the binding of anti-CD antibodies to the red cells resulted in a stimulus to the formation of anti-E autoantibodies. In this situation, the autoantibodies were directed against determinants different from those with which the transferred antibodies reacted. In the anti-TBM model, it is not possible to investigate this question, since the nature of the relevant TBM antigens is unknown and purified TBM antigens are not available.

Another possible example of autoimmune amplification is in a model of experimental thyroiditis that can be transferred by isologous murine antisera to thyroglobulin (Tomazic and Rose, 1975). An early and a late (20 day) phase of cellular infiltration were observed. The late phase was postulated to be due to an active response by the recipient. However, no antibody production against thyroid antigens by the recipients was evident. Although it has been suggested that autoantibodies are produced and play a role in the second phase of nephrotoxic serum nephritis (Lange *et al.,* 1961), there is compelling evidence against this possibility (Unanue and Dixon, 1965).

It would be difficult to determine whether autoimmune amplification occurs during the course of autoimmune diseases in man. In some instances, such diseases are self-limited, and automimmune amplification either does not develop or in time can be inactivated. It is suggested that this phenomenon may provide a mechanism for the intensification and prolongation of some autoimmune diseases, a process that might be interrupted by procedures that cause depletion of autoantibodies, such as plasmapheresis (Lockwood *et al.,* 1976).

2.1.2. *Immunogenetics of Anti-TBM Nephritis in Guinea Pigs*

Susceptibility to anti-TBM nephritis is influenced by at least two types of genetic control: (1) expression of the relevant TBM antigen(s); and (2) production of an effective immune response. Both guinea pig and rat strains differ in their immune response to exogenous TBM preparations. The most detailed studies are in guinea pigs and these will be elaborated here.

Strain 13 and strain 2 guinea pigs show marked differences in susceptibility to anti-TBM nephritis when immunized with rabbit TBM (Hyman *et al.,* 1976a,b) or with bovine TBM (Colvin and Bhan, unpublished data). In Table 2 are summarized the results obtained in strain 13, strain 2, F_1 and F_2 backcross animals (Hyman *et al.,* 1976). Several conclusions can be drawn from these data. The strain 13 animals have significantly more disease (mean extent of disease in the cortex 83.7%) and have higher titers of anti-TBM antibody (mean titer of 10.2, $\log_2$) than do strain 2 animals (mean disease of 2.5% and mean titer 2.5). F_1 (2 × 13) have intermediate anti-TBM levels and extent of disease. The difference in antibody titers clearly shows that the immune response to TBM antigens differs in these strains.

Table 2. Immunogenetic Studies of Anti-TBM Nephritis in Guinea Pigs

Strain	Ia phenotype[a]	*n*	Extent of anti-TBM nephritis[b] (mean % ± S.E.M.)	Anti-TBM titer[c] ($\log_2$ ± S.E.M.)
13	13/13	27	83.7 ± 3.9	10.2 ± 0.2
$(F_1 \times 13)F_2$	13/13	3	83.3 ± 9.5	8.8 ± 1.1
2	2/2	22	2.5 ± 0.1	2.5 ± 0.5
$(F_1 \times 2)F_2$	2/2	12	5.0 ± 2.1	1.9 ± 0.6
$(2 \times 13)F_1$	2/13	26	27.5 ± 5.2	6.9 ± 0.8
$(F_1 \times 2)F_2$	2/13	11	37.1 ± 11.2	7.3 ± 0.7
$(F_1 \times 13)F_2$	2/13	3	19.3 ± 8.5	5.3 ± 0.9

[a] Lymph node cells from F_1 and F_2 animals typed by strain 13 and strain 2 reciprocal antisera. Homozygotes were typed as having either 2 or 13 antigens but not both (data from Hyman *et al.*, 1976b).
[b] Animals were immunized with 1 mg of rabbit TBM in Freund's complete adjuvant. The kidneys were studied 21–30 days later and the percentage of cortex that was diseased was measured by a morphometric technique using light microscopy.
[c] Titers measured by indirect immunofluorescence.

The lack of anti-TBM nephritis in strain 2 animals is not absolute, although it may appear to be so with certain immunization schedules. Further studies (Colvin and Bhan, unpublished; see also Rudofsky and Pollara, this volume) have shown that when anti-TBM nephritis develops in strain 2 animals, it has a slower pace than in strain 13 guinea pigs. The fact that some strain 2 animals eventually do develop anti-TBM antibodies and anti-TBM disease following certain types of immunization is not surprising because similar observations have been made with respect to certain other immune responses under genetic control (Benacerraf and McDevitt, 1972).

The genetic basis of the anti-TBM immune response was elucidated by F_1 backcrosses to either parental strain (Hyman *et al.*, 1966). Backcross animals were immunized with rabbit TBM and their lymph node cells typed for the train 2 and 13 Ia antigens by immunofluorescence. Those F_2 animals that had a parental Ia phenotype (2/2 and 13/13) had anti-TBM disease and antibody levels that were indistinguishable from those in the analogous parental strain. This demonstrates that a *single* genetic linkage group (but not necessarily a single gene) is the principal determinant of the anti-TBM disease and that these genes are linked with those controlling the 2/13 Ia antigens, as are several other immune response genes in the guinea pig. Genes on other strain 2 or 13 chromosomes have no measurable effect on the development of anti-TBM nephritis and antibodies.

Those F_2 animals that had a 2/13 Ia phenotype had intermediate antibody levels and disease similar to that in F_1 animals. This is also consistent with a single genetic linkage group and suggests that the anti-TBM nephritis trait is either dominant or codominant. It was not determined whether or not the strain 13 anti-TBM immune response gene, termed Ir-TBM, actively favors anti-TBM antibody production and/or whether the corresponding gene in strain 2, termed Ir-tbm, may exert a suppressive effect. Finally, the data show a very close correlation between anti-TBM titers and the extent of the disease ($p < 0.001$), providing further evidence that anti-TBM antibodies are a prime pathogenetic factor.

Recent studies (Colvin, Carey, and Rappaport, unpublished) were undertaken in outbred Hartley guinea pigs to determine whether the Ir-TBM and Ir-tbm genes were separable from the genes determining the strain 2/13 Ia antigens and from the genes that determine the immune response to dinitrophenol linked to guinea pig albumin (DNP_5GSA). Animals were immunized with rabbit TBM and DNP_5GSA. After 3 weeks, the extent of anti-TBM disease, the delayed-type skin reaction to DNP_5GSA, and the 2/13 Ia phenotype were determined. The results for the animals typed as 2 or 13 (Table 3) indicate a significant but not perfect correlation between the strain 13 and 2 Ia phenotype and the development of anti-TBM nephritis ($p < 0.05$). However, two animals that typed similarly to strain 13 (13+, 2−) failed to develop disease (< 3% of cortex diseased) and two animals that typed as strain 2 (13−, 2+) developed severe disease (> 50% of cortex involved). Thus, the strain 2 and 13 Ia phenotypes are not the determinants of the anti-TBM nephritis and the corresponding genes are different from the Ir-TBM/tbm genes. The data indicate a genetic disequilibrium and are consistent with a close linkage between the Ia and Ir-TBM loci. Six of eleven animals that developed anti-TBM nephritis had delayed reactions to DNP_5GSA, while four of eight that did not develop nephritis reacted to DNP_5GSA ($p > 0.5$). Therefore, the Ir genes that determine the immune response to DNP_5GSA are different from the Ir-TBM/tbm.

Curiously, even when anti-TBM antibodies are given to strain 2 animals in passive transfer experiments, they usually do not develop disease, in contrast to strain 13 recipients. The antibodies are deposited in strain 2 kidneys, which apparently do not lack the relevant TBM antigens. The nature of the deficient "second factor" in strain 2 animals is not clear. As discussed earlier, we have recently obtained evidence that passive transfer of anti-TBM antibody stimulates strain 13 recipients to produce their own anti-TBM antibodies (Hall *et al.*, 1977). Such B-cell reactivity (perhaps T cell dependent) may be the missing factor in strain 2 animals, although this has not been tested.

It is concluded from these studies that anti-TBM nephritis in the guinea pig is largely, if not exclusively, determined by one or more immune response

Table 3. Relationship between Ia Phenotype and Anti-TBM Nephritis in Outbred Hartley Guinea Pigs

Ia phenotype	Anti-TBM nephritis[a]
2	3/9
13	9/11

[a] Number > 10% of cortex diseased/total number of animals. The probability that the differences between the groups are due to chance is $p = 0.04$, Fisher exact test.

genes linked to the genes controlling the Ia antigens. The genetic simplicity of this autoimmune disease contrasts with the genetic complexity of murine lupus and further study may provide insight into the genetic mechanisms of autoimmunity. Rat strains also differ in their anti-TBM immune response (Lehman *et al.*, 1974), but the genetic basis has not been explored (see Section 2.2.2). Identification of genetic factors in man in anti-TBM and perhaps anti-GBM disease will be more difficult, but may be fruitful.

2.1.3. *Cellular Infiltrate in Guinea Pig Experimental Anti-TBM Nephritis*

The cellular infiltrate in guinea pig anti-TBM nephritis is composed predominantly of mononuclear cells, although multinuclear giant cells are generally conspicuous and plasma cells are often present, especially in later stages. In 1-μm sections prepared from Epon-embedded tissue, occasional mast cells may be seen, but basophils are lacking (Van Zwieten *et al.*, 1976). Neutrophils are usually not seen, or are found only in small numbers. Several other lesions that are apparently mediated by antibodies have a predominantly mononuclear cell infiltrate, but in these situations either there has been recognized an earlier phase during which neutrophils predominate, or the lesions have not been examined at sufficiently early intervals to exclude such a possibility (Tomazic and Rose, 1975; Oldstone and Dixon, 1970; Porter *et al.*, 1972). In order to see if neutrophil infiltration occurs at any stage of guinea pig anti-TBM disease, careful histological studies of the kidneys of guinea pigs were performed at frequent intervals following transfer of anti-TBM antiserum, beginning at 4 hr (Van Zwieten *et al.*, 1976). At no stage was there an appreciable increase in neutrophils. Thus, although anti-TBM nephritis is initiated by antibodies, mononuclear cells represent the principal reacting cell. (The possibility that cell-mediated mechanisms participate in the production of lesions is discussed below.)

The mononuclear cells in the infiltrate consist of several cell types, whose proportions appear to vary among different individual guinea pigs and probably at various stages of the disease (although this has not been studied systematically). In the fully developed lesion, mononuclear phagocytes predominate, as shown by several lines of evidence. First, the morphologic appearance of the majority of the cells in histologic preparations is that of monocytes or macrophages. Second, many of the cells possess Fc receptors, as shown by their reactivity in frozen sections with IgG-coated sheep erythrocytes (IgGEA) (Van Zwieten *et al.*, 1976). Third, strain 13 guinea pigs with anti-TBM disease given intravenous injections of carbon on days 10, 11, and 12 were found at sacrifice on day 13 to have 20 to 40% of carbon-containing mononuclear cells in the infiltrate (Bhan, unpublished). Fourth, irradiation of guinea pigs with early established anti-TBM disease, produced by serum transfer, usually failed to inhibit progression of the lesions, presumably because radioresistant macrophages were already present in the infiltrate (Rudofsky and Pollara, 1975). Fifth, as shown by Rudofsky and Pollara (1976), reconstitution of irradiated guinea pigs by bone marrow cells, but not by spleen cells, restores their capacity to develop infiltrates after transfer of anti-TBM serum. It is probable that this results from transfer of monocytes, although this was not directly shown.

The mononuclear phagocytes give rise to many, if not all, of the multinuclear giant cells in the infiltrates of guinea pig anti-TBM disease, as shown by the presence of carbon in some of the giant cells on day 13 following injections of colloidal carbon on days 10, 11, and 12 (Bhan, unpublished). However, as suggested by Rudofsky and Pollara elsewhere in this volume, some giant cells may result from proliferation of tubular cells.

Although mononuclear phagocytes appear to be the most numerous, many of the cells in the infiltrate of guinea pig anti-TBM disease have the appearance of lymphocytes. The nature of these cells has not been thoroughly defined, but some information is available from rosetting studies on tissue sections and from analysis of cells recovered in suspensions from the kidneys. In frozen tissue sections, the IgMEAC reagent reacts principally with B cells, via receptors for activated C3. This reagent failed to adhere to cells in the infiltrate of guinea pigs with anti-TBM disease at day 14 (Van Zwieten *et al.*, 1976). However, this finding does not exclude participation of B cells: first, because the lesions were examined only at one interval; second, because the C3 receptors may have been blocked or lost; and third, because either very immature or highly differentiated B cells lack receptors for C3. Indeed, plasma cells are found in small numbers at various stages of the disease. It is of interest that plasma cells are found not only in actively immunized guinea pigs, but also in recipients of anti-TBM antibodies, apparent evidence of participation in the autoimmune amplification response.

In other studies, cells were obtained from the kidneys of guinea pigs with actively induced anti-TBM disease at day 14 and studied in suspension after Ficoll–Hypaque separation (Bhan, unpublished). In five experiments, each using two or three animals, 10 to 50% of the recovered cells formed rosettes with IgGEA (indicating mononuclear phagocytes). In most cases, fewer than 1% of the cells formed rosettes with IgMEAC. However, in one experiment, 13% of the cells reacted. Eleven to twenty-seven percent formed rosettes with rabbit erythrocytes (indicating T cells). Further evidence for the presence of T cells was provided by the demonstration that delayed-onset reactions could be initiated in syngeneic recipients by local (intradermal) transfer of cells recovered from the kidneys, when given together with the immunizing TBM preparation or, less regularly, with syngeneic guinea pig TBM preparations (Bhan, unpublished).

2.2. Anti-TBM Nephritis in Rats

Sugisaki *et al.* (1973) showed that anti-TBM disease could be induced in Brown Norway (BN) or Lewis × BN rats by injections of homologous kidney preparations in Freund's complete adjuvant, plus an injection of pertussis vaccine. Later, these animals also developed autologous immune complex glomerular disease (Heymann nephritis). Lehman *et al.* (1974) described the production of anti-TBM nephritis without accompanying glomerular disease in BN or Lewis × BN rats by immunization with bovine TBM preparations in Freund's complete adjuvant or pertussis vaccine (the latter adjuvant being more effective). More recently, Robertson *et al.* (1977) reported on the induction of anti-TBM nephritis in BN rats by a single injection of a lyophilized bovine GBM preparation. Anti-GBM nephritis developed at a later stage.

The main features of anti-TBM disease in the rat are similar to those in the guinea pig. Thus, there is linear accumulation of IgG along the TBM, accompanied by severe tubulointerstitial nephritis with basement membrane disruption and tubular cell damage. Anti-TBM antibodies are found in the circulation and in eluates of kidneys. Transfer of anti-TBM antiserum to BN rats leads to linear accumulation of IgG along the TBM and interstitial inflammation. There are, however, certain distinctive aspects of rat anti-TBM disease that warrant comment, notably with respect to the nature of the cellular infiltrate and the lack of susceptibility of certain strains of rats.

2.2.1. *Nature of the Cellular Infiltrate*

Unlike the guinea pig model, rat anti-TBM disease in actively immunized animals is characterized in its earliest stages by neutrophil accumulation and, as seen with the electron microscope, by platelet aggregation in peritubular vessels (Sugisaki *et al.,* 1973). These features appear to coincide with the appearance of C3 and IgG along the TBM. In the guinea pig model, C3 is frequently not demonstrable by immunofluorescence in our experience (see discussion by Rudofsky and Pollara, this volume). Lymphocytes and mononuclear phagocytes appear in appreciable numbers only later, together with multinuclear giant cells. In the fully developed stage, mononuclear cells constitute the bulk of the infiltrate. Plasma cells and eosinophils also may be seen (Robertson *et al.,* 1977). As in the guinea pig model, mononuclear cells can be found invading tubules, sometimes apparently penetrating through gaps in the TBM. Most of the mononuclear cells appear to be lymphocytes, as judged by electron microscopy, but the cells have not been characterized by studies of cell surface markers.

Based on electron microscopic observations, it appears that the multinuclear giant cells develop from the fusion of macrophages (Sugisaki *et al.,* 1973). These cells often are found surrounding disrupted fragments of basement membranes.

2.2.2. *Strain Susceptibility to Anti-TBM Disease in Rats*

Sugisaki *et al.* (1973) reported that sera from BN or L × BN rats with anti-TBM nephritis reacted with the basement membranes of proximal convoluted tubules of several strains of rats, or of man, rabbit, guinea pig, and mouse, as shown by immunofluorescence. Curiously, there was one exception. No reaction was seen with the TBM of Lewis rats. These results were confirmed and extended by Lehman *et al.* (1974), who showed that Wistar Furth and Maxx strains of rats also lack the TBM antigen with which anti-TBM antibodies react. This allotypic specificity is not determined by the major histocompatibility locus (Ag-B). Fisher 344 and Lewis rats are Ag-B identical, yet discordant in the expression of the TBM antigen. The rat strains lacking the TBM antigen are incapable of developing anti-TBM nephritis, although they do produce antibodies.

Two other strains of rats (F344 and August) fail to develop anti-TBM disease, not because they lack the relevant TBM antigen(s), but because they fail to produce anti-TBM antibodies following immunization with bovine TBM and adjuvant (Lehman *et al.*, 1974). Certain other strains of rats [ACI, DA, Buffalo, W/F (*fz*), and Wistar] possess the TBM antigen and produce anti-TBM antibodies, yet fail to develop the disease, presumably because insufficient amounts of antibodies are produced (Lehman *et al.*, 1974). While this explanation may be adequate, it is also possible that the failure of these animals to develop anti-TBM nephritis is due to the lack of essential and as yet undefined secondary pathogenetic mechanisms.

2.3. *Possible Role of Sensitized Cells in Experimental Anti-TBM Nephritis*

A possible pathogenetic role of sensitized cells in anti-TBM nephritis is suggested by the predominance of mononuclear cells in the infiltrate. This finding is not definitive and may represent an unusual response to an antibody-mediated reaction. Obviously, helper T cells may participate in the production of anti-TBM antibodies and in this way indirectly contribute to the disease. This discussion addresses the possibility of direct participation of sensitized lymphocytes in the production of tissue damage in the kidney, as through development of a delayed sensitivity reaction or through cytotoxic effects. The presence of numerous T cells in the infiltrate (see above) provides evidence for the involvement of sensitized cells. Furthermore, as noted above, cells recovered from the kidneys of strain 13 guinea pigs with anti-TBM disease are sometimes capable of mediating delayed-onset reactions following local transfer with syngeneic TBM preparations. The most compelling evidence against a role of cell-mediated immunity in anti-TBM nephritis is the finding that the disease is readily transferable with anti-TBM antibodies. As noted above, the lesions develop slowly and progressively in the recipients. Although this may be explicable by the requirement for autoantibody production by the recipient, it is possible that concomitant cell-mediated reactivity against TBM (or altered TBM) constituents also develops, and is involved in the renal lesions.

Neilson and Phillips (1978) recently have reported in abstract form that peritoneal exudate cells from guinea pigs with anti-TBM nephritis exhibit cytotoxic activity against fetal guinea pig kidney cell monolayers. However, it was not demonstrated that the reactivity was directed against TBM antigens.

The best evidence for a pathogenetic role of sensitized cells in anti-TBM nephritis would be provided by successful transfer of lesions with lymphocytes. Attempts to induce the disease in guinea pigs by systemic transfer of lymphocytes from sensitized donors have been unsuccessful so far (Van Zwieten *et al.,* 1976). Lehman and Wilson (1976) have reported that the injection of lymphocytes from rats that had been immunized with bovine TBM directly into the kidneys of syngeneic recipients results in local destructive lesions. Nevertheless, the lesions were generally mild. The authors concluded that cell-mediated immunity played at best a minor role in anti-TBM disease. Although there is suggestive evidence for the participation of cell-mediated mechanisms in experimental anti-TBM nephritis, further studies are needed to clarify this situation.

3. Human Anti-TBM Disease

Following descriptions of experimental models, evidence has been obtained for the participation of anti-TBM antibodies in human renal diseases, but only in a relatively small number of cases (Andres and McCluskey, 1975; McCluskey and Colvin, 1978). Anti-TBM antibodies have been found in association with anti-GBM antibodies, in some renal allograft recipients, in a few cases of glomerulonephritis presumably mediated by immune complexes, in some cases of drug-induced acute interstitial nephritis, and in isolated disease. The presence of anti-TBM antibodies is indicated by linear TBM staining for IgG and C3. Usually only proximal tubules are involved and in some cases not all proximal tubules are affected. There is usually no difficulty in distinguishing the characteristic linear pattern of IgG accumulation from the type of granular deposits that are seen along the TBM or in the interstitium in many patients with lupus nephritis and certain other disorders (McCluskey and Colvin, 1978). These deposits presumably represent immune complexes. Staining for C3 alone in an interrupted linear pattern is not regarded as evidence for anti-TBM antibodies as this often is found in normal kidneys and is of uncertain significance. Further evidence for anti-TBM antibodies can be provided by the demonstration by indirect immunofluorescence of anti-TBM antibodies in the circulation, or when adequate tissue is available, in eluates of kidney. It is probable that improved techniques, in particular radioimmunoassay procedures, will provide more reliable and more sensitive means for detecting and measuring anti-TBM antibodies.

Based on the findings in experimental models, it seems likely that anti-TBM antibodies in man are often of pathogenetic significance. Attempts to induce tubulointerstitial nephritis in animals by transfer of human serum containing anti-TBM antibodies have not been successful (Border *et al.,* 1974; Ooi *et al.,* 1978). Nevertheless, some evidence that anti-TBM antibodies have injurious properties in man has been provided by the study of Andres *et al.* (1978) in which the nature and severity of the tubulointerstitial damage seen histologically was compared in two groups of patients: (1) those with anti-GBM antibodies with associated anti-TBM antibodies (Group I), and (2) those with anti-GBM antibodies without evidence of associated anti-TBM antibodies (Group II). In Group I there was appreciably greater tubulointerstitial damage than in Group II. There were certain histological features that were present only in the kidneys of Group I, namely multinuclear giant cells in the interstitium, proliferation of proximal convoluted tubular cells, gaps and extensive destruction of the TBM, and proliferation of adventitial cells in juxtamedullary veins. Although these findings provide evidence that anti-TBM antibodies exert damaging effects, they do not exclude the possibility that associated cell-mediated reactivity against TBM constituents also participates. This mechanism is worth considering in view of the observation that lymphocytes from patients with anti-GBM disease have been shown to produce macrophage migration inhibitory factor in the presence of GBM antigens (which were probably contaminated with TBM antigens and certainly contained antigens cross-reactive with the TBM) (Rocklin *et al.*, 1970).

The situation in which anti-TBM antibodies are most likely to be found is in association with anti-GBM disease. In fact, half or more of patients with anti-GBM antibody-mediated glomerular disease have evidence of anti-TBM antibodies (Wilson and Dixon, 1973). In some cases, eluates of renal tissue have been shown to contain antibodies that react both with the GBM and with the TBM (and occasionally with pulmonary basement membranes as well).

Anti-TBM antibodies have also been described in some patients with renal allografts. The first report (Klassen *et al.*, 1973) described two patients with chronic glomerulonephritis who received renal allografts. Both patients developed progressive renal functional impairment following transplantation. The allograft was found to contain linear TBM deposits of IgG. In the one patient whose kidneys had not been removed prior to transplantation, similar staining for IgG was present in the patient's own kidneys, showing that the anti-TBM antibodies, in fact, were autoantibodies. It was suggested that chronic rejection acted as a nonspecific adjuvant, or injured TBM so as to render them immunogenic. In a subsequent study (Wilson *et al.*, 1974), a renal transplant recipient was found to have developed antibodies reactive with the TBM of two successive renal allografts. In this case, antibodies eluted from the transplanted kidney failed to react with the patient's own kidney, although they did react with the TBM of all other human kidneys studied. It was proposed that the patient may have reacted to a TBM alloantigen present in the allograft but not in his own kidney, as has been observed experimentally when kidneys are transplanted from strains of rats possessing the relevant TBM antigen into rats lacking this antigen (Wilson *et al.*, 1974).

It is not known why some patients with immune complex-mediated glomerular disease develop anti-TBM antibodies (which has been observed more often than one would expect on a chance basis) (McCluskey and Colvin, 1978). A plausible explanation is that the damage to the GBM stimulates the production of autoantibodies that are principally directed against cross-reacting antigens in the TBM.

Several drugs or antibiotics (in particular methicillin) are known to be capable of inducing acute tubulointerstitial nephritis in man. There is reason to believe that such renal lesions are caused by hypersensitivity mechanisms rather than by toxic effects (Baldwin *et al.,* 1968; McCluskey and Colvin, 1978). The lesions are characterized by severe interstitial inflammation. It appears that the tubular cell damage is secondary to leukocyte invasion, rather than primary, as would be anticipated if a direct toxic action were responsible. Acute interstitial nephritis is seen in only a minority of patients receiving the drug in question and is not dose related. The patients generally exhibit other manifestations of drug hypersensitivity, including fever, arthralgia, skin rash, and eosinophilia. The underlying immunological mechanisms have not been elucidated and appear to be heterogeneous. No experimental model of drug-induced interstitial nephritis has been described. The concern here is to examine to what extent anti-TBM antibodies are involved in drug-induced interstitial nephritis. Other evidence suggests that IgE antibodies or delayed sensitivity may play a role (Baldwin *et al.,* 1968; McCluskey and Colvin, 1978).

Border *et al.* (1974) described a patient with methicillin-induced interstitial nephritis with anti-TBM antibodies. Immunofluorescent studies revealed linear TBM deposits of IgG, C3, and a methicillin derivative which is assumed to be dimethoxyphenylpenicilloyl. Circulating antibodies reactive with human TBM were demonstrable by indirect immunofluorescence. The antibodies could be removed by incubation with normal TBM preparations, but not by methicillin. The authors postulated that a conjugate of TBM with a methicillin derivative stimulated the formation of anti-TBM antibodies.

Since that report, several other cases of drug-induced interstitial nephritis with anti-TBM antibodies have been described (Ooi *et al.,* 1978; Hyman *et al.,* 1978).

However, it appears that in most patients, evidence of anti-TBM antibodies is lacking. Ooi and colleagues found evidence of anti-TBM antibodies in two of nine patients with drug-induced acute interstitial nephritis. The sera of 10 patients with clinically diagnosed drug-induced interstitial nephritis were examined and anti-TBM antibodies by indirect immunofluorescence were not found (A. B. Collins, N. Hyslop, and R. T. McCluskey, unpublished). It would appear that anti-TBM antibodies do not provide the usual mechanism for renal damage in this condition. However, when they develop, anti-TBM antibodies could intensify and perpetuate the renal damage.

Finally, anti-TBM antibodies have been described in a case of otherwise unexplained interstitial nephritis (Bergstein and Litman, 1975). In addition, one of the patients studied by Andres *et al.* (1978) suffered predominantly from anti-TBM antibody-mediated damage, with only a very slight anti-GBM component.

In summary, it is clear that although anti-TBM antibodies do occur in man, they are quite rare. Even allowing for the possibility that in some instances anti-TBM disease might become burned out, leaving only nonspecific histologic findings without linear TBM deposits of IgG, it seems likely that anti-TBM antibodies account for only a small fraction of cases of unexplained interstitial nephritis.

4. Summary

Experimental studies have demonstrated that a form of tubulointerstitial nephritis in guinea pigs and rats is mediated by antibodies to the TBM. The anti-TBM response can be elicited with immunization in heterologous (guinea pig, rat) or isologous (rat) TBM preparations. Of interest, the autoantibody response against TBM antigens can also be evoked by passive transfer of anti-TBM antibodies, as shown in strain 13 guinea pigs, a phenomenon termed *autoimmune amplification.* This process may be an important mechanism for the intensification and perpetuation of certain other autoimmune diseases.

The anti-TBM immune response has been shown to be controlled by a gene(s) found to be linked to but separate from the Ia genes in strain 13 and strain 2 guinea pigs. The expression of the TBM antigen(s) is also under genetic control. Some rat strains lack this antigen and do not develop anti-TBM nephritis.

Although apparently initiated by antibodies, the lesions in the guinea pig are characterized by a predominantly mononuclear cell infiltrate, without appreciable neutrophil participations. In the rat, neutrophils are found in early lesions. The infiltrating cells are chiefly mononuclear phagocytes, but numerous lymphocytes, including many T cells, are present. The importance of cell-mediated hypersensitivity in the renal damage has not been established.

In man, anti-TBM antibodies have been found in a few cases of renal disease, including in association with anti-GBM antibodies, renal allografts, immune complex-mediated glomerulonephritis, drug-induced interstitial nephritis, and idiopathic interstitial nephritis.

References

Andres, G. A., and McCluskey, R. T., 1975, Tubular and interstitial renal disease due to immunologic mechanisms, *Kidney Int.* **7:**211.

Andres, G., Brentjens, J., Kohli, R., Anthone, R., Anthone, S., Baliah, T., Montes, M., Mookerjee, B. K., Prezyna, A., Sepulveda, M., Venuto, R., and Elwood, C., 1978, Histology of human tubulo-interstitial nephritis associated with antibodies to renal basement membranes, *Kidney Int.* **13:**480.

Baldwin, D. S., Levine, B. B., McCluskey, R. T., and Gallo, G. R., 1968, Renal failure and interstitial nephritis due to penicillin and methicillin, *N. Engl. J. Med.* **279:**1245.

Benacerraf, B., and McDevitt, H. O., 1972, Histocompatibility linked immune response genes, *Science* **175:**273.

Bergstein, J. M., and Litman, N., 1975, Interstitial nephritis with antitubular basement membrane antibody, *N. Engl. J. Med.* **292:**875.

Bloch, K. H., Kourilsky, F. M., Ovary, Z., and Benacerraf, B., 1963, Properties of guinea pigs 7S antibodies. III. Identification of antibodies involved in complement fixation and hemolysis, *J. Exp. Med.* **117:**965.

Border, W. A., Lehman, D. H., Egan, J. D., Sass, H. J., Glode, J. E., and Wilson, C. B., 1974, Antitubular basement membrane antibodies in methicillin-associated interstitial nephritis, *N. Engl. J. Med.* **291:**381.

Hall, C. L., Colvin, R. B., Carey, K., and McCluskey, R. T., 1977, Passive transfer of autoimmune disease with isologous IgG_1 and IgG_2 antibodies to the tubular basement membrane in strain XIII guinea pigs, *J. Exp. Med.* **146:**1246.

Hyman, L. R., Colvin, R. B., and Steinberg, A. D., 1976a, Immunopathogenesis of autoimmune tubulointerstitial nephritis. I. Demonstration of differential susceptibility in strain II and strain XIII guinea pigs, *J. Immunol.* **116:**327.

Hyman, L. R., Steinberg, A. D., Colvin, R. B., and Bernard, E. F., 1976b, Immunopathogenesis of autoimmune tubulointerstitial nephritis. II. Role of an immune response gene linked to the major histocompatibility locus, *J. Immunol.* **117:**1894.

Hyman, L. R., Ballow, M., and Knieser, M. R., 1978, Diphenylhydantoin interstitial nephritis: Roles of cellular and humoral immunologic injury, *J. Pediatr.* **92:**915.

Klassen, J., Kano, K., Milgrom, F., Menno, A. B., Anthone, S., Anthone, R., Sepulveda, M., Elwood, C. M., and Andres, G. A., 1973, Tubular lesions produced by autoantibodies to tubular basement membrane in human renal allografts, *Int. Arch. Allergy Appl. Immunol.* **45:**675.

Lange, K., Wachstein, M., and McPherson, E. St., 1961, Immunological mechanism of transmission of experimental glomerulonephritis in parabiotic rats, *Proc. Soc. Exp. Biol. Med.* **106:**13.

Lehman, D. H., and Wilson, C. B., 1976, Role of sensitized cells in antitubular basement membrane interstitial nephritis, *Int. Arch. Allergy Appl. Immunol.* **51:**168.

Lehman, D. H., Wilson, C. B., and Dixon, F. J., 1974, Interstitial nephritis in rats immunized with heterologous tubular basement membrane, *Kidney Int.* **5:**187.

Lockwood, C. M., Rees, A. J., Pearson, T. A., Evans, D. J., Peters, D. R., and Wilson, C. B., 1976, Immunosuppression and plasma-exchange in the treatment of Goodpasture's syndrome, *Lancet* **1:**711.

McCluskey, R. T., and Colvin, R. B., 1978, Immunological aspects of renal tubular and interstitial diseases, *Annu. Rev. Med.* **29:**191.

Milgrom, F., and Dubiski, S., 1957, Mecanisme de l'autoimmunisation au cours des anemies hemolytique, *Vox Sang.* **27:**11.

Mohn, J. R., Lambert, R. M., Bowman, H. S. and Brason, F. W., 1965, Experimental production in man of autoantibodies with Rh specificity, *Ann. N.Y. Acad. Sci.* **124:**477.

Neilson, E. G., and Phillips, S. M., 1978, Cell-mediated lymphocytotoxicity in interstitial nephritis: *In vitro* and *in vivo* observations, *Kidney Int.* (abstract).

Oldstone, M. B. A., and Dixon, F. J., 1970, Pathogenesis of chronic disease associated with persistent lymphocytic choriomeningitis viral infection. II. Relationship of the anti-lymphocytic choriomeningitis immune response to tissue injury in chronic lymphocytic choriomeningitis disease, *J. Exp. Med.* **131:**1.

Ooi, B. S., Ooi, Y. M., Mohini, R., and Pollak, V. E., 1978, Humoral mechanisms in drug induced acute interstitial nephritis, *Clin. Immunol. Immunopathol.* **10:**330.

Porter, D. D., Larsen, A. E., and Porter, H. G., 1972, The pathogenesis of Aleutian disease of mink. II. Enhancement of tissue lesions following the administration of a killed virus vaccine or passive antibody, *J. Immunol.* **109:**1.

Robertson, J. L., Hill, G. S., and Rowlands, D. T., 1977, Tubulointerstitial nephritis and glomerulonephritis in Brown Norway rats immunized with heterologous glomerular basement membrane, *Am. J. Pathol.* **88:**53.

Rocklin, R. E., Lewis, E. J., and David, J. R., 1970, *In vivo* evidence for cellular hypersensitivity to glomerular basement membrane antigens in human glomerulonephritis, *N. Engl. J. Med.* **283**:497.

Rudofsky, U. H., and Pollara, B., 1975, Studies on the pathogenesis of experimental autoimmune renal tubulointerstitial disease in guinea pigs. I. Inhibition of tissue injury in leukocyte-depleted passive transfer recipients, *Clin. Immunol. Immunopathol.* **4**:425.

Rudofsky, U. H., and Pollara, B., 1976, Studies on the pathogenesis of experimental autoimmune renal tubulointerstitial disease in guinea pigs. II. Passive transfer of renal lesions to leukocyte-depleted recipients by anti-tubular basement membrane autoantibodies and non-immune bone marrow cells, *Clin. Immunol. Immunopathol.* **6**:107.

Steblay, R. W., and Rudofsky, U. H., 1973, Transfer of experimental autoimmune renal cortical tubular and interstitial disease in guinea pigs by serum, *Science* **180**:966.

Sugisaki, T., Klassen, J., Milgrom, F., Andres, G. A., and McCluskey, R. T., 1973, Immunopathologic study of an autoimmune tubular and interstitial renal disease in Brown Norway rats, *Lab. Invest.* **28**:658.

Tomazic, V., and Rose, N. R., 1975, Autoimmune murine thyroiditis. VII. Induction of the thyroid lesions by passive transfer of serum, *Clin. Immunol. Immunopathol.* **4**:511.

Unanue, E. R., and Dixon, F. J., 1965, Experimental glomerulonephritis: VI. The autologous phase of nephrotoxic serum nephritis, *J. Exp. Med.* **121**:715.

Van Zwieten, M. J., Bhan, A. K., McCluskey, R. T., and Collins, A. B., 1976, Studies on the pathogenesis of experimental anti-tubular basement membrane nephritis in the guinea pig, *Am. J. Pathol.* **83**:531.

Vuagnat, P., 1974, Further studies on the biological properties of guinea pigs IgG_1 antibodies: Antilymphocytic antibodies, *Immunology* **27**:351.

Wilson, C. B., and Dixon, F. J., 1973, Anti-glomerular basement membrane antibody-induced glomerulonephritis, *Kidney Int.* **3**:74.

Wilson, C. B., Lehman, D. H., McCoy, R. C., Gunnels, J. C., Jr., and Stickel D. L., 1974, Antitubular basement membrane antibodies after renal transplantation, *Transplantation* **18**:447.

21

Autoimmunity to Tamm–Horsfall Protein

John R. Hoyer, J. Friedman, and Marcel W. Seiler

1. Immune Complex-Mediated Tubulointerstitial Nephritis

Although interstitial inflammation and fibrosis, and tubular damage are prominent pathologic features in a variety of renal diseases, the pathogenesis of these lesions has received much less attention than have mechanisms of glomerular injury. Recently, clinical and experimental studies have shown that, in addition to well-established roles of immunologic mechanisms in glomerulonephritis, such immune mechanisms can cause tubulointerstitial nephritis also. Primary antibody-mediated tubular and interstitial lesions may be caused by either antibodies to tubular basement membranes (TBM) or by immune complexes. Anti-TBM-mediated nephritis is characterized by a smooth linear pattern of immunoglobulin fixed along the TBM, and the pathogenesis of these lesions has been discussed in detail (McCluskey and Colvin, 1978). In this discussion, features of tubulointerstitial nephritis mediated by immune complexes and having a granular staining pattern will be presented with emphasis on the pathogenesis of renal lesions produced by antibodies to Tamm–Horsfall protein (TH), a urinary glycoprotein of renal origin.

Evidence for immune complex-mediated tubulointerstitial nephritis in man has been derived primarily from immunofluorescent studies of renal tissue and from demonstration by indirect immunofluorescence of antibodies to tubular epithelium in serum of such patients. Granular deposits of IgG

John R. Hoyer, J. Friedman, and Marcel W. Seiler · Departments of Pediatrics and Pathology, Harvard Medical School, Boston, Massachusetts 02155. Supported by grants from the National Institutes of Health (AM 27122) and the American Heart Association. Dr. Hoyer was an Established Investigator of the American Heart Association. Dr. Friedman was a Massachusetts Heart Association Fellow.

and C3 have been identified along proximal and/or distal TBM in human diseases, including many patients with systemic lupus erythematosus (SLE) (Brentjens *et al.*, 1975; Lehman *et al.*, 1975) and also patients with Sjögren's syndrome (Winer *et al.*, 1977) and in patients having renal allografts (Andres *et al.*, 1970). DNA has been demonstrated to be present in these deposits in some patients with SLE (Brentjens *et al.*, 1975). However, in most cases of human tubulointerstitial nephritis, the antigenic component of these presumed immune complexes has not been identified. Autoantibodies reacting with distal tubular epithelium have been demonstrated in human diseases, particularly in those considered to be of immune etiology. The studies have included patients with renal tubular acidosis (Pasternack and Linder, 1970; Ford, 1973; Chanarin *et al.*, 1974).

Granular deposits of IgG and C3 also have been identified along proximal and/or distal TBM in rabbits and in rats immunized with homologous renal tissue (Unanue *et al.*, 1967; Klassen *et al.*, 1971a,b, 1977), in rabbits with chronic serum sickness (Brentjens *et al.*, 1974), in renal allografts (Klassen and Milgrom, 1969), and in rats immunized with TH (Hoyer, 1980). The serum of such rats and rabbits has been shown to contain autoantibodies to proximal and/or distal tubular epithelium. The antigens involved in most of the above instances have not been defined. TH is readily isolated from urine, and is the best characterized of the antigens involved in models of immune complex-mediated tubulointerstitial nephritis.

2. *TH Protein*

TH protein was isolated nearly three decades ago during studies of inhibitors of viral hemagglutination in human urine (Tamm and Horsfall, 1950). TH is the primary constituent of urinary casts (McQueen, 1962). Daily TH urinary excretion by normal adults is approximately 50 mg (McKenzie *et al.*, 1964). Remarkable changes in the physical state of TH are caused by variations in the ranges of ionic environment observed in urine or within the kidney. Aggregation of TH leading to gel formation is caused by increasing concentrations of TH, electrolytes, or hydrogen ions (McQueen and Engel, 1966). Formation of hyaline casts is a direct result of the aggregation of urinary TH. TH has been identified immunochemically in urine produced by isolated perfused kidneys (Cornelius *et al.*, 1965) and in hamster kidney cells grown in culture (Dunstan *et al.*, 1974).

2.1. *Morphologic Localization*

Immunofluorescent studies indicate that TH is localized exclusively in renal tissue. These studies have demonstrated TH in the initial segment of the distal nephron, the thick ascending limb of the loop of Henle (ALH), and immediately beyond the macula densa (McKenzie and McQueen, 1969; Schenk *et al.*, 1971; Hoyer *et al.*, 1974). Recent ultrastructural studies of rat kidney (Allen and Tisher, 1976; Kaissling *et al.*, 1977) have shown that the morphologic transition from cells with features characteristic of the ALH to distal convoluted tubular cells occurs beyond, rather than at the macula densa, the traditionally defined transition point. Thus, the renal localization of TH corresponds precisely to the morphologic limits of the ALH. Ultrastructural studies of the cellular distribution of TH in the normal rat kidney using peroxidase-labeled antibodies to TH have been completed recently (Hoyer *et al.*, 1979). TH was demonstrated by immunoelectron microscopy along the basal, lateral, and luminal surface membranes of ALH cells, as well as in the Golgi apparatus and in the interstitial spaces between basal membrane infolding of ALH cells. It is noteworthy that TH is not present on the basal and lateral membranes of macula densa cells which are negative for TH by immunofluorescence. The additional presence of TH on the luminal surface membranes of the nephron segments distal to the ALH probably reflects adsorption related to urinary excretion of TH. In contrast, the presence of TH with its unusual physical properties of electrolyte-dependent reversible aggregation on all of the extensive surface membranes of ALH cells may influence the permeability characteristics of the ALH which allow the net movement of ions in excess of water. The factors favoring such a potential functional role in the "diluting segment" (Burg, 1976) for TH have been discussed recently (Hoyer and Seiler, 1979). Surface localization also exposes TH to plasma proteins reaching the peritubular interstitial space of ALH cells. In the juxtaglomerular region, TH on ALH surface membranes also has the potential for interacting with macromolecules transported to the extraglomerular portion of the glomerular mesangial pathway. Already, iron dextran particles in normal mice (Leiper *et al.*, 1977), immunoglobulin deposits in diabetic mice (Mauer *et al.*, 1976) and in rats with anti-GBM nephritis (Hoyer and Seiler, 1979) have been shown to extend from the glomerular mesangium to the base of ALH cells.

2.2 TH in Human Disease

Several immunologic responses to TH have been reported. These include antibodies to TH in the serum of patients with pyelonephritis (Hanson *et al.*, 1976), abnormal cellular immunity to TH in patients with liver disease and in patients with distal renal tubular acidosis (Cochrane *et al.*, 1976). Strong evidence defining the role of immunologic responses to TH in the pathogenesis of tubulointerstitial nephritis in man is not currently available.

Extratubular deposits of TH in several human tubulointerstitial diseases including medullary cystic disease, obstructive uropathy with vesicoureteral reflux, and chronic pyelonephritis have been demonstrated in recent reports (Resnick *et al.*, 1978; Zager *et al.*, 1978; Solez and Heptinstall, 1978). In this laboratory's immunofluorescent studies, these TH deposits were shown to be identical in distribution, size, shape, and fine detail with the interstitial PAS-positive deposits seen by light microscopy. These TH deposits appear to result from the following pathogenetic sequence. There is disruption of tubular integrity causing release of urine into the interstitial space. As water is osmotically removed, TH in urine becomes less soluble, and is converted into extratubular aggregates. Once formed, the ionic environment in the interstitium greatly favors aggregation of TH and therefore prolonged persistence of these deposits. Whether the inflammatory infiltrates which were occasionally seen to surround interstitial TH deposits represent a specific response to TH remains uncertain. However, in experimental obstructive uropathy in pigs (reflux nephropathy), interstitial deposits of TH, similar to those seen in human renal disease, are present (Cotran, 1979) and autoantibodies to TH have been described (Hodson *et al.*, 1975).

3. Experimental Anti-TH Antibody-Mediated Tubulointerstitial Nephritis in Rats

The renal lesions produced in rats actively and passively immunized to TH (Hoyer, 1980; Seiler and Hoyer, 1981; Friedman, *et al.*, 1982) have been studied in order to better define the pathogenetic potential for TH suggested by the above studies. Rats were immunized actively by 1–8 monthly intradermal injections of rat TH along with Freund's complete adjuvant and pertussis vaccine. Characteristic granular and nodular IgG, C3, and TH deposits at the base of ALH cells and selective infiltration of leukocytes around this distal nephron segment were present in the kidneys of these rats, whereas there were no tubular deposits in rats injected with adjuvants only. The antigenic components of these deposits, TH, were readily demonstrated (Fig. 1) without prior elution of sections. Although the most

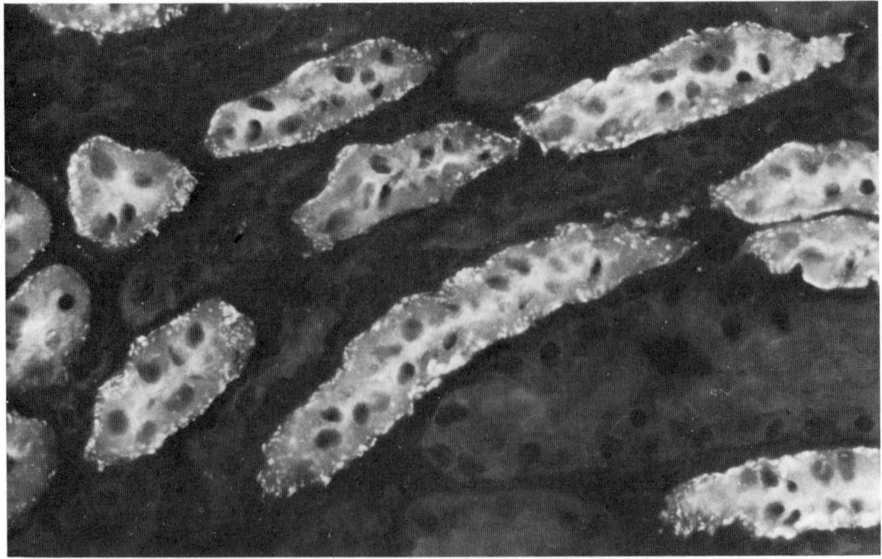

Figure 1. Section of kidney from rat immunized with TH and stained with a fluorescein-labeled antiserum to TH. Numerous granular deposits of TH are present along the TBM of ALH cells as well as staining of ALH cells.

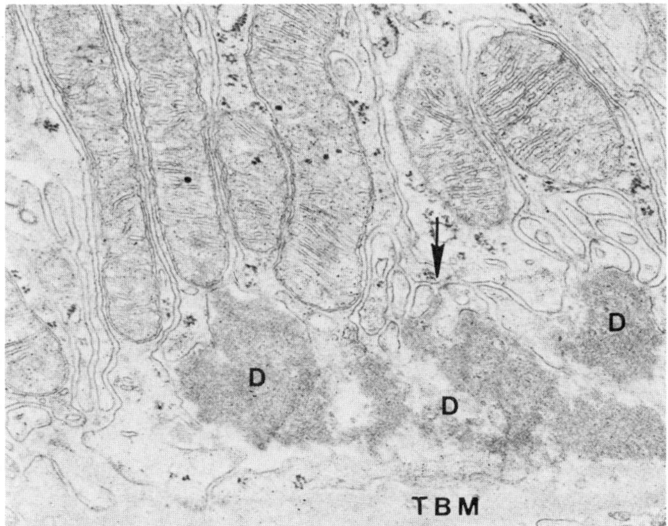

Figure 2. Electron micrograph of kidney of rat immunized with TH. Electron-dense deposits (D) are present between the TBM and the surface membranes of an ALH cell. These deposits displace this cell from the TBM and extend into the space between tubular cell membranes (arrow).

numerous and largest deposits most frequently were seen after several monthly injections, there was no direct correlation between number of injections and quantity of deposits. IgG deposits were mildly decreased in kidneys studied more than 1 month after the last TH injection but persisted for prolonged periods. These deposits were detected as late as 12 months after the last TH injection. The largest deposits were concentrated in the outer stripe of the outer medulla and in the inner cortex. In severe lesions, basal IgG, C3, and TH deposits were present along the entire course of the ALH. In the juxtaglomerular region, ALH cells opposite and beyond the macula densa had basal immune deposits, while macula densa cells lacked these deposits. Ultrastructural analysis of these renal lesions showed that the frequency, size, and distribution of electron-dense deposits at the base of ALH cells closely correlated with immune deposits of IgG and C3 (Seiler and Hoyer, 1981). The earliest deposits were subepithelial and present in the extracellular space between basal cell membrane infoldings and the TBM. In more advanced lesions, deposits were larger and confluent (Fig. 2). These deposits extended between tubular cell membranes and displaced tubular cells and also were present within adjacent TBM. PAS-positive deposits at the base of ALH cells were seen by light microscopy in these advanced lesions. The pathogenetic role of IgG antibodies to TH in this model was supported by the direct correlation shown between serum anti-TH titers determined by indirect immunofluorescence and the extent of immune deposits and histologic changes in kidneys of these rats (Hoyer, 1980). These serum antibodies that fixed to ALH cells in sections of normal kidney were demonstrated by absorption studies using highly purified TH to be antibodies to TH.

4. Pathogenesis of in Situ Immune Complex Formation

A critical question in immune complex-mediated injury is the mechanism of tissue deposition. Although the antigens involved in most of the instances of tubulointerstitial nephritis cited above have not been identified, recent evidence supports the concept that many of these immune complexes are formed *in situ* by the combination of circulating antibody and an antigenic component already present within renal tissue by a process similar to that which occurs in thyroiditis (Clagtet *et al.*, 1974) and in orchitis (Bigazzi *et al.*, 1976). The mechanism of *in situ* immune complex formation in the TH model diagrammatically shown in Fig. 3 is consistent with several experimental observations. As noted above, the electron-dense deposits in this model have an appearance similar to other immune complexes. These deposits are subepithelial and located between TBM and infoldings of the cell surface membranes. Immunoglobulin molecules must be able to pass through TBM prior to complex formation. This is the case, since ultrastructural tracer studies using ferritin (molecular weight 500,000) and catalase (molecular weight 240,000) have shown that peritubular capillaries are much less restrictive to the movement of macromolecules than the glomerular capillary wall (Venkatachalam and Karnovsky, 1972). Considerable diffusion of IgG antibodies across TBM will occur without prior injury. The absence of IgG deposits on the luminal surface of ALH cells and in glomeruli indicates that these immune complexes are not the consequence of alternative mechanisms of anti-TH antibodies passing into the urine prior to complex formation or the deposition of circulating immune complexes. Furthermore, similar immune complexes of IgG and TH at the base of ALH cells are formed in rats given heterologous antisera to TH (Friedman *et al.*, 1982. Accessibility of tubular antigens to circulating antibodies is a crucial requirement for *in situ* complex formation to be the primary step in initiating tubular injury. It is known that many tissue-specific autoantibodies directed against intracellular antigens do not have access and, therefore, do not cause immune complex formation and injury. The distribution of immunofluorescent staining within tubules suggested that some of the tubular antigens involved in the above models were cytoplasmic. Therefore, it was postulated that these antigens must "leak out" of the cells (Klassen *et al.*, 1971a) in order to participate in local complex formation. Although such a process of release into the extravascular space may contribute to complex formation, recent ultrastructural immunoperoxidase studies suggest that such a mechanism of exit is not essential. Ultrastructural localization has shown that antigens may be present on surface membranes rather than in the cytoplasm of the normal ALH (Hoyer *et al.*, 1979) and proximal tubule (Van Damme *et al.*, 1978) and only appear to be cytoplasmic because of the extensive infoldings of cell

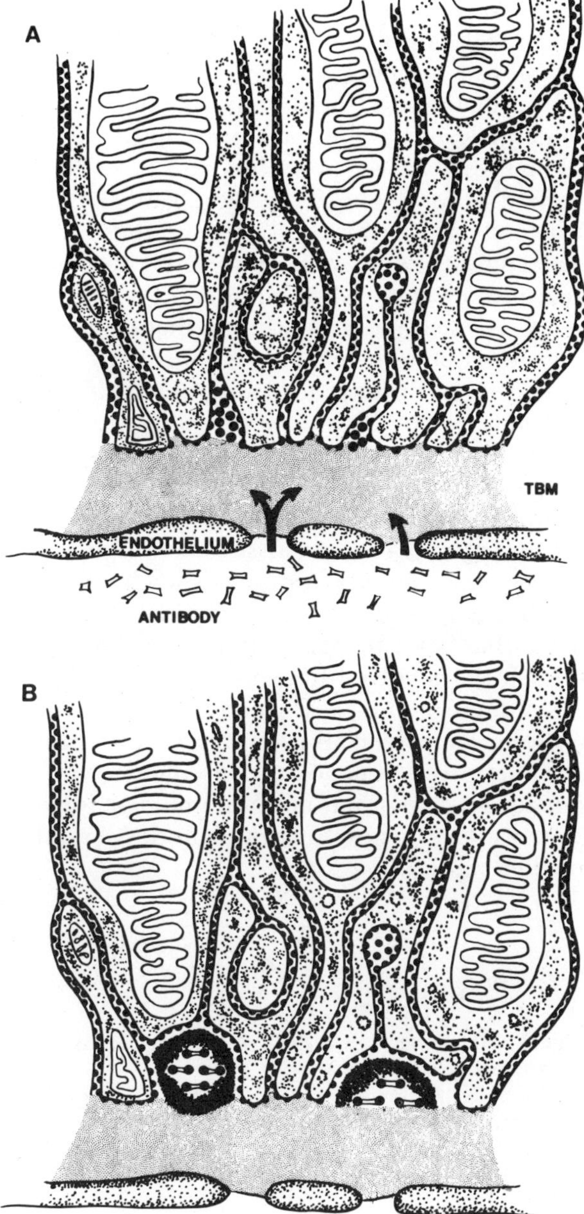

Figure 3. Diagrammatic representation of the mechanism of *in situ* formation of immune complexes involving a tubular antigen. The normal distribution of TH, a surface membrane glycoprotein of ALH cells, is shown by the solid half-circles along surface membranes and by solid circles between these membranes. (A) Circulating IgG antibodies to TH diffuse through TBM (arrows) prior to complex formation. (B) Immune complexes formed by the combination of IgG antibodies and TH in the subepithelial space displace the tubular cell membranes from the TBM and have a discrete electron-dense appearance. (Combination of anti-TH antibodies with surface membrane TH molecules has not been illustrated in this simplified design.) (Reprinted from Seiler and Hoyer, 1981, with permission of the publisher.)

surface membranes. These surface antigens, such as TH, are thus normally accessible to antibody reaching the extravascular space. The regular presence of TH in these deposits probably reflects the large quantities of TH, a surface membrane glycoprotein with rapid turnover (Grant and Neuberger, 1973), that are available for combining with antibodies that have diffused across the TBM. Double label studies showing that IgG and TH are present within the same deposits provide additional evidence that these deposits are immune complexes. Support for the pathogenetic role of IgG antibodies to TH in the formation of these immune deposits was also given by analysis of sequential studies in rats given heterologous antisera to TH. The basal tubular deposits of rabbit IgG and of rat TH were maximal during the first week after intravenous injection. Coincident with the disappearance of anti-TH antibodies from the serum of these rats, these deposits decreased and were almost gone by 28 days after injection (Friedman, *et al.*, 1982). The clearance of basal ALH immune deposits formed after injection of antisera to TH is much more rapid than that of glomerular immune deposits formed after injection of heterologous antisera to proximal tubular antigens (Feenstra *et al.*, 1975; Van Es *et al.*, 1977). Although the mechanism of rapid clearance of immune complexes from the interstitial space has not been defined, these observations have important implications. The relatively infrequent presence of basal tubular deposits in human renal biopsies could be related to rapid clearance of immune complexes from the interstitial space. It may be necessary to obtain renal tissue early in the course of human tubulointerstitial diseases in order to demonstrate such immune deposits.

Since primary tubulointerstitial nephritis mediated by immune complexes has been recognized only recently, many aspects of the pathogenetic mechanism involved have not yet been clarified. These include the kinetics of immune complex formation and clearance, determinants of antibody responses involved, the nature of the antigens, the role of cell-mediated immunity, the functional consequences of the lesions produced, and the relationships to other, nonimmunologic forms of renal injury and to immune glomerulonephritis. Improved understanding of these aspects is a goal for further studies.

References

Allen, F., and Tisher, C. C., 1976, Morphology of the ascending thick limb of the loop of Henle, *Kidney Int.* **9:**8.

Andres, G. A., Accinni, L., Hsu, K. C., Penn, I., Porter, K. A., Randall, J. M., Seegal, B. C., and Starzl, T. E., 1970, Human renal transplants. III. Immunopathologic studies, *Lab. Invest.* **22:**588.

Bigazzi, P. E., Kosuda, L. L., Hsu, K. C., and Andres, G. A., 1976, Immune complex orchitis in vasectomized rabbits, *J. Exp. Med.* **143:**382.

Brentjens, J. R., O'Connell, D. W., Pawlowski, I. B., and Andres, G. A., 1974, Extraglomerular lesions associated with deposition of circulating antigen–antibody complexes in kidneys of rabbits with chronic serum sickness, *Clin. Immunol. Immunopathol.***3:**112.

Brentjens, J. R., Sepulveda, M., Baliah, T., Bentzel, C., Erlanger, B. F., Elwood, C., Montes, M., Hsu, K. C., and Andres, G. A., 1975, Interstitial immune complex nephritis in patients with systemic lupus erythematosus, *Kidney Int.* **7:**342.

Burg, M. B., 1976, Tubular chloride transport and the mode of action of some diuretics, *Kidney Int.* **9:**189.

Chanarin, I., Loewi, G., Tavill, A. S., Swain, C. P., and Tidmarsh, E., 1974, Defect of renal tubular acidification with antibody to loop of Henle, *Lancet* **2:**317.

Clagett, J. A., Wilson, C. B., and Weigle, W. O., 1974, Interstitial immune complex thyroiditis in mice: The role of autoantibody to thyroglobulin, *J. Exp. Med.* **140:**1439.

Cochrane, A. M. G., Tsantoulos, D. C., Moussouros, A., McFarlane, I. G., Eddleston, A. L. W. F., and Williams, R., 1976, Lymphocyte cytotoxicity for kidney cells in renal tubular acidosis of autoimmune liver disease, *Br. Med. J.* **2:**276.

Cornelius, C. E., Min, A. S., and Rosenfeld, S., 1965, Ruminant urolithiasis. VII. Studies on the origin of Tamm–Horsfall urinary mucoprotein and its presence in ovine calculous matrix, *Invest. Urol.* **2:**453.

Cotran, R. S., and Hodson, C. J., 1979, Extratubular localization of Tamm–Horsfall protein in experimental reflux nephropathy in the pig, in: *Reflux Nephropathy* (Hodson, C. J., and Kinaid-Smith, P., eds.) Masson, New York, p. 213.

Dunstan, D. R., Grant, A. M. S., Marshall, R. D., and Neuberger, A., 1974, A protein immunologically similar to Tamm–Horsfall glycoprotein produced by cultured baby hamster kidney cells, *Proc. R. Soc. London Ser. B* **186:**297.

Feenstra, K., Lee, R. V. D., Greben, H. A., Arends, A., and Hoedemaeker, P. J., 1975, Experimental glomerulonephritis in the rat induced by antibodies directed against tubular antigens. I. The natural history: A histologic and immunohistologic study at the light microscopic and ultrastructural level, *Lab. Invest.* **32:**235.

Ford, P. M., 1973, Naturally occurring human antibody to loops of Henle, *Clin. Exp. Immunol.* **14:**569.

Friedman, J., Hoyer, J. R., and Seiler, M. W., 1982, Formation and clearance of tubulointerstitial immune complexes in kidneys of rats immunized with heterologous antisera to Tamm–Horsfall protein, *Kidney Int.* **21:**575.

Grant, A. M. S., and Neuberger, A., 1973, The turnover rate of rabbit urinary Tamm–Horsfall glycoprotein, *Biochem. J.* **136:**659.

Hanson, L. A., Fasth, A., and Jodal, U., 1976, Auto-antibodies to Tamm–Horsfall protein, a tool for diagnosing the level of urinary infections, *Lancet* **1:**226.

Hodson, J., Maling, T. M. J., McManomon, P. J., and Lewis, M. G., 1975, Reflux nephropathy, *Kidney Int.* **8:**550.

Hoyer, J. R., 1980, Tubulointerstitial immune nephritis in rats immunized with Tamm–Horsfall protein, *Kidney Int.* **17:**284.

Hoyer, J. R., and Seiler, M. W., 1979, Pathophysiology of Tamm–Horsfall protein, *Kidney Int.* **16:**279.

Hoyer, J. R., Sisson, S., Vernier, R. L., 1979, Tamm–Horsfall glycoprotein; ultrastructural immunoperoxidase localization in rat kidney, *Lab. Invest* **41:**168.

Hoyer, J. R., Resnick, J. S., Michael, A. F., and Vernier, R. L., 1974, Ontogeny of Tamm–Horsfall urinary glycoprotein, *Lab. Invest.* **30:**757.

Kaissling, B., Peter, S., and Kriz, W., 1977, Transition of the thick ascending limb of Henle's loop into the distal convoluted tubule in the nephron of the rat kidney, *Cell Tissue Res.* **182:**111.

Klassen, J., and Milgrom, F., 1969, Autoimmune concomitants of renal allografts, *Transplant Proc.* **1:**605.

Klassen, J., McCluskey, R. T., and Milgrom, F., 1971a, Nonglomerular renal disease produced in rabbits by immunization with homologous kidney, *Am. J. Pathol.* **63:**333.

Klassen, J., Sugisaki, T., Milgrom, F., and McCluskey, R. T., 1971b, Studies on multiple renal lesions in Heymann nephritis, *Lab. Invest.* **25:**577.

Klassen, J., Milgrom, F. M., and McCluskey, R. T., 1977, Studies of the antigens involved in an immunologic renal tubular lesion in rabbits, *Am. J. Pathol.* **88:**135.

Lehman, D. H., Wilson, C. B., and Dixon, F. J., 1975, Extraglomerular immune deposits in human nephritis, *Am. J. Med.* **58:**765.

Leiper, J. M., Thompson, D., and MacDonald, M. K., 1977, Uptake and transport of imposil by the glomerular mesangium in the mouse, *Lab. Invest.* **37:**526.

McCluskey, R. T., and Colvin, R. B., 1978, Immunological aspects of renal tubular and interstitial diseases, *Annu. Rev. Med.* **29:**191.

McKenzie, J. K., and McQueen, E. G., 1969, Immunofluorescent localization of Tamm–Horsfall mucoprotein in human kideny, *J. Clin. Pathol.* **22:**334.

McKenzie, J. K., Patel, R., and McQueen, E. G., 1964, The excretion rate of Tamm–Horsfall urinary mucoprotein in normals and in patients with renal disease, *Aust. Ann. Med.* **13:**32.

McQueen, E. G., 1962, The nature of urinary casts, *J. Clin. Pathol.* **15:**367.

McQueen, E. G., and Engel, G. B., 1966, Factors determining the aggregation of urinary mucoprotein, *J. Clin. Pathol.* **19:**392.

Mauer, S. M., Steffes, M. W., Michael, A. F., and Brown, D. M., 1976, Studies of diabetic nephropathy in animals and man, *Diabetes* **25:**850.

Pasternack, A., and Linder, E., 1970, Renal tubular acidosis: An immunopathologic study on four patients, *Clin. Exp. Immunol.* **7:**115.

Resnick, J. S., Sisson, S., and Vernier, R. L., 1978, Tamm–Horsfall protein: Abnormal localization in renal disease, *Lab. Invest.* **38:**550.

Schenk, E. A., Schwartz, R. H., and Lewis, R. A., 1971, Tamm–Horsfall mucoprotein. I. Localization in the kidney, *Lab. Invest.* **25:**92.

Seiler, M. W., and Hoyer, J. R., 1981, Ultrastructural studies of tubulointerstitial immune complex nephritis in rats immunized with Tamm–Horsfall protein, *Lab. Invest.* **45:**321.

Solez, K., and Heptinstall, R. H., 1978, Intrarenal urinary extravasation with formation of venous polyps containing Tamm–Horsfall protein, *J. Urol.* **119:**180.

Tamm, I., Horsfall, F. L., Jr., 1950, Characterization and separation of an inhibitor of viral hemagglutination present in urine, *Proc. Soc. Exp. Biol. Med.* **74:**108.

Unanue, E. R., Dixon, F. J., and Feldman, J. D., 1967, Experimental allergic glomerulonephritis induced in the rabbit with homologous renal antigens, *J. Exp. Med.* **125:**163.

Van Damme, B. J. C., Fleuren, G. J., Bakker, W. W., Vernier, R. L., and Hoedemaeker, P. J., 1978, Experimental glomerulonephritis in the rat induced by antibodies directed against tubular antigens. V. Fixed glomerular antigens in the pathogenesis of heterologous immune complex glomerulonephritis, *Lab. Invest.* **38:**502.

Van Es, L. A., Blok, A. P. R., Schoenfeld, L., and Glassock, R. J., 1977, Chronic nephritis induced by antibodies reacting with glomerular bound immune complexes, *Kidney Int.* **11:**106.

Venkatachalam, M. A., and Karnovsky, M. J., 1972, Extravascular protein in the kidney: An ultrastructural study of its relation to renal peritubular capillary permeability using protein tracers, *Lab. Invest.* **27:**435.

Winer, R. L., Cohen, A. H., Sawhney, A. S., and Gorman, J. T., 1977, Sjögren's syndrome with immune complex tubulointerstitial renal disease, *Clin. Immunol. Immunopathol.* **8:**494.

Zager, R. A., Cotran, R. S., and Hoyer, J. R., 1978, Pathologic localization of Tamm–Horsfall protein in interstitial deposits in renal disease, *Lab. Invest.* **38:**52.

22

Renal Antigens in Experimental Immune Complex Glomerulonephritis

P. J. Hoedemaeker, J. J. Weening, J. Grond, W. W. Bakker, and G. J. Fleuren

1. Introduction

The study of experimental glomerulonephritis has greatly extended our knowledge and understanding of human glomerulopathies. One of the models in experimental glomerulonephritis is the autologous immune complex glomerulonephritis (AIC), which was originally described by Heymann *et al.* (1959) and was given its present name by Edgington *et al.* (1967). They elucidated its pathogenesis and demonstrated glomerular deposition of immune complexes, consisting of an antigen normally present in the brush border of the proximal tubules of rat kidney and its specific antibody. The glomerulopathy can be induced in certain rat strains by immunization with a crude antigen fraction from the brush border (Fx1A) or with the purified nephritogenic antigen (RTEα5) in Freund's complete adjuvant (Edgington *et al.*, 1968). This procedure results after 6 weeks in glomerular deposition of immune complexes, which are localized exclusively at the epithelial side of the GBM. Morphologically and clinically the disease resembles human membranous glomerulopathy.

In earlier studies it was shown that Fx1A-like antigens are present in the normal GBM (Van Damme *et al.*, 1978) and that glomerular immune deposits in heterologous immune complex glomerulonephritis (HIC), a variant of the AIC (Feenstra *et al.*, 1975), originate from *in situ* formation rather than from deposition from the circulation (Van Damme *et al.*, 1978). Therefore, it seemed worthwhile to investigate whether in AIC a similar mechanism of glomerular immune complex formation exists.

P. J. Hoedemaeker, J. J. Weening, J. Grond, W. W. Bakker, and G. J. Fleuren · Department of Pathology, State University, Groningen, 9713 EZ Groningen, The Netherlands.

This study was performed with unilateral renal perfusion using IgG eluted from kidneys with AIC. The eluted IgG was also used in an indirect immunoperoxidase technique to demonstrate the presence of the nephritogenic antigen in the glomerular structures. Since the assumed pathogenetic mechanism implies an antigen-sharing between the GBM and the tubular brush border, induction of AIC was tried indirectly by applying a chronic injury to the tubular cells. A liberation of Fx1A antigens by this injury might lead to an autoimmune reaction and subsequently to glomerulonephritis. To study this, the glomerulopathy model in rats induced by chronic mercury intoxication as described by Weening *et al.* (1978) was used. Finally, characterization of the nephritogenic antigens involved in this model as well as in AIC and HIC, was tried by using lectins and their specific inhibitors α-D-methylmannoside and α-D-methylgalactoside (Brown and Hunt, 1978).

The results of the studies presented here give evidence in favor of an *in situ* formation of glomerular immune deposits in AIC. A binding between Fx1A-like antigens in the GBM and autologous anti-Fx1A antibody seems to be the pathogenetic mechanism in this model rather than a deposition of circulating immune complexes from the serum. Although in AIC and in mercury-induced glomerulopathy different antigens apparently are involved, the results show that they are related chemically at least.

2. Materials and Methods

2.1. Animals

Throughout the study female PVG/c rats weighing approximately 200 g were used. The rats were fed RMH-B (Hope Farms, Woerden, The Netherlands) and received water *ad libitum*.

2.2 Induction of Glomerulonephritis

AIC was induced through immunization with 10 weekly injections containing 4 mg diazotized Fx1A antigens (Gribnau, 1975) in Freund's complete adjuvant.

HIC was induced with one intravenous injection of 10 mg rabbit anti-Fx1A IgG. Immune complex depositions in the glomeruli were checked after 24 hr with immunofluorescence.

Mercury glomerulopathy was induced as described by Bariéty *et al.* (1971).

2.3 Immunological Procedures

Antisera to rat serum proteins and horseradish peroxidase were prepared in rabbits as described by Fleuren *et al.* (1978).

Acid elution of IgG from glomeruli with AIC or mercury glomerulopathy was performed according to the two-step method of Bartolotti (1977).

Purification of the IgG fraction from antisera, normal and diseased rat sera, or from eluates was performed as described by Feenstra *et al.* (1975).

The presence of antibodies to tissue antigens in the sera of diseased rats was assessed by indirect immunofluorescence using normal rat kidney or rat liver as a target.

Ex vivo perfusion of a normal left rat kidney was performed as described by Van Damme *et al.* (1978). After the procedure the perfused kidney was reconnected to the circulation for periods varying from 4 hr to 4 days.

Heterologous anti-Fx1A IgG, and antinuclear rat IgG eluted from rat kidneys in which mercury glomerulopathy had been induced were absorbed with mannane and galactane. Ten milligrams of IgG was added to 10 mg of the absorbent and allowed to incubate for 1 hr at 37°C. Subsequently the mixture was centrifuged for 1 hr at 14,000 rpm. The supernatant was used directly in immunofluorescence or for the induction of HIC.

Immunohistology at the light microscopic and ultrastructural level was performed as described before (Hoedemaeker *et al.*, 1976). In some cases the cryostat sections were preincubated with Con A (1 mg/ml). These incubations took place for 30 min at room temperature, and were followed by a rinse in phosphate buffer pH 7.4. Cryostat sections also were incubated with a mixture of Con A and α-D-methylmannoside or with Con A and α-D-

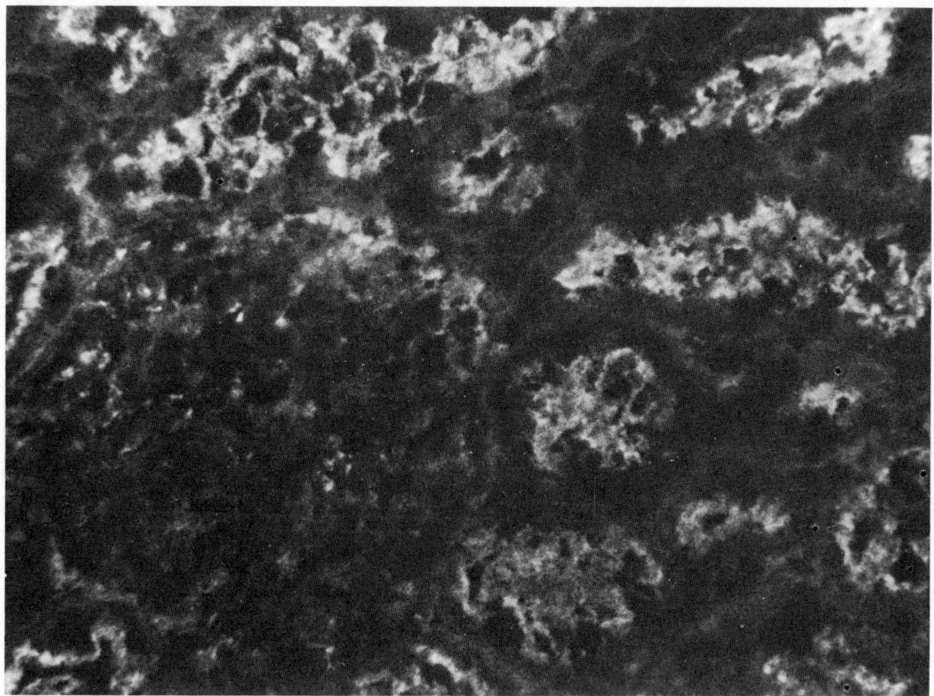

Figure 1. Indirect immunofluorescence of normal rat kidney with rat IgG eluted from kidneys with AIC. Binding of IgG is observed in brush borders and to a lesser extent in the glomerulus. × 500.

methylgalactoside under the same conditions. Con A and the sugar were preincubated for 30 min at room temperature.

3. Results

3.1. Immunofluorescence

1. Indirect immunofluorescence using eluted IgG from kidneys with AIC showed a binding to tubular brush border. Some binding in glomeruli was observed also (Fig. 1). Normal rat IgG did not show any binding to the renal tissues. Indirect immunofluorescence with serum of rats suffering from mercury glomerulopathy with normal rat kidney or rat liver as a target demonstrated a binding to nuclei in a granular peripheral pattern (Fig. 2). This antinuclear activity also was present in the IgG fraction eluted from kidneys with mercury glomerulopathy. Some affinity for the glomeruli could be demonstrated but no binding to the brush border was observed. The nuclear and glomerular staining of the circulating autologous antinuclear antibody was blocked completely when the sections were preincubated with

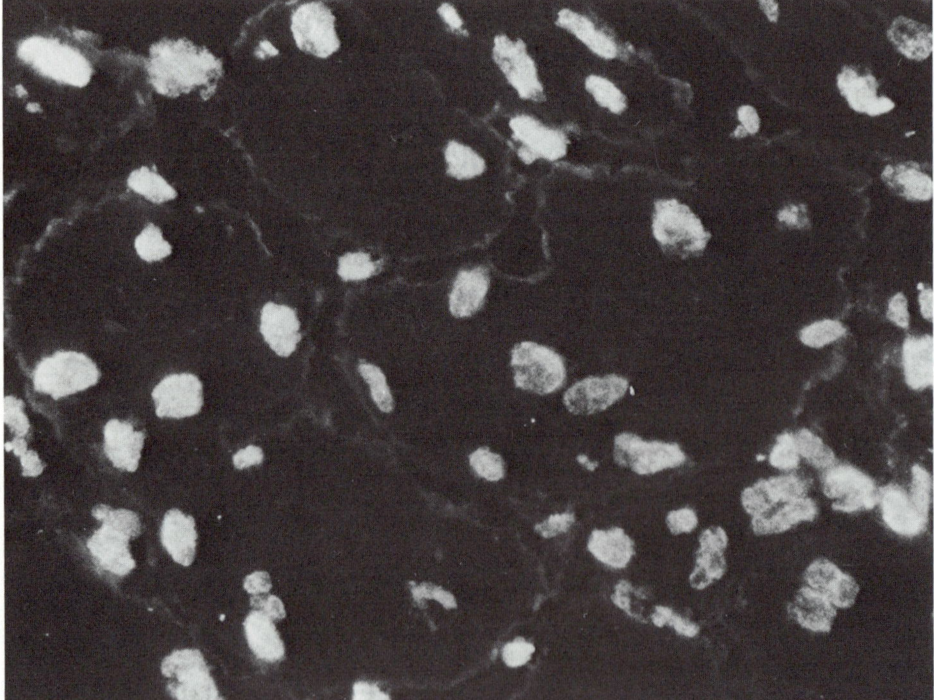

Figure 2. Indirect immunofluorescence of normal rat kidney with serum of rats suffering from mercury glomerulopathy. A binding to nuclei is observed in a granular and peripheral pattern. The brush border is negative. × 900.

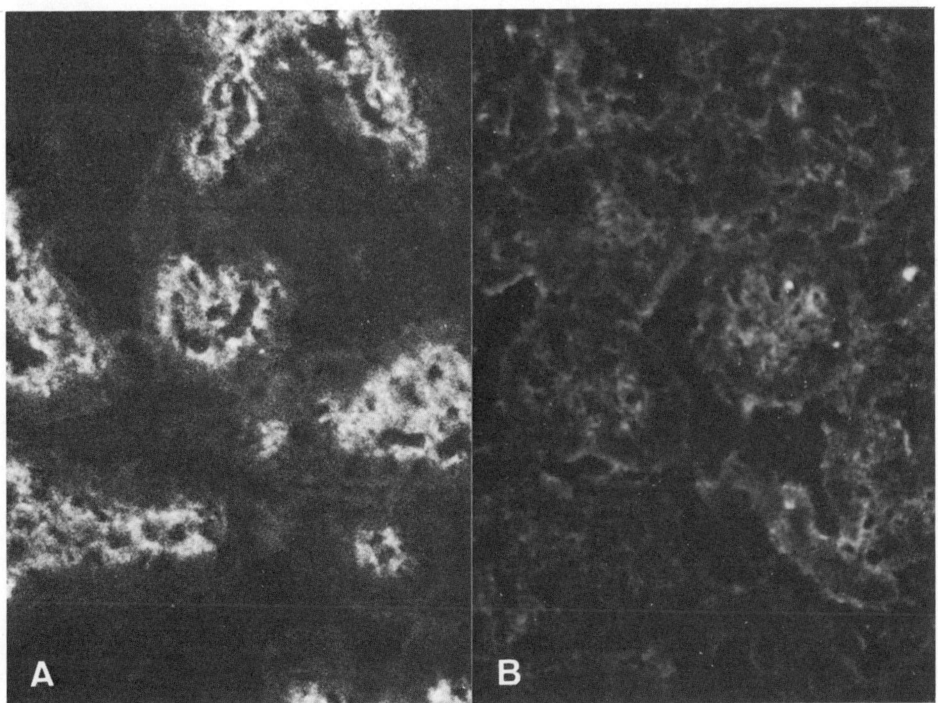

Figure 3. Indirect immunofluorescence of normal rat kidney with heterologous anti-Fx1A antibody. × 500. (A) A binding of the antibody to the brush border of the proximal tubular cells is present. (B) Preincubation of the section with Con A blocked the binding of this antibody partially.

Con A. This blocking was not seen when Con A was mixed with α-D-methylmannoside. However, α-D-methylgalactoside could not abolish the blocking capacity of Con A. Other lectins like peanut agglutinin or *Ricinus communis* did not show blocking of the binding of antinuclear antibody to nuclei. Con A partially blocked the binding of heterologous anti-Fx1A antibody to the brush border (Fig. 3). This blocking was annulled when Con A was mixed with α-D-methylmannoside but not with α-D-methylgalactoside.

2. Absorption of heterologous anti-Fx1A antibodies with mannane abolished their capacity to bind the brush border. Absorption with galactane did not have this effect. Moreover, immunofluorescence studies showed that no glomerular immune complex localization was present in HIC induced with the mannane-absorbed antibody fraction (Fig. 4). Injection with galactane-absorbed anti-Fx1A IgG resulted after 24 hr in a granular localization of IgG in the glomeruli (Fig. 4). Absorption of the antinuclear antibody with either mannane or galactane had no effect on their nuclear-binding capacity. The results of the immunofluorescence studies before and after incubation are summarized in Table 1.

Table 1. Immunofluorescence of IgG of Rats with Mercury Glomerulopathy (ANF), AIC (Autologous Anti-Fx1A), and HIC (Heterologous Anti-Fx1A) on Normal Rat Kidney, or Rat Kidney Preincubated with Peanut Agglutinin, Con A, Con A + α-D-Methylmannoside, Con A + α-D-Methylgalactoside. Also, Results of Immunofluorescence on Normal Rat Kidney and Capacity to Induce HIC, of Sera Absorbed with Mannane or Galactane

		+ mannane	+ galactane	+ dextran	Con A	Peanut agglutinin	Con A + α-D-methylmannoside	Con A + α-D-methylgalactoside
ANF nuclei	++	++	++	++	−	++	++	−
Autologous anti-Fx1A brush border	++	−	++	++	±	++	++	±
Heterologous anti-Fx1A brush border	++	−	++	++	±	++	++	±
Heterologous anti-Fx1A HIC	++	−	++	ND[a]	ND	ND	ND	ND
ANF GBM	++	ND	ND	ND	−	ND	++	−

[a] ND, not determined.

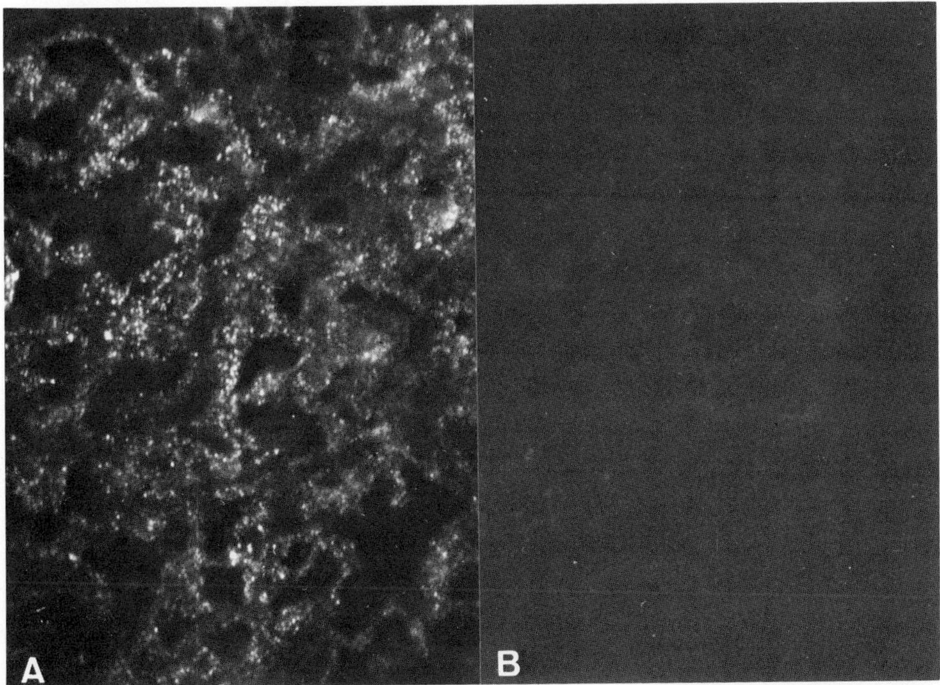

Figure 4. Direct immunofluorescence of a rat kidney injected 24 hr previously with heterologous anti-Fx1A antibody. × 900. (A) Heterologous IgG binds in a granular pattern along the GBM. (B) Absorption of the heterologous antibody with mannane inhibited this binding completely.

3.2. *Immunoelectron Microscopy*

Using eluted IgG from kidneys with AIC in a concentration of 0.1 mg/ml, binding to normal glomerular structures was observed (Fig. 5). This binding was strongest in that part of the cell membrane of the epithelial foot processes bordering the GBM. To a lesser extent, binding was observed throughout the GBM and to the cell membranes of epithelial and of endothelial cells. Immunohistology with IgG from animals with mercury glomerulopathy also showed binding to glomerular structures. The binding was present in cell membranes of epithelial and endothelial cells and throughout the GBM (Fig. 6). Four hours after perfusion of normal rat kidney, the IgG eluted from kidneys with AIC showed binding to parts of the cell membrane of the epithelial foot processes bordering the GBM. To a lesser extent, binding throughout the width of the GBM was observed (Fig. 7). Perfusion with normal rat IgG did not result in a binding to glomerular structures (Fig. 8). The nonperfused right kidney also did not show bound IgG.

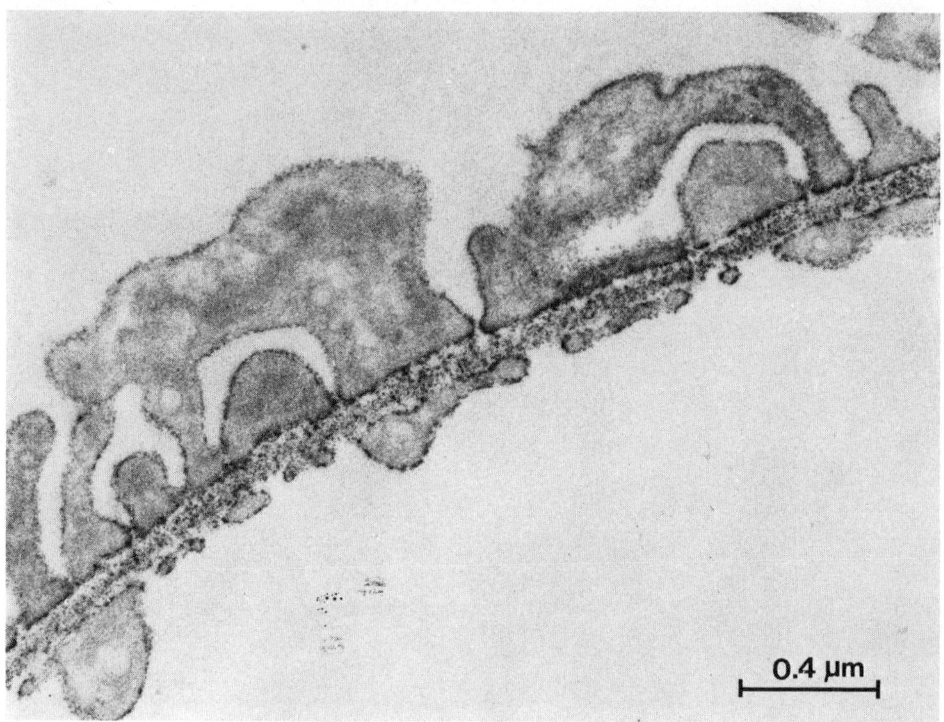

Figure 5. Indirect immunoperoxidase technique of a normal rat glomerulus with IgG eluted from kidneys with AIC. A binding of the IgG is observed in parts of the cell membranes of epithelial foot processes bordering the GBM and throughout the GBM. To a lesser extent, binding is also seen to the cell membranes of epithelial and endothelial cells. Unstained.

4. *Discussion*

1. Recently, evidence was presented in favor of *in situ* formation of immune complexes in HIC (Van Damme *et al.*, 1978). This model is related closely to AIC and in both models Fx1A antigens are involved. Therefore, this investigation into the pathogenesis of AIC was performed with emphasis upon the possibility of *in situ* formation of immune complexes in this model. Perfusion experiments with normal rat kidneys were performed using acid eluates from kidneys with AIC. The eluted IgG was preferred over circulating autologous anti-Fx1A IgG because this latter antibody probably contains many specificities, all directed against different antigenic fractions of the Fx1A antigens. Using eluted IgG, one could be certain that one was dealing with an antibody directed against the nephritogenic antigen. The results of these perfusion studies show clearly that in the absence of circulating antigen, autologous anti-Fx1A antibody can bind to glomerular structures. The strongest binding is seen in those parts of the epithelial cell membranes bordering the GBM. Also, some binding was observed within the GBM. An identical localization of rat IgG is seen in the early phase of AIC, i.e., in

week 6, before immune complexes are present (Fig. 8). An essentially similar binding pattern results when the eluate is used in an indirect immunoperoxidase technique with normal rat kidney as a target.

The results of these experiments indicate that the presence of immune deposits in AIC is the result of a binding of autologous anti-Fx1A antibody to Fx1A-like antigens present at the epithelial side of the GBM. These antigens were shown to be present in the normal rat GBM by Van Damme *et al.* (1978). The binding of rat anti-Fx1A to these antigens is specific because perfusion with normal rat IgG did not result in a binding, nor did normal rat IgG bind to glomerular structures in the indirect immunoperoxidase technique. It seems unlikely that the binding occurred because of the ischemic conditions, which are indisputably present during perfusion, since after 4 days a similar binding of the rat IgG was seen. Moreover, recent studies involving perfusion procedures not associated with ischaemia led to the same results (Fleuren *et al.*, 1981). The reason why no immune aggregates are observed in the GBM following perfusion with the eluted IgG, could be a quantitative one. In the perfusion experiments, only 10 mg IgG was perfused through a kidney, of which amount probably only a minor part bound to the GBM. If a larger amount of antibody is perfused (Couser *et al.*, 1978;

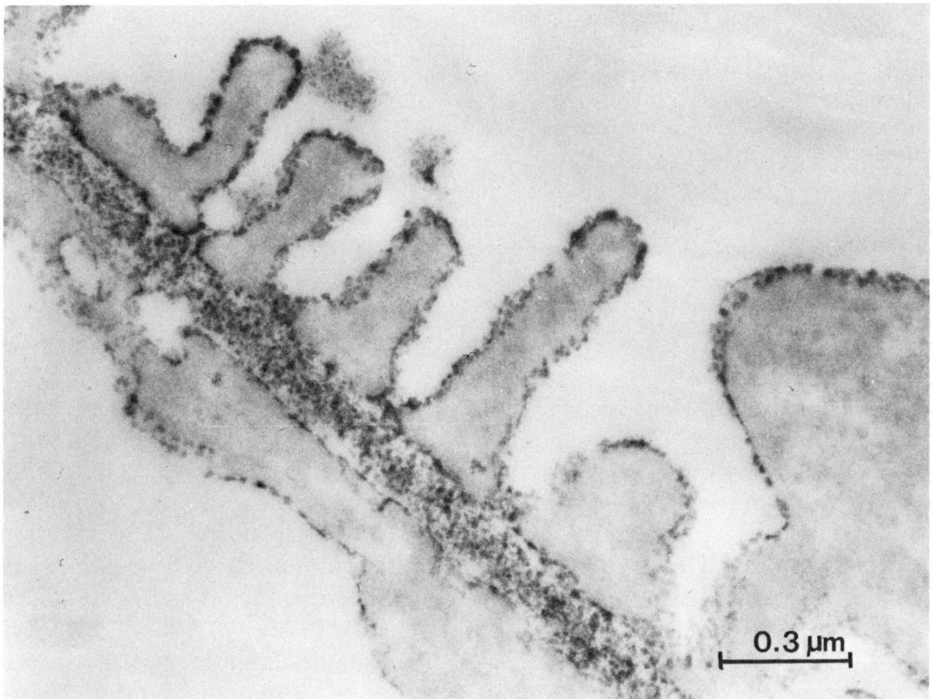

Figure 6. Indirect immunoperoxidase technique of a normal rat glomerulus with rat IgG from animals with mercury glomerulopathy. Binding is seen to epithelial and endothelial cell membranes and throughout the GBM. Unstained.

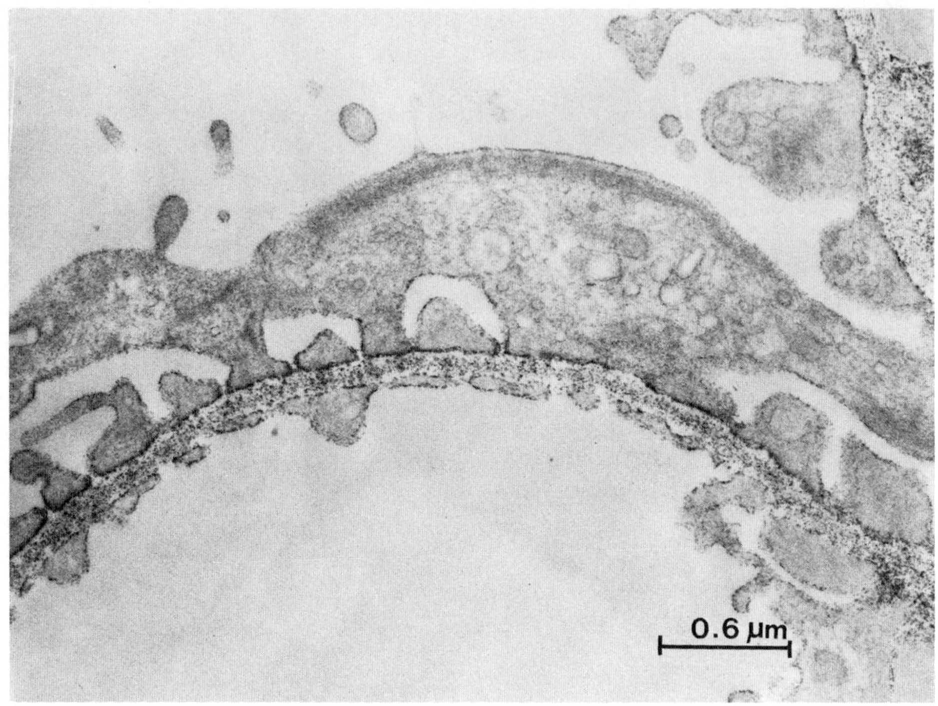

Figure 7. Indirect immunoperoxidase of a normal rat glomerulus with rat IgG eluted from kidneys with AIC. Binding is observed to the part of the cell membranes of the epithelial foot processes and to a lesser extent throughout the GBM and to the endothelial cell membrane. Unstained.

Hoedemaeker *et al.*, 1981) immune aggregates could be found at the epithelial side of the GBM. The idea that in AIC *in situ* formation of immune complexes is the major pathogenetic mechanism is further strengthened by the finding of Fleuren (1976, 1980) who demonstrated a major role for free-circulating anti-Fx1A antibody.

The possibility that, in AIC immune complexes containing Fx1A, antigens are circulating in the serum, as suggested by Abrass *et al.* (1979), is not excluded. However, it is hard to believe that these immune complexes are deposited in the GBM because injection of preformed immune complexes consisting of Fx1A and heterologous anti-Fx1A never resulted in a localization in the GBM but rather in a mesangial localization (Van Damme *et al.*, 1978). Furthermore, a crossing of the GBM by immune complexes in the course of AIC could not be observed (Hoedemaeker *et al.*, 1976).

2. Fx1A antigens are present also in other cell membranes of the rat organs associated with absorption or secretion (Mietinen and Linder, 1976). This could mean that in situations in which such antigen is liberated, an autoimmunization to these antigens could occur possibly resulting in a glomerulonephritis. An effort to mimic this situation in an experiment by using the mercury-induced glomerulopathy as published by Weening *et al.*

(1978) was made. In this model chronic mercury intoxication was believed to cause damage to proximal tubular cells, which could be associated with liberation of Fx1A antigen. Subsequently, autoimmunization to this antigen might occur resulting in glomerulonephritis. Although a glomerulopathy did occur which showed many characteristics of AIC like epimembranous immune complex depositions, as shown by Bariéty *et al.* (1971), it was not possible to demonstrate the participation of Fx1A antigens in this model. Instead an antinuclear antibody was found in the serum of the diseased animals. This activity, which also could be eluted from the glomeruli of kidneys with mercury glomerulopathy. (Weening *et al.*, 1978).

The fluorescence pattern of the nuclei and the fact that an increase of the intensity of the fluorescence could be induced by pretreatment of the sections with acid buffer (Tan *et al.*, 1976; Weening *et al.*, 1980) suggested a nonhistone character of the antigens involved. Recent studies revealed a direct effect of mercury on immune competent T cells, resulting in immunodysregulation (Weening *et al.*, 1981) and polyclonal stimulation of B cells (Hirsch *et al.*, 1981).

According to Rizzo and Bustin (1977) we tried to determine the nature of the antigen involved by using preincubation of the cryostat sections with lectins in the immunofluorescence procedure. The results show that the affinity of the antibody for nuclei was completely abolished by preincubation

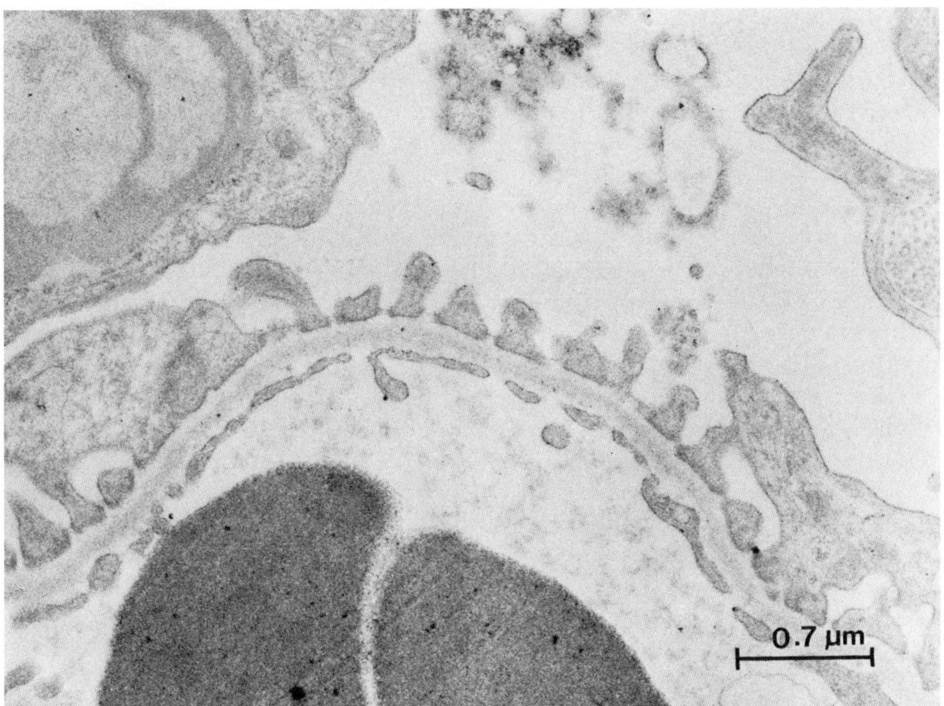

Figure 8. Indirect immunoperoxidase with normal rat IgG. No binding of rat IgG to glomerular structures is seen. Two erythrocytes show endogenous peroxidase activity. Unstained.

of the sections with Con A. Preincubation with other lectins did not have this effect. Moreover, the inhibition by Con A was annulled by pretreatment of the sections with a mixture of Con A and α-D-methylmannoside. This sugar which is a specific inhibitor of Con A, apparently competed with antigen binding of Con A. Specific inhibitors of other lectins like α-D-methylgalactose did not have this effect. This finding confirms the nonhistone protein character of the nuclear antigen that binds the autologous antibodies in mercury glomerulopathy (Rizzo and Bustin, 1977). As the binding to the GBM can be blocked in the same way as the nuclear binding, it seems likely that common antigenic determinants are shared by both structures, although competitive inhibition of the respective bindings by glycoproteins like mannane could not be demonstrated (Table 1).

Preincubation with Con A also blocked partially the binding of heterologous and autologous anti-Fx1A antibody to brushborder antigens. This blocking, which could not be achieved with other lectins, could again be annulled by adding α-D-methylmannoside to Con A. Moreover, absorption of heterologous anti-Fx1A antibody with mannane completely abolished its capacity to induce HIC. Absorption with galactane, however, did not have this effect. These results indicate that the nephritogenic antigen in HIC is a (glyco) protein containing mannosyl groups which is possibly related to the antigen involved in mercury glomerulopathy. Since AIC and HIC are closely related models of glomerulopathy and in both models Fx1A antigens are involved, it is tempting to think that in AIC the nephritogenic antigen also consists of a (glyco) protein bearing α-D-methylmannosyl groups. Indirect evidence for this thesis is provided by Shibata et al. (1977) who were able to induce an immune complex glomerulopathy with a Con A binding antigen which they purified from the GBM.

From the results described it appears that experimental immune complex glomerulopathy may be induced by antigens which are localized at different sites but may have mannosyl groups in common. Although it is not necessary for these antigens to be identical, the results suggest that "antigen sharing" between GBM and other structures in the body is very important in the pathogenesis of experimental epimembranous immune complex glomerulopathy.

An immune reaction to an antigen in some organ or another could result in an immune complex glomerulopathy if this antigen or its antigenic determinants are also present in the GBM.

A similar mechanism could also be operating in human glomerulonephritis the more because in regard with the distribution of Fx1A-like antigens, in humans a similar situation is found as in the rat (Miyakawa et al., 1976). The pathogenesis of *in situ* formation of immune complexes which was described for the experimental models could be working especially in membranous glomerulopathy associated with epithelial malignancies. In several of these cases, tumour membrane antigens have been demonstrated in the immune complex deposits in the GBM (Eagen and Lewis, 1977), suggesting an antigen-sharing between tumour cell membranes and GBM.

Further studies will have to clarify the exact character of the antigens involved in experimental immune complex glomerulonephritis and prove whether such antigens may also play a role in human membranous glomerulopathy.

References

Abrass, C. K., Border, W. A., and Glassock, R. J., 1978, The pathogenesis of autologous immune complex glomerulonephritis in rats, in: *Proceedings, Conference on Immune Mechanisms in Renal Disease.*

Bariéty, J., Druet, P., Laliberté, F., and Sapin, C., 1971, Glomerulonephritis with γ and β 1C-globulin deposits induced in rats by mercuric chloride, *Am. J. Pathol.* **65:**293.

Bartolotti, S. R., 1977, Quantitative elution studies in experimental immune complex and nephrotoxic nephritis, *J. Clin. Exp. Immunol.* **29:**334.

Brown, J. C., and Hunt, R. C., 1978, Lectins, in: *International Review of Cytology* (G. H. Bourne and J. F. Danielli, eds.), Vol. 52, pp. 277–349, Academic Press, New York.

Couser, W. G., Steinmuller, D. R., Stilmant, M. M., Salant, D. J., and Lowenstein, L. M., Experimental glomerulonephritis in the isolated perfused rat kidney, *J. Clin. Invest.* **62:**1275–1287.

Eagen, J. W., and Lewis, E. J., 1977, Glomerulopathies of neoplasia, *Kidney Int.* **11:**297.

Edgington, T. S., Glassock, R. J., and Dixon, F. J., 1967, Autologous immune-complex pathogenesis of experimental allergic glomerulonephritis, *Science* **155:**1432.

Edgington, T. S., Glassock, R. J., and Dixon, F. J., 1968, Autologous immune complex nephritis induced with renal tubular antigen. I. Identification and isolation of the pathogenetic antigen, *J. Exp. Med.* **127:**555.

Feenstra, K., van der Lee, R., Greben, H. A., Arends, A., and Hoedemaeker, P. J., 1975, Experimental glomerulonephritis in the rat induced by antibodies directed against tubular antigens. I. The natural history: A histologic and immunohistologic study at the light microscopic and the ultrastructural level, *Lab. Invest.* **32:**235.

Fleuren, G. J., 1976, Studies on pathogenesis and treatment of experimental immune complex glomerulonephritis, Academic Thesis, Groningen, The Netherlands.

Fleuren, G. J., van der, Lee, R., Greben, H. A., Van Damme, B. J. C., and Hoedemaeker, P. J., 1978, Experimental glomerulonephritis in the rat induced by antibodies directed aganist tubular antigens. IV. Investigations into the pathogenesis of the model, *Lab. Invest.* **38:**496.

Fleuren, G. J., Grond J., Hoedemaeker Ph. J., 1980, The pathogenetic role of free-circulating antibody in autologous immune complex glomerulonephritis, *Clin. Exp. Immunol.* **41:**205–217.

Fleuren, G. J., Moons W. M., Slegers J. F. G., Hoedemaeker P. J., 1981, *In situ* formation of subepithelial immune aggregates is independent of ischaemia. Abstract 8th Int. Congr. of Nephrol. Athens.

Gribnau, F. W. J., 1975, Indomethacin in experimental nephritis: Studies in Heymann-type nephritis and in puromycin aminonucleoside nephropathy, Academic Thesis, Nijmegen, The Netherlands.

Heymann, W., Hackel, D. B., Harwood, S., Wilson, S. G. F., and Hunter, J. L. P., 1959, Production of nephrotic syndrome in rats by Freund's adjuvant and kidney suspensions, *Proc. Soc. Exp. Biol. Med.* **110:**660.

Hirsch, F., Couderc, J., Sapin, C., Fournié G., Druet, P., 1981, Polyclonal effect of $HgCl_2$ in the rat. Its possible role in mercury induced glomerulonephritis. Abstract 8th Int. Congr. Nephrol. Athens.

Hoedemaeker, P. J., Donga, J., and Fleuren, G. J., 1976, Immuno electron microscopic studies of experimental glomerulonephritis, using peroxidase as a label, in: *Proceedings of the First International Symposium on Immunoenzymatic Techniques* (G. Feldmann, ed.), North-Holland, Amsterdam.

Hoedemaeker Ph. J., Grond J., Fleuren G. J., 1981, Renal Tubular Antigens. *In*: Proc. 8th Int. Congr. Nephrol. Athens, pp. 896–902.

Mietinen, A., and Linder, E., 1976, Membrane antigens shared by renal proximal tubules and other epithelia associated with absorption and excretion, *Clin. Exp. Immunol.* **23**:568.

Miyakawa, Y., Kitamura, K., Shibata, S., and Naruse, T., 1976, Demonstration of human nephritogenic tubular antigen in the serum and organs by radio immunoassay, *J. Immunol.* **117**:1203.

Rizzo, W. B., and Bustin, M., 1977, Lectins as probes of chromatin structure: Binding of concanavalin A to purified rat liver chromatin, *J. Biol. Chem.* **252**:7062.

Shibata, S., Nagasawa, T., and Miura, K., 1977, Nephritogenoside, the receptor glycoprotein for concanavalin A in rat glomerular basement membrane: Demonstration of α-**D**-glucopyranosyl unit at the non-reducing terminus, *Biochim. Biophys. Acta* **499**:392.

Tan, E. M., Robinson, J., and Robitaille, P., 1976, Studies on antibodies to histones by immunofluorescence, *Scan. J. Immunol.* **5**:1076.

Van Damme, B. J. C., Fleuren, G. J., Bakker, W. W., Vernier, R. L., and Hoedemaeker, P. J., 1978, Experimental glomerulonephritis in the rat induced by antibodies directed against tubular antigens. V. Fixed glomerular antigens in the pathogenesis of heterologous immune complex glomerulonephritis, *Lab. Invest.* **38**:502.

Weening, J. J., Fleuren, G. J., and Hoedemaeker, P. J., 1978, Demonstration of anti-nuclear antibodies in mercuric chloride-induced glomerulopathy in the rat, *Lab. Invest* **39**:405.

Weening J. J., Grond J., van de Top D., Hoedemaeker Ph. J., 1980, Identification of the nuclear antigen involved in mercury-induced glomerulopathy in the rat. *Invest. Cell. Path.* **3**:129–134.

Weening J. J., Hoedemaeker P. J. Bakker W. W., 1981, Immunoregulation and anti-nuclear antibodies in mercury-induced glomerulopathy in the rat. *Clin. Exp. Immunol.* **45**:64–71.

23

Mechanisms of Proteinuria Induced by Antikidney Antibodies in Noninflammatory Experimental Glomerulonephropathy

William G. Couser, David J. Salant, and Magda M. Stilmant

1. Introduction

A number of studies carried out largely in the past 5 years have contributed to a significant increase in our understanding of the determinants which regulate the permeability of the normal glomerulus to various macromolecules (Rennke and Venkatachalam, 1977; Brenner *et al.*, 1978). These morphologic and physiologic studies have been well summarized elsewhere in this volume (Chapters 1, 2, and 6). The topic of this chapter is renal disease mediated by antikidney antibodies. To link the material presented earlier on glomerular permeability with diseases induced by antikidney antibodies, the present discussion will review some of the recent studies of immunologic mechanisms of proteinuria carried out largely in two models of experimental nephropathy in Couser's laboratory.

It is well established that complement–neutrophil (PMN)-mediated inflammatory glomerular injury results in structural damage to the glomerular capillary wall (Kuhn *et al.*, 1977). This discussion will focus on proteinuria

William G. Couser · Division of Nephrology, University of Washington, Seattle, Washington 98195. ***David J. Salant*** · Evans Memorial Department of Clinical Research and Departments of Medicine and Pathology, Boston University Medical Center, Boston, Massachusetts 02118. ***Magda M. Stilmant*** · Mallory Institute of Pathology, Boston City Hospital, Boston, Massachusetts 02118. Portions of this work were supported by Research Grants AM 17722, AM 17713, HL 18313, AM 19097, AM 16749, and National Research Service Award AM 07053 from the U.S. Public Health Service. Dr. Couser is a recipient of a Research Career Development Award (AM 00102) from the U.S. Public Health Service.

mediated by glomerular antibody deposition in the absence of detectable inflammatory changes or structural alterations in the proximal layers of the glomerular filtration barrier. A full understanding of the mechanisms of immunologically induced proteinuria requires that a much better correlation be established between the immunologic agents and mediator systems which induce glomerular disease and the determinants of glomerular permselectivity defined by physiologic and ultrastructural studies than is possible at the present time.

2. *Complement-Independent Nephrotoxic Nephritis in the Guinea Pig*

Injection of outbred guinea pigs with sheep antibody to guinea pig glomerular basement membrane (GBM) induces an initial oliguric period lasting for 1–2 hr followed by a marked but transient increase in urine protein excretion which reaches a peak value of over 25 mg/hr within 5–6 hr but returns to essentially normal values within 36 hr (Fig. 1). (Couser *et al.*, 1977). Electrophoretic studies have shown the urine protein to be composed of over 90% albumin. This dramatic change in GBM permeability is accompanied by linear deposition of both γ_1 and γ_2 subgroups of sheep IgG on the GBM. However, there is no detectable deposition of guinea pig C3 or C4 *in vivo,* and these glomerular antibody deposits do not fix guinea pig or human C3 *in vitro* (Couser *et al.*, 1977).

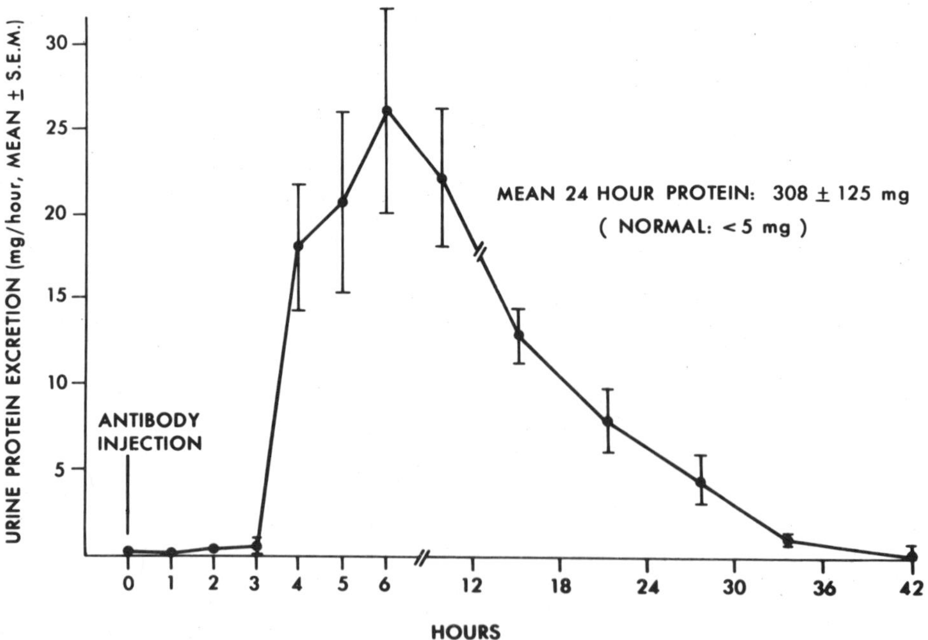

Figure 1. Time course of proteinuria induced by administration of sheep antibody to guinea pig GBM.

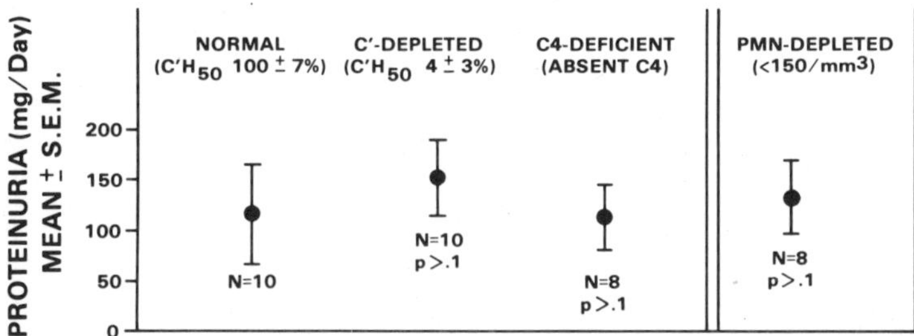

Figure 2. Proteinuria induced by injection of a standard dose of nephrotoxic serum in normal guinea pigs and guinea pigs depleted of C3–C9 by cobra venom factor, genetically deficient in C4, and depleted of PMNs by nitrogen mustard.

Hourly biopsies performed after antibody injection revealed no significant glomerular histopathology. Specifically, there were no PMNs, mononuclear cells, or other signs of inflammation seen at any time prior to or during the course of proteinuria. Ultrastructural studies demonstrated only widespread epithelial cell foot process fusion with no demonstrable abnormalities in endothelium or GBM. No endothelial or epithelial cell detachment was seen. When native anionic ferritin was injected as an ultrastructural tracer molecule at the peak of proteinuria, ferritin molecules were confined largely to the capillary lumen, and no increase in permeability to this molecule could be demonstrated (Couser *et al.*, 1977).

In contrast to the findings in classical complement–PMN-dependent nephrotoxic nephritis (NTN) in rats (Cochrane *et al.*, 1965), proteinuria in the guinea pig model is not diminished when C3 is depleted to less than 5% of normal values by injection of cobra venom factor prior to administration of nephrotoxic serum or when nephrotoxic serum is administered to animals genetically deficient in C4 (Couser *et al.*, 1977) (Fig. 2). Moreover, both complement- and noncomplement-fixing subgroups of IgG and equimolar amounts of the $F(ab)_2$ portion of nephrotoxic IgG are equally effective in producing proteinuria (Simpson *et al.*, 1975).

With regard to the mechanism of proteinuria induced by nephrotoxic antibody, Bennett *et al.* (1976) have demonstrated that proteinuria late in NTN reflects in part a loss of net negative charge on the glomerular capillary wall as evidenced by reduced histochemical staining for glomerular polyanion and increased fractional clearance of anionic dextran sulfate compared to neutral dextran. However, these studies were carried out 1–3 weeks after the initial deposition of nephrotoxic antibody, and the conclusions are therefore applicable only to the autologous phase of NTN when a second antigen–antibody reaction is occurring within the glomerulus. The mechanism by which the initial anti-GBM antibody deposits induce proteinuria has not been clearly defined.

Attempts to study the role of altered capillary wall charge in the guinea pig NTN model using histochemical staining techniques revealed no change in colloidal iron staining at the peak of proteinuria at 6 hr (Couser *et al.*,

Table 1. *Results of Colloidal Iron Staining in Guinea Pig NTN*

Time[a] (hr)	n	Proteinuria (mg/hr)	Colloidal iron staining		
			Normal	Reduced	Absent
0 (control	12	< 0.2	12	0	0
6	24	25 ± 8	24	0	0
12	12	16 ± 9	10	2	0
24	24	6 ± 6	12	12	0
120	12	< 0.4	12	0	0

[a] Hours after injection of proteinuric dose of nephrotoxic serum.

1977) (Table 1). Glomerular permeability to anionic ferritin also was not increased. At 24 hr, reduced colloidal iron staining was demonstrable in 12 of 24 animals studied, but the reductions in staining seen were minimal and correlated poorly with urine protein excretion. Thus, at present, there is little evidence directly supporting either structural changes or an alteration in the charge on the glomerular capillary wall as the basis for immediate proteinuria induced by nephrotoxic antibody in this model. The mechanism for altered GBM permeability induced acutely by IgG antibody interacting with GBM antigens is unclear.

3. *Experimental Membranous Nephropathy Induced by Antibodies to Renal Tubular Epithelial Cell Antigens*

3.1. *General*

A second model of noninflammatory glomerular disease with heavy proteinuria is induced in rats by deposition of autologous or heterologous antibodies against a kidney antigen termed fraction 1A (Fx1A) which is apparently associated with the brush border of proximal tubular epithelial cells (Edgington *et al.*, 1968). Rats actively immunized with Fx1A develop proteinuria within 6–8 weeks and have a glomerular lesion characterized by diffuse, finely granular subepithelial deposits of IgG and C3 which is indistinguishable from membranous nephropathy in man (Heymann nephritis, autologous immune complex nephropathy, AICN) (Fig. 3) (Couser *et al.*, 1976). In this model, tubular brush border antigen can be demonstrated in glomerular immune deposits, and the deposits have been thought to result from glomerular trapping of soluble immune complexes containing tubular antigen and antibody to it (Edgington *et al.*, 1967).

Intravenous administration of sheep antibody to rat Fx1A induces apparently identical deposits of sheep IgG within minutes (Fig. 3). Although we have been unable to demonstrate tubular antigen deposits in glomeruli in this passive Heymann nephritis model (PHN) by immunofluorescence, the pathogenesis of this model has been said to involve soluble complex trapping. In contrast to NTN in the rat and guinea pig, in the PHN model,

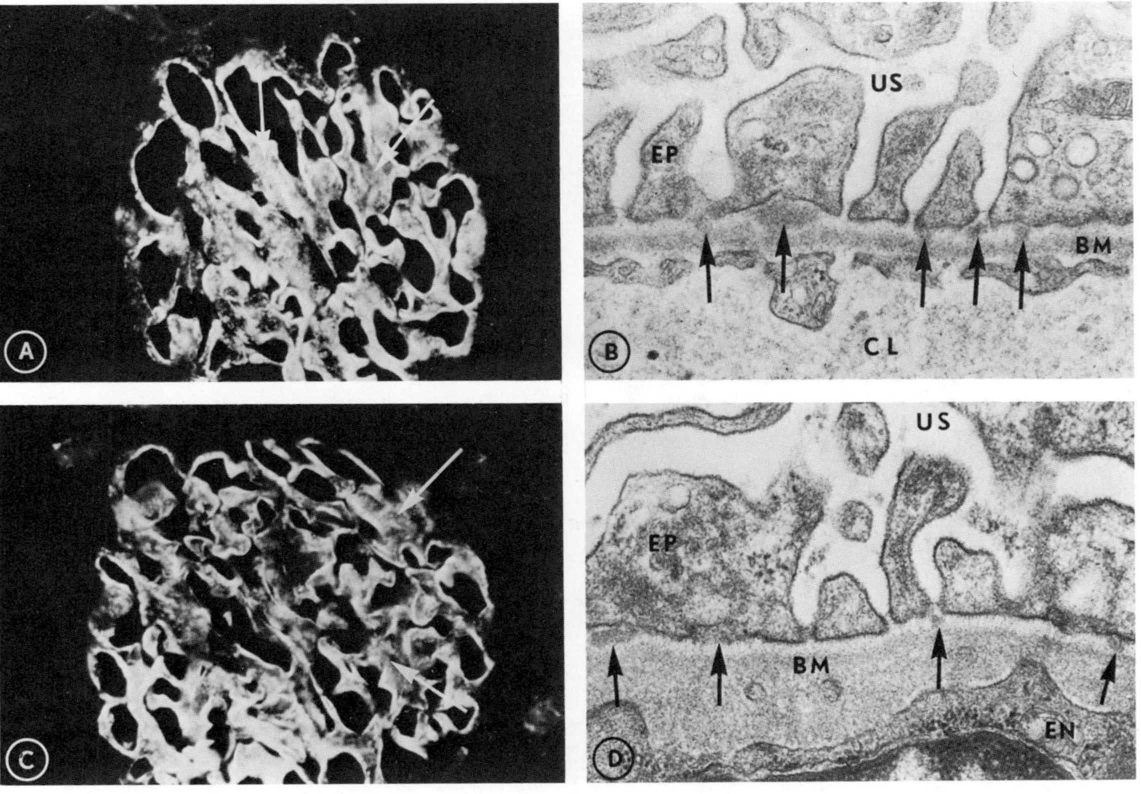

Figure 3. Glomeruli of rat with AICN 4 weeks after immunization with Fx1A (A and B) and rat with PHN 4 days after injection of 10 mg sheep anti-rat Fx1A (C and D). Immunofluorescence shows very finely granular deposits of rat IgG (A) and sheep IgG (C) on the capillary loops with more homogeneous staining in capillary walls cut tangentially (white arrows). Electron micrographs from the same animals (B and D) show discrete granular deposits in the subepithelial space and slit pores (dark arrows). BM, basement membrane; CL, capillary lumen; EN, endothelial cell; EP, epithelial cell; US, urinary space. Original magnification: A, C, × 630; B, D, × 45,000. (From Couser *et al.*, 1978c.)

proteinuria is delayed and appears 4–5 days after the injection of antibody to tubular antigen (Fig. 4).

3.2. Mechanisms of Subepithelial Complex Formation in PHN

To study the role of circulating immune complexes versus alternate mechanisms of complex formation in the PHN model, nephritogenic quantities of purified antibody to rat Fx1A were added directly to the reservoir of a modified isolated perfused rat kidney system shown schematically in Fig. 5. Perfusions were carried out for up to 2 hr with a medium that contained only oxygenated 6.7 g% bovine serum albumin in bicarbonate buffer and IgG antibody (or control nonantibody IgG) maintained at constant temperature, pressure, pH, and flow rate (Couser *et al.*, 1978c). In this system, renal venous effluent was run to waste to exclude any possibility that immune complexes formed in the perfusate due to release of tubular antigen from the perfused kidney (Fig. 5). Finely granular deposits of antibody on the capillary wall identical to those seen in the intact animal were produced within minutes and increased with the duration of perfusion to appear characteristically membranous within 2 hr (Fig. 6). By conventional electron microscopy, deposits could be readily visualized at 2 hr in the subepithelial space and slit pores exactly as seen in early AICN or membranous nephropathy (Fig. 6). Perfusions carried out with equal amounts of nonantibody IgG produced no deposits (Fig. 6), thus demonstrating that the formation of subepithelial deposits in this model reflects antibody interaction with some

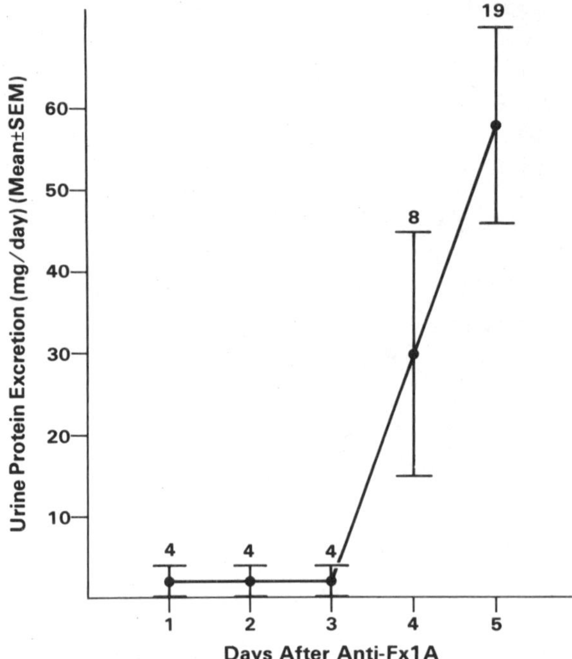

Figure 4. Time course of proteinuria induced by administration of sheep antibody to rat Fx1A.

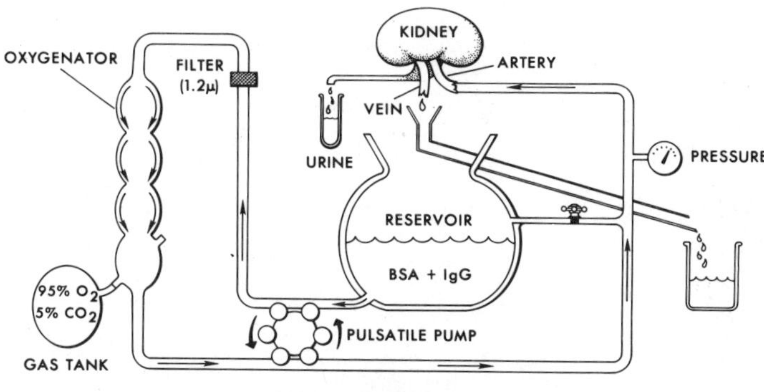

ISOLATED PERFUSED RAT KIDNEY
(nonrecirculating system)

Figure 5. Schematic depiction of modified single-pass kidney perfusion system in which filtered, oxygenated perfusate is delivered to an isolated rat kidney at constant temperature, pressure, pH, and flow rate, and renal venous effluent is discarded.

component of the glomerular capillary wall rather than deposition of circulating immune complexes.

Moreover, in PHN induced by injections of anti-Fx1A antibody radiolabeled with ^{125}I, treatment with agents which might be expected to alter glomerular deposition of circulating immune complexes, including steroids and the vasoactive amine antagonists cyproheptadine and chlorpheniramine, had no significant effect on the amount or site of antibody deposition at 5 days compared to untreated controls (Belok *et al.*, 1977; Salant *et al.*, 1978b). As anticipated, these same agents also had no effect on the development of proteinuria at 5 days (Belok *et al.*, 1977).

On the basis of these studies, as well as the work presented by Hoedemaeker and previously published by Van Damme and associates (1978), Couser's group believes that these models of experimental membranous nephropathy induced by antibody to rat tubular antigen represent examples of glomerulonephritis resulting from formation of glomerular immune deposits locally within the glomerulus rather than from circulating immune complex deposition.

3.3. *Effect of Properties of the Glomerulus on Subepithelial Deposit Formation in AICN and PHN*

In addition to the apparent lack of effect of systemic factors on epimembranous complex formation, it has been shown in both the AICN and PHN models that when physical properties and permeability of the glomerular capillary wall are altered by treatment of the animal with aminonucleoside of puromycin (PA) to induce proteinuria prior to complex formation in AICN (Couser *et al.*, 1978a) or prior to anti-Fx1A antibody injection in PHN (Couser *et al.*, 1978b), immune deposits fail to develop in

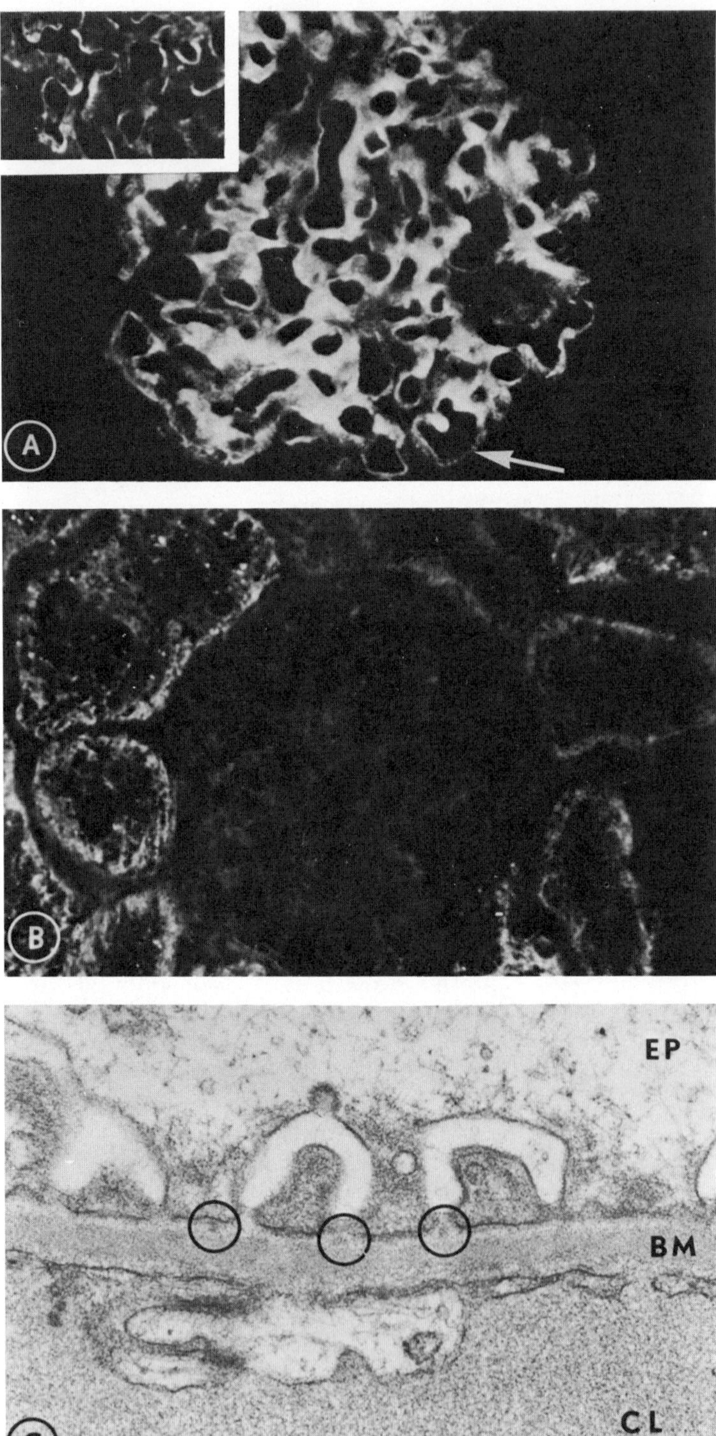
A
B
EP
BM
CL
C

PA nephrotic glomeruli despite intense tubular brush border staining indicating adequate glomerular delivery and filtration of antibody. An identical reduction in subepithelial deposits occurs when proteinuria is induced by pretreatment with nephrotoxic serum prior to anti-Fx1A administration (Couser *et al.*, 1978b). This finding is in direct contrast to results recently reported by Trevillian and Cameron (1978) who showed that pretreatment with nephrotoxic serum increased rather than decreased glomerular deposition of circulating immune complexes in the acute serum sickness model in rabbits.

To exclude any possible systemic effect of PA in causing the reduction in GBM deposits observed, additional studies were carried out in rats with unilateral proteinuria produced by selective perfusion of the left renal artery with PA before induction of PHN (Belok *et al.*, 1977) or development of deposits in AICN (Couser *et al.*, 1978a). In both models, subepithelial deposits developed as usual in the nonperfused right kidneys but were reduced markedly in the proteinuric left kidneys of these same animals (Fig. 7).

Of further interest is the observation that when PA nephrosis was induced in AICN rats actively immunized with tubular antigen, in addition to the marked reduction in capillary wall deposits there was an increase in mesangial deposits of both IgG and Fx1A in a granular pattern (Fig. 7) (Couser *et al.*, 1978a). These deposits were interpreted to indicate increased mesangial uptake of immune complexes derived from the circulation. The presence of such circulating complexes in AICN rats has subsequently been confirmed by Abrass *et al.* (1977) but their pathogenetic significance has not been established. However, no such mesangial deposits have been seen in rats with PA nephrosis given anti-Fx1A antibody (Belok *et al.*, 1977), suggesting that similar circulating complexes are not present in the PHN model, although an identical glomerular lesion develops.

3.4. Kinetics of Glomerular Antibody Binding in Relation to Proteinuria in PHN

Studies in which PHN is induced using anti-Fx1A IgG trace-labeled with ^{125}I and renal antibody deposition is quantitated by counting kidneys from individual rats have revealed a unique time course of antibody deposition in

Figure 6. Representative immunofluorescent and electron micrographs from glomeruli of isolated rat kidneys perfused for 2 hr with 30 mg/100 ml of anti-Fx1A IgG (A and C) or nonantibody IgG (B). (A) Immunofluorescence in antibody-perfused kidneys shows diffuse, very finely granular deposition of sheep IgG along all capillary walls. In some loops, closely spaced deposits along the epithelial surface of the capillary wall are clearly apparent (white arrow). Original magnification: × 600. Inset demonstrates finely granular deposits along the epithelial surface of the capillary loops in a biopsy obtained only 10 min after initiation of antibody perfusion. Original magnification: × 630. (B) Kidney perfused with normal sheep IgG for 2 hr shows no glomerular deposition of sheep IgG. Original magnification: × 630. (C) Electron micrograph of the same antibody-perfused kidney shown in (A) demonstrates multiple small electron-dense deposits in the subepithelial space and slit pores (circles). Original magnification: × 38,000. Abbreviations as in Fig. 3. (From Couser *et al.*, 1978c.)

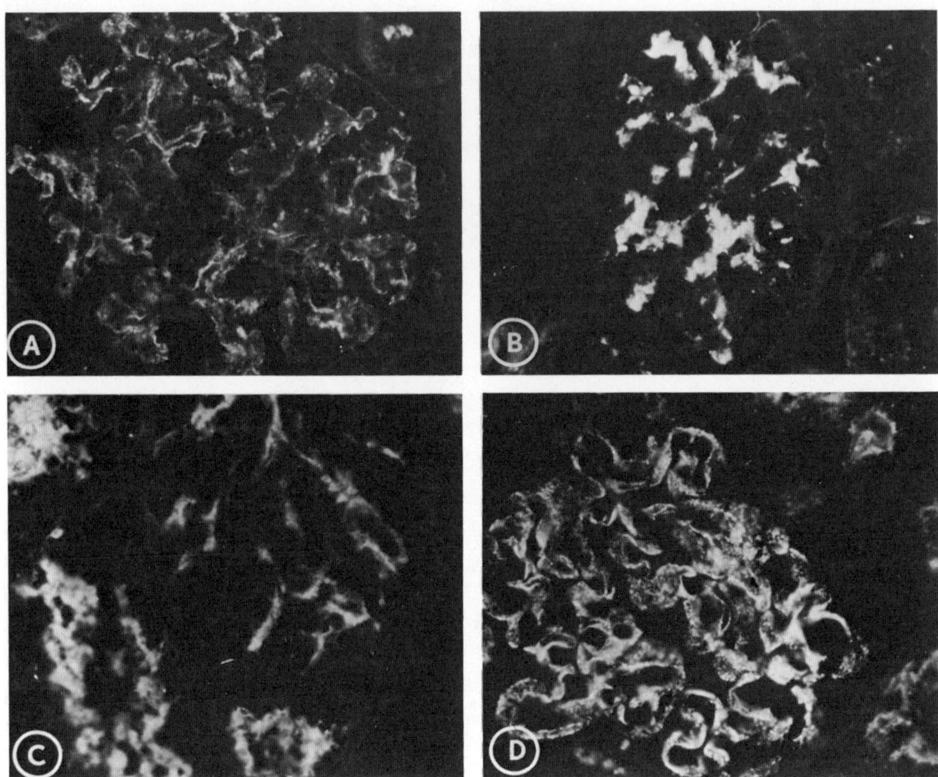

Figure 7. Immunofluorescent photomicrographs from AICN rats unilaterally perfused with PA. (A) IgG on GBM at day 28 in nonperfused right kidney. (B) PA-perfused left kidney at day 28 showing marked reduction in GBM deposits and increased mesangial localization of IgG. (C) Same biopsy as in (B) stained for Fx1A showing absence of deposits on capillary wall and granular staining in the mesangium. (D) Same kidney as in (B) at day 49 showing development of typical membranous deposits of IgG after cessation of proteinuria and disappearance of mesangial deposits. Residual tubular brush border staining is present. Original magnification: all × 450. (From Couser *et al.*, 1978a.)

PHN (Fig. 8). A similar curve is obtained when glomerular deposits are quantitated by isolating and counting glomeruli from each rat. Glomerular deposits consistently represented about 45% of total kidney bound antibody (Salant *et al.*, 1978b). Antibody binding in the subepithelial space occurs immediately. However, unlike NTN where antibody binding is maximal at 10 min and proteinuria occurs immediately (Unanue and Dixon, 1965), in the PHN model antibody continues to deposit for several days and deposits enlarge progressively before a change in glomerular permeability sufficient to induce proteinuria develops at 4–5 days (Fig. 8). At the onset of proteinuria, a proteinuric threshold can be defined from these data (Salant *et al.*, 1978b) which is about 100 μg IgG/kidney or 45 μg glomerular bound IgG/kidney, a figure comparable to that of about 100 μg IgG/kidney reported as the proteinuric threshold for anti-GBM antibody in the rat by Unanue and Dixon (1965).

3.5. Role of Complement in Proteinuria in PHN

Subepithelial antibody deposits in PHN fix autologous and heterologous C3 *in vivo* and *in vitro*. When cobra venom factor is injected daily to deplete C3 to less than 10% of normal values starting before anti-Fx1A injection and for 5 days thereafter, C3 deposition *in vivo* is abolished. Complement depletion does not alter the quantity of ^{125}I-labeled antibody deposited in glomeruli at 5 days compared to controls (Fig. 9). However, despite deposition of nephritogenic quantities of antibody, the depletion of C3 totally prevents development of proteinuria at 5 days (Fig. 9). Moreover, when PHN is induced by injection of equimolar amounts of the $F(ab')_2$ portion of antibody IgG, epimembranous deposits of $F(ab')_2$ are readily demonstrable by immunofluorescence, but no rat C3 is fixed and no proteinuria occurs at 5 days. Of note is the finding that rats injected with $F(ab)_2$ fragments of anti-Fx1A IgG manifest an initial proteinuria on day 1 (13 ± 6 mg/day, normal 3 ± 2 mg/day) which is not seen when whole IgG antibody is administered. This proteinuria in 95+% endogenous albumin and thus resembles the proteinuria induced transiently by guinea pig nephrotoxic antibody (Couser *et al.*, 1977).

3.6. Role of Neutrophils (PMNs) in Proteinuria in PHN

Careful glomerular PMN counts in biopsies obtained from 10 min to 5 days after anti-Fx1A administration to normal rats have never revealed more

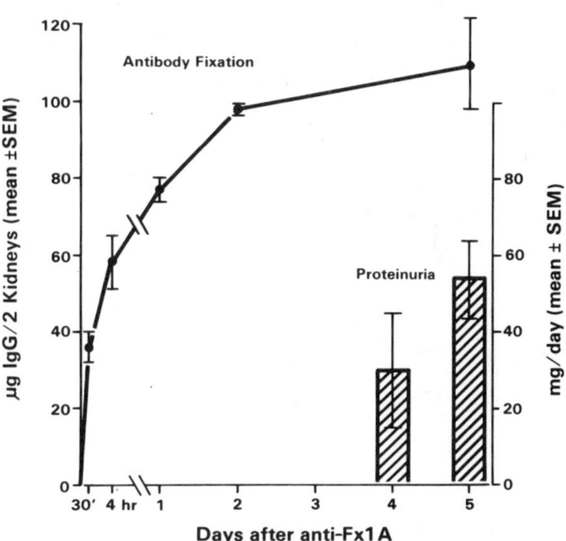

Figure 8. Time course of kidney uptake of anti-Fx1A and development of proteinuria in rats with PHN induced with antibody radiolabeled with ^{125}I.

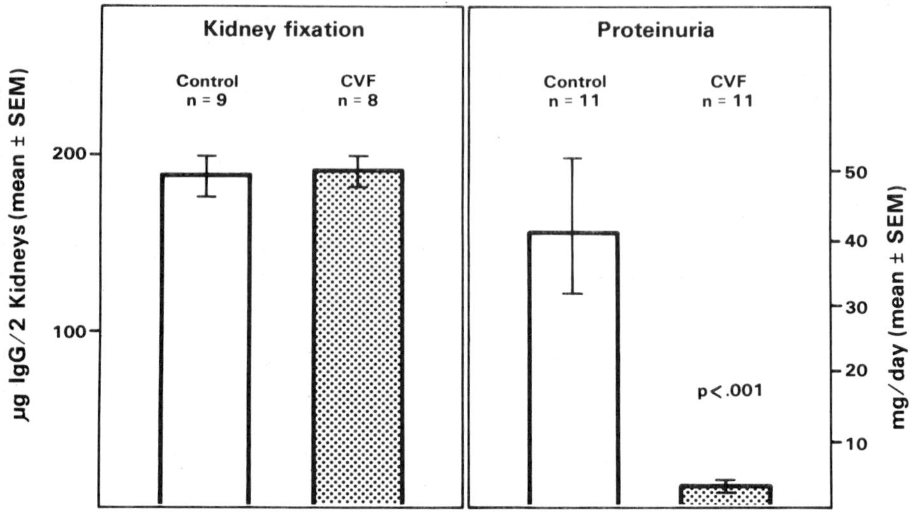

Figure 9. Kidney fixation of ^{125}I-labeled antibody and urine protein excretion 5 days after anti-Fx1A administration in normal rats (open bars) and rats depleted of C3–C9 with cobra venom factor (CVF) for 5 days (stippled bars).

than 1 PMN per 10 glomeruli at any time prior to or during the course of proteinuria. When selective PMN depletion is induced by repeated administration of rabbit antibody to rat PMNs, proteinuria of equal severity developed in 2 of 3 rats consistently depleted to less than 500 PMNs/mm^3 for 5 days, in 3 of 5 rats depleted to less than 500 PMNs/mm^3 for 4 of the 5 days, and in 6 of 8 control rats with normal PMN counts of over 1300/mm^3 (Table 2) (Salant *et al.*, 1978a).

3.7. Mechanisms of Proteinuria in AICN

Histochemical studies in AICN have shown no reduction in glomerular affinity for polycationic stains before or during development of proteinuria in AICN, although some reduced staining was seen after 4–6 weeks of sustained heavy proteinuria (Couser *et al.*, 1976). Similar studies in the PHN model have shown no reduction in colloidal iron staining in heavily proteinuric animals at 5 days. Recent physiologic studies, done in collaboration with Rennke and co-workers, have measured the fractional clearances, compared

Table 2. Effects of PMN Depletion on Proteinuria in PHN

Group	PMN counts	Proteinuric at 5 days	Urine protein (mg/day) (mean ± S.E.M.)
Controls	> 1300/mm^3	6/8	18 ± 7
Partial PMN depletion[a]	< 500/mm^3	3/5	12 ± 4
PMN depleted	< 500/mm^3	2/3	14 ± 6

[a] PMN counts > 500/mm^3 for 1 or more of 5 days after anti-Fx1A injection.

to inulin, of a positively charged, neutral, and negatively charged protein molecule, horseradish peroxidase (HRP), in proteinuric AICN rats. HRP was chemically modified to produce tracers with isoelectric points of about 9, 7.4, and less than 4, respectively, without significant alteration in the molecular radius of about 30 Å or molecular weight of about 40,000 (Rennke *et al.*, 1978b). If proteinuria in AICN resulted from a reduction in net negative charge on the capillary wall, as shown in late NTN (Bennett *et al.*, 1976) and PA nephrosis (Bohrer *et al.*, 1977), an increase in fractional clearance of negatively charged HRP and a decrease in fractional clearance of positively charged HRP would have been anticipated. Instead, these studies demonstrated an increase in fractional clearance of all three tracers compared to controls, a finding consistent with the hypothesis that the complement-dependent mechanism of glomerular injury in these models induces proteinuria primarily by altering the sieving properties rather than the negatively charged components of the glomerular capillary wall (Rennke *et al.*, 1978a).

4. Summary

Two models of experimental glomerulonephritis induced by antibodies to renal antigens are both characterized by diffuse deposition of specific IgG antibody along the glomerular capillary walls in a linear (guinea pig NTN) or finely granular (PHN) pattern. In both models, antibody deposits induce a marked increase in glomerular permeability to albumin but do not result in any histologic changes in the glomerulus or accumulation of PMNs or mononuclear cells, and no structural damage to the proximal layers of the glomerular filter is demonstrable.

In the guinea pig NTN model, antibody binding and proteinuria occur immediately. Proteinuria occurs independently of the complement–neutrophil system. Some evidence for a reduction in negative charge on the capillary wall has been obtained, but this is a late and inconsistent finding. Therefore, the mechanism of proteinuria induced by initial IgG binding to GBM antigens alone is still undefined.

In the experimental membranous nephropathy models in rats induced by antibody to renal tubular antigens, antibody deposits develop slowly and proteinuria occurs when a proteinuric threshold is finally reached days to weeks later. These subepithelial deposits, like antibody deposits in NTN, apparently form *in situ* and then enlarge through a poorly understood mechanism that may be initiated by antibody binding to fixed or planted glomerular antigens. The proteinuria which follows is complement-dependent but PMN-independent, thus demonstrating an apparently new role for the complement system in mediating glomerular injury. Current evidence favors a change in sieving properties rather than charge characteristics of the glomerular capillary wall in the genesis of proteinuria in the *in situ* immune complex nephropathy models.

5. *Brief Overview—Immunologic Mechanisms of Proteinuria*

Currently established consequences of antikidney antibody binding to the glomerular capillary wall are summarized schematically in Fig. 10. Nephritogenic quantities of anti-GBM antibody may bind in a linear pattern to GBM and induce no apparent glomerular injury (Henson, 1971; Couser *et al.*, 1973) even when C3 is deposited (Kobayashi *et al.*, 1973). This finding is similar to that reported when antibody to GBM collagen alone is injected (Rothbard and Watson, 1959). Proteinuria may be PMN-dependent but complement-independent as reported in the autologous phase of NTN in rabbits (Naish *et al.*, 1975; Thompson *et al.*, 1976). More commonly, nephrotoxic antibody induces proteinuria and glomerular inflammation by mechanisms that are both complement- and PMN-dependent (Unanue and Dixon, 1965; Cochrane *et al.*, 1965; Hawkins and Cochrane, 1968; Cochrane, 1969). It is now clear that anti-GBM antibody alone also can effect a marked increase in glomerular permeability independently of the complement–neutrophil system and without causing glomerular inflammation (Couser *et al.*, 1973; Simpson *et al.*, 1975; Couser *et al.*, 1977). Finally, a similar noninflammatory glomerular lesion associated with heavy proteinuria is

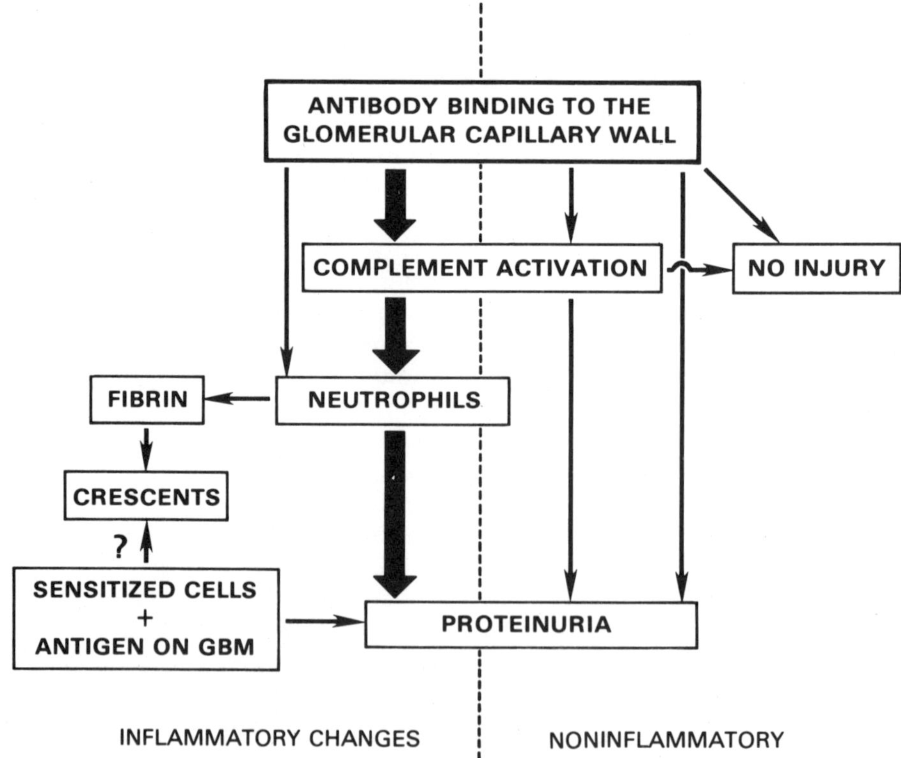

Figure 10. Currently established immunologic mechanisms of proteinuria.

induced by glomerular subepithelial deposition of antibody to rat tubular antigen and C3. Proteinuria in this lesion is complement-dependent but PMN-independent and apparently reflects a new role for the complement system in mediating noninflammatory glomerular injury (Salant *et al.*, 1978a). In addition to these various proteinuric glomerular lesions induced by antibody deposition, evidence presented here for the first time by Unanue now suggests that in addition to the apparent role of circulating mononuclear cells in crescent formation, sensitized T cells, reacting with specific antigens on the GBM, may also increase glomerular permeability.

Much work remains to be done to define how proteinuria is induced by these various immunologic events and to correlate these disease mechanisms with changes in the physiologic and structural determinants of glomerular permselectivity defined by other studies. Further clarification of the molecular basis of proteinuria induced by antikidney antibodies should prove relevant to understanding the pathogenesis of the nephrotic syndrome seen in a variety of noninflammatory human renal diseases.

ACKNOWLEDGMENTS. The authors are grateful to Christine Darby, Vita Sliogeris, Neva Capparell, Mary Moran, and Audrey Levine for expert technical assistance and to Lisa Medoff for secretarial support in preparation of the manuscript.

References

Abrass, C. K., Border, W. A., and Glassock, R. J., 1977, Demonstration of circulating immune complexes in autologous immune complex nephritis in rats, *Kidney Int.* **12:**508 (abstract).

Belok, S., Steinmuller, D. R., Salant, D. J., Darby, C., Stilmant, M. M., and Couser, W. G., 1977, Determinants of glomerular localization of subepithelial immune deposits, *Kidney Int.* **2:**510 (abstract).

Bennett, C. M., Glassock, R. J., Chang, R. L. S., Deen, W. M., Robertson, C. R., and Brenner, B. M., 1976, Permselectivity of the glomerular capillary wall: Studies of experimental glomerulonephritis in the rat using dextran sulfate, *J. Clin. Invest.* **57:**1287.

Bohrer, M. P., Baylis, C., Robertson, C. R., and Brenner, B. M., 1977, Mechanisms of puromycin-induced defects in the transglomerular passage of water and macromolecules, *J. Clin. Invest.* **60:**152.

Brenner, B. M., Hostetter, T. H., and Humes, H. D., 1978, Molecular basis of proteinuria of glomerular origin, *N. Engl. J. Med.* **298:**836.

Cochrane, C. G., 1969, Mediation of immunologic glomerular injury, *Transplant. Proc.* **1:**949.

Cochrane, C. G., Unanue, E., and Dixon, F. J., 1965, A role of polymorphonuclear leukocytes and complement in nephrotoxic nephritis, *J. Exp. Med.* **122:**99.

Couser, W. G., Stilmant, M. M., and Lewis, E. J. 1973. Experimental glomerulonephritis in the guinea pig. I. Glomerular lesions associated with anti-glomerular basement membrane antibody deposits, *Lab. Invest.* **29:**236.

Couser, W. G., Stilmant, M. M., and Darby, C., 1976, Autologous immune complex nephropathy. I. Sequential study of immune complex deposition, ultrastructural changes, proteinuria and alterations in glomerular sialoprotein, *Lab. Invest.* **34:**23.

Couser, W. G., Stilmant, M. M., and Jermanovich, N. B., 1977, Complement-independent nephrotoxic nephritis in the guinea pig, *Kidney Int.* **11:**170.

Couser, W. G., Hoyer, J. R., Stilmant, M. M., Jermanovich, N. B., and Belok, S., 1978a, The effect of aminonucleoside nephrosis on subepithelial immune complex localization in autologous immune complex nephropathy in rats, *J. Clin. Invest.* **61:**561.

Couser, W. G., Salant, D. J., Stilmant, M. M., Arbeit, L. A., and Darby, C., 1978b, The effect of aminonucleoside of puromycin and nephrotoxic serum on subepithelial immune deposits in "in situ" immune complex glomerulonephropathy, Abstracts of the American Society of Nephrology, 1978, p. 75A.

Couser, W. G., Steinmuller, D. R., Stilmant, M. M., Salant, D. J., and Lowenstein, L. M., 1978c, Experimental glomerulonephritis in the isolated perfused rat kidney, *J. Clin. Invest.* **62:**1275.

Edgington, T. S., Glassock, R. J., and Dixon, F. J., 1967, Autologous immune complex pathogenesis of experimental allergic glomerulonephritis, *Science* **155:**1432.

Edgington, T. S., Glassock, R. J., and Dixon, F. J., 1968, Autologous immune complex nephritis induced with renal tubular antigen. I. Identification and isolation of the pathogenetic antigen, *J. Exp. Med.* **127:**555.

Hawkins, D., and Cochrane, C. G., 1968, Glomerular basement membrane damage in immunological glomerulonephritis, *Immunology* **14:**665.

Henson, P. M., 1971, Release of biologically active constituents from blood cells and its role in antibody mediated tissue injury, in: *Progress in Immunology* (B. Amos, ed.), pp. 155–171, Academic Press, New York.

Kobayashi, Y., Shigematsu, H., and Tada, T., 1973, Nephritogenic properties of nephrotoxic guinea pig antibodies. I. Glomerulonephritis induced by guinea pig IgG antibody in rats, *Virchows Arch. Path. Anat.* **14:**259.

Kuhn, K., Ryan, G. C., Hein, S. J., Galoske, R. G., and Karnovsky, M. J., 1977, An ultrastructural study of the mechanism of proteinuria in rat nephrotoxic nephritis, *Lab. Invest.* **36:**375.

Naish, P. F., Thompson, N. M., Simpson, I. J., and Peters, D. K., 1975, The role of polymorphonuclear leucocytes in the autologous phase of nephrotoxic nephritis, *Clin. Exp. Immunol.* **22:**102.

Rennke, H. G., and Venkatachalam, M. A., 1977, Structural determinants of glomerular permselectivity, *Fed. Proc.* **36:**3619.

Rennke, H. G., Couser, W. G., Patel, Y., and Venkatachalam, M. A., 1978a, Membranous nephropathy: Fractional clearances of anionic, neutral and cationic horseradish peroxidase in Lewis rats with autologous immune complex nephritis, Abstracts of the Seventh International Congress of Nephrology, Montreal, 1978,

Rennke, H. G., Patel, Y., and Venkatachalam, M. A., 1978b, Glomerular filtration of proteins: Clearance of anionic, neutral and cationic horseradish peroxidase in the rat, *Kidney Int.* **13:**324.

Rothbard, S., and Watson, R. F., 1959, Renal glomerular lesions induced by rabbit anti-rat collagen serum in rats prepared with adjuvant, *J. Exp. Med.* **109:**633.

Salant, D. J., Belok, S., Stilmant, M. M., and Couser, W. G., 1978a, A new role for complement in experimental glomerulonephritis, *Clin. Res.* **26:**384.

Salant, D. J., Darby, C., and Couser, W. G., 1978b, A quantitative analysis of subepithelial immune deposits in "in situ" immune complex glomerulonephropathy, Abstracts of the American Society of Nephrology, 1978, p. 83A.

Simpson, I. J., Amos, N., Evans, D. J., Thompson, N. M., and Peters, D. K., 1975, Guinea pig nephrotoxic nephritis. I. The role of complement and polymorphonuclear leukocytes and the effect of antibody subclass and fragments in the heterologous phase, *Clin. Exp. Immunol.* **19:**499.

Thompson, N. M., Naish, P. F., Simpson, I. F., and Peters, D. K. 1976, The role of C3 in the autologous phase of nephrotoxic nephritis, *Clin. Exp. Immunol.* **24:**464.

Trevillian, P., and Cameron, J. S., 1978, Interaction of anti-GBM antibody and immune complexes in rabbits, *Kidney Int.* **14:**295 (abstract).

Unanue, E. R., and Dixon, F. J., 1965, Experimental glomerulonephritis. V. Studies on the interaction of nephrotoxic antibodies with tissues of the rat, *J. Exp. Med.* **121:**697.

Unanue, E., and Dixon, F. J., 1969, Experimental glomerulonephritis. IV. Participation of complement in nephrotoxic nephritis, *J. Exp. Med.* **119:**965.

Van Damme, B. J. C., Fleuren, G. J., Bakker, W. W., Vernier, R. L., and Hoedemaeker, P. J., 1978, Experimental glomerulonephritis in the rat induced by antibodies directed against tubular antigens. V. Fixed glomerular antigens in the pathogenesis of heterologous immune complex glomerulonephritis, *Lab. Invest.* **38:**502.

24

The Pathogenesis of Autologous Immune Complex Glomerulonephritis in Rats

Christine K. Abrass, Wayne A. Border, and Richard J. Glassock

1. Introduction

Over 11 years has elapsed since the term *autologous immune complex nephritis* (AICN) was initially proposed to describe the pathogenetic mechanisms operative in an experimental membranous glomerulopathy induced in rats by *active* immunization with renal tubular epithelial (RTE) antigens in Freund's complete adjuvant. In this experimental model, which was originally described by Heymann and co-workers (Heymann *et al.*, 1959), it was envisaged that circulating immune complexes (CIC) composed of autoantibodies to a specific proximal RTE antigen (designated RTE α_5) and autologous RTE α_5 deposited continuously in the glomerular capillaries (Edgington *et al.*, 1967a). These CIC ultimately localized in the subepithelial space and provoked the typical morphologic and clinical features of membranous glomerulopathy including granular deposits of immunoglobulin and subepithelial electron-dense deposits in glomeruli (Glassock *et al.*, 1968). Since then, a number of additional *autologous* antigen–antibody systems capable of evoking glomerular injury have been described in both animals and man (Naruse *et al.*, 1973; Couser *et al.*, 1974; O'Regan *et al.*, 1976).

The recent development of a model of glomerular disease induced by *passive* administration of *heterologous* anti-RTE antibodies to otherwise normal animals has challenged the traditional concepts concerning the actively

---

Christine K. Abrass, Wayne A. Border, and Richard J. Glassock · Division of Nephrology and Hypertension, Los Angeles County Harbor/UCLA Medical Center, Torrance, California 90502.
Dr. Abrass was supported as a Fellow of The National Kidney Foundation.

induced model of AICN (Barabas *et al.*, 1974; Feenstra *et al.*, 1975). Studies of the heterologous antibody-induced model (passive Heymann nephritis, PHN) have suggested that immune complexes are formed instead *in situ* in the subepithelial space as circulating anti-RTE antibody reacts with fixed, RTE-like antigen native to some component of the glomerular capillary wall (Van Damme *et al.*, 1978). Thus, the reaction of passively administered heterologous anti-RTE antibody with the native RTE-like glomerular antigen can be viewed in the same context as classical nephrotoxic serum nephritis (NSN) induced by the passive administration of heterologous antibody to the major glomerular basement membrane (GBM) glycopeptide, except that the antigen in the case of PHN is *not* uniformly distributed along the capillary wall. Consequently, the antibody is deposited in a discontinuous fashion along the GBM rather than the smooth linear pattern characteristically seen in NSN (Hammer and Dixon, 1963). An *autologous* phase of PHN, analogous in most respects to the autologous phase of NSN, also has been clearly delineated by Van Es *et al.* (1977).

Although circulating antibody to RTE antigens clearly develops in the actively immunized rat with AICN, it remains controversial whether *in situ* formation of immune complexes or glomerular localization of CIC is responsible primarily for the glomerular lesions observed in AICN.

The evidence favoring these two alternative views of pathogenesis are summarized below.

1. *Evidence favoring a CIC pathogenesis for AICN.* Eluates of diseased glomeruli and circulating autoantibody from rats with AICN react with isologous proximal RTE antigens but not with normal glomeruli *in vitro*, by indirect immunofluorescent methods (Grupe and Kaplan, 1969). RTE antigen (RTE α_5) is present in the circulation and its concentration diminishes as the glomerular disease develops (Glassock *et al.*, 1968; Naruse *et al.*, 1973). Species-specific RTE antigen accumulates in the glomerular immunoglobulin deposits with time following immunization (Edgington *et al.*, 1967a). Similar morphologic findings are found in other spontaneous and experimentally induced models of glomerular disease believed to be caused by the deposition of CIC (Naruse *et al.*, 1973; Couser *et al.*, 1974; O'Regan *et al.*, 1976).

2. *Evidence which is ambiguous with respect to pathogenetic mechanism.* Granular deposits of IgG, complement components, and RTE antigens are found in diseased glomeruli (Glassock *et al.*, 1968). The disease recurs in renal isografts (Edgington *et al.*, 1969). The disease may be transferred by lymphoid cells and by parabiosis (Glassock *et al.*, 1969). The interpretation of reports (Barabas *et al.*, 1974; Sugisaki *et al.*, 1973) that the disease may be transferred by serum harvested from diseased animals is complicated by the recent observations of Hall *et al.* (1977) that passively administered homologous autoantibody may facilitate the development of autoantibodies on the part of the recipient animal. Finaly, the pattern of immunoglobulin deposition seen in diseased animals is drastically altered by the concomitant induction of heavy proteinuria due to the administration of aminonucleoside of puromycin (Couser *et al.*, 1978a).

3. *Evidence favoring in situ immune complex formation.* Heterologous antibody to RTE binds to glomeruli in a discontinuous pattern in the subepithelial space *in vivo* in the absence of circulating RTE (Couser *et al.*, 1978b). Heterologous antibody to RTE binds *in vitro* to GBM as detected after neuraminidase treatment of the kidney section substrate (Van Damme *et al.*, 1978). Circulating antibody to RTE in actively induced Heymann nephritis correlates with the appearance of glomerular deposits of immunoglobulins (Grupe and Kaplan, 1969). Hoedemaeker and colleagues recently reported that eluates of diseased kidneys harvested from animals with AICN bind to normal glomeruli *in vivo* using the immunoperoxidase method. This has not been confirmed by all investigators using *in vitro* methodology.

One additional piece of evidence, and one which would help to distinguish the importance of the circulating versus *in situ* immune complex mechanism, would be the demonstration of CIC in animals with actively induced disease. Efforts to identify and characterize CIC in the actively induced model of AICN have been made. Two questions were asked in these studies: (1) What is the prevalence of CIC in AICN? and (2) if present, what is the immunochemical composition of CIC?

2. Materials and Methods

Kidneys from normal Sprague–Dawley rats (Microbiological Associates) were used to prepare RTE antigens (as fraction Fx1A) according to previously described methods (Edgington *et al.*, 1967b). A crude, low-speed homogenate was prepared from the Sprague–Dawley livers and used as a liver antigen. Crystalline bovine serum albumin (BSA) was purchased from a commercial laboratory (Miles).

3. Experimental Groups

3.1. Immunizations

Male Lewis rats (Microbiological Associates) weighing 200–250 g were used exclusively. Antigens were emulsified in Freund's complete adjuvant (FCA) containing 4 mg *Mycobacterium tuberculosis* H37 Ra/ml adjuvant (Difco). Animals were immunized once with 0.25 ml divided into each rear footpad.

Five groups, 10 animals each, were studied. Group I received 10 mg Fx1A in FCA; Group II received FCA only; Group III received 10 mg liver homogenate in FCA; Group IV received 10 mg BSA in FCA; Group V received 1 mg Fx1A in FCA.

3.2. Experimental Procedure

Prior to and at weekly intervals for 14 weeks, 24-hr urine samples and 1 to 1.5 ml of blood from the tail vein was collected in all animals. Urine was analyzed for protein by the Kingsbury–Clark method (1926). Normal Lewis rats excrete < 5.6 mg/day by this method. Blood was allowed to clot at room temperature and the sera separated by centrifugation and stored at −70°C.

3.3. Circulating Antibody to RTE

Circulating antibody to RTE was determined by indirect immunofluorescence using twofold dilutions of test sera and fluorescein-conjugated rabbit anti-rat IgG (Cappel Laboratories, Cochranville, Pa.) and normal Lewis rat kidney as the substrate. Antibody titer was defined as the highest dilution which exhibited positive immunofluorescence on the proximal renal tubule of the rat kidney. Antibody to liver antigens was sought by similar techniques using normal Lewis rat liver as the substrate. Antibody to BSA was estimated semiquantitatively by double diffusion in agarose gels using crystalline BSA at concentrations ranging from 0.01 to 1.0 mg/ml as the antigen.

3.4. Analysis of CIC

CIC were determined in duplicate on all sera of Groups I, II, III, and IV by previously reported techniques of fluid-phase (Nydegger *et al.*, 1974) and solid-phase Clq binding (Hay *et al.*, 1976), modified for measurement of rat IgG-containing immune complexes. Group V animals were studied only with the fluid-phase Clq binding assay. Samples were selected for assay on any given day on a random basis. The Clq utilized for both assays was isolated from fresh normal human serum (NHS) by the method of Yonemasu and Stroud (1971). Aggregated rat IgG (ARG) was prepared by heating 5 ml of 2% rat IgG (Miles Laboratories) in phosphate-buffered saline (PBS) at 63°C for 30 min. Insoluble aggregates were removed by centrifugation and the preparation stored in small aliquots at −70°C. Hyperimmune rabbit anti-rat IgG was prepared by repeated immunization of New Zealand rabbits with purified rat IgG and FCA. Proteins were made radioactive with ^{125}I using the chloramine-T method (McConahey and Dixon, 1966). Gelatin (0.1%) was substituted for BSA in all solutions used for CIC detection in the sera of rats immunized with BSA in FCA.

The fluid-phase Clq binding assay (FClq) was modified from the method of Nydegger *et al.* (1974), in which precipitation of the [^{125}I]-Clq bound to CIC was carried out at 2.5% polyethylene glycol (PEG). The means of duplicates were calculated as a percent of maximum binding and expressed as μg/ml ARG equivalents. The lower limit of detection in the FClq was 30 μg/ml ARG in normal rat serum. Intra- and interassay coefficients of variation were 3.6 and 8.1%, respectively.

The solid-phase Clq binding assay (SClq) was modified from the method of Hay *et al.* (1976). Freshly isolated human Clq was incubated with polystyrene tubes which were then washed with 1% BSA in PBS or 0.1% gelatin in PBS. Following incubation of tubes with test serum or ARG, the tubes were washed and ^{125}I-labeled rabbit anti-rat IgG was used to indicate the extent of binding of rat IgG to the Clq-coated tubes. The means of duplicates were calculated as the percent maximum binding and expressed as μg/ml ARG equivalents in normal rat serum. The lower limit of detection was 5 μg/ml ARG in normal rat serum. Intra- and interassay coefficients of variation were 2.3 and 5.2%, respectively.

3.5. *Histology and Immunofluorescene*

Renal cortex was obtained at sacrifice, 14 weeks after initial immunization, and samples were studied by light microscopy and immunofluorescence using fluorescein-conjugated anti-rat IgG (Cappell Laboratories).

3.6. *Size Characteristics of CIC*

Gradient ultracentrifugation of the Clq-reactive material was carried out in linear 10–40% sucrose density gradients centrifuged at 180,000 g for 20 hr at 4°C. One hundred nanograms of[^{125}I]-Clq in 100 μl of 1% BSA in Veronal-buffered saline was added to 200 μl of test serum and the mixture incubated for 30 min followed by the ultracentrifugation run. Sedimentation markers included ^{131}I-labeled BSA, and human thyroglobulin (courtesy of Dr. Gildon Beall). Heavily sedimenting ^{125}I-containing fractions were pooled, concentrated, and analyzed for rat IgG by double diffusion in agarose gels using rabbit anti-rat IgG.

3.7. *Detection of RTE Antigens in CIC*

The PEG precipitate of an FClq-positive serum from an RTE-immunized animal in Group I, 10 weeks following immunization, and a PEG precipitate from an animal immunized with FCA alone from Group II were redissolved in PBS and emulsified in FCA. Each of two New Zealand White rabbits were immunized with each of the redissolved PEG precipitates at two intervals 1 week apart. The animals were bled on the seventh day following the second immunization. The antibody binding characteristics of these antisera were evaluated by indirect immunofluorescence using *in vitro* complement fixation (Weir, 1973), utilizing fresh NHS as the source of complement, fluorescein-conjugated goat anti-human C3 (Meloy Laboratories), and normal Lewis rat kidney as the substrate. Controls including direct immunofluorescence with fluorescein-conjugated anti-human C3, indirect immunofluorescence with NHS, normal rabbit serum, normal rat serum, and the rabbit antisera to the PEG precipitates absorbed with normal rat serum, liver homogenate, rat GBM, and rat RTE antigens.

3.8. *Statistical Analysis*

The frequency of positive assay for CIC among experimental and control animals was compared by χ^2 analysis. The frequency of positive results per animal was compared by Student's *t* test for unpaired data. The temporal pattern of the positivity was compared by the sign test. Correlation between assays was analyzed by χ^2.

4. Results

4.1. Documentation of Nephritis

All animals in Groups I and V demonstrated typical granular deposits of rat IgG along the glomerular capillary wall at the time of sacrifice. No animals in Groups II, III, and IV had similar rat IgG deposits at sacrifice. Abnormal proteinuria (> 5.7 mg/day) developed in 9 of the 10 animals in Group I, 10 of 10 in Group V, and 0 of 10 in Groups II, III, and IV.

4.2. Circulating Antibody Studies

A total of 130 individual serum samples were examined in each group. All animals in Groups I and V developed circulating antibody to RTE as demonstrated by indirect immunofluorescence. No animals in Groups II, III, and IV developed anti-RTE antibody. Circulating anti-RTE antibody in animals from Groups I and V showed no reaction with normal glomeruli in any dilution (neat to 1:512) by indirect immunofluorescence. Circulating anti-RTE antibody was first detected at day 7 and peak titers (1:32–1:256) were observed at 49–63 days, thereafter slowly declining. Weakly reactive antinuclear antibody (titer 1:4) was found in 0 of 130 sera in Group I, 7 of 130 in Group II, 11 of 130 in Group III, 0 of 130 in Group IV, and 0 of 130 in Group V animals. Low levels of precipitating antibody to BSA were detected in all animals in Group IV at 14 days and peak antibody levels were noted at 8–10 weeks following immunization. No antibody to liver antigens was detectable in Group III by indirect immunofluorescence.

4.3. CIC

The preimmune sera from normal Lewis rats were examined in FClq and SClq binding assays. The mean value of binding activity for FClq was 12.0 ± 8.5% (3 S.D.) and for SClq, 32.8 ± 10.7% (3 S.D.). Thus, the upper limit of normal for FClq was established at 20.5% of maximum bound and was equivalent to 100 μg/ml ARG equivalents. The upper limit of normal for SClq was established at 53.2% of maximum bound and was equivalent to 11 μg/ml ARG equivalents.

Table 1 summarizes the prevalence of CIC as detected by FClq and SClq. Clq-reactive immune complexes were more prevalent in sera from Group I as compared to Group III (χ^2 7.88, $p < 0.005$) and Group II (χ^2 12.60, $p < 0.01$). Further, there was no decrease in the prevalence of positive samples in the FClq in Group V which were immunized with 1/10th the antigen dose of Group I. All animals in Group IV developed positive serum

Table 1. Circulating Immune Complexes in Autologous Immune Complex Nephritis in Rats

		Group				
	(*n*)	I FCA + Fx1A (10 mg)	II FCA	III FCA + liver (10 mg)	IV FCA + BSA (10 mg)	V FCA + Fx1A (1 mg)
Animals positive	10	10	8	6	10	10
Samples positive						
FCl$_q$[a]	120	25	13	20	21	35
SCI$_q$[b]	120	29	15	5	87	41
Any	120	48[c]	27	22	100	64
Mean of frequency of positivity score		4.8[c]	2.7	2.2	10.0	6.4

[a] Fluid-phase C1q assay.
[b] Solid-phase C1q assay.
[c] Different from FCA control, $p < 0.01$.

samples for FClq and served as an internal control group. There were no correlations found between the results in the FClq and SClq assays in Groups I, II, III, and IV.

The level of Clq binding activity varied among the groups and is summarized in Fig. 1. In Group I the levels of Clq-reactive material measured by the FClq assay varied from barely above the upper limits of normal to over 400 μg/ml ARG equivalents. The majority of positive samples (20 of 25 in FClq and 23 of 30 in SClq) ranged from 100 to 200 μg/ml ARG equivalents.

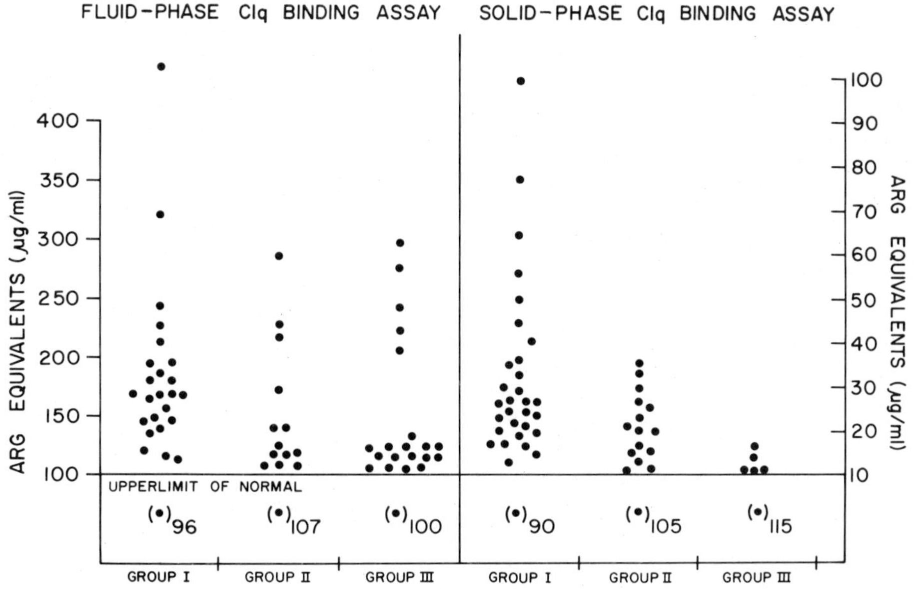

Figure 1. Range of positivity in both assays for all samples in Groups I, II, and III plotted as μg/ml ARG equivalents. $(\cdot)_n$ denotes number in each group with normal values in each assay.

There was no difference in the level of Clq-reactive materials found in Groups I, II, and III.

Serum samples positive for Clq-reactive material in Groups II and III occurred in a random pattern versus time following immunization. However, the positive serum samples found in Groups I, V, and IV demonstrated a temporal relationship to the level of circulating antibody to RTE and BSA, respectively. In Group I, positive serum assays for FClq clustered early following immunization when antibody levels were rising and later when antibody levels were falling. On the other hand, positive SClq samples clustered in the periods associated with peak titers of circulating antibody to RTE.

4.4. *Characteristics of the Clq-Reactive Material*

Sucrose density ultracentrifugation of selected sera positive in the CIC assays revealed that Clq-reactive material in a Group I animal, 49 days

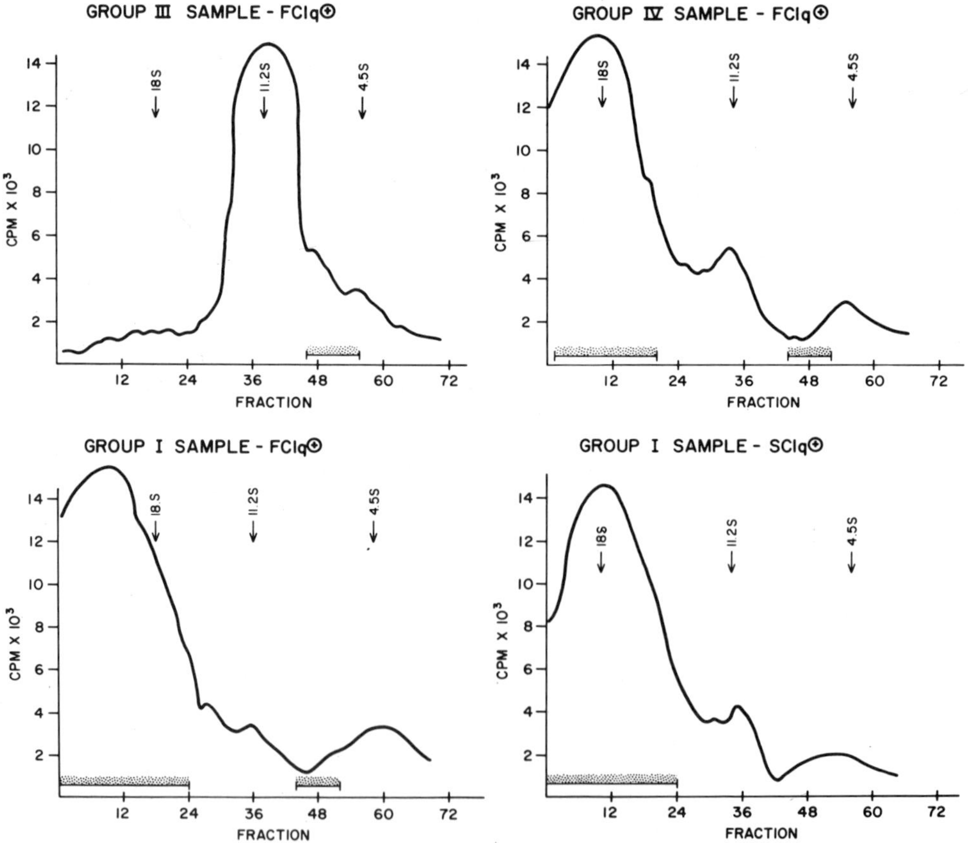

Figure 2. Patterns of sucrose gradient ultracentrifugation analysis. Amount of [^{125}I]-Clq (expressed as cpm $\times$ 10^3) plotted as a function of fraction number. Cross-hatched area denotes fractions which contained rat IgG.

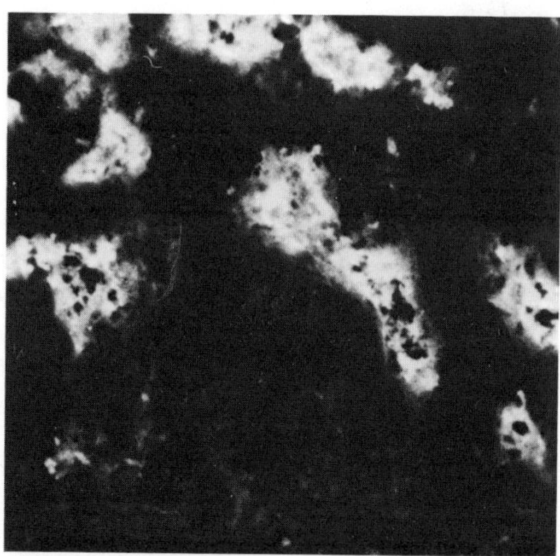

Figure 3. Positive staining of the brush border of the proximal renal tubule with rabbit anti-PEG precipitate (Group I) by indirect immunofluorescence with *in vitro* complement fixation. × 312.

postimmunization, had a sedimentation coefficient of 14–23 S with major peaks in the 20 S range (Fig. 2). This heavily sedimenting material also contained rat IgG. No such heavily sedimenting peaks of Clq-reactive material could be found in an FClq-positive serum examined from an animal from Group II, whereas heavily sedimenting material greater than 19 S containing rat IgG could be found readily in Group IV animals 21 days following immunization with BSA in FCA.

4.5. Demonstration of RTE Antigens in CIC

The rabbit antiserum developed against a PEG precipitate of a Clq-reactive material in a rat from Group I, 10 weeks following immunization, contained antibody to RTE as revealed by indirect immunofluorescence using *in vitro* complement fixation (Fig. 3). No binding to normal glomeruli was observed. The pattern of binding was the same as that observed with homologous rat anti-rat RTE. All controls were negative, and the anti-RTE reactivity could be absorbed completely with insoluble rat Fx1A, but not normal rat serum, rat liver, or rat GBM (Table 2). No such reactivity could

Table 2. Antibodies to PEG Precipitates Induced in Rabbits: Immunofluorescence Demonstration of Antibody Binding

	Substance used for absorption				
	Unabsorbed	GBM	Fx1A	Liver	Normal rat serum
Normal rat serum	–	–	–	–	–
Rabbit anti-rat Fx1A	+	+	–	+	+
Rabbit-anti-PEG ppt.	+	+	–	+	+

be demonstrated in rabbit serum raised against the PEG precipitate from a control animal in Group II.

5. Discussion

Rats with actively induced AICN develop circulating Clq-reactive material of a macromolecular nature which contains rat IgG. This material has been demonstrated by two different assays. Using a combination of two assays, about 40% of samples were positive. Control animals immunized with FCA alone or in combination with liver homogenate but without nephritis or glomerular deposits of autologous IgG also developed C1q-binding material, but significantly less frequent than in the RTE-immunized animals. The Clq-reactive material in the control groups is of unknown composition and could not be demonstrated to be of macromolecular nature or contain rat IgG. There was no correlation of the FClq and SClq assays among the experimental groups. A pattern of assay positivity that was related to the time postimmunization and the levels of circulating antibody was apparent. It is possible that these observations reflect changing relationships of free antibody and available antigen. The FClq assay is more sensitive in detecting CIC formed in mild antigen excess, whereas the SClq may be more sensitive in detecting CIC formed in slight antibody excess.

The Clq-reactive material found in an actively immunized rat with AICN contained an RTE antigen and probably represented a CIC. The design of these experiments does not permit a definitive conclusion regarding the autologous or exogenous source of the antigen in these CIC, but since the prevalence of CIC was not greatly modified by a log difference in the dose of immunizing antigens, an autologous source is suggested. The inability to detect CIC in up to 60% of animals with AICN is unexplained but may reflect the relatively low levels of CIC attained and the low sensitivity of the assays used. The circulating anti-RTE autoantibody found in actively induced disease shows no reactivity with normal isologous glomerular capillary wall *in vitro*, at least by indirect immunofluorescence. This observation does not support a role of circulating antibody in the *in situ* production of immune complexes; however, it is possible that the circulating anti-RTE antibody may not be truly representative of the total population of antibody produced following immunization due to a selective absorption by the diseased kidneys of a subpopulation of RTE antibodies of particular specificities. It is also possible that circulating anti-RTE antibody participates in some way in the accretion and growth of immune complex material already deposited in the glomerular capillary bed. Further studies will be required in order to define the specificities of the antibody present in the deposited immune complexes in the actively induced model. Hoedemaeker and co-workers have recently demonstrated that eluates from diseased kidneys of actively induced AICN show reactivity with *normal* glomerular capillary wall antigens as studied by the immunoperoxidase method. These findings require confirmation, but would not support a role for the CIC described in this study in the production of glomerular disease.

6. Summary

These studies demonstrate the presence of circulating macromolecular Clq-reactive materials, presumably immune complexes, containing autologous IgG and RTE antigens in rats with actively induced AICN, and support the traditional view that in AICN, autologous RTE–RTE autoantibody complexes are continuously formed at low levels in the circulation and subsequently deposit in the glomerular capillary bed to evoke chronic membranous glomerulopathy.

ACKNOWLEDGMENTS. The authors greatly appreciate the technical assistance of Peggy Miles and David Strong and the secretarial help of Mary Norton and Kay Anderson.

References

Barabas, A. Z., Nagi, A. H., and Lannigan, R., 1974, Induction of an autologous immune complex nephritis in rats by intravenous injection of heterologous anti-rat kidney tubular antibody, *Br. J. Exp. Pathol.* **55:**47.

Couser, W. G., Wagonfeld, J. B., Spargo, B. H., and Lewis, E. J., 1974, Glomerular deposition of tumor antigen in membranous nephropathy associated with colonic carcinoma, *Am. J. Med.* **57:**962.

Couser, W. G., Jermanovich, N. B., Belok, S., and Stilmant, M. M., 1978a, Effect of aminonucleoside nephrosis on immune complex localization in autologous immune complex nephropathy in rats, *J. Clin. Invest.* **61:**561.

Couser, W. G., Steinmuller, D. R., Stilmant, M. M., Salant, D. J., and Lowenstein, L. M., 1978b, Experimental glomerulonephritis in the isolated perfused rat kidney, *J. Clin. Invest.* **62:**1275.

Edgington, T. S., Glassock, R. J., and Dixon, F. J., 1967a, Autologous immune complex pathogenesis of experimental allergic glomerulonephritis, *Science* **155:**1432.

Edgington, T. S., Glassock, R. J., and Dixon, F. J., 1967b, Characterization and isolation of specific renal tubular epithelial antigens, *J. Immunol.* **99:**1199.

Edgington, T. S., Lee, S., and Dixon, F. J., 1969, Persistence of the autoimmune pathogenetic process in experimental autologous immune complex nephritis, *J. Immunol.* **103:**528.

Feenstra, K., Lee, R., Greben, H. A., Arends, A., and Hoedemaeker, P. J., 1975, Experimental glomerulonephritis in the rat induced by antibodies directed against tubular antigens. I. The natural history: A histologic and immunohistologic study at the light microscopic and ultrastructural level, *Lab. Invest.* **32:**235.

Glassock, R. J., Edgington, T. S., Watson, J., and Dixon, F. J., 1968, Autologous immune complex nephritis induced with renal tubular antigen. II. The pathogenetic mechanism, *J. Exp. Med.* **127:**573.

Glassock, R. J., Watson, J., Edgington, T. S., and Dixon, F. J., 1969, Autologous immune complex glomerulonephritis. III. Studies in cellular and parabiotic transfer, *J. Immunol.* **102:**194.

Grupe, W. E., and Kaplan, M. H., 1969, Demonstration of an antibody to proximal tubular antigen in the pathogenesis of experimental autoimmune nephrosis in rats, *J. Lab. Clin. Med.* **74:**400.

Hall, C. L., Colvin, R. B., Carey, K., and McCluskey, R. T., 1977, Passive transfer of autoimmune disease with isologous IgG_1 and IgG_2 antibodies to the tubular basement membrane in strain XIII guinea pigs, *J. Exp. Med.* **146:**1246.

Hammer, D. K., and Dixon, F. J., 1963, Experimental glomerulonephritis. II. Immunologic events in the pathogenesis of nephrotoxic serum nephritis in the rat, *J. Exp. Med.* **117:**1019.

Hay, F. C., Nineham, L. J., and Roitt, I. M., 1976, Routine assay for the detection of immune complexes of known immunoglobulin class using solid phase Clq, *Clin. Exp. Immunol.* **24:**396.

Heymann, W., Hackel, D. B., Harwood, S., Wilson, S. G. F., and Hunter, J. L. P., 1959, Production of nephrotic syndrome in rats by Freund's adjuvants and rat kidney suspensions, *Proc. Soc. Exp. Biol. Med.* **100:**660.

Kingsbury, F. B., and Clark, C. P., 1926, The rapid determination of albumin in urine, *J. Lab. Clin. Med.* **11:**981.

McConahey, P. H., and Dixon, F. J., 1966, A method for trace iodination of proteins for immunologic studies, *Int. Arch. Allergy Appl. Immunol.* **29:**185.

Naruse, T., Kitamura, K., Miyakawa, Y., and Shibata, S., 1973, Deposition of renal tubular epithelial antigen along the glomerular capillary walls of patients with membranous glomerulonephritis, *J. Immunol.* **110:**1163.

Nydegger, U. E., Lambert, P. H., Geber, H., and Miescher, P. A., 1974, Circulating immune complexes in the serum in systemic lupus erythematosus and in carriers of hepatitis-B antigen: Quantitation by binding to radiolabeled Clq, *J. Clin. Invest.* **34:**297.

O'Regan, S., Fong, J. S. C., Kaplan, B. S., De Chardarevian, J. P., Lapointe, N., and Drummond, K. N., 1976, Thyroid antigen–antibody nephritis, *Clin. Immunol. Immunopathol.* **6:**341.

Sugisaki, S., Klassen, J., Andres, G. A., Milgrom, F., and McCluskey, R. T., 1973, Passive transfer of Heymann nephritis with serum, *Kidney Int.* **3:**66.

Van Damme, B. J. C., Fleuren, G. J., Bakker, W. W., Vernier, R. L., and Hoedemaeker, P.J, 1978, Experimental glomerulonephritis in the rat induced by antibodies directed against tubular antigens in the pathogenesis of heterologous immune complex glomerulonephritis, *Lab. Invest.* **38:**502.

Van Es, L. A., Blok, A. P. R., Schoenfeld, L., and Glassock, R. J., 1977, Chronic nephritis induced by antibodies reacting with glomerular bound immune complexes, *Kidney Int.* **11:**106.

Weir, D. M. (ed.), *Handbook of Experimental Immunology*, Vol. I, Sect. 18.5.

Yonemasu, K., and Stroud, R. M., 1971, Clq: Rapid purification method for preparation of monospecific antisera and for biochemical studies, *J. Immunol.* **106:**304.

25

Immunopathogenesis of Murine SLE

Frank J. Dixon

1. Introduction

An SLE-like disease has been investigated extensively in the (NZB × NZW) F_1 mouse for well over a decade (Howie and Helyer, 1968). Clearly, these mice demonstrate many immunologic, virologic, and other abnormalities and it has been extremely difficult to determine which, if any of these, are primary etiologic factors of the SLE-like syndrome and which are secondary to the disease or even merely peculiarities of New Zealand mice. Among postulated etiologic factors of this murine disease are: retroviruses or their products (Dixon *et al.*, 1974; Yoshiki *et al.*, 1974), thymic atrophy or failure (Burnet and Holmes, 1964), antithymocyte antibodies (Shirai and Mellors, 1971; Klassen *et al.*, 1977), immunologic hyperreactivity (Playfair, 1968; Evans *et al.*, 1968), deficiency in suppressor T cells (Barthold *et al.*, 1974; Krakauer *et al.*, 1976) and other subsets of T cells (Cantor *et al.*, 1978), abnormalities of phagocytic cells (Morgan and Steward, 1976), and abnormal T-cell cytotoxicity (Botzenhardt *et al.*, 1978).

2. Comparison of SLE in NZB × W, MRL/l, and BXSB Mice

In order to help identify the essential elements in the genesis of murine SLE, a comparison was made of immunologic, virologic, and genetic features of NZB × W mice with those of two newly described murine strains, MRL/l and BXSB (Murphy and Roths, 1976, 1978), which also develop an SLE-like disease. It was hoped that these very similar syndromes in the several different kinds of mice might represent a single disease and that one might

Frank J. Dixon · Department of Immunopathology, Research Institute of Scripps Clinic, Scripps Clinic and Research Foundation, La Jolla, California 92037. Supported by U. S. Public Health Service Grants AI 07007, NO1 CP 71018, CA 16600, and The Elsa U. Pardee Foundation.

expect to find the essential etiologic and pathogenetic factors present in all strains. The elements of the SLE-like disease shared by all the mice include: B-cell polyclonal activation apparent very early in life, increased levels of immunoglobulin, autoantibodies, circulating immune complexes (IC), depressed levels of complement, extensive thymic cortical atrophy, and severe IC-type degenerative vascular disease and glomerulonephritis.

2.1. *Genetic Background*

The several strains of mice developing an SLE-like syndrome have very different genetic backgrounds and no apparent genetic trait or traits in common which would account for their aberrant immunologic behavior. The NZB × W hybrid mouse is derived from a cross betwee NZB and NZW mice originally inbred in New Zealand and the female has a 50% SLE-related mortality by 8.5 months. The MRL/l mouse has a genome derived 75% from the LG strain, 13% from the AKR, 12% from the C3H, and 0.2% from the C57BL/6 and has a 50% SLE-related mortality by 5.5 months in both males and females (Murphy and Roths, 1978). The BXSB mouse was derived from a cross between a C57BL/6J female and and SB/Le male with the hybrids being brother × sister mated and selected for color over many generations (Murphy and Roths, 1978). BXSB male mice have a 50% SLE-related mortality by 5 months. Since the H-2 region of the 17th chromosome of the mouse determines many aspects of immunologic behavior, these mice with a similar immunologic disease might be expected to have similarities in this region of the genome. However, the NZB × W mouse is H-2 type e/z, the MRL/l is H-2^k, and the BXSB is H-2^b, indicating no commonality in these major determinants of the H-2 region. Genetic analyses of these several strains of mice suggest that the important genetic determinants of disease are located differently in the genome of each type of mouse. In the NZB × W, at least three dominant genes have been defined, all linked more or less closely with H-2 on the 17th chromosome (Knight *et al.*, 1977). A major contributor to the disease of the MRL/l mouse is a lymphoproliferative gene, an autosomal recessive located on chromosome 5 (Murphy and Roths, 1976). The disease of the BXSB mouse is apparently determined by a dominant Y-linked gene with perhaps a Y-linked accelerator factor (Murphy and Roths, 1978). The possibility that the variously located genetic determinants of the SLE-like syndrome might be complementary was checked by crossing BXSB, MRL/l, NZB and NZW mice in all combinations to obtain F_1 offspring. Those F_1's with a BXSB male parent plus the NZB × W female F_1 developed an early SLE syndrome, while all other combinations showed little or no early disease. Thus, there was no complementarity evident in the genetic backgrounds of SLE in most of these strains. Taken together, the results of these genetic observations would suggest that a number of quite different immunologically related genetic backgrounds are capable of or compatible with the spontaneous development of a severe SLE-like disease.

2.2. *Immunologic Features of SLE Syndrome in Mice*

Of those immunologic elements common to the SLE syndrome in all mice, the one detected earliest in life is a spontaneous polyclonal B-cell activation (Izui *et al.*, 1978). By testing for splenic plaque-forming cells producing antibody to a variety of haptens including TNP, it was found that NZB, MRL/l, NZB × W females, and BXSB males all had abnormally high levels of plaque-forming cells. By 2 months of age, autoantibodies against ssDNA were also evident at increased levels in the circulation of the same strains while all normal strains tested had only background activity. This polyclonal B-cell activation as measured by plaque-forming cells in some instances was detectable as early as 2 weeks of life and increased for the next several weeks to maximum values at 1–2 months of age which were either maintained or declined gradually over the next several months. As would be expected with increased B-cell activation, the serum levels of IgG were elevated in all strains with lupus. IgG levels in normal adult mice averaged 3–4 mg/ml; in the strains with SLE, values were from 2 to 4 times normal by 3 months of age and 4 to 8 times normal when the mice reached 4–5 months of age (Andrews *et al.*, 1978).

A variety of autoantibodies were detected in the mice with SLE. The most prominent and consistent autoantibodies were those to dsDNA, ssDNA (Andrews *et al.*, 1978), and retroviral gp70 (Izui *et al.*, 1979). The anti-nucleic acid antibodies were evident as early as 2 months of age and increased to a maximum shortly before the animal's demise. Antibodies to retroviral gp70 appeared along with other immunologic abnormalities and persisted throughout the course of the disease. Since all mice have within their genomes the information necessary for the production of one or more retroviruses, and since all mice normally have in their circulation some retroviral gp70, it would seem appropriate to consider such antibodies against retroviral gp70 as autoantibodies. In these studies, the antibodies to retroviral gp70 were detected by observing a heavy form of gp70 in which the viral molecule was bound to immunoglobulin and was precipitated by either anti-immunoglobulin antibodies or by staphylococcal A protein (Izui *et al.*, 1979).

As a result of the autoantibody formation, the mice with SLE developed increasing amounts of circulating IC as detected by the Raji assay (Andrews *et al.*, 1978). In all SLE strains, increased IC levels were detected as early as 3 months of age and increased thereafter until the animal's demise. In most strains, the mean IC levels approached 200 μg/ml serum, but in the MRL/l strain the levels averaged nearly 900 μg/ml. As measured by the Raji technique, these complexes contained IgG antibody as well as bound complement. With the increasing amounts of IC, there was, as would be expected, a decrease in serum complement, reaching very low levels shortly before the animals expired. Also present in the serum of all of the SLE mice were increased amounts of cryoglobulins.

The most important and consistent histopathologic expression of IC disease in the SLE mice was glomerulonephritis, which tended to be acute or early subacute in the BXSB and MRL/l mice and subacute to chronic in the NZB × W (Andrews *et al.*, 1978). The glomerular lesions were characterized by deposition of immunoglobulin, C3, and, in many animals, gp70. Earlier studies, in which only the NZB × W mice were observed, revealed deposition of dsDNA along with immunoglobulin and C3 in their glomeruli (Lambert and Dixon, 1968). In view of the several different kinds of autoantibodies in mice with SLE, it is likely that the IC deposits in the tissue lesions of these animals involve a number of different antigen–antibody systems. A second histopathologic lesion associated with IC deposition was degenerative vascular change in the systemic vessels particularly evident in the coronaries where it was associated with significant myocardial infarction in approximately one-quarter of the animals late in their disease (Andrews *et al.*, 1978). Immunofluorescent observations indicated the deposition of immunoglobulin, C3, and, in some cases, gp70 in the walls of vessels which showed no inflammatory changes but did have degenerative changes in the media and intima. Also, in some of the affected vessels, there were platelet aggregation and thrombus formation presumably related to the myocardial infarcts.

These degenerative, noninflammatory vascular lesions associated with the deposition of IC in vessel walls have not been described previously and are quite distinct from the well-recognized acute necrotizing and inflammatory vasculitides that may accompany circulating IC. Since such changes are not marked by an inflammatory exudate, they are not likely to be detected unless immunohistologic study is made. The occurrence of such lesions in the lupus mice and their relationship with myocardial infarction suggests that similar events may be occurring in man. As a matter of fact, myocardial infarcts are being found in increasing numbers in humans with SLE (Bulkley and Roberts, 1975; Meller *et al.*, 1975; Urowitz *et al.*, 1976). While the vascular lesions associated with myocardial infarcts in humans have been described as atherosclerotic, it is entirely possible that they were contributed to or triggered by deposits of IC. This certainly would tend to make the vessels in which they lodged increasingly susceptible to atherogenesis.

Finally, much has been made of the virologic abnormalities of the lupus mouse and of the possible role of retroviruses in the etiology of this disease in both mice and man (Dixon *et al.*, 1974; Yoshiki *et al.*, 1974; Mellors and Mellors, 1976). It is clear that all mice developing SLE have modestly to greatly elevated levels of gp70 in the serum throughout life. However, these levels are not greater than those found in a number of murine strains which do not develop SLE or any other immunologic abnormality (Andrews *et al.*, 1978). Thus, it would appear that any involvement of retroviral gp70 in murine SLE is not determined by the mere presence or amount of this protein in the circulation but rather that the host destined to develop SLE makes an antibody to the gp70. Inasmuch as the SLE mice make autoantibodies to many endogenous components, it is not entirely unexpected that they would also make antibodies to the ever-present retroviral gp70. That this anti-gp70 antibody response is a component of murine SLE seems clear. The importance and quantitative significance of gp70 and anti-gp70 complexes that occupy serum and tissues in the pathogenesis of the disease are still unknown. Another possible role of gp70 in the genesis of murine SLE would be its action as a lymphocyte activator. Preliminary evidence suggests that gp70 at concentrations found in the sera of SLE mice has a modest stimulating effect on both B and T cells *in vitro* (J. E. Bubbers, personal communication). However, if such stimulation were a factor in SLE, it would appear that lymphocytes from SLE mice must be affected differently by gp70 than lymphocytes from immunologically normal mice.

Three of the several immunologic abnormalities which appear in some but not all of the kinds of SLE mice and therefore are apparently not essential to the development of SLE, are worth mentioning. Antithymocyte antibodies are found in high titers and in high incidence in the New Zealand mice but are found in at best modest titers in BXSB mice and in very low titers in MRL/l mice. Again, even the high values for antithymocyte antibodies in the New Zealand mice are not unique to immunologically abnormal strains since several non-SLE murine strains show as high or higher levels of antithymocyte antibodies as do the New Zealand mice and yet demonstrate no thymic or other immunologic abnormalities. The preponderance of SLE in the female NZB × W mouse has been emphasized and the relationship of the disease to female hormones has been demonstrated (Roubinian *et al.*, 1978). Such a sex relationship, however, is not found in the other murine strains since MRL/l mice of both sexes develop their disease early and in the BXSB mice it is the male which is most severely involved. Finally, the MRL/l mice are unique in their development of IgM rheumatoid factor in relatively high levels. These mice also develop swelling of the joints of their lower extremities which is evident in approximately one-quarter of older mice late in their disease. Histopathologic studies of these swollen joints reveal a chronic proliferative and destructive inflammatory process not too dissimilar from that seen in human rheumatoid arthritis. However, it has not been possible to demonstrate a correlation between the levels of rheumatoid factor in the serum of these mice and their joint lesions to date.

3. Summary

MRL/l and BXSB male mice have an SLE-like disease similar to but more acute than that occurring in NZB × W mice. The common elements of B-cell hyperreactivity, autoantibodies, circulating IC, complement consumption, IC glomerulonephritis and degenerative vascular disease, and thymic atrophy are found in all three kinds of SLE mice. On the basis of these common elements, SLE seen in these mice can be considered a single disease in the same sense that human SLE is one disease. The earliest and apparently the primary immunologic abnormality in all murine SLE is a polyclonal B-cell hyperreactivity of as yet undetermined etiology. The significant differences in genetic backgrounds and in immunogenetic characteristics in the various kinds of SLE mice indicate that different constellations of factors, genetic and/or pathophysiologic, may operate in the three murine strains and that each constellation is capable of leading, via its particular effect of the lymphoid system, to the activation of common immunopathologic effector mechanisms that cause quite similar SLE-like syndromes.

References

Andrews, B. S., Eisenberg, R. A., Theofilopoulos, A. N., Izui, S., Wilson, C. B., McConahey, P. J., Murphy, E. D., Roths, J. B., and Dixon, F. J., 1978, Spontaneous murine lupus-like syndromes: Clinical and immunopathological manifestations in several strains, *J. Exp. Med.* **148:**1198.

Barthold, D. R., Kysela, S., and Steinberg, A. D., 1974, Decline in suppressor T cell function with age in female NZB mice, *J. Immunol.* **12:**9.

Botzenhardt, U., Klein, J., and Ziff, M., 1978, Cytotoxic reactions of NZB spleen cells with lymphocytes of MHC identical strains, *Fed. Proc.* **37:**1373 (abstract).

Bulkley, B. H., and Roberts, W. C., 1975, The heart in systemic lupus erythematosus and the changes induced in it by corticosteroid therapy, *Am. J. Med.* **58:**243.

Burnet, F. M., and Holmes, M. C., 1964, Thymic changes in the mouse strain NZB in relation to the autoimmune state, *J. Pathol. Bacteriol.* **88:**229.

Cantor, H., McVay-Boudreau, L., Hugenberger, J., Naidorf, K., Shen, F. W., and Gershon, R. K., 1978, Immunoregulatory circuits among T cell sets. II. Physiologic role of feedback inhibition in vivo: Absence in NZB mice, *J. Exp. Med.* **147:**1116.

Dixon, F. J., Croker, B., Del Villano, B., Jensen, F. C., and Lerner, R. A., 1974, Oncornavirus infection and "auto" immune complex disease of mice, *Prog. Immunol. II* **5:**49.

Evans, M. M., Williamson, W. G., and Irvine, W. J., 1968, The appearance of immunological competence of an early age in New Zealand Black mice, *Clin. Exp. Immunol.* **3:**375.

Howie, J. B., and Helyer, B. J., 1968, The immunology and pathology of NZB mice, *Adv. Immunol.* **9:**215.

Izui, S., McConahey, P. J., and Dixon, F. J., 1978, Increased spontaneous polyclonal activation of B lymphocytes in mice with spontaneous autoimmune disease, *J. Immunol.* **121:**2213.

Izui, S., McConahey, P. J., Theofilopoulos, A. N., and Dixon, F. J., 1979, Association of circulating retroviral gp70–anti-gp70 immune complexes with murine systemic lupus erythematosus, *J. Exp. Med.* **149:**1099.

Klassen, L. W., Lynell, W., Krakauer, R. S., and Steinberg, A. D., 1977, Selective loss of suppressor cell function in New Zealand mice induced by NTA, *J. Immunol.* **119:**830.

Knight, J. G., Adams, D. D., and Purves, H. D., 1977, The genetic contribution of the NZB mouse to the renal disease of the NZB × NZW hybrid, *Clin. Exp. Immunol.* **28:**352.

Krakauer, R. S., Waldmann, T. A., and Strober, W., 1976, Loss of suppressor T cells in adult NZB/NZW mice, *J. Exp. Med.* **144:**662.

Lambert, P. H., and Dixon, F. J., 1968, Pathogenesis of glomerulonephritis of NZB/NZW mice, *J. Exp. Med.* **127:**507.

Meller, J., Conde, C. A., Deppisch, L. M., Donoso, E., and Dack, S., 1975, Myocardial infarction due to coronary atherosclerosis in three young adults with systemic lupus erythematosus, *Am. J. Cardiol.* **35**309.

Mellors, R. C., and Mellors, J. W., 1976, Antigen related to mammalian type-C RNA viral p30 proteins is located in renal glomeruli in human systemic lupus erythematosus, *Proc. Natl. Acad. Sci. US A* **73:**233.

Morgan, A. G., and Steward, M. W., 1976, Macrophage clearance function and immune complex disease in New Zealand Black/White F_1 hybrid mice, *Clin. Exp. Immunol.* **26:**133.

Murphy, E. D., and Roths, J. B., 1976, A single gene model for massive lymphoproliferation with immune complex disease in new mouse strain MRL, in *Proceedings of the 16th International Congress in Hematology*, p. 69, Excerpta Medica, Amsterdam.

Murphy, E. D., and Roths, J. B., 1978, New inbred strains, *Mouse News Letter* **58:**51.

Playfair, J. H. L., 1968, Strain differences in the immune response of mice. I. The neonatal response to sheep red cells, *Immunology* **15:**35.

Roubinian, J. R., Talal, N., Greenspan, J. S., Goodman, J. R., and Siiteri, P. K., 1978, Effect of castration and sex hormone treatment on survival, anti-nucleic acid antibodies, and glomerulonephritis in NZB/NZW F_1 mice, *J. Exp. Med.* **147:**1568.

Shirai, T., and Mellors, R. C., 1971, Natural thymocytotoxic autoantibody and reactive antigen in New Zealand Black and other mice, *Proc. Natl. Acad Sci. USA* **68:**1412.

Urowitz, M. B., Bookman, A. A. M., Koehler, B. E., Gordon, D. A., Smythe, H. A., and Ogryzlo, M. A., 1976, The bimodal mortality pattern of systemic lupus erythematosus, *Am. J. Med.* **60:**221.

Yoshiki, T., Mellors, R. C., Strand, M., and August, J. T., 1974, The viral envelope glycoprotein of murine leukemia virus and the pathogenesis of immune complex glomerulonephritis of New Zealand mice, *J. Exp. Med.* **140:**1011.

26

Studies on Detection of Nephritogenic Immune Complexes

Felix Milgrom

Three procedures have been successfully used in this laboratory for detection and for identification of immune complexes deposited in the kidney and/or appearing in a soluble form in the circulation.

1. "Hot" Immunoelectrophoresis

In 1965, a procedure was described for the separation of immune complexes, based on immunoelectrophoresis conducted at 56°C (Milgrom *et al.*, 1965). At this temperature, many antigen–antibody complexes dissociate (Landsteiner and Miller, 1925) and therefore, when electrophoresis is conducted at this temperature, antigen and antibody separate physically, provided that they differ in electrophoretic mobility.

More recently, this principle was employed for study of immune complexes in kidney (Milgrom *et al.*, 1976). The test can be performed with as little as 20 mg of kidney tissue and accordingly it can be applied to biopsy material. Minced kidney tissue is incorporated into a center well of an agar or agarose plate. The washing of the tissue may be conducted either before its incorporation into the plate or it may be conveniently achieved by soaking the plate with the tissue in an excess of buffer.

Electrophoresis is conducted in a routine way except that it is performed in a laboratory incubator with the temperature adjusted to 56°C. After the electrophoresis, antibody is detected in the cathodal part of the field by means of a reaction with the proper anti-immunoglobulin serum raised in a foreign species. Antigen, if it has fast electrophoretic mobility, is detected in

---

Felix Milgrom · Department of Microbiology, School of Medicine, State University of New York, Buffalo, New York, 14214. Supported by NIAMDD Grant AM 17317.

the anodal part of the electrophoretic field in reaction with its corresponding antibody. In many instances, detection of the antigen may be facilitated by using counterimmunoelectrophoresis principle, which increases significantly the sensitivity of the reaction.

Studying renal tissues by means of this procedure allowed (Milgrom *et al.*, 1976) detection of BSA–anti-BSA complexes in experimental chronic serum sickness in rabbits and of DNA–anti-DNA complexes in human nephritis accompanying SLE. Other investigators also employed this procedure successfully in their studies (Houba *et al.*, 1977; Carella *et al.*, 1977).

2. *Dissolving Immune Complexes in Excess of Antigen*

In recent experiments (Penner *et al.*) immune complexes were dissolved in microtome sections of kidneys of rabbits suffering from a chronic serum sickness elicited by injections of BSA. The dissolving effect was judged by comparing immunofluorescent staining for antigen, antibody, and complement in untreated and treated sections. In recent cases of serum sickness, immune complexes were dissolved readily by soaking the sections in BSA only. On the other hand, in sections from "old" cases of several months' duration, immune complexes were only partially dissolved by BSA. Interestingly, a mixture of BSA with heat-denatured rabbit IgG dissolved such complexes completely. Apparently, in "old" serum sickness cases, immune complexes also contained antibodies resembling rheumatoid factor, which combined with denatured autologous IgG.

Immune complexes deposited in human kidneys (Andres *et al.*, 1976) were dissolved. The kidney investigated came from a patient who died of heart failure in an early phase of infectious mononucleosis. Immunofluorescence study of his kidney showed mesangial deposits staining for IgM. It was thought that these deposits might be composed of Paul–Bunnell antigen and its antibody. Soaking of sections in an extract of bovine erythrocyte stromata containing soluble Paul–Bunnell antigen resulted in disappearance of mesangial staining for IgM. Control experiments in which the sections were soaked in an extract of human erythrocyte stromata did not affect the immunofluorescent staining.

3. *Neutralization and Absorption of Anti-antibody*

It is obvious that the pathogenicity of immune complexes depends to a great extent on the molecular transformation of the antibody part of the complex (Dixon, 1971). In the mid-1950s, denaturation of antibodies in the course of serologic reaction was suspected by some investigators and denied by others. Those studies were initiated on the assumption that antibody suffers molecular transformation during its reaction with the antigen and that this transformation results in creation or exposure of novel configurations which may be antigenic to the antibody producer itself.

Because of this (Milgrom *et al.*, 1956a,b), human sera were screened for the presence of anti-antibody (AA), i.e., an antibody combining specifically with antibody molecules modified in serologic reactions. Rh-positive erythrocytes sensitized by incomplete Rh antibodies were used for this screening. In about 0.5% of sera from random hospital populations, serum factor fulfilling these criteria was detected in that it agglutinated sensitized erythrocytes, but it did not react with any unaltered human serum, normal or immune. However, only 1 of 10 AA-containing sera had a titer higher than 100, a property helpful in practical application of such sera.

The reaction of AA with sensitized erythrocytes did not require any washing of erythrocytes to remove extraneous serum proteins. Such washing is critical for the reaction of erythrocyte-bound antibodies with Coombs' reagent. This reagent would combine with extraneous, unbound gamma globulin, preventing agglutination of erythrocytes. Furthermore, a mixture of AA-containing serum with an anti-Rh serum could be preserved for several weeks at 4°C without losing its activity. Upon addition of Rh-positive erythrocytes, such a mixture agglutinated them. The first reaction to occur was sensitization of erythrocytes by incomplete anti-Rh antibodies followed by the molecular transformation of these antibodies and creation of "novel" antigenic sites. The second reaction was between AA and the denatured anti-Rh, which resulted in agglutination of the cells. There was no evidence for any reaction between AA and anti-Rh in the serum mixture prior to the addition of erythrocytes.

A few years later, AA was discovered in rabbit sera (Milgrom, 1962). Rabbit AA had properties quite analogous to human AA. AA was the first reagent which could recognize molecular transformation of antibodies in serologic reaction. Further support of this thesis came from immunochemical studies by Robert and Grabar (1957) and Ishizaka and Campbell (1959). With the progress in studies on rheumatoid factor (RF), it became important to compare AA with this factor (Milgrom, 1963; Fudenberg *et al.*, 1964). Both AA and RF are presumably produced in response to antigen–antibody complexes formed *in vivo*. AA is IgM and RF is most frequently but not always IgM. AA and RF combine with IgG but AA acts upon the Fd fragment of IgG while RF acts upon the Fc fragment. AA gives a weak reaction with heat-aggregated human IgG, whereas RF gives a strong reaction with such IgG.

AA has the potential to serve as an exquisite reagent for detection of immune complexes. Studies along these lines (Milgrom, 1977; Milgrom and Kano, 1978; Kano *et al.*, 1978) demonstrated that soluble complexes in human pathological sera may be readily detected by neutralization of AA. This neutralization can be recognized by demonstration that, after addition of the tested serum, the AA-containing serum lost its ability to agglutinate sensitized Rh-positive erythrocytes. Sera tested for immune complexes may be evaluated quantitatively by simple titration and establishing the highest dilution at which such sera neutralize a standard concentration of AA, e.g., three agglutinating units. These studies demonstrated immune complexes with a frequency of over 30% in sera of patients suffering from SLE, rheumatoid arthritis, malaria, and chronic active hepatitis.

Sera of 70 renal graft recipients also were studied for immune complexes. In 16 recipients, pretransplantation sera were negative while their posttransplantation sera were positive. This suggests that immune complexes were formed by these patients as a consequence of transplantation and possibly composed of transplantation antigens and antibodies. In eight of these recipients, immune complexes became detectable within 1–6 months posttransplantation, and in the remaining eight, after more than 10 months posttransplantation. Once they appeared, immune complexes were detectable for the rest of the observation period in some recipients. However, in other recipients, disappearance and reappearance of immune complexes was noted.

AA combines best with immune complexes formed at or close to the equivalence zone, while hardly any reaction is observed with immune complexes formed in excess of antigen. This feature has been used to develop a convenient method for identifying the antigen in the soluble immune complexes. By adding the proper antigen in excess to an inhibitory serum, one may observe its conversion into a noninhibitory preparation. A high degree of specificity of this reaction was shown. By using this procedure, it was demonstrated that immune complexes encountered in rheumatoid arthritis sera frequently are composed of Hanganutziu–Deicher antigen and its corresponding antibody (Nishimaki *et al.*, 1978).

AA also could be used for demonstration of "sessile" immune complexes present in the tissues. The absorption test performed resembles the test of anti-gamma globulin consumption described by Steffen *et al.* (1955). In the latter test, however, the tissue has to be submitted to repeated washing to avoid neutralization of anti-gamma globulin reagent by extraneous gamma globulin trapped in the tissue. In contrast, AA reacts only with IgG antibodies that entered previously into reaction with their corresponding antigen(s) and it is not influenced by extraneous IgG. The procedure of absorption of AA may be conducted with as little as 10 mg of tissue and, therefore, it may be employed for examination of tissue biopsies.

Using this procedure in the study on experimental animal material, it was possible to absorb rabbit AA by renal tissue from animals with chronic serum sickness induced by injections of BSA. In studies with human material, human AA was absorbed by kidney tissue from patients with SLE and by renal graft tissues. The latter study included 19 grafts from 18 recipients. Twelve grafts absorbed AA. This was interpreted as evidence for the presence of serologically bound IgG in the tissue. In five instances, serum of the recipient obtained at the time of graft removal had no circulating immune complexes as evidenced by negative AA inhibition test. This provided additional evidence that the procedure used detected the complexes produced between sessile antigens and their antibodies. Otherwise, only firmly bound complexes that had been brought from the circulation were detected while circulating complexes that were loosely trapped in the tissue were not detectable.

References

Andres, G. A., Kano, K., Elwood, C., Prezyna, A., Sepulveda, M., and Milgrom, F., 1976, Immune deposit nephritis in infectious mononucleosis, *Int. Arch. Allergy Appl. Immunol.* **52:**136.

Carella, G., Digeon, M., Feldmann, A., Jungers, P., Drouet, J., and Bach, JF., 1977, Detection of hepatitis B antigen in circulating immune complexes in acute and chronic hepatitis, *Scand. J. Immunol.* **6:**1297.

Dixon, F. J., 1971, Experimental serum sickness, in: *Immunological Diseases* (M. Santer, ed.), pp. 253–264, Little, Brown, Boston.

Fudenberg, H. H., Goodman, J. W., and Milgrom, F., 1964, Immunochemical studies on rabbit anti-antibody, *J. Immunol.* **92:**227.

Houba, V., Sturrock, R. F., and Butterworth, A. E., 1977, Kidney lesions in baboons infected with *Schistosoma mansoni, Clin. Exp. Immunol.* **30:**439.

Ishizaka, K., and Campbell, D. H., 1959, Biologic activity of soluble antigen–antibody complexes. V. Change of optical rotation by the formation of skin reactive complexes, *J. Immunol.* **83:**318.

Kano, K., Nishimaki, T., Palosuo, T., Loza, U., and Milgrom, F., 1978, Detection of circulating immune complexes by the inhibition of anti-antibody, *Clin. Immunol. Immunopathol.* **9:**425.

Kano, K., Nishimaki, T., and Milgrom, F., 1979, Detection of immune complexes in human renal transplantation by using anti-antibody, in: *Protides of the Biological Fluids,* 26th Colloquium (H. Peeters, ed.), Pergamon Press, Oxford.

Landsteiner, K., and Miller, C. P., Jr., 1925, Serological studies on the blood of the primate. II. The blood groups in anthropoid apes, *J. Exp. Med.* **42:**853.

Milgrom, F., 1962, Rabbit sera with "anti-antibody," *Vox Sang.* **7:**545.

Milgrom, F., 1963, Discussion, *Arthritis Rheum.* **6:**408.

Milgrom, F., 1977, Immune complex disease, in: *An International Symposium on the Nature and Significance of Complement Activation*, pp. 49–56, Ortho Research Institute of Medical Sciences, Raritan, N. J.

Milgrom, F., and Kano, K., 1978, Comparison of various procedures for the detection of antigen–antibody complexes, *Int. Arch. Allergy Appl. Immunol.* **56:**224.

Milgrom, F., Dubiski, S., and Wozniczko, G., 1956a, Human sera with "anti-antibody," *Vox Sang.* **1:**172.

Milgrom, F., Dubiski, S., and Wozniczko, G., 1956b, A simple method of Rh determination, *Nature (London)* **178:**539.

Milgrom, F., Tuggac, Z. M., and Campbell, W. A., 1965, Analysis of antigen–antibody complexes by immunoelectrophoresis, *Immunology* **8:**406.

Milgrom, F., Campbell, W. A., and Andres, G. A., 1976, Antigen in immune complex nephritis. V. Recovery and identification by gel precipitation, *Immunology* **30:**277.

Nishimaki, T., Kano, K., and Milgrom, F., 1978, Studies on immune complexes in rheumatoid arthritis, *Arthritis Rheum.* **21:**639.

Penner, E., Albini, B., Glurich, I., Andres, G. A., and Milgrom, F., 1982, Dissociation of immune complexes in tissue sections by excess of antigen, *Int. Arch. Allergy Appl. Immunol.* **67:**245.

Robert, B., and Grabar, P., 1957, Dosage des groupements thiol protéiques dans des réactions immunochimiques, *Ann. Inst. Pasteur, Paris* **92:**56.

Steffen, C., 1955, Untersuchungen über Verwendung Antihumanglobulinablenkungs-Methode zum Nachweis von Thrombozyten-Antikörpern, *Wien. Z. Inn. Med. Ihre Grenzgeb.* **36:**246.

27

The Significance of Cryoimmunoglobulinemia in Immunologically Mediated Kidney Diseases

John J. McPhaul, Jr., W. R. Montgomery, and J. Shorey

1. Introduction

Immunologically mediated glomerulonephritis generally is acknowledged to result from one of two basic immunopathogenetic mechanisms: (1) antibodies directed against antigens associated with the glomerular basement membrane (GBM); or (2) circulating immune complexes (Dixon, 1978). Recent data have broadened this concept by suggesting that immune complex-mediated disease is the major mechanism by which clinical human glomerulonephritis operates (Morel-Maroger *et al.*, 1972; McPhaul and Mullins, 1976; Wilson and Dixon, 1973). In contrast to experimental models in which the inducing antigen is known, recognition and identification of putative antigens in spontaneous clinical glomerulonephritis remains enigmatic. With uncommon exceptions, the offending immunogen is unknown in most cases (Combes *et al.*, 1971; Koffler *et al.*, 1967; Krishnan and Kaplan, 1967; Naruse *et al.*, 1973).

Cryoimmunoglobulinemia (CIG) is a phenomenon associated with varying disease states and is accompanied by an important glomerulonephritis in many patients, particularly those with the syndrome of mixed cryoglobuli-

John J. McPhaul, Jr. · Departments of Medicine and Pathology, University of Texas Southwestern Medical School, Dallas, Texas, 75235 ***W. R. Montgomery*** · Department of Medicine, Wilford Hall USAF Medical Center, San Antonio, Texas 78236
J. Shorey · Department of Medicine, University of Texas Southwestern Medical School, Dallas, Texas 75235. Supported in part by Veterans Administration General Medical Research Funds and Biomedical Research Support Grant 5 S07 RR 05426 15.

nemia (Levo *et al.*, 1977; Meltzer *et al.*, 1966). Immune complex-mediated glomerulonephritis is the principal expressed pathogenetic disorder noted in CIG. In addition, cryoimmunoglobulins have been detected in some patients with glomerulonephritis due to specific etiologic agents or to defined antigen–antibody immunological systems, and in some patients with idiopathic glomerulonephritis unassociated with systemic disease. In these latter situations, glomerular disease apparently results from immune complex deposits also (Adam *et al.*, 1973; Brouet *et al.*, 1974; McIntosh *et al.*, 1970).

The studies reported here were initiated because: (1) cryoimmunoglobulins are thought by many to be a species of circulating immune complexes; (2) immune complex glomerulonephritis may be associated with circulating cryoimmunoglobulins; and (3) the specific antigen–antibody immune complex system is unidentified in the majority of patients with glomerulonephritis. Initially, the investigations surveyed a consecutive series of patients evaluated for glomerulonephritis to estimate the frequency of detectable CIG and to establish some of the immunological characteristics of the proteins. Later studies, which constitute the major positive observations reported herein, were undertaken to examine the potential autoantibody and antigen content of the cryoprotein (CP) isolates and their apparent relationship to glomerular immunoglobulin deposits.

2. *Materials and Methods*

Consecutive adult patients with suspected medical renal disease admitted to Wilford Hall USAF Medical Center and to the Dallas VA Medical Center for diagnostic and/or therapeutic evaluation including renal biopsy were studied.

Cryoimmunoglobulins were isolated from freshly drawn blood clotted at 37°C for 2 hr in a water bath. Serum was decanted and centrifuged twice at room temperature for 30 min at 2500 rpm. Supernatant serum was placed in an acid-washed, conical glass test tube and refrigerated at 5°C for 5–7 days. Harvest of precipitates detected visually was done by centrifugation and resuspension of packed precipitates 4–5 times in cold phosphate-buffered saline (PBS).

Coprecipitations of fresh sera were done as follows: to duplicate 2-ml samples of test and of control sera were added 1 ng or 1 μg deaggregated radiolabeled protein (McPhaul, 1978); reactants were mixed, incubated at 37°C for 30–40 min, and stored at 5°C for 5–7 days. After formation of cryoprecipitates, tubes were centrifuged, decanted, and precipitates washed. All samples were counted in a well detector with thallium-activated sodium iodide crystal. Percent binding was calculated as cpm in precipitates as a fraction of total cpm. Coprecipitations using previously isolated, washed cryoprecipitates generally were done in the same way, but CP were solubilized at 50°C, and incubations with radiolabeled reactant were done at 50°C for 30 min before refrigeration.

Radial immunodiffusion analyses were done on cryoprecipitates to test for component proteins using commercial antisera to IgG, IgM, IgA, B_1C (C′3) component of complement, fibrinogen, and albumin. Some were tested also for κ and λ light chains. All immunodiffusions were done in 1% agarose. Plates were prewarmed to 37°C and CP were solubilized at 50°C prior to filling wells. Immunoelectrophoresis (IEP) was done on cryoprecipitates prepared in a similar manner. Quantitative immunodiffusions of serum and cryoprecipitates to measure Ig concentrations were done using standard and low-level commercial kits (Meloy Laboratories, Springfield, Va.; Hyland Division, Travenol., Inc., Costa Mesa, Calif.). All analyses were done at 37°C (McPhaul, 1978).

Human, rabbit, and sheep IgG were isolated from normal serum. IgM and IgA were isolated from human myeloma sera. Fractionations utilized ammonium sulfate salting, DEAE cellulose gradient elution chromatography, preparative electrophoresis on Pevikon, and gel filtration. Bovine serum albumin (BSA) was purchased from Armour Laboratories (Kankakee, Ill.) and DNA from Worthington. Human IgG subclass proteins were the gift of Dr. Howard Grey (National Jewish Hospital, Denver, Colo.) as were sera from which they were isolated. Digestions of human IgG and preparation of human Fc and Fab′ were done as described by Franklin (1960) using mercuripapain. Radioiodination of proteins was done by the method of McConahey and Dixon (1966). Immunizations were done as follows: (1) antisera to soluble protein antigens isolated as above were induced by immunization of New Zealand White rabbits (McPhaul and Dixon, 1970) using 0.5 to 1.0 mg protein in Freund's incomplete adjuvant; (2) antisera to CP were induced by immunizing rabbits with washed, resolubilized CP isolates in Freund's complete adjuvant. Animals were bled out at 21 days, or boosted on day 21 and bled out on day 28. Antisera were heat-inactivated at 56°C for 40 min.

Antisera to CP were absorbed with lyophilized, pooled, normal human sera (NHS) and subsequently absorbed one or more times using pooled NHS insolubilized by the technique of Avrameas and Ternynck (1967). Prior to use, all antisera were absorbed with mouse liver powder.

Immunofluorescent microscopy was done by methods described below. (1) Direct immunohistochemical staining of human tissues was done as described (McPhaul and Dixon, 1970) and using conventional controls. (2) Indirect immunohistochemical staining was done using target substrates incubated with sera or isolated CP and subsequently stained with fluorescein-conjugated sheep anti-rabbit IgG or rabbit anti-human globulin (F II). For assay of autoantibodies in CP isolates, tissue sections were fixed in ether–alcohol, washed with PBS at 37°C, incubated with solubilized CP isolates for 30 min at 37°C, and washed twice with warm PBS (37°C) prior to incubation with the fluoresceinated antisera. Human tissues for target substrates were obtained from fresh surgical or autopsy specimens. Routinely tested were: thyroid, lung, kidney, liver, pancreas, lymph node, spleen, testicle, skin, gut, stomach, skeletal muscle, and heart. (3) Binding of antisera to CP against autologous tissues were done both by: (a) two-step procedure incubating autologous tissues with absorbed rabbit antiserum to CP and secondarily staining with sheep anti-rabbit IgG, and (b) incubation of autologous tissue with fluoresceinated globulin fraction of the rabbit anti-CP serum. Controls available were nonimmune rabbit serum and preimmunization bleedings from rabbits used to produce antisera to CP.

Antibody activity to hepatitis B surface antigens (HBsAg) ad and ag was tested by incubating dilutions of rabbit sera with purified radiolabeled HBsAg for 72 hr, followed by precipitation with hyperimmune goat anti-rabbit IgG. Binding at any dilution was calculated as percent radiolabeled antigen precipitated and compared to immune sera standards. A battery of normal rabbits constituted the negative controls; positive results were confirmed by appropriate absorption studies.

Concordance or discordance of data regarding CIG and glomerular immunoglobulin deposits was assessed by five general criteria: (1) presence or absence of apparent immunologically mediated disease; (2) identity of composition of CP and glomerular immunoglobulin deposits; (3) CIG in patients with glomerular immunoglobulin deposits; (4) relationship established between glomerular immunoglobulin and CP by anti-CP serum; (5) specificity of renal eluates and CP.

3. Results

The overall frequency of CIG detected in patients with renal disease was 17% as compared to an incidence of 2% in an immunized control population of apparently healthy Air Force recruits. The incidence was higher in patients with systemic lupus erythematosus (SLE) whether or not they had clinical evidence of renal involvement; and in dialysis and in renal allograft patients (McPhaul, 1978).

CP isolated from most patients were composed of IgG, IgM, and IgA, although some contained IgG and IgM or IgA, and a few comprised IgG, or IgA only.

The amount of CP isolated from sera of these patients was variable, ranging from 0.2 μg/ml to 830 μg/ml. In general, patients with the syndrome of mixed essential CIG and active SLE with glomerulonephritis tended to have the larger amounts.

Virtually all CP forming spontaneously in the cold from freshly separated serum bound homologous IgG in coprecipitation experiments. All CP isolates also bound homologous IgG by coprecipitation both in saline and canine serum. Greater amounts of heat-aggregated and freeze–thaw-aggregated homologous IgG, were bound than were deaggregated IgG. Homologous IgG was bound in higher percentage than were equal concentrations of sheep or rabbit IgG. Fc fractions were bound in preference to Fab fractions of homologous IgG.

Resolubilized CP from five patients were tested. Two patients had IgG binding to human tissue sections as detected by indirect immunofluorescence. One, isolated from a youngster with rapidly progressive glomerulonephritis, bound to vascular smooth muscle. No binding was demonstrable to visceral smooth muscle, cardiac, or skeletal muscle. The other CP isolated from a young man with muscle pain, elevated serum CPK enzyme activity, and proliferative glomerulonephritis, contained IgG which bound only to autologous skeletal muscle. No binding was demonstrable to homologous skeletal muscle. Eighty- to 160-fold greater concentrations of antitissue antibodies were present in isolated CP than in whole serum IgG in these two cases. Papain digestions of CP isolates indicated that IgG binding was by Fab fractions. No other autoantibody activity was noted with either CP as tested on tissue sections.

Anti-CP antisera were induced using 16 CP isolates. The antisera, extensively absorbed with soluble and insoluble homologous serum, showed no binding to autologous kidney glomerular immune deposits in any of the nine cases tested. However, 3 of the 16 antisera contained rabbit IgG antibody activity against tissue antigens in sections of human organs: skeletal muscle (1 antiserum), and nuclear antigen (1 antiserum) and fibrillar material (probably reticulin) found in many human tissue sections (1 antiserum). CP used for inducing these three antisera were not tested by indirect immunofluorescence for autoantibody content. All three of these antisera were tested against autologous kidneys which were known to contain glomerular granular immunoglobulin deposits. All were unreactive.

Eleven antisera made against CP isolates were tested for antibody activity to HBsAg. Two antisera contained apparently specific antibody activity. None of the sera from which the CP were isolated had detectable HBsAg using a commercial radioimmunoassay. CP isolates themselves were not tested for HBsAg.

Nineteen consecutive patients with CIG constituted the group analyzed for concordance of observations (Table 1). Most of the patients also were tested for autoantibody specificity and for apparent antigen content of CP. (1) Immunologically mediated disease was noted in 15 of 19 patients with CIG. In 4 of 19 patients in whom CIG was detected, nonimmunologic disease was thought to be present. (2) In 13 patients with CIG in whom technically

Table 1. Relationship Established by Antisera to Autologous CP

		Observations judged to be:	
Points of comparison	No. of patients	Concordant	Discordant
Immunological disease clinically	19	15	4
Both CIG and glomerular Ig deposits detected	13	9	4
Composition of CP and glomerular Ig deposits	8	0	8
Anti-CP relationship	9	0	9

adequate renal biopsies were done, only 9 had renal immunoglobulin deposits detected. (3) In none of the eight patients in whom composition of CP and renal immune deposits were tested simultaneously was the immunoglobulin identical. (4) Anti-CP antisera, induced by immunization of rabbit hosts with CP isolates, did not react with autologous renal immunoglobulin deposits in any of the nine cases tested. (5) No concrete immunological identity could be constructed from renal eluates, CP isolates, and antisera to CP in the two cases tested extensively.

4. *Discussion*

The nature of the relationship between cryoimmunoglobulins and the glomerular immunoglobulin deposits observed in some cases of glomerulonephritis in patients with CIG is not completely clear. Glomerular deposits which occur in patients with monoclonal paraproteinemias are inferred to result from local precipitation of the abnormal protein due to concentration gradients, hemodynamic alterations, and physicochemical characteristics of the protein. On the other hand, glomerular immunoglobulin deposits occurring in the presence of systemic disease in patients with mixed cryoglobulinemia may be in the form of immune complexes, with all the pathophysiologic consequences attendant on tissue deposition of immune complexes. It may be hypothesized in such cases that glomerular immunoglobulin is locally (glomerular) deposited CP, and that in fact, CP causes glomerulonephritis.

Experimental data supporting the relationship between glomerular immunoglobulin deposits and CP have been offered by Agnello *et al.* (1971) and data relating a circulating monoclonal paraprotein to glomerular immunoglobulin deposits have been described by Avasthi *et al.* (1977). These investigators established an immunological relationship between circulating cryoimmunoglobulins or paraprotein and glomerular immunoglobulin deposits by using a heterologous antiserum to the cryoimmunoglobulin protein component IgM in the former case and to the IgG paraprotein in the latter. Similar parallel relationships between circulating CP and glomerular immunoglobulin deposits have been made by Pardo *et al.* (1975), who showed that glomerular immunoglobulin deposits contained renal tubular epithelial (RTE) antigen and that CP isolated from the same patients contained both RTE antigen and anti-RTE antibodies.

Studies performed on patients in the Dallas VA confirmed results reported by others suggesting the regular, albeit infrequent, occurrence of CIG in patients with idiopathic, apparently immune complex-mediated glomerulonephritis. Moreover, these investigations have confirmed the immunologic similarity of CP isolated in these patients with renal disease to CP isolated from patients with CIG due to other causes: anti-IgG binding, binding to Fc fragments, and to homologous IgG subclasses (Grey and

Kohler, 1973). However, coprecipitation studies done using radiolabeled homologous IgG have suggested that CP bind limited amounts of immunoglobulin, and that binding may be limited both by substrate concentration and by antibody content (McPhaul, 1978). Such suggestions are compatible with the idea that CP may represent heterogeneous mixtures of diverse antigen–antibody systems.

In efforts to define the relationship between glomerular disease and CIG, studies in 17 patients with both were done and in two other patients with CIG but no clinically apparent renal disease. Renal biopsy tissue was available for immunological studies in 13 of these patients. Although these 13 had clinical and pathological evidence of kidney disease, only 9 had renal immunoglobulin deposits, and 3 had no immunohistochemical evidence of immunologically mediated kidney disease. Moreover, kidney biopsies from 9 patients tested with heterologous anti-CP antisera induced in rabbits with autologous, isolated CP failed to show reactivity.

Despite these discordant immunological data relating CIG and autologous renal immunoglobulin deposits, the isolated CP surprisingly showed reactivity to defined tissue antigens. Analysis of binding to homologous and/or autologous tissue sections by CP from 5 patients, and binding of heterologous antisera induced by CP isolated from 16 patients, both to human tissue sections and to HBsAg, showed positive results with one or the other in 7 of the total 16 patients tested in all systems.

These data permit several inferences regarding cryoimmunoglobulins in renal disease:

1. These observations do not rule out a relationship between CP and renal immunoglobulin deposits in most patients with CIG, but they do not confirm or support an immunopathogenetic relationship in the patients we studied.

2. Isolated cryoimmunoglobulins have multifaceted immunological reactivity: anti-IgG (rheumatoid factor) activity in most, DNA binding *in vitro*, and demonstrable autoantibody content in some. The reactivity of heterologous antisera induced by CP suggests that several others contain covert antigens, presumably as components of hitherto unidentified soluble immune complexes.

3. Available data from these as well as previous studies support the hypothesis that CIG in clinical states other than those associated with monoclonal paraproteinemias is an immunologically induced phenomenon. However, this phenomenon may be independent of concomitant nonimmunologically mediated renal disease.

Although these investigations have provided no support directly relating CIG to immunologically mediated renal disease, the surprisingly frequent reactivity of isolated CP, and of heterologous antisera induced by CP, to defined, homologous tissue or unsuspected microbial antigens indicates that this approach to CP analysis may be a fruitful technique to explore further for putative antigens in immunologically mediated diseases.

References

Adam, C., Morel-Maroger, L., and Richet, G., 1973, Cryoglobulins in glomerulonephritis not related to systemic disease, *Kidney Int.* **3:**334.

Agnello, V., Koffler, D., Eisenberg, J. W., Winchester, R. J., and Kunkel, H. G., 1971, C1q precipitins in the sera of patients with systemic lupus erythematosus and other hypocomplementemic states: Characterization of high and low molecular weight types, *J. Exp. Med.* **134:**228s.

Avasthi, P. S., Erickson, D. G., Williams, R. C., Jr., and Tung, K. S. K., 1977, Benign monoclonal gammaglobulinemia and glomerulonephritis, *Am. J. Med.* **62:**324.

Avrameas, S., and Ternynck, T., 1967, Biologically active water-insoluble protein polymers. I. Their use for isolation of antigens and antibodies, *J. Biol. Chem.* **242:**1651.

Brouet, J. C., Clauvel, J. P., Danon, F., Klein, M., and Seligmann, M., 1974, Biological and clinical significance of cryoglobulins: A report of 86 cases, *Am. J. Med.* **57:**775.

Combes, B., Stastny, P., Shorey, J., Eigenbrodt, E. H., Barrera, A., Hull, A. R., and Carter, N. W., 1971, Glomerulonephritis with deposition of Australia antigen–antibody complexes in glomerular basement membrane, *Lancet* **2:**234.

Dixon, F. J., 1978, The pathogenesis of glomerulonephritis, *Am. J. Med.* **64:**493.

Franklin, E. C., 1960, Structural units of human 7S gamma globulin, *J. Clin. Invest.* **39:**1933.

Grey, H. M., and Kohler, P. F., 1973, Cryoimmunoglobulins, *Sem. Hematol.* **10:**87.

Koffler, D., Schur, P. H., and Kunkel, H. G., 1967, Immunological studies concerning the nephritis of systemic lupus erythematosus, *J. Exp. Med.* **126:**607.

Krishnan, C., and Kaplan, M. H., 1967, Immunopathologic studies of systemic lupus erythematosus. II. Antinuclear reaction of γ-globulin eluted from homogenates and isolated glomeruli of kidneys from patients with lupus nephritis, *J. Clin. Invest.* **46:**569.

Levo, Y., Gorevic, P. D., Kassab, H., Zucker-Franklin, D., Gigli, I., and Franklin, E. C., 1977, Mixed cryoglobulinemia—An immune complex disease often associated with hepatitis B virus infection, *Trans. Assoc. Am. Physicians* **90:**167.

McConahey, P. J., and Dixon, F. J., 1966, A method of trace-iodination of proteins for immunologic studies, *Int. Arch. Allergy Appl. Immunol.* **79:**185.

McIntosh, R. M., Kaufman, D. B., Kulvinskas, C., and Grossman, B. J., 1970, Cryoglobulins. I. Studies on the nature, incidence, and clinical significance of serum cryoproteins in glomerulonephritis, *J. Lab. Clin. Med.* **75:**566.

McPhaul, J. J., Jr., 1978, Cryoimmunoglobulinaemia in patients with primary renal disease and systemic lupus erythematosus. I. IgG- and DNA-binding assessed by co-precipitation, *Clin. Exp. Immunol.* **31:**131.

McPhaul, J. J., Jr., and Dixon, F. J., 1970, Characterization of human antiglomerular basement membrane antibodies eluted from glomerulonephritic kidneys, *J. Clin. Invest.* **49:**308.

McPhaul, J. J., Jr., and Mullins, J. D., 1976, Glomerulonephritis mediated by glomerular basement membrane antibodies: Immunological, clinical, and histopathological characteristics, *J. Clin. Invest.* **57:**351.

Meltzer, M., Franklin, E. C., Elias, K., McCluskey, R. T., and Cooper, N., 1966, Cryoglobulinemia. A clinical and laboratory study. II. Cryoglobulins with rheumatoid factor activity, *Am. J. Med.* **40:**837.

Morel-Maroger, L., Leathem, A., and Richet, G., 1972, Glomerular abnormalities in nonsystemic diseases: Relationship between finding by light microscopy and immunofluorescence in 433 renal biopsy specimens, *Am. J. Med.* **53:**170.

Naruse, T., Kitamura, K., Miyakawa, Y., and Shibata, S., 1973, Deposition of renal tubular epithelium antigen along the glomerular capillary walls of patients with membranous glomerulonephritis, *J. Immunol.* **110:**1163.

Pardo, V., Strauss, J., Kramer, H., Ozawa, T., and McIntosh, R. M., 1975, Nephropathy associated with sickle cell anemia: An autologous immune complex nephritis. II. Clinicopathologic study of seven patients, *Am. J. Med.* **59:**650.

Wilson, C. B., and Dixon, F. J., 1973, Anti-GBM antibody induced glomerulonephritis, *Kidney Int.* **3:**74.

28

Relationship of Serum Cryoglobulins and Their Composition to Glomerulonephritis in Systemic Lupus Erythematosus

John B. Winfield and H. Alexander Wilson

1. Introduction

For nearly a quarter-century, glomerulonephritis in systemic lupus erythematosus (SLE) has been the prototype of immune complex-mediated renal injury in man. Through investigation in many laboratories, most notably that of Dr. Henry Kunkel at The Rockefeller University, steady progress in our understanding has ensued. Certain important issues remain to be clarified. As a sign of sustained interest and vigor in this area, new observations continue to force changes in thinking about the mechanisms operant in this type of tissue injury. Therefore, it is appropriate to review briefly the lines of evidence which are important in the evolution of current concepts, and which may be relevant to interpretation of the experimental data obtained by immunochemical analysis of cryoprecipitates.

2. Evidence Implicating DNA/Anti-DNA Complexes in SLE Glomerulonephritis

2.1. Immunofluorescent and Glomerular Elution Studies

A large variety of antibodies to host-tissue constituents have been identified in the serum of patients with SLE. Only certain of these are

John B. Winfield and H. Alexander Wilson · Division of Immunology and Rheumatology, University of North Carolina, Chapel Hill, North Carolina 27514.

associated with tissue injury and with clinical manifestations. The DNA/anti-DNA system is involved predominantly in the pathogenesis of glomerulonephritis. Initial information came from immunofluorescent studies of kidney biopsy sections from patients with SLE in the late 1950s by Mellors *et al.* (1957) and Vasquez and Dixon (1957) which identified immunoglobulin in deposits along the glomerular basement membrane. Subsequent investigation localized complement components and DNA in a distribution similar to that of immunoglobulin in the kidney (Freedman and Markowitz, 1962; Koffler *et al.*, 1974). A fundamental advance was provided by the observation that immunoglobulin eluted from isolated glomeruli from cadaver kidneys contained anti-DNA antibody (Krishnan and Kaplan, 1967; Koffler *et al.*, 1967, 1974). Anti-DNA activity is specifically concentrated in such eluates relative to the serum level. This strongly suggests that anti-DNA antibody and DNA antigen localize in the kidney as an immune complex. An indication of the potential importance of qualitative characteristics of antibody in the glomerular deposits was the demonstration that anti-native DNA (nDNA) antibody in glomerular eluates is of much higher binding avidity than that in serum of patients with glomerulonephritis (Winfield *et al.*, 1977). The evidence presented thus far clearly implicates the DNA/anti-DNA system in the pathogenesis of glomerulonephritis in SLE and is persuasive because the data were obtained by study of immunoglobulin and DNA localized at the actual site of tissue injury.

2.2. *Serologic Studies*

Although the data are less direct, much useful information has come from study of patient serum. Increased levels of anti-nDNA and, to a lesser extent, of anti-single-stranded DNA (ssDNA) antibodies are found in patients with active glomerulonephritis (Tan *et al.*, 1966; Schur and Sandson, 1968; Koffler *et al.*, 1969). The hypocomplementemia characteristic of active nephritis in SLE (Vaughn *et al.*, 1951) parallels closely the associated elevation of anti-DNA antibodies (Schur and Sandson, 1968; Davis *et al.*, 1977). The third line of evidence basic to the concept that DNA and anti-DNA antibody constitute a circulating immune complex system derived from the work of Tan *et al.* (1966) and Koffler *et al.* (1973), who showed that free DNA persists in the circulation and alternates with anti-DNA antibody in patients with nephritis who are followed over a period of time.

In the past several years, some question regarding the *in vivo* significance of DNA detected in serum of patients with SLE has arisen. In experimental animal systems, DNA is cleared extremely rapidly from the circulation even in the absence of specific antibody (Tsumita and Iwanaga, 1963; Natali and Tan, 1972; Chused *et al.*, 1972). Such rapid clearance of DNA has provoked the question of why rather large amounts of DNA should persist in the circulation of patients with SLE. Of significance are recent studies of Frank and his associates (Frank *et al.*, 1977; Hamburger *et al.*, 1978; see also Frank, this volume) which show defects in the reticuloendothelial system clearance of immune complexes in patients with active SLE. In addition, data of Emlen and Mannik (1978a,b) indicate that clearance mechanisms for ssDNA are easily saturable in mice, and that by altering clearance kinetics, immune complexes may contribute to the persistence of DNA in the circulation.

A second difficulty with studies of free DNA in the circulation relates to the demonstration that DNA may be released into serum from leukocyte nuclei during clotting (Tan *et al.*, 1966; Davis and Davis, 1973; Steinman, 1975). As nearly all work has been done with serum and not with plasma, doubt remains concerning what is real and what is artifact. Against *in vitro* artifact being the entire explanation is the demonstration of much larger amounts of DNA in SLE sera than might be expected to be released through clotting (Tan *et al.*, 1966; Koffler *et al.*, 1973). Furthermore, recent studies by Steinman (1975) using plasma and not serum have confirmed both the persistence of circulating DNA in patients with SLE for prolonged periods of time and the alternation of free DNA with anti-DNA in patients with nephritis (Steinman, personal communication).

Another observation which has provoked considerable interest is the finding of Izui *et al.* (1976) that DNA, particularly ssDNA, binds with high avidity to collagen and collagen-like material in the glomerular basement membrane. These investigators speculate that DNA/anti-DNA complex deposition in the kidney may be largely a local phenomenon with initial binding of free DNA and secondary binding of anti-DNA antibody. This concept represents a distinct departure from the dogma that DNA/anti-DNA complexes are deposited in the glomerulus from the circulation. The possibility that DNA/anti-DNA complexes might form locally has received support from studies failing to demonstrate DNA complexes in the circulation (Izui *et al.*, 1977). This issue, however, is controversial (Harbeck *et al.*, 1973; Bruneau *et al.*, 1977; Cano *et al.*, 1977).

The great amount of recent work directed toward measuring immune complexes in patient serum with various quantitative assays has provided further indirect evidence for a circulating immune complex pathogenesis for SLE nephritis. Immune complex levels rise and fall in concert with anti-DNA antibody and complement activity, and correlate with exacerbation and remission of nephritis (Theofilopoulos *et al.*, 1976; Davis *et al.*, 1977; Zubler *et al.*, 1978; Abrass *et al.*, 1978). There are two major problems with this type of work at the present time. It is unclear whether or not these assays, in all cases, actually measure immune complexes which circulate *in vivo*. Thus far, little information has been forthcoming concerning the nature of the material being detected in these assays.

3. Relationship between Cryoglobulinemia and Glomerulonephritis

Interest in serum cryoproteins as possibly having pathogenetic significance for nephritis in SLE has been stimulated by observations in individual patients such as those shown in Fig. 1. Early in her course, this patient

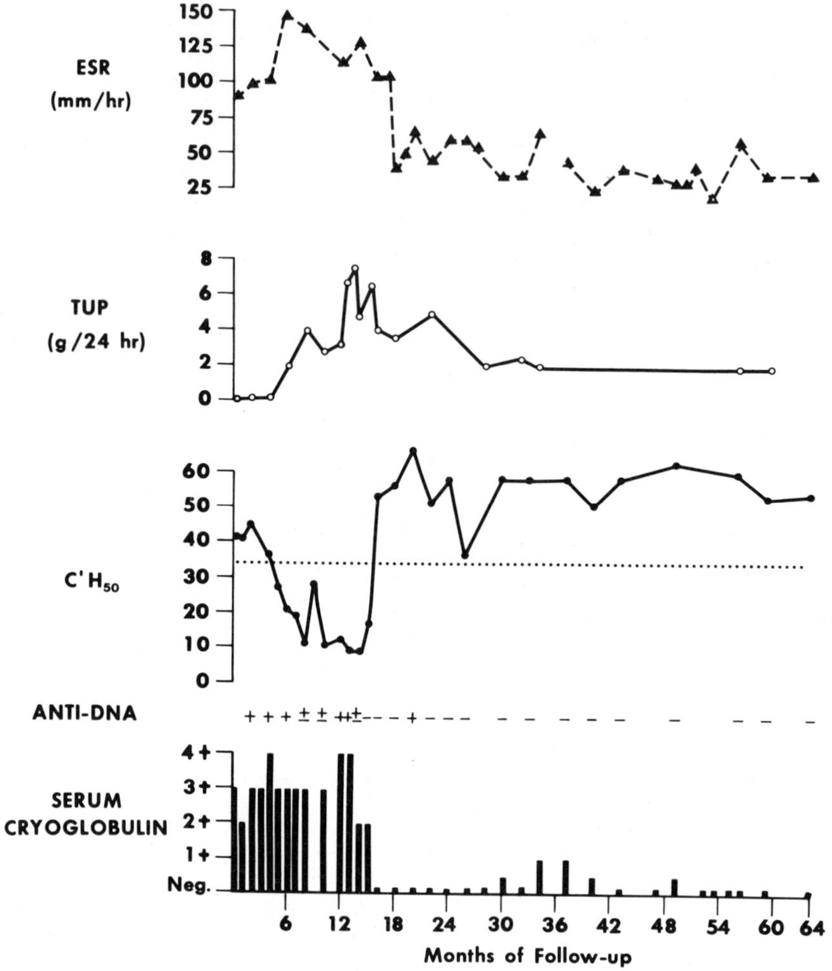

Figure 1. Relationship between cryoglobulinemia, hypocomplementemia, and anti-nDNA antibodies in a patient with SLE and diffuse, proliferative glomerulonephritis.

developed diffuse proliferative glomerulonephritis manifested by rising 24-hr urine protein excretion. During this phase of active nephritis, there was marked hypocomplementemia with associated DNA antibody and cryoglobulins in serum. Therapy with cyclophosphamide in the 14th month resulted in complete remission of her nephritis with disappearance of cryoglobulins and anti-DNA antibodies, and return of total hemolytic complement activity to normal levels.

This type of serial study has been extended to the total population of patients with SLE followed in the Lupus Clinic at the University of Virginia. At the Lupus Clinic, both clinical and laboratory data are collected in a uniform fashion at each patient visit and for the past 5 years have been entered into a computer. These data were analyzed to answer the question,

Table 1. Patients with SLE Attending the Lupus Clinic at the University of Virginia, 1973–1978

SLE patients	No.	Follow-up: Months/patient Mean	Median	Range	Visits/patient Mean	Median	Range
-Nephritis positive	33	61	65	15–106	27	22	11–57
-Nephritis negative	68	45	48	16–124	18	15	6–53
Total	101	50	50	15–124	21	19	6–57

"What is the relationship between cryoglobulinemia and the development of glomerulonephritis?" As shown in Table 1, 33 of 101 patients followed for 15–124 months developed glomerulonephritis which was defined by a progressive increase in 24-hr protein excretion; and either decreased creatinine clearance or increased serum creatinine. Renal biopsy confirmed the presence of glomerulonephritis in 28 patients.

Four patterns of cryoglobulinemia were seen in the serial studies of these 101 patients (Table 2). Cryoglobulinemia which varied inversely with the total hemolytic complement level was associated with the development of glomerulonephritis in 24 of 32 patients. Nephritis developed in only 7 of 30 patients with cryoglobulinemia either persistent throughout the period of follow-up or present sporadically without any relationship to the complement level. Thirty-two patients never exhibited cryoglobulins in their serum and only two of these developed glomerulonephritis. Viewed another way, 24 of 33 (72%) patients with active glomerulonephritis had associated cryoglobulinemia and hypocomplementemia, whereas only 8 of 68 (12%) patients without glomerulonephritis exhibited this serologic pattern.

Hypocomplementemia alone would be expected to be associated with glomerulonephritis in SLE and, indeed, was present in 27 of 33 (80%) patients with this type of tissue injury. Only 3 of 8 patients with hypocom-

Table 2. Relationship between Cryoglobulinemia and Glomerulonephritis in 101 Patients with SLE

Cryoglobulinemia	Glomerulonephritis: Present[a]	Absent
Persistent	2	12
Varies inversely with CH_{50}	24	8
Sporadic	5	18
Absent	2	30

[a] Histopathologic diagnoses: persistent cryoglobulinemia—focal (2); cryoglobulinemia varying inversely with CH_{50}—diffuse proliferative (12), focal (7), membranous (1), no biopsy (4); sporadic cryoglobulinemia—diffuse proliferative (2), focal (2), membranous (1); absent cryoglobulinemia—diffuse proliferative (1), no biopsy (1).

plementemia and absence of associated cryoglobulinemia developed glomerulonephritis. Thirteen of fifty-five (24%) patients who did not develop glomerulonephritis were hypocomplementemic at various periods, suggesting that additional information of predictive value vis-à-vis clinically apparent glomerulonephritis may be obtained by considering both the complement level and serum cryoglobulins in the serologic assessment of patients with SLE. In other studies, the relationship between the concentration of cryoprecipitate in serum and the total hemolytic complement level was examined for 23 patients by linear regression analysis. A highly significant inverse correlation between the degree of hypocomplementemia and the concentration of cryoprecipitate in serum was found ($r = 0.8501$, $p < 0.0001$). These data confirm those of a number of other laboratories (Christian *et al.*, 1963; Stastny and Ziff, 1969; Agnello *et al.*, 1971; Druet *et al.*, 1973), and indicate a special relationship between cryoglobulinemia and glomerulonephritis in SLE.

4. Immunochemical Analysis of Cryoprecipitates

4.1. Methodology

The various techniques used to collect, isolate, fractionate, and characterize the cryoprecipitates in SLE have been described in detail (Winfield *et al.*, 1975a,b; Davis *et al.*, 1978). Cryoprecipitates were isolated from 50 ml of serum kept at 4°C under sterile conditions or with added sodium azide for 1 to 2 weeks. After exhaustive washing with cold phosphate-buffered saline, the cryoprecipitate was resolubilized at 37°C or, for fractionation studies, in acid buffers. Fractionation of serum cryoprecipitates was performed by sucrose density gradient ultracentrifugation in glycine acetate buffer, pH 3.5. Protein content was determined by the Folin–Ciacolteau method. IgM- and IgG-containing fractions were identified by quantitative radial immunodiffusion. Anti-IgG antibody was determined by hemagglutination of chromic chloride-sensitized type O human erythrocytes coated with human IgG. Antibodies to ssDNA or nDNA were quantitated by hemagglutination of DNA-coated erythrocytes or by a modified Farr assay using radiolabeled DNA. DNA antigen was sought by diphenylamine assay or, in more recent experiments, by counterimmunoelectrophoresis after exhaustive digestion of the cryoprecipitate with Pronase (Davis *et al.*, 1978). Anti-double-stranded RNA (dsRNA) and antiribonucleoprotein (anti-RNP) were determine by hemagglutination.

In all experiments, an aliquot of supernatant serum from which the cryoprecipitate had been collected was fractionated and studied in parallel. By quantitating the specific antibody activity or antigen content in both cryoprecipitate and supernatant serum, enrichment of antibody or antigen in the cryoprecipitate relative to the serum level was assessed. Significant enrichment in the cryoprecipitate argues against nonspecific coprecipitation of antibody from serum during isolation of the cryoprecipitate, and suggests the participation of that antibody in a circulating immune complex system. As a control, certain cryoprecipitates were studied for "nonsense" antibody activity, i.e., anti-tetanus toxoid, which would not be expected to be enriched in the cryoprecipitate.

4.2. *Anti-immunoglobulins*

Typical immunoglobulin composition of a cryoprecipitate from a patient with SLE fractionated by sucrose density gradient ultracentrifugation using acid buffers is shown in Fig. 2. Both IgM and IgG are present, with IgG representing the greater proportion. The 19 S fractions (IgM concentration 100 μ/ml) from five cryoprecipitates prepared in this fashion contained anti-IgG in a titer of 32–1024 by hemagglutination at cold temperatures (Winfield *et al.*, 1975a). Titers obtained with IgM isolated from supernatant serum under identical conditions were much lower, 2–4. Enrichment of anti-IgG in the cryoprecipitates relative to supernatant serum was calculated to be 16- to 256-fold. These data together with observations from earlier studies (Agnello *et al.*, 1971; Hanauer and Christian, 1967) indicate that cold-reactive IgM anti-IgG is an important factor in the cryoprecipitation of complexes in SLE.

4.3. *Antipolynucleotide Antibodies*

Because of the evidence implicating DNA/anti-DNA complexes in the pathogenesis of glomerulonephritis in SLE, cryoprecipitates from hypocomplementemic patients were isolated from serum and examined for polynucleotide antigens and antibodies as described above (Winfield *et al.*, 1975b). The data in Fig. 3 indicate the presence of anti-nDNA and anti-ssDNA antibodies in the majority. The mean enrichment of these antibodies relative to serum levels was 90- and 130-fold, respectively. Similar enrichment for anti-DNA was obtained in other experiments using a Farr assay and ^{3}H-

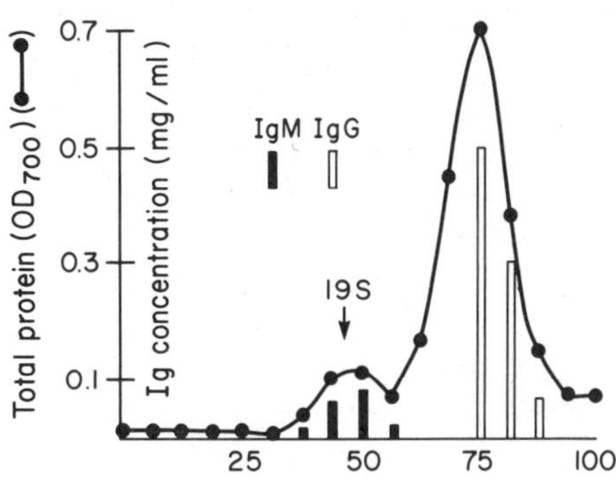

Figure 2. Sucrose gradient fractionation of an SLE serum cryoprecipitate using acid buffers.

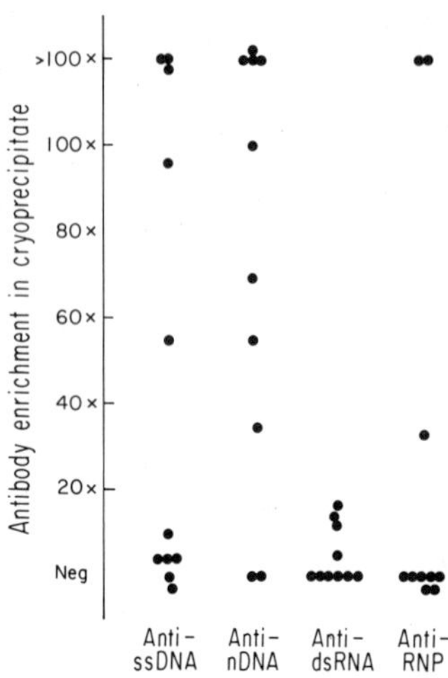

Figure 3. Enrichment of antipolynucleotide antibodies in cryoprecipitates relative to serum levels. Each datum for each antipolynucleotide represents the maximum enrichment in cryoprecipitates from single, different patients. Enrichment was calculated from relative hemagglutination titers of serum and cryoprecipitates: [(serum IgM + IgG)/(cryo IgM + IgG)] × 2(cryo titer − serum titer). Titers in this calculation were expressed as $\log_2$ of the reciprocal (from Winfield *et al.*, 1975b).

labeled HeLa DNA as antigen (Winfield *et al.*, 1975b; Davis *et al.*, 1978). A minority of cryoprecipitates were found to be enriched for anti-RNP antibody. Anti-dsRNA was not concentrated. Fifteen non-SLE cryoprecipitates also were examined for anti-DNA antibody. Two of these cryoprecipitates exhibited low-titer agglutination of DNA-coated erythrocytes. None bound ^{3}H-labeled HeLa DNA in the Farr assay.

The demonstration of specific concentration of anti-DNA antibodies in serum cryoprecipitates is similar to the findings of Koffler *et al.* (1974) from the study of glomerular eluates. The data suggest that cryoprecipitates in SLE may be composed of the same immune complexes which are found in the kidney.

4.4 DNA

In our original analyses of cryoprecipitates from patients with SLE, rather large quantities of DNA-like material (2.2–109.8 μ/mg cryoimmunoglobulin) were found using the diphenylamine assay (Winfield *et al.*, 1975b). The demonstration of similar amounts of "DNA" in non-SLE cryoprecipitates raised doubt concerning the specificity of this assay for DNA. Additional confusion resulted from repeated failures to detect DNA directly by immunologic techniques. Certain data were obtained to indicate that this latter discrepancy might be explained by the low molecular weight of DNA circulating in these patients. Thus, when serum from patients with SLE containing large amounts of DNA in antigen excess was fractionated by sucrose density gradient ultracentrifugation in acid pH, DNA always was demonstrable only in 7 S (IgG) fractions. We hypothesized that following dialysis of cryoprecipitate fractions against neutral buffers, DNA/anti-DNA complexes re-formed, and that antibody blocked the antigenic sites on the DNA molecules. Efforts to demonstrate increased DNA-binding activity in cryoprecipitates following deoxyribonuclease digestion were also unsuccessful (Davis *et al.*, unpublished data).

For these reasons, additional experiments to demonstrate DNA were performed following exhaustive digestion of cryoprecipitates with Pronase to destroy anti-DNA antibody (Davis *et al.*, 1978). With this approach, serum cryoprecipitates from 15 of 28 patients contained DNA by counterimmunoelectrophoresis using an SLE serum containing a high titer of anti-DNA antibody as a detection reagent (Table 3). The mean concentration of DNA was estimated to be 1.0 ± 1.2 μg/mg cryoimmunoglobulin. Supernatant sera were uniformly negative for DNA, both before and after Pronase digestion. Cryoprecipitates from 4 of 20 patients with a variety of disorders other than SLE also contained DNA, but in approximately 10-fold lower amounts, 0.03–0.2 μg/mg cryoimmunoglobulin.

In other experiments, Clq-binding material in serum was eluted from Clq-Sepharose columns and analyzed for immunoglobulin, anti-DNA antibody, and DNA antigen by counterimmunoelectrophoresis following digestion with Pronase (Davis *et al.*, 1978). Three of four such eluates contained both DNA and anti-DNA antibody enriched relative to the serum level.

This finding has been interpreted as providing additional evidence for the existence of DNA/anti-DNA complexes in the circulation of patients with SLE. An ambiguity of these findings is that the experiments were performed with serum and not with plasma. As the concentration of DNA found in the cryoprecipitates and the Clq-Sepharose eluates is within the range that could be released *in vitro* during the clotting process, absolute proof that DNA/anti-

Table 3. SLE Cryoprecipitates Containing Detectable DNA (μg/mg Ig)[a]

Patient	Before Pronase digestion	After Pronase[c] digestion	Ig (mg/ml)	Anti-DNA (% DNA bound)[b]
Ed	—	4.4	0.48	91%
Br	1.2	2.6	0.91	3%
Sh	—	2.4	0.5	37%
Gr	—	2.2	0.54	11%
Di	0.3	0.54	1.86	ND
Ga	—	0.50	0.59	33%
Be	—	0.41	0.73	16%
Pa	—	0.40	0.37	67%
Ay	—	0.30	0.50	0%
Es	—	0.30	0.56	ND
Ca	—	0.27	0.55	4%
Jo	—	0.20	1.48	63%
Co	—	0.19	0.77	6%
Hi	—	0.16	0.94	92%
Bl	—	(> 0.15)	ND	29%

[a] From Davis *et al.* (1978).
[b] Determination by Farr assay using 10 ng [^{3}H]nDNA per assay.
[c] Mean DNA concentration, when expressed as μg/mg of resolubilized cryoprecipitate, was 0.78 ± 0.85 after Pronase digestion.

DNA complexes in SLE cryoprecipitates actually circulate *in vivo* will require additional experiments in which this potential artifact is avoided.

5. Comment

There is no longer any serious doubt that anti-DNA antibodies and DNA comprise the predominant immune complex system underlying glomerulonephritis in SLE. Large gaps in our knowledge remain. Although considerable information has been obtained concerning the characteristics of anti-DNA antibody, almost nothing is known about the endogenous DNA with which it is complexed. Because of difficulty in isolating this endogenous DNA, its source, antigenicity, and molecular weight remain conjectural. Indeed, to establish even the existence of circulating DNA is problematic because patients with SLE encountered today rarely present with florid, advanced illness. Nor has the immunogen been identified. Future research in this area will be especially challenging and interesting.

Increased understanding of the antigen in the DNA/anti-DNA system will be required to resolve important questions about the complexes themselves. For example, recent studies of the dissociation kinetics of artificial DNA/anti-DNA complexes indicate that those containing nDNA are extremely stable even at physiologic temperatures (Taylor *et al.*, 1979). This high stability of nDNA/anti-DNA complexes may have important implications for the kinetic control of complex size and for the clearance of complexes by the reticuloendothelial system or the kidney. Further work to define the nature of defective reticuloendothelial clearance mechanisms, and the direct binding of free DNA to basement membranes in the glomerulus obviously is important in this regard.

Clinical investigation of patients with SLE and other diseases has provided persuasive, albeit indirect, evidence that cryoglobulinemia and hypocomplementemia are related to the development of glomerulonephritis. Skeptics may consider analytic studies of cryoproteins as a backward step of modern immunology toward the ice age or perhaps a discarding of sophisticated technology in favor of the ice bath. Nevertheless, cryoprecipitation of serum remains the easiest technique for collecting large amounts of relatively pure immune complexes for analysis. The data generated thus far in SLE, and in a number of other diseases, have provided useful information about the types of complexes which may localize in the kidney. The direction for further studies should be to eliminate artifactual ambiguities and to define the relationship between immune complexes in cryoprecipitates and those detected in the circulation by other techniques.

ACKNOWLEDGMENTS. Gratitude is due my colleagues who have made major contributions to the experimental work summarized in this paper: Henry G. Kunkel, David Koffler, Robert J. Winchester, and John S. Davis and to

Dennis Brinkmann, Lydia LeGrand, Virginia Estabrook, and Stephanie Godfrey for technical assistance. We are grateful to Ms. Brenda Cherry for typing the manuscript.

References

Abrass, C. K., Nies, K. M., Louis, J. S., Borden, W. A., White, B. S., and Glassock, R. J., 1978, Correlations of circulating immune complexes (CIC) and disease activity in patients with systemic lupus erythematosus (SLE), *Arthritis Rheum.* **21:**539 (abstract).

Agnello, V., Koffler, D., Eisenberg, J. W., Winchester, R. J., and Kunkel, H. G., 1971, Clq precipitins in the sera of patients with systemic lupus erythematosus and other hypocomplementemic states: Characterization of high and low molecular weight types, *J. Exp. Med.* **134:**228S.

Bruneau, C. O., Edmonds, J. P., Hughes, G. R. V., and Aarden, L., 1977, Detection and characterization of DNA/anti-DNA complexes in a patient with systemic lupus erythematosus, *Clin. Exp. Immunol.* **28:**433.

Cano, P. O., Jerry, L. M., Sladowski, J. P., and Osterland, C. K., 1977, Circulating immune complexes in systemic lupus erythematosus, *Clin. Exp. Immunol.* **29:**197.

Christian, C. L., Hatfield, W. B., and Chase, P. H., 1963, Systemic lupus erythematosus: Cryoprecipitation of sera, *J. Clin. Invest.* **42:**823.

Chused, T. M., Steinberg, A. D., and Talol, N., 1972, The clearance and localization of nucleic acids by New Zealand and normal mice, *Clin. Exp. Immunol.* **12:**465.

Davis, G. L., Jr., and Davis, J. S., IV, 1973, Detection of circulating DNA by counterimmunoelectrophoresis (CIE), *Arthritis Rheum.* **16:**52.

Davis, J. S., Godfrey, S. M., and Winfield, J. B., 1978, Direct evidence for circulating DNA/anti-DNA complexes in systemic lupus erythematosus, *Arthritis Rheum.* **21:**17.

Davis, P., Cumming, R. H., and Verrier-Jones, J., 1977, Relationship between anti-DNA antibodies, complement consumption, and circulating immune complexes, *Clin. Exp. Immunol.* **28:**226.

Druet, P., Letonturier, P., Contet, A., and Mandet, C., 1973, Cryoglobulinemia in human renal diseases: A study of seventy-six cases, *Clin. Exp. Immunol.* **15:**483.

Emlen, W., and Mannik, M., 1978a, Kinetics and mechanisms for removal of circulating single-stranded DNA in mice, *J. Exp. Med.* **147:**684.

Emlen, W., and Mannik, M., 1978b, Effect of immune complexes on clearance of single-stranded DNA in mice, *Arthritis Rheum.* **21:**555.

Frank, M. M., Jaffe, C. J., Kimberly, R. P., Lawley, T. J., and Plotz, P. H., 1977, An immunospecific clearance deficit in patients with systemic lupus erythematosus (SLE) related to the levels of circulating immune complexes (IC), *Clin. Res.* **25:**375A.

Freedman, P., and Markowitz, A. S., 1962, Globulin and complement in the diseased kidney, *J. Clin. Invest.* **41:**328.

Hamburger, M. I., Lawley, T. L., Plotz, P. H., and Frank, M. M., 1978, A serial study of reticuloendothelial (RES) Fc receptor function in patients with systemic lupus erythematosus, *Arthritis Rheum.* **21:**563 (abstract).

Hanauer, L. B., and Christian, C. C., 1967, Studies of cryoproteins in systemic lupus erythematosus, *J. Clin. Invest.* **46:**400.

Harbeck, R. J., Bardana, E. J., Kohler, P. F., and Carr, R. I., 1973, DNA/anti-DNA complexes: Their detection in systemic lupus erythematosus sera, *J. Clin. Invest.* **52:**789.

Izui, S., Lambert, P. H., and Miescher, P. A., 1976, *in vitro* demonstration of a particular affinity of glomerular basement membrane and collagen for DNA, *J. Exp. Med.* **144:**428.

Izui, S., Lambert, P.-H., and Miescher, P. A., 1977, Failure to detect circulating DNA/anti-DNA complexes by four radioimmunological methods in patients with systemic lupus erythematosus, *Clin. Exp. Immunol.* **30:**384.

Koffler, D., Schur, P., and Kunkel, H. G., 1967, Immunological studies concerning the nephritis of systemic lupus erythematosus, *J. Exp. Med.* **126:**607.

Koffler, D., Carr, R. I., Agnello, V., Fiezi, T., and Kunkel, H. G., 1969, Antibodies to polynucleotides: Distribution in human serums, *Science* **166:**1648.

Koffler, D., Agnello, V., Winchester, R., and Kunkel, H. G., 1973, The occurrence of single-stranded DNA in the serum of patients with systemic lupus erythematosus and other diseases, *J. Clin. Invest.***52:**198.

Koffler, D., Agnello, V., and Kunkel, H. G., 1974, Polynucleotide immune complexes in serum and glomeruli of patients with systemic lupus erythematosus, *Am. J. Pathol.* **74:**109.

Krishnan, C., and Kaplan, M. H., 1967, Immunopathological studies of systemic lupus erythematosus. II. Anti-nuclear reaction of γ-globulin eluted from homogenates and isolated glomeruli of kidneys from patients with lupus nephritis, *J. Clin. Invest.* **46:**569.

Mellors, R. C., Ortega, L. G., and Holman, H. R., 1957, Role of gamma globulin in pathogenesis of renal lesions in systemic lupus erythematosus and chronic membranous glomerulonephritis, with an observation on lupus erythematosus cell reaction, *J. Exp. Med.* **106:**191.

Natali, P. G., and Tan, E. M., 1972, Experimental renal disease induced by DNA/anti-DNA immune complexes, *J. Clin. Invest.* **51:**345.

Schur, P. H., and Sandson, J., 1968, Immunologic factors and clinical activity in systemic lupus erythematosus, *N. Engl. J. Med.* **278:**533.

Stastny, P., and Ziff, M., 1969, Cold-insoluble complexes and complement level in systemic lupus erythematosus, *N. Engl. J. Med.* **280:**1376.

Steinman, C. R., 1975, Free DNA in serum and plasma from normal adults, *J. Clin. Invest.* **56:**512.

Tan, E. M., Schur, P. H., Carr, R. I., and Kunkel, H. G., 1966, Deoxyribonucleic acid (DNA) and antibodies to DNA in the serum of patients with systemic lupus erythematosus, *J. Clin. Invest.* **45:**1732.

Taylor, R. P., Weber, D., Broccoli, A. V., and Winfield, J. B., 1979, DNA/anti-DNA complexes, *J. Immunol.* **122:**115.

Theofilopoulos, A. N., Wilson, C. B., and Dixon, F. J., 1976, The Raji cell radioimmune assay for detecting immune complexes in human sera, *J. Clin. Invest.* **57:**169.

Tsumita, T., and Iwanaga, M., 1963, Fate of injected deoxyribonucleic acid in mice, *Nature (London)* **198:**1088.

Vasquez, J. J., and Dixon, F. J., 1957, Immunohistochemical study of lesions in rheumatic fever, systemic lupus erythematosus, and rheumatoid arthritis, *Lab. Invest.* **6:**205.

Vaughn, J. H., Bayles, T. B., and Favour, C. B., 1951, Response of serum gamma globulin level and complement titer to adrenocorticotropic hormone (ACTH) therapy in lupus erythematosus disseminates, *J. Lab. Clin. Med.* **37:**698.

Winfield, J. B., Winchester, R. J., Wernet, P., and Kunkel, H. G., 1975a, Specific concentration of anti-lymphocyte antibodies in the serum cryoprecipitates of patients with SLE, *Clin. Exp. Immunol.* **19:**399.

Winfield, J. B., Koffler, D., and Kunkel, H. G., 1975b, Specific concentration of polynucleotide immune complexes in the cryoprecipitates of patients with systemic lupus erythematosus, *J. Clin. Invest.* **56:**563.

Winfield, J. B., Faiferman, I., and Koffler, D., 1977, Avidity of anti-DNA antibodies in serum and IgG glomerular eluates from patients with systemic lupus erythematosus, *J. Clin. Invest.* **50:**90.

Zubler, R. H., Lange, G., Lamberg, P. H., and Miescher, P. A., 1978, Detection of immune complexes in unheated sera by a modified ^{125}I-Clq binding test, *J. Immunol.* **116:**232.

29

Cryoprecipitable Immunoglobulins with Native DNA Reactivity in the Glomerulopathies

Edmund J. Lewis and Jimmy L. Roberts

1. *Introduction*

During the course of studies of the composition of antigen–antibody systems in disease states associated with cryoglobulinemia, a method which appeared to allow us to examine cold-precipitable immunoglobulins for antibody specificity was developed. Presuming that cryoglobulins represent immune reactants, it was reasoned that it would be necessary to dissociate intact antigen–antibody complexes prior to examining them for antibody content. The approach adopted was to first solubilize the cryoprecipitates in acid buffer. The material then was tested for antibody activity against nuclear antigens. In addition, cryoglobulins were examined for antibodies reactive with the mitochondrial double-stranded DNA (dsDNA) of the kinetoplast of *Crithidia luciliae* as evidence of anti-native DNA activity. The results of these studies of the anti-DNA and native DNA content of the serum cryoglobulins of patients within several diagnostic categories are presented.

2. *Methods*

2.1. *Patients*

Serum was obtained from the following: four patients with systemic lupus erythematosus with glomerulonephritis; four patients with mixed essential cryoglobulinemia; four patients with glomerulonephritis [membra-

Edmund J. Lewis and Jimmy L. Roberts · Department of Medicine, Rush Medical College, Rush–Presbyterian–St. Luke's Medical Center, Chicago, Illinois 60612.

nous glomerulopathy (1), membranoproliferative glomerulonephritis (1), rapidly progressive glomerulonephritis (1), and chronic proliferative glomerulonephritis (1)]; and four patients with active bacterial infection [subacute bacterial endocarditis with nephritis (2), klebsiella sepsis (1), and anaerobic cutaneous abscess (1)]. No patients in this study were receiving procainamide, hydralazine, isoniazid, or phenytoin.

2.2 *Cryoprecipitation of Serum*

Serum and plasma were collected and processed under conditions which minimized blood cell trauma using previously described methods (Roberts and Lewis, 1978). Under these conditions, serum cryoglobulin concentrations in normal subjects were less than 10μg/ml. DNA was not detectable in normal serum processed by this technique, using either the ethidium bromide or counterimmunoelectrophoresis (CIE) assays (see below). Cryoglobulins were assayed for content of total protein, immunoglobulins, Clq, and rheumatoid factor. The details of these procedures are provided in a previous publication (Roberts and Lewis, 1978).

2.3. *Antinuclear and Antinative DNA Assays*

Antinuclear and anti-native DNA antibody titers were determined on supernatant serums and warm-solubilized cryoprecipitates using serial dilutions in phosphate-buffered saline (PBS), pH 7.4. Antinuclear antibodies were assayed using indirect immunofluorescence with normal mouse kidney as antigen substrate. Anti-native DNA antibody titers were measured by indirect immunofluorescence staining of the kinetoplast of C. luciliae which had been airfixed to microscopic slides (Stienert, 1965; Aarden *et al.*, 1975). In this laboratory a significant serum anti-native DNA titer using this substrate is > 1:8. All antibody titers in this study are expressed as $\log_2$ of the reciprocal ($1/\log_2$), i.e., 1:2 . . .q 1; 1=:4 = 2; 1:8 = 3, etc.

In order to determine whether antinuclear and anti-native DNA antibodies were present in cryoglobulins in a complexed state, which could preclude reactivity at neutral pH, cryoprecipitates were examined after acidification. Cryoprecipitates were diluted in acid citrate-buffered saline (CBS), pH 3.2. The solubilized precipitates were applied to a substrate containing DNA (mouse kidney or C luciliae). The pH of the reaction medium was then restored to neutrality by the addition of a specific volume of PBS (pH 7.4). After incubation for 30 min, the slides were washed with PBS and stained with monospecific conjugated antiserums to human IgG, M and A heavy chains, and κ and λ light chains. Each antiserum used in this study produced a single line on immunoelectrophoresis and double diffusion in gel when tested against serum or plasma, and a single line of complete identity with reference antiserums directed against the appropriate antigen.

2.4. Control Studies

A number of control studies of the acidification technique were undertaken in order to verify that exposure of immunoglobulins or DNA substrate to acid pH and subsequent neutralization did not result in artifactual results.

2.4.1. *Reaction Specificity*

In order to determine whether serum proteins or immune complexes were capable of nonspecifically reacting with the antigen substrates, the following reactants were tested at neutral pH, acid pH, and after acidification followed by neutralization to pH 7.4.: (1) normal human serum; (2) IgG isolated from normal human serum; (3) heat-aggregated IgG isolated from normal human serum; (4) PBS-washed human albumin–anti-human albumin complexes cryoprecipitated at equivalence from a goat anti-human albumin antiserum.

2.4.2. *Substrate Controls*

In order to determine whether substrate native DNA was altered by the acidification or incubation procedures, the following controls were undertaken. (1) Anti-single-stranded DNA (ssDNA) was produced in rabbits injected with heat-denatured calf thymus DNA and was adsorbed with insolubilized native DNA prior to us (Plescia *et al.*, 1964). *C. luciliae* smears were tested with this antiserum before and after acid incubation. (2) Mouse tissue and *Crithidia* were reacted with ethidium bromide, a substance which reacts only with dsDNA (Plescia *et al.*, 1964), in order to detect the latter's presence in substrate after alcohol fixation or acid incubation. The intensity of ethidium bromide kinetoplast fluorescence of untreated *Crithidia* smears was compared with smears incubated with (a) acid buffer, (b) DNase, (c) RNase, and (d) *Neurospora crassa* endonuclease (Linn and Lehman, 1965a,b). (3) Mouse tissue or *Crithidia* were pretreated with DNase or RNase in order to determine whether these digestions abolished the subsequent reaction with immunoglobulins in cryoprecipitates. (4) Substrates were incubated with *N. crassa* endonuclease, which is capable of digesting single-stranded polynucleotides but has no effect on dsDNA (Linn and Lehman, 1965a,b,). Cryoglobulins were then tested for their ability to bind to these endonuclease-digested substrates. (5) Mouse kidney sections and *Crithidia* were incubated with CBS (pH 3.2.) and then with (a) normal human serum, (b) test serum supernatants, (c) cryoprecipitates, in order to determine whether acidification of the antigenic material caused nonspecific protein binding or altered reactivity with the cryoprecipitates. (6) Substrates were extracted with 0.1 N HCl according to the method published by Fritzler and Tan (1978) in order to extract histones and nucleoproteins. These substrates were then reacted with selected cryoprecipitates in order to determine whether the immunoglobulins were reacting with native DNA or histone nucleoprotein antigens.

2.4.3. *Studies of Antibody–Antigen Interaction*

In order to determine whether the reaction between cryoprecipitable immunoglobulins and dsDNA in the substrates was antibody–antigen, rather than a nonantibody interaction, the following studies were performed. (1) An attempt to ascertain whether Clq which could be attached to the Fc portion of IgG could be binding the IgG to DNA was made. Cryoprecipitates were tested after pretreatment at 56°C for 30 min in order to remove Clq and after exposure to bacterial collagenase in order to destroy the collagen portion of Clq (Agnello *et al.*, 1970; Knobel *et al.*, 1974).(2) In order to further determine that DNA-reactivity of the immunoglobulin represented antibody, cryoprecipitates were pepsin-digested to yield $F(ab')_2$ immunoglobulin fragments and tested for anti-DNA activity (Lachman, 1971).

2.5. *Native DNA Content of Cryoprecipitates*

Native DNA concentrations in supernatant serum and solubilized cryoprecipitates were measured fluorimetrically using ethidium bromide (Le-Peca, and Paoletti; 1967; Kamm and Smith, 1972). DNase- and RNase-pretreated aliquots of each patient's serum were used for preparation of serum native DNA standards. A Farrand filter fluorometer, Model A, with an 85-W mercury vapor light source, a 5–57 excitation filter with a 420-nm peak transmittance, 2–63 emission filter with a sharp cut below 580 nm, and a 5-mm slit diameter were used to measure samples in 10 × 75-mm borosilicate glass tubes. In this laboratory, native DNA concentrations in normal serum and plasma, obtained and processed in the same manner, are less than 0.1 μg/ml. Quantitation of native DNA concentrations in simultaneously obtained sera and plasma from nine of the patients in this study also was performed to ascertain whether there were differences between native DNA concentrations in pathologic serum and plasma.

Representative cryoglobulin specimens also were studied using the CIE method for seimquantitative estimation of DNA content (Davis and Davis, 1973; Steinman, 1975). In addition, The DNA content of selected cryoglobulin samples was measure by both the ethidium bromide and CIE techniques before and after incubation of the samples with Pronase type IV (Sigma), DNase, and Pronase followed by DNase (Davis *et al.*, 1978; Shepard *et al.*, 1978). The latter experiments were carried out in order to determine the degree to which the interaction between DNA and anti-DNA might cause spatial interference with enzyme or reagent which is normally capable of combining with DNA.

3. *Results*

3.1. *Cryoglobulin Protein Content*

In addition to the data in Table 1, 7 of 16 isolates also contained Clq.

Table 1. Cryoglobulin Protein, Immunoglobulins, and Rheumatoid Factor (RF)

Group	Protein (μg/ml serum)	IgG (μg/ml serum)	IgM (μg/ml serum)	IgA (μg/ml serum)	RF titer/ml serum[a]
Lupus erythematosus					
1	140	16.3	6.5	2.1	Neg
2	166	19.1	13.7	< 0.1	Neg
3	209	51.1	46.6	3.8	4
4	62	23.6	< 0.1	< 0.1	Neg
Essential cryoglobulinemia					
1	440	112.0	2.6	< 0.1	1
2	1250	253.0	207.4	611.3	Neg
3	270	38.2	82.6	21.5	4
4	775	334.0	132.2	21.4	6
Glomerulonephritis					
1 Rapidly progressive	52	17.7	6.5	< 0.1	Neg
2 Membranous	44	10.0	1.7	< 0.1	Neg
3 Membranoproliferative	150	< 0.1	< 0.1	< 0;1	Neg
4 Chronic proliferative	150	41.3	8.2	1.3	Neg
Bacterial infection					
1 Endocarditis	88	16.9	19.5	< 0.1	Neg
2 Endocarditis	290	45.9	23.7	14.0	1
3 Anaerobic abscess	64	9.4	34.2	1.6	Neg
4 Klebsiella sepsis	55	3.1	13.0	0.9	Neg

[a] Titer expressed as $1/\log_2$.

3.2. Control Studies

Normal human sera, isolated IgG, heat-aggregated IgG, and albumin–antialbumin immune complexes failed to react with mouse kidney nuclei or *Crithidia* kinetoplasts at neutral pH or when either the test material or the substrate had been subjected to acidification.

Rabbit antibody to ssDNA reacted with mouse nuclei, but did not react with *Crithidia* kinetoplasts before or after acid incubation. Pretreatment of *Crithidia* with DNase abolished ethidium bromide fluorescence of the kinetoplasts, whereas pretreatment with RNase and *N. crassa* endonuclease did not alter ethidium bromide fluorescence, confirming that this antigen substrate was dsDNA. The fluorescence observed after ethidium bromide reactivity with kinetoplasts was unchanged by incubation of the kinetoplasts in acid citrate buffer for up to 1 hr.

DNase pretreatment of both nuclear and *Crithidia* substrates abolished antinuclear rim-staining patterns and kinetoplast staining by the cryoprecipitates, indicating that immunoglobulin in the cryoglobulins was binding to DNase-sensitive antigens. This reaction was not altered by acid extraction of histones and nucleoproteins from the substrate, indicating reactivity of the immunoglobulin with DNA, not DNA–histone or –nucleoprotein complex. Pretreatment of substrates with *N. crassa* endonuclease caused a reduction of antinuclear antibody titers, but no decrease in immunoglobulin reactivity with kinetoplasts. Antinuclear and antikinetoplast titers were not altered

Table 2. Summary of Control Study Titers[a] Using Cryoglobulin Acidification Technique

	Antikinetoplast (native DNA) antibody titer[a]			
	IgG		L-Chain	
Control conditions	Phosphate buffer	Citrate buffer	Phosphate buffer	Citrate buffer
Untreated cryoglobulin[b], untreated substrate	Neg	3	1	5
$F(ab')_2$ cryoglobulin, untreated substrate	Neg	0	1	5
56°C heated cryoglobulin, untreated substrate	Neg	3		
Untreated cryoglobulin, RNase-treated substrate	Neg	3		
Untreated cryoglobulin, DNase-treated substrate	Neg	0		
Untreated cryoglobulin, endonuclease-treated substrate	Neg	3		
Untreated cryoglobulin, 0.1 N HCl-extracted substrate	Neg	3		

[a] Titer expressed as $1/\log_2$.
[b] Comparably diluted aliquots of the same cryoglobulin were used for each of the control studies shown in this table.

Table 3. Comparison of Cryoglobulin Antinuclear Antibody (ANA) and Anti-Native (NDNA) Titers[a] at Neutral pH (PBS) and after Acid (CBS) Treatment[b]

	Peripheral pattern ANA						Anti-NDNA IgG	
	IgG		IgM		IgA			
Group	PBS	CBS	PBS	CBS	PBS	CBS	PBS	CBS
Lupus erythematosus								
1	Neg	9	3	7	1	5	Neg	8
2	Neg	8	Neg	Neg	Neg	Neg	Neg	7
3	8	9	2	8	1	8	3	7
4	Neg	6	1	Neg	Neg	3	Neg	5
Essential cryoglobulinemia								
1	Neg	11	Neg	4	Neg	Neg	Neg	9
2	Neg	12	2	11	9	17	Neg	12
3	4	10	3	11	3	11	3	9
4	7	19	6	12	3	9	5	11
Glomerulonephritis								
1 Rapidly progressive	Neg	6	Neg	5	Neg	Neg	Neg	5
2 Membranous	Neg	5	Neg	Neg	Neg	Neg	Neg	4
3 Membrano-proliferative	Neg	Neg	Neg	Neg	Neg	Neg	Neg	Neg
4 Chronic proliferative	Neg	9	Neg	7	Neg	5	Neg	7
Bacterial infection								
1 Endocarditis	Neg	6	Neg	8	Neg	Neg	Neg	7
2 Endocarditis	1	11	1	9	3	9	1	9
3 Anaerobic abscess	Neg	8	Neg	8	Neg	5	Neg	8
4 Klebsiella sepsis	Neg	6	Neg	8	Neg	3	Neg	5

[a] Titer expressed as $1/\log_2$.
[b] Cryoprecipitate resuspended in one-eighth the original serum volume.

when the test substrate was pretreated by acid citrate buffer incubation, alcohol fixation, RNase, or acid extraction with 0.1 N HCl (see Table 2).

3.3. Antinuclear and Antikinetoplast (Native DNA) Antibody Content of Cryoglobulins

Antinuclear antibody titers were recorded according to the production of a peripheral (rim) nuclear staining pattern (Fig. 1). Reactivity of the cryoprecipitable immunoglobulins with nuclear antigens was slightly reduced when sections were predigested with *N. crassa* endonuclease, abolished when predigested with DNase, and unaffected by preincubation with 0.1 N HCl to remove histone and nucleoprotein from DNA (Table 2). Incubation of solubilized cryoprecipitate at pH 7.4 resulted in a positive staining pattern in 2 of 4 SLE, 3 of 4 MEC, 1 of 4 infection, and 0 of 4 glomerulonephritis patients (Table 3). Preincubation of the cryoglobulin in acid citrate buffer

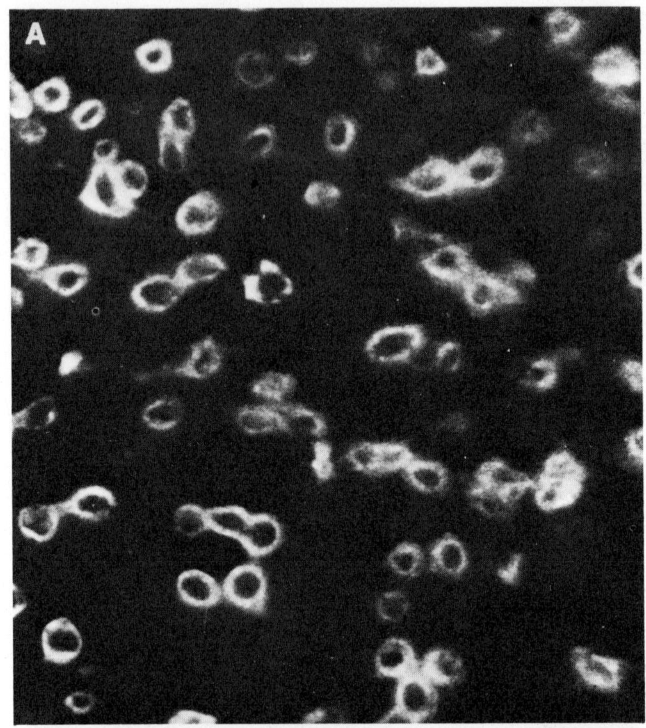
A

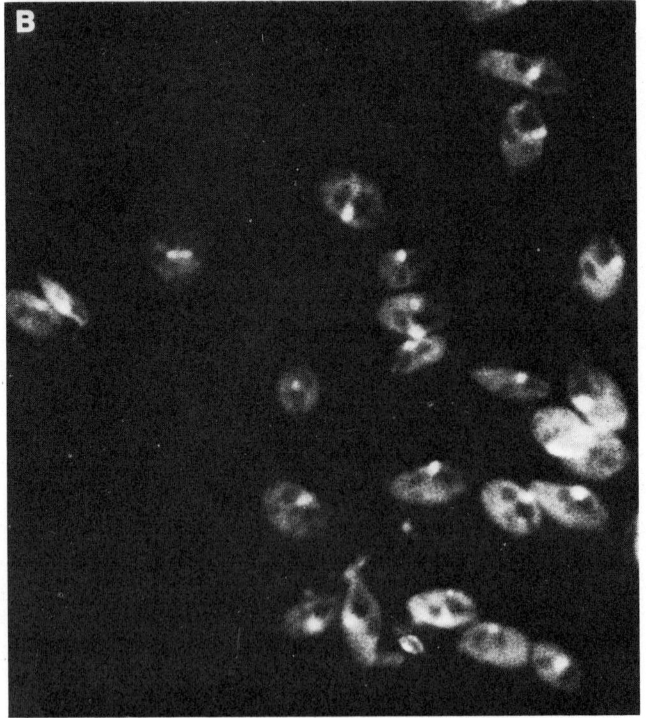
B

Table 4. Comparison of Acid-Dissociated Cryoglobulin and Supernatant Serum Anti-Native DNA Titers and IgG Concentrations

Group	Cryo titer[a,b]	Serum titer[a]	Cryo IgG (μg/ml serum)	Serum IgG (μg/ml)	Cryo anti-native DNA enrichment over serum
Lupus erythematosus					
1	5	6	16.3	36,500	1866
2	4	3	19.1	35,200	2457
3	4	3	51.1	12,200	318
4	2	4	23.6	18,100	383
Essential cryoglobulinemia					
1	6	5	112.0	24,700	265
2	9	3	253.0	11,700	139
3	6	2	38.2	11,600	911
4	8	1	334.0	5,200	125
Glomerulonephritis					
1 Rapidly progressive	2	1	17.7	34,000	3842
2 Membranous	1	3	10.0	9,600	320
3 Membrano-proliferative	Neg	Neg	< 0.1	870	—
4 Chronic proliferative	4	5	41.3	13,000	251
Bacterial infection					
1 Endocarditis	4	2	16.9	11,100	1314
2 Endocarditis	5	4	45.9	33,000	899
3 Anaerobic abscess	5	5	9.4	12,000	1277
4 Klebsiella sepsis	2	3	3.1	14,800	3183

[a] Titer expressed as $1/\log_2$.
[b] Titer of cryoprecipitate when resuspended in the same volume as the serum volume from which it was precipitated.

resulted in positive staining in all samples but one and enhancement of the titers in those samples which had been positive at pH 7.4. Anti-native DNA titers were carried out for IgG and the results were virtually identical to those noted for antinuclear reactivity (Fig. 1, Table 3).

3.4. IgG Anti-native DNA in Cryoglobulins and in Supernatant Serum (Table 4)

In order to determine whether anti-native DNA antibodies were concentrated in the cryoglobulin relative to the serum, an estimate of anti-native

←

Figure 1. Antinuclear and antikinetoplast (native DNA) antibody immunofluorescence. (A) A typical peripheral (rim) antinuclear staining pattern for IgG is produced with normal mouse kidney by acid preincubation and subsequent neutralization of this cryoglobulin. (B) The kinetoplasts of *Crithidia luciliae* are positively stained for IgG by this cryoglobulin after incubation of the precipitate in acid buffer. This staining of kinetoplasts is specific for anti-native DNA antibodies. (A: Glomerulonephritis cryoprecipitate #1, 1:8/goat anti-human IgG, FITC; B: same as A except titer 1:4. Both × 160.)

Table 5. Cryoglobulin and Supernatant Serum Native DNA Concentrations

Group	Cryo[a] native DNA (μg/ml serum)	Serum native DNA (μg/ml)	Native DNA in cryo[a] (%)
Lupus erythematosus			
1	0.72	0.20	78.3
2	1.70	1.00	63.0
3	0.28	< 0.10	93.0
4	1.10	3.60	23.4
Essential cryoglobulinemia			
1	0.24	0.40	37.5
2	1.20	7.20	14.6
3	0.14	4.00	3.4
4	1.65	8.40	16.4
Glomerulonephritis			
1 Rapidly progressive	ND[b]	1.20	—
2 Membranous	0.87	7.60	10.4
3 Membranoproliferative	< 0.10	< 0.10	—
4 Chronic proliferative	1.90	6.00	24.1
Bacterial infection			
1 Endocarditis	ND	1.60	—
2 Endocarditis	1.31	0.20	86.6
3 Anaerobic abscess	0.12	0.10	54.5
4 Klebsiella sepsis	1.25	7.20	14.8

[a] Cryo, cryoprecipitate.
[b] ND, not determined.

DNA enrichment was constructed. The ratio of the relative anti-native DNA in the cryoglobulin to that of the supernatant serum was multiplied by the ratio of IgG in supernatant serum to that in cryoglobulin. In all cases in which anti-native DNA was detectable in the cryoglobulin, this antibody appeared to be selectively concentrated in the cryoglobulin.

3.5. Native DNA Content of Cryoglobulins

Concentrations of native DNA in cryoglobulins and in supernatant serum are shown in Table 5. Simultaneous serum and plasma DNA determinations in these specimens did not differ significantly. There was no correlation between the DNA content of the cryoglobulin and the presence or quantity of Clq in the specimen.

The amount of measurable DNA in cryoglobulins by either the ethidium bromide or CIE methods was enhanced by predigestion of the protein component of the sample with Pronase (Table 6). In addition, DNase incubation with the cryoglobulins resulted in total digestion of DNA only after the sample had been previously incubated with Pronase (Table 6).

Table 6. DNA Concentrations of Isolated Cryoglobulins

	DNA (ethidium bromide)[a,b]				DNA (CIE)[c]	
Diagnosis	Untreated sample	After Pronase digestion	After DNase digestion	After Pronase + DNase digestion	Untreated sample	After Pronase digestion
Lupus erythematosus	0.8	1.8	0.4	0.0	> 0.3 < 0.7	> 1.3 < 2.6
Lupus erythematosus	1.0	2.1	0.5	0.0	> 0.3 < 0.7	> 0.7 < 1.3
Essential cryoglobulinemia	1.8	2.3	0.6	0.0	> 0.3 < 0.7	> 2.7 < 5.3
Essential cryoglobulinemia	1.6	3.4	0.3	0.0	> 0.3 < 0.7	> 0.7 < 1.3
Glomerulonephritis	0.5	1.6	0.1	0.0	> 0.3 < 0.7	> 0.3 < 0.7

[a] DNA concentrations expressed as micrograms of DNA in cryoprecipitate per milliliter of original serum specimen.
[b] All untreated samples comparably diluted in same buffer used for Pronase digestion.
[c] CIE (counterimmunoelectrophoresis) results are semiquantitative, based upon the concentration of standard serial dilutions.

4. Discussion

These findings reveal that immunoglobulins present in cryoprecipitates taken from the serum of patients with diseases other than systemic lupus erythematosus are capable of binding to antigens in mouse nuclei and in the kinetoplast of *C. luciliae*. That the antigen to which the immunoglobulins are bound is native DNA is supported by the finding that incubation of substrate with DNase abolishes the reaction. Incubation with *N. crassa* endonuclease, which would abolsih reactivity with ssDNA, or with 0.1 N HCl, which would abolish reactivity with histone or necleoprotein antigens, has no effect upon antikinetoplast titers.

Evidence that the interaction between cryoprecipitable immunoglobulins and native DNA in the substrates represents antibody–antigen activity is supported by the observation of $F(ab')_2$ fragment reactivity with DNA substrate. The inability to demonstrate Clq immunochemically in half of the specimens, making DNA–Clq–immunoglobulin coprecipitation an unlikely explanation of the phenomenon, and the failure to alter reactivity by maneuvers which dissociate Clq from immunoglobulins or which destroy the part of the Clq molecule which is presumed to interact with DNA, lend further evidence against the phenomenon being a nonantibody interaction between IgG and DNA.

Data suggesting that anti-native DNA antibodies present in cryoglobulins exist as components of immune complexes include: (1) the demonstration of enhanced anti-native DNA antibody titers after acidification of the cryoprecipitates, a procedure which dissociates antigen–antibody complexes; (2) the demonstration of native DNA as well as anti-DNA in cryoprecipitates; (3) the enhancement of measurable DNA in the specimens after Pronase digestion (this observation indicates an intimate spatial relationship between the DNA and immunoglobulin components of cryoprecipitates); (4) the observation that DNase does not completely digest the DNA present in cryoprecipitates unless the immunoglobulin component is first digested with Pronase further suggests intimate binding between DNA and immunoglobulins, as would be present in antigen–antibody complexes.

These studies of patients with systemic lupus erythematosus reveal similar results to those of others who have studied cryoglobulins in this disease state (Winfield *et al.*, 1973; Koffler *et al.*, 1968, 1971a, 1974). Patients in other disease categories in this study revealed findings strikingly comparable with regard to the detection of native DNA and anti-native DNA antibodies in cryoprecipitate. Previous efforts to demonstrate anti-native DNA and DNA in immune complexes from patients with diseases other than lupus have been inconclusive (Harbeck *et al.*, 1973; Stingl *et al.*, 1976). Bluestone *et al.* (1970) were able to demonstrate DNA in the cryoprecipitates of patients with essential mixed cryoglobulinemia, but they did not demonstrate that the immunoglobulin in the precipitates had specific anti-DNA activity. Similarly, Davis *et al.* (1978) demonstrated DNA in cryoglobulins isolated from four patients with shunt nephritis, Sjögren's syndrome, hyperlipoproteinemia, and another connective tissue disorder, but did not report whether or not DNA-reactive immunoglobulin could be detected in the cryoprecipitates. McPhaul (1978) studied the tendency of radiolabeled DNA to reprecipitate with solubilized cryoglobulins taken from patients with glomerulonephritis and with lupus. His results indicated that the coprecipitation of DNA with cryoglobulins did not appear to be explained by nonspecific DNA–protein interactions.

These findings therefore deserve consideration regarding the classic concepts of native DNA as a self antigen. Although the response to DNA in the circulation is not well understood, native DNA has not been considered to be highly immunogenic (Plescia *et al.*, 1964; Koffler *et al.*, 1971b; Christian *et al.*, 1965). In some animal experiments, induction of anti-DNA antibodies has required carrier-bound denatured DNA, other hapten–carrier stimulation, or stimulation with a B-cell mitogen (Plescia *et al.*, 1964; Christian *et al.*, 1965; Fournié *et al.*, 1974; Izui *et al.*, 1977; Yamauchi *et al.*, 1975).

Antibodies to denatured DNA are seen in a variety of human disease states, but antibodies to native DNA have been considered specific for systemic lupus erythematosus (Harbeck *et al.*, 1973; Stingl *et al.*, 1976; Koffler *et al.*, 1971b; Tan *et al.*, 1966; Jain *et al.*, 1976). However, in a few instances these antibodies have been described in other disease states. Anti-native DNA antibodies have been reported to develop in patients with chronic hepatic disease as well as in a small number of patients with immunologic disease other than systemic lupus erythematosus (Davis and Read, 1975; Jain *et al.*, 1976; Pincus *et al.*, 1969; Epstein *et al.*, 1971; Rochmis *et al.*, 1974). In addition, it has been demonstrated recently that a small percentage of B lymphocytes from normal persons have surface receptors for native DNA (Bankhurst and Williams, 1975). Hence, the cells presumed to be required for the development of a humoral immune response to DNA are present in the normal state.

It is conceivable that the development of anti-native DNA antibodies can be a normal response to the release of DNA into the circulation. In mice, the injection of bacterial lipopolysaccharides or the lipid A fraction of these lipopolysaccharides results in the release of DNA into the circulation and the subsequent development of antibodies to both native and denatured DNA (Fournié *et al.*, 1974). In addition to the bacterial endotoxin-induced release of DNA from leukocytes, other mechanisms of DNA release may pertain in inflammatory or immune disease states. *In vitro*, stimulated human lymphocytes can also release DNA, without associated cell death (Anker *et al.*, 1975). These mechanisms could explain the presence of DNA in serum and plasma from patients with a variety of inflammatory states (Davis and Davis, 1973; Bluestone *et al.*, 1970; Tan *et al.*, 1966; Hughes *et al.*, 1971b). The development of anti-native DNA antibodies, therefore, could represent a response to the release of unusual amounts of native DNA into the circulation in otherwise normal subjects.

5. Summary

Anti-native DNA antibodies and DNA are present in cryoprecipitates from patients with systemic lupus erythematosus and some other cryoglobulinemic states. The data suggest that these antibodies may be bound in immune complexes. The demonstration of native DNA in these precipitates raises the likelihood that they represent specific antigen in these complexes. Whether or not these complexes play a pathogenetic role in nonlupus inflammatory diseases remains to be demonstrated.

References

Aarden, L. A., de Groot, E. R., and Feltkamp, T. E. W., 1975, Immunology of DNA. III. *Crithidia luciliae*, a simple substrate for the determination of anti-dsDNA with the immunofluorescence technique, *Ann. N.Y. Acad. Sci.* **254:**505.

Agnello, V., Winchester, R. J. and Kunkel, H. G., 1970, Precipitin reactions of the Clq component of complement with aggregated γ-globulin and immune complexes in gel diffusion, *Immunology* **19:**909.

Anker, P., Stroun, M., and Maurice, P. A., 1975, Spontaneous release of DNA by human blood lymphocytes as shown in an in vitro system, *Cancer Res.* **35:**2375.

Bankhurst, A. D., and Williams, R. C., 1975, Identification of DNA-binding lymphocytes in patients with systemic lupus erythematosus, *J. Clin. Invest.* **56:**1378.

Bluestone, R., Goldberg, L. S., Cracchiolo, A., and Barrett, E. V., 1970, Detection and characterization of DNA in mixed (IgG-IgM) cryoglobulins, *Int. Arch. Allergy Appl. Immunol.* **39:**16.

Christian, C. L., DeSimone, A. R., and Abruzzo, J. L., 1965, Anti-DNA antibodies in hyperimmunized rabbits, *J. Exp. Med.* **121:**309.

Davis, G. L. Jr., and Davis, J. S., IV, 1973, Detection of circulating DNA by counterimmunoelectrophoresis (CIE), *Arthritis Rheum.* **16:**52.

Davis, J. S., Godfrey, S. M., and Winfield, J. B., 1978, Direct evidence for circulating DNA/anti-DNA complexes in systemic lupus erythematosus, *Arthritis Rheum.* **21:**17.

Davis, P., and Read, A. E., 1975, Antibodies to double-stranded (native) DNA in active chronic hepatitis, *Gut* **16:**413.

Epstein, W. V., Tan, M., and Easterbrook, M., 1971, Serum antibody to double-stranded RNA and DNA in patients with idiopathic and secondary uveitis, *N. Engl. J. Med.* **285:**1502.

Fournié, G. J., Lambert, P. H., and Miescher, P. A., 1974, Release of DNA in circulating blood and induction of anti-DNA antibodies after injection of bacterial lipopolysaccharides, *J. Exp. Med.* **140:**1189.

Fritzler, M. J., and Tan, E. M., 1978, Antibodies to histones in drug-induced and idiopathic lupus erythematosus, *J. Clin. Invest.* **62:**560.

Harbeck, R. J., Bardana, E. J., Kohler, P. F., and Carr, R. I., 1973, DNA/anti-DNA complexes: Their detection in systemic lupus erythematosus sera, *J. Clin. Invest.* **52:**789.

Hughes, G. R. V., Cohen, S. A., and Christian, C. L., 1971a, Anti-DNA activity in systemic lupus erythematosus: A diagnostic and therapeutic guide, *Ann. Rheum. Dis.* **30:**259.

Hughes, G. R. V., Cohen, S. A., Lightfoot, R. W., Meltzer, J. I., and Christian, C. L., 1971b, The release of DNA into serum and synovial fluid, *Arthritis Rheum.* **14:**259.

Izui, S., Lambert, P. H., Fournié, G. J., Türler, H., and Miescher, P. A., 1977, Features of systemic lupus erythematosus in mice injected with bacterial lipopolysaccharides: Identification of circulating DNA and renal localization of DNA–anti-DNA complexes, *J. Exp. Med.* **145:**1115.

Jain, S., Markham, R., Thomas, H. C., and Sherlock, S., 1976, Double-stranded DNA-binding capacity of serum in acute and chronic liver disease, *Clin. Exp. Immunol.* **26:**35.

Kamm, R. C., and Smith, A. G., 1972, Nucleic acid concentrations in normal human plasma, *Clin. Chem.* **18:**519.

Knobel, H. R., Heusser, C., Rodrick, M. L., and Isliker, H., 1974, Enzymatic digestion of the first component of human complement (Clq), *J. Immunol.* **112:**2094.

Koffler, D., Schur, P. H., and Kunkel, H. G., 1968, Immunological studies concerning the nephritis of systemic lupus erythematosus, *J. Exp. Med.* **126:**607.

Koffler, D., Agnello, V., Thoburn, R., and Kunkel, H. G., 1971a, Systemic lupus erythematosus: Prototype of immune complex nephritis in man, *J. Exp. Med.* **134:**169s.

Koffler, D., Carr, R., Agnello, V., Thoburn, R., and Kunkel, H. G., 1971b, Antibodies to polynucleotides in human sera: Antigenic specificity and relation to disease, *J. Exp. Med.* **134:**294.

Koffler, D., Agnello, V., and Kunkel, H. G., 1974, Polynucleotide immune complexes in serum and glomeruli of patients with systemic lupus erythematosus, *Am. J. Pathol.* **74:**109.

Lachman, P. J., 1971, The purification of specific antibody as $F(ab')_2$ by the pepsin digestion of antigen–antibody precipitates, and its application to immunoglobulin and complement antigens, *Immunochemistry* **8:**81.

LePecq, J. B., and Paoletti, C., 1967, A fluorescent complex between ethidium bromide and nucleic acids: Physical-chemical characterization, *J. Mol. Biol.* **27:**87.

Linn, S., and Lehman, I. R., 1965a, An endonuclease from *Neurospora crassa* specific for polynucleotides lacking an ordered structure. I. Purification and properties of the enzyme, *J. Biol. Chem.* **240:**1287.

Linn, S., and Lehman, I. R., 1965b, An endonuclease from *Neurospora crassa* specific for polynucleotides lacking an ordered structure. II. Studies of enzyme specificity, *J. Biol. Chem.* **240:**1294.

McPhaul, J. J., Jr., 1978, Cryoimmunoglobulinemia in patients with primary renal disease and systemic lupus erythematosus. I. IgG- and DNA-binding assessed by co-precipitation, *Clin. Exp. Immunol.* **31:**131.

Pincus, T., Schur, P. H., Rose, J. A., Decker, J. L., and Talal, N., 1969, Measurement of serum DNA-binding activity in systemic lupus erythematosus, *N. Engl. J. Med.* **281:**701.

Plescia, O. J., Braun, W., and Palczuk, N. E., 1964, Production of antibodies to denatured deoxyribonucleic acid (DNA), *Proc. Natl. Acad. Sci. USA* **52:**279.

Roberts, J. L., and Lewis E. J., 1978, Identification of antinative DNA antibodies in cryoglobulinemic states, *Am. J. Med.* **65:**437.

Rochmis, P. G., Palefsky, H., Becker, M., Roth, H., and Zvaifler, N. J., 1974, Native DNA binding in rheumatoid arthritis, *Ann. Rheum. Dis.* **33:**357.

Shepard, J. D., Fritzler, M. J., Watson, J. H., and van de Sande, J. H., 1978, Anti-DNA antibody binding as measured by the inhibition of ethidium bromide fluorescence, *Arthritis Rheum.* **21:**591.

Steinman, C. R., 1975, Free DNA in serum and plasma from normal adults, *J. Clin. Invest.* **56:**512.

Stienert, M., 1965, L'absence d'histone dans le kinetonucleus des trypanosomes: Etude cytochimique, *Exp. Cell Res.* **39:**69.

Stingl, Meingassner, J. G., Swelty, P., 1976, An immunofluorescence procedure for the demonstration of antibodies to native, double-stranded DNA and of circulating DNA–anti-DNA complexes, *Clin. Immunol. Immunopathol.* **6:**131.

Tan, E. M., Schur, P. H., Carr, R. I., and Kunkel, H. G., 1966, Deoxyribonucleic acid (DNA) and antibodies to DNA in the serum of patients with systemic lupus erythematosus, *J. Clin. Invest.* **45:**1732.

Winfield, J. B., Koffler, D., and Kunkel, H. G., 1973, Specific concentration of polynucleotide immune complexes in the cryoprecipitates of patients with systemic lupus erythematosus, *J. Clin. Invest.* **56:**563.

Yamauchi, Y., Litwin, A., Adams, L., Zimmer, H., and Hess, E. V., 1975, Induction of antibodies to nuclear antigens in rabbits by immunization with hydralazine–human serum albumin conjugates, *J. Clin. Invest.* **56:**958.

30

The Role of Streptococcal and Glomerular Basement Membrane Antigens in Glomerulonephritis

H. M. Fillit, H. Villarreal, Jr., and J. B. Zabriskie

1. General Introduction

The association of the group A streptococcus with the subsequent development of acute poststreptococcal glomerulonephritis (APSGN) is now well established (Rammelkamp, 1954). However, there are enormous gaps in our knowledge concerning the mechanisms of interaction between the host and the organism which finally results in the acute disease. Specifically, one would like to know what streptococcal antigens are involved in the acute process, where they are localized in the organism, and by what mechanism they exert their noxious stimuli (i.e., complex formation, activation of complement components, alteration of host gamma globulin, binding to renal glomerular cells, or a combination of all these factors).

The most important question which is still unanswered with respect to progressive idiopathic glomerulonephritis is how the disease progresses in the apparent absence of a continuing exogenous stimulus. Specifically, these investigations have centered around the concept that bacterial antigens, in particular streptococcal antigens which are cross-reactive with native or altered glomerular basement membrane (GBM) antigens, have a predisposing and/or exacerbating role in the continuation of the disease. Furthermore, altered basement membrane antigens may play an important primary role in the progression of the chronic disease.

H. M. Fillit, H. Villarreal, Jr., and J. B. Zabriskie · The Rockefeller University, New York, New York 10021. This work was supported by Grant HL 03919 from the National Institutes of Health and Grant 1019 from the New York State Health Research Council. Drs. Fillit and Villarreal are the recipients of National Kidney Foundation fellowships.

This discussion centers about the most recent findings concerning the pathogenesis of APSGN and introduces some new evidence about possible mechanisms of progression to chronic disease. For the sake of clarity, these areas of investigation will be divided into two sections. The first will be concerned with recent investigations concerning the presence of a nephritis strain-associated protein isolated from the extracellular products of these strains. The second will discuss the cellular reactions in chronic nephritis to altered GBM antigens.

2. A Streptococcal Extracellular Protein Unique to Nephritogenic Strains

2.1. Introduction

Reports of the presence of both IgG and complement components in the glomeruli of patients with streptococcal nephritis has been well-documented. A number of investigators have reported the presence of streptococcal antigens in these biopsy specimens. The localization of these antigens in the organism has been the subject of some dispute. Seegal *et al.* (1965) indicated that the antigen in question is part of the streptococcal cell wall

Table 1. Presence of the Nephritis Strain-Associated Protein (NSAP) in Various Streptococcal Strains

Group	Type	Source of strains			
		APSGN patients		Non-APSGN patients	
		$NSAP^+$	$NSAP^-$	$NSAP^+$	$NSAP^-$
A	1	F203D			D480
	2	A207			B931
	3				A830, A868
	4	B512, B905, B974			A915, A990
	5		B743		A964, B434
	9				A552, A728
	12	A374, B281, B923, Gt7940, Gt7899, t12		D313, L92541	D897, L02407, L01596
	18	8438			A992
	19				1GL362
	30				1GL22
	36				A456
	49	B915, B920, Gt8760			B737, A834
	50				A315
	55		A928		D438
	57	A995			
	NT[a]	B515, A218, A547			
D					B272, B443
No. of strains		19	2	2	23

[a] Nontypeable strains.

and is sensitive to the action of trypsin. In contrast, Lange *et al.* (1976) reported that the antigen lies within the cytoplasmic contents of the streptococcal cell and is unrelated to specific serotypes of streptococci. An important factor in both of these investigations has been the finding that the antigen appears in the glomerulus early during the acute stages of the disease and often is seen in those areas of the glomerulus which do not have similar deposits of IgG and complement.

While the investigations described above have concentrated on identification of the streptococcal antigen *in situ,* another approach has been the structural and biological differences between those strains which are associated with nephritis (nephritogenic) and those strains which do not appear to cause the disease (nonnephritogenic). The majority of these studies have either been inconclusive or controversial (Noble and Vosti, 1973). The possible reasons for these discrepancies might be the complex nature of the streptococcal cell (McCarty, 1964), the excretion of many different extracellular products (Halbert and Keatinge, 1961), and the marked variation in the production of these extracellular proteins by a given strain (Wannamaker, 1958).

There are difficulties inherent in comparing multiple extracellular products in various streptococcal strains, but it was decided to reexplore the question of whether nephritis-producing strains of streptococci preferentially excreted an antigen(s) unique to these strains for the following reasons. The appearance of new biochemical methods capable of detecting minute differences in the protein composition of microbial products (Maizel, 1971) was encouraging. These techniques could provide a powerful tool with which to examine the differences in the extracellular proteins of those strains which do not cause APSGN. Secondly, an analysis of the antigen(s) in its naturally occurring form might provide valuable insight into the biological and structural properties of the protein in question. This assumes some importance since many of the current methods of protein extraction from streptococcal cells (Fox, 1974) could destroy the antigen under study or produce a larger molecule in which the relevant antigenic sites were buried (Krause, 1958).

A total of 46 group A streptococcal strains were used for this study. Twenty-one were isolated from patients with clinical and/or pathological diagnoses of acute streptococcal nephritis, and 25 were isolated from patients with suppurative and nonsuppurative sequelae other than acute nephritis. In addition, three strains isolated from patients with nephritis were mouse passed, and two other strains (originally isolated from nephritic patients) were repeatedly subcultured in rabbit blood neopeptone broth.

2.2. *Methods of Isolation*

Without going into elaborate details, the method for the growth and isolation of the extracellular products of these strains was as follows. Lyophilized stocks of each strain were grown and successively passed through several culture cycles of Todd–Hewitt dialysate broth (van de Rijn *et al.*, 1977) in order to eliminate any contaminating blood proteins from the original culture. The strain was then grown for varying periods of time in individual flasks of the dialysate medium; centrifuged to remove the organisms and the supernatant fluid brought to 80% saturation with ammonium sulfate. The resulting precipitate was then centrifuged. It was dialyzed against 0.005 M sodium phosphate buffers and concentrated approximately 200-fold. The protein content was equalized for each preparation, and 50-ml aliquots of each strain were placed on a polyacrylamide 7–30% gradient discontinuous slab gel electrophoresis system and run for 18 hr at 50 V. Appropriate standards of varying molecular weights were run simultaneously as markers in the system.

2.3. *Polyacrylamide Gel Electrophoresis Pattern*

When the SDS gels containing the streptococcal extracellular products (SEP) of 44 group A strains were compared, a marked variability in the number of protein bands was observed. Figure 1 shows a representative gel where it can be seen that SEP of some strains showed numerous protein bands while in others only a few were detected. The molecular weights of these protein bands ranged from about 80,000 to 10,000. It was not possible to assess the presence of SEP below 10,000 molecular weight due to the presence of contaminating low-molecular-weight media peptides.

To determine whether variation existed within a single streptococcal serotype, several group A strains of similar serotypes were compared. Eight type 12 strains, six type 4 strains, and four type 49 strains were examined. Figure 2 shows the SEP of six type 12 strains. Once again, marked differences in the number of protein bands present were observed. Strain-to-strain variation of the SEP persisted even when the number of streptococci in the cultures as measured by the optical density was kept constant or the protein concentration of each strain studied was equalized. These differences also occurred in samples taken at specific times (5, 18, 48 hr) after inoculation.

While it was not possible to demonstrate that strains commonly labeled "nephritogenic" excreted proteins that were different from "nonnephritogenic" strains, the possibility arose that consistent differences might exist in strains directly isolated from patients with APSGN irrespective of serotype. Figure 3 illustrates the results of these experiments. While the variation in protein bands between these group A strains is again apparent, an examination of the gels showed that a protein band of molecular weight about 46,000 (nephritis strain-associated protein, NSAP) (arrows) occurred mainly in the SEP of the strains recovered from patients with APSGN. This band was not present in the SEP of those strains of similar serotypes recovered from patients without this disease.

Table 1 shows that of 21 strains isolated from patients with APSGN, 19 had the NSAP; the only exceptions were one type 5 and one type 55 strain obtained from patients with clinical diagnoses of APSGN. Of 25 group A

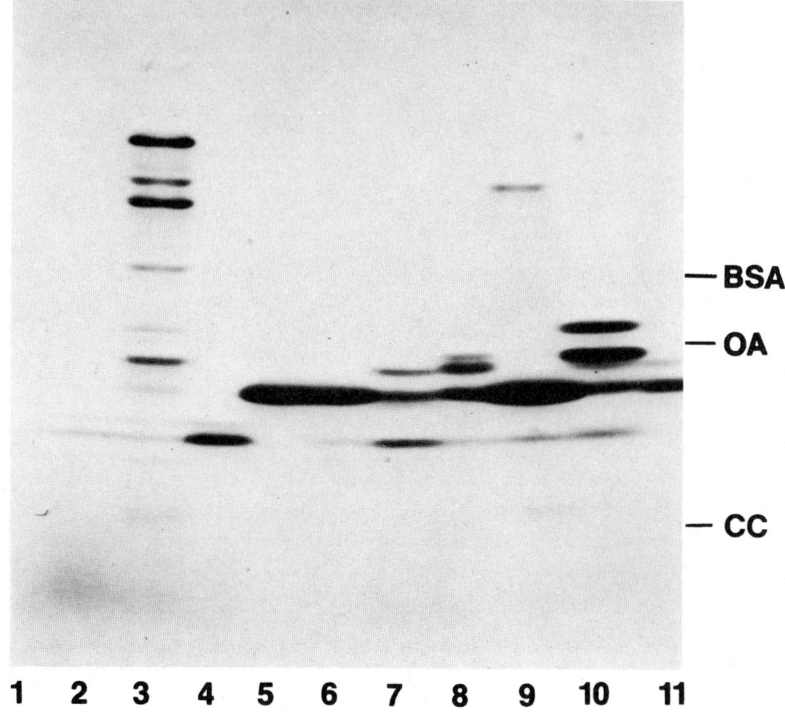

Figure 1. SEP patterns of eleven group A strains of different serotypes. One hundred microliters of each preparation isolated from 5-hr grown cells was loaded onto an SDS gel as described in text. Note the marked variation in the number of proteins produced by the different types of streptococci. Strains: 1, A547; 2, A456; 3, B281; 4, A992; 5, B434; 6, 1GL362; 7, A552; 8, A728; 9, B737; 10, A207; 11, D480. Positions of migration of the protein standards [bovine serum albumin (BSA), ovalbumin (OA), and cytochrome *c* (CC)] are noted.

strains recovered from patients without APSGN (16 of which were similar in serotype to those isolated from patients with APSGN), only 2 showed the NSAP, and both were type 12 strains. Five hours of culture was usually sufficient for the NSAP to be detected by SDS-PAGE in the SEP of the throat strains studied. Further incubation (up to 48 hr) generally did not result in an increased production of NSAP. However, the prolonged incubation of the 48-hr cultures resulted in the appearance of new protein bands. The NSAP was not detected in the negative strains even when the SEP were concentrated 2000-fold at various times of growth (up to 48 hr).

It has been well established that mouse passage results in the selection of high producers of type-specific M protein (Todd and Lancefield, 1928). To determine if this procedure also increased the production of the NSAP, three streptococcal strains were mouse passed. These experiments resulted in the disappearance of the NSAP (Fig. 4). In contrast, certain other proteins increased after mouse passage. In a similar manner, repeated subcultures in the growth medium also resulted in the disappearance of the NSAP.

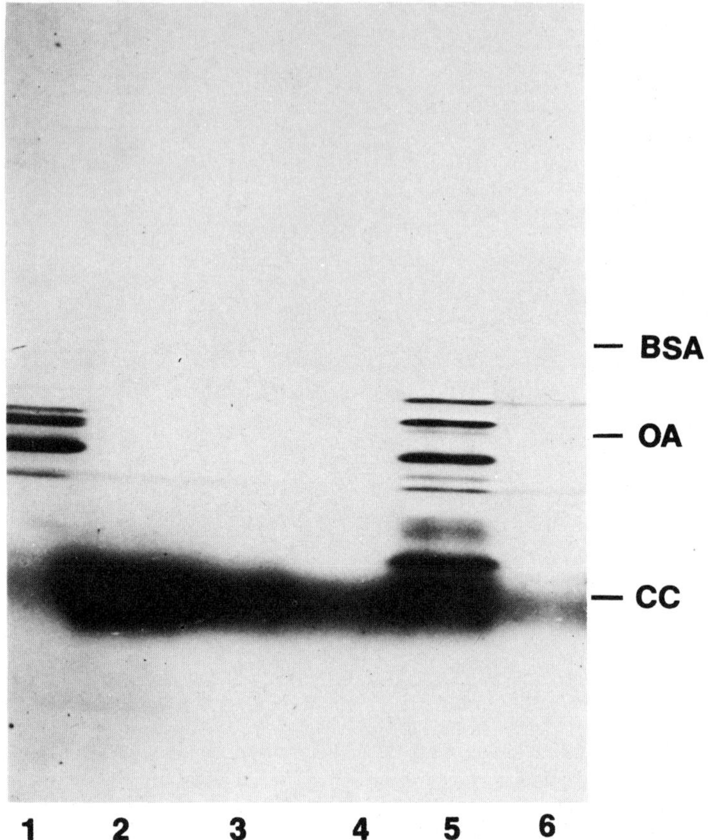

Figure 2. SEP of six group A type 12 strains. One hundred microliters of each preparation isolated from a constant culture density was loaded onto an SDS gel as noted in text. Note the marked variation in the number of proteins excreted by these strains. Strains: 1, t12; 2, t12 M+; 3, t12 M−; 4, t12/126/4; 5, B923; 6, A374. Positions of migration of the protein standards are noted.

2.4. *Purification of the Protein*

While the protein band was clearly visible in each of the nephritis-associated strains, many other protein bands were also present. After a series of purification steps involving ion-exchange and molecular sieve chromatography, a pure protein line was demonstrated on SDS gels. This material was then used for the production of antisera and subsequent absorption studies.

In order to determine whether the protein band noted in each of the strains isolated from patients with acute streptococcal nephritis were indeed similar, double-diffusion studies in agar were carried out. The antisera used in these experiments were prepared in the following manner. The crude extracellular products from a nephritis-associated strain contained the protein

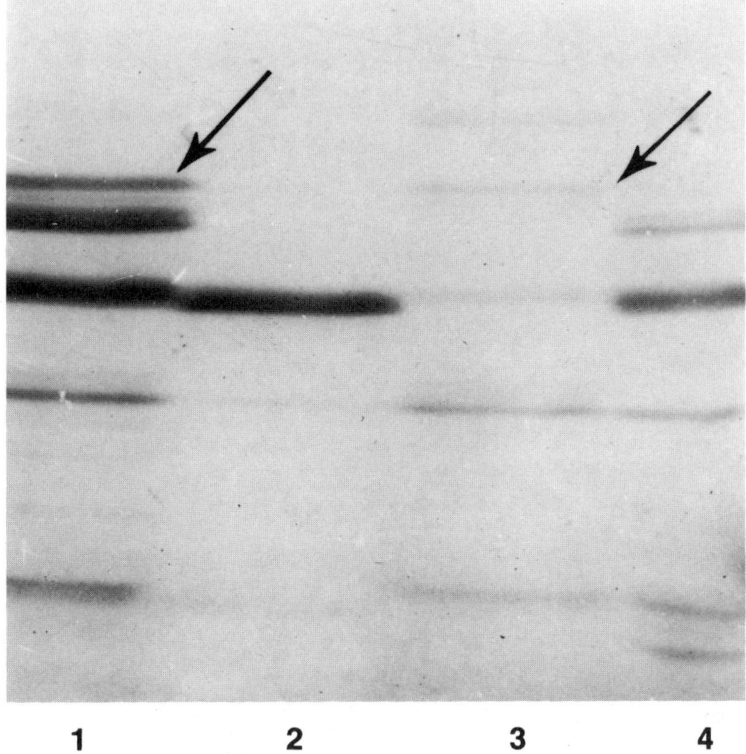

Figure 3. SEP of four group A streptococcal strains. One hundred microliters of each preparation was loaded onto an SDS gel as noted in text. Lanes 1 (type 2) and 3 (type 12) are extracellular products obtained from strains isolated from patients with APSGN. Lanes 2 (type 2) and 4 (type 12) are SEP recovered from strains obtained from patients without APSGN. Note (arrows) the presence of a protein band with molecular weight of 46,000 (NSAP) only in the strain isolated from patients with APSGN.

band ingestates which were injected into rabbits. The resulting antiserum then was absorbed with several extracellular products obtained from strains which did not contain the protein of 46,000 molecular weight. Packing double-diffusion experiments with the purified protein demonstrated that only a single line of precipitation occurred with the protein. This antiserum was then reacted against the extracellular products of several strains which were or were not associated with nephritis.

Figure 5 is illustrative of one of these double-diffusion studies. Antiserum specific for the NSAP was added to the center well. In wells 1–3 were placed the crude SEP of three group A streptococcal strains isolated from patients with APSGN. These SEP were obtained from strains B281 (type 12), Gt8760 (type 49), and A995 (type 57), respectively. Wells 4–6 contained the crude SEP of three group A strains obtained from patients without APSGN or

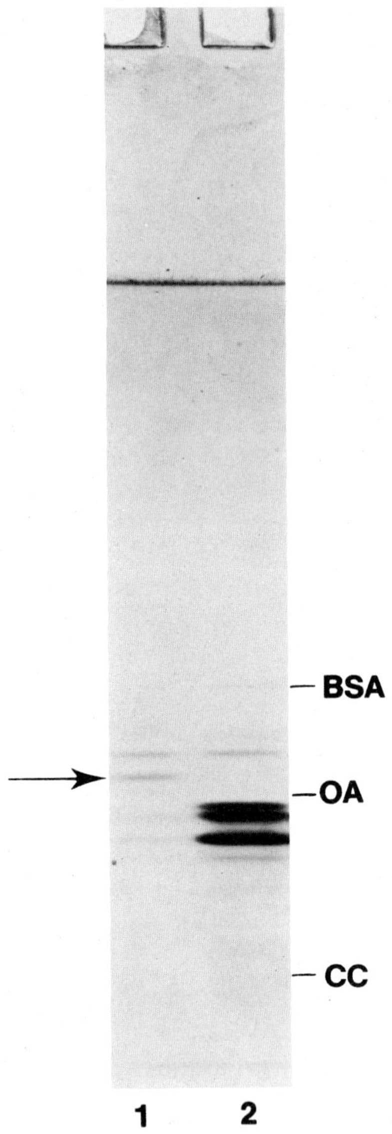

Figure 4. SEP of strain A995 isolated from a patient with APSGN. One hundred microliters of SEP obtained from the strain before (lane 1) and after (lane 2) mouse passage. Note the loss of NSAP (arrow) after 91 mouse passages. Positions of migration of the molecular weight standards are noted.

mouse-passed strains (no NSAP present)—strains A995/91/1 (type 57), A834 (type 49), and D897 (type 12), respectively. A line of identity was formed by the SEP of the three strains isolated from APSGN patients. No precipitin line formed with the SEP of strains recovered from patients without APSGN or mouse-passed strains.

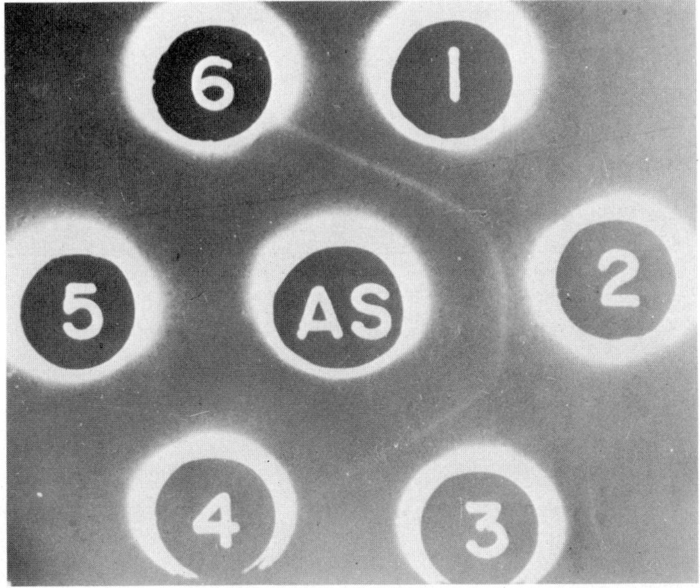

Figure 5. Immunodiffusion analysis of the NSAP in various streptococcal extracellular products. The center well contains antiserum specific to the NSAP. Wells 1–3 contain the SEP of three group A strains isolated from patients with APSGN. Well 4 contains the SEP of a mouse-passed strain. Wells 5 and 6 contain the SEP of strains obtained from patients without APSGN. Note the line of identity formed only by those strains isolated from patients with APSGN (for details, see text).

2.5. *Presence of the Protein in Human Kidney Biopsies*

Since the NSAP was found primarily in the extracellular products of streptococci isolated directly from patients with APSGN, it was decided to examine 21 kidney biopsies of patients with APSGN for the presence or absence of this protein. These were also studied for the presence of IgG, IgM, C3, and fibrinogen.

Fourteen of twenty-one biopsies from patients with APSGN showed deposits of moderate fluorescence when fluoresceinated antiserum specific to the NSAP was employed. The fluorescence increased markedly when an indirect immunofluorescence method was used. The deposits were finely granular and found both along the GBM and mesangium (Fig. 6). The positive biopsies of patients with APSGN were usually those that also had deposits of IgG. In contrast, 5 kidney biopsies of patients with acute rheumatic fever and 11 from other nonstreptococcal glomerulonephritis patients, such as membranous nephritis, lupus nephritis, and minimal change disease, were all negative for the NSAP. The antiserum to crude SEP containing NSAP produced similar fluorescence in the kidney biopsies of patients with APSGN as did the antiserum to the purified NSAP. In contrast, antiserum to crude SEP without the NSAP failed to exhibit fluorescence in the same biopsies.

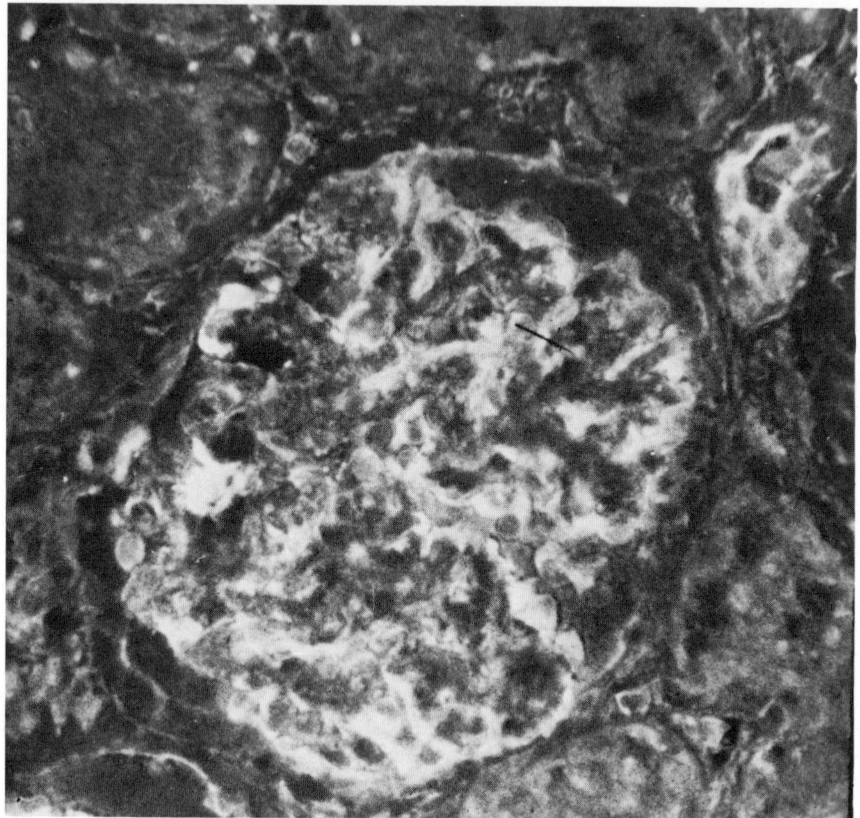

Figure 6. Glomerulus of a patient with early well-documented APSGN stained with antiserum specific to the NSAP. Note the presence of granular deposits of this antigen along the GBM and mesangium. × 384.

The fluorescence was abolished from the APSGN biopsies when the rabbit anti-NSAP gamma globulin was absorbed with crude, partially purified, or purified NSAP. Absorptions with crude SEP which did not contain the NSAP or lyophilized Todd–Hewitt media did not abolish the fluorescence. While it was not determined whether or not this protein also exists within the cell, the present observations could explain a number of discrepancies noted in the past (Zabriskie *et al.*, 1970). The presence of the NSAP in the extracellular products of those serotypes commonly associated with streptococcal nephritis (McCluskey *et al.*, 1966; Feldman *et al.*, 1966), coupled with its production predominantly by strains isolated from patients with this disease, could explain why APSGN follows infection with only a limited number of streptococcal strains even within the same serotype. For example, many group A type 12 strains induce pharyngitis, but only those producing the NSAP would be of potential pathogenetic significance in poststreptococcal glomerulonephritis.

2.6. *Discussion*

With respect to the discrepancies noted in different immunofluorescent studies, attempts to detect streptococcal antigens in the kidney biopsies of patients with APSGN would have failed for the following reasons. First, the antisera prepared against streptococcal strains which did not produce the NSAP (even if of "nephritogenic" types) would not have contained antibodies to the NSAP and therefore would have failed to detect this streptococcal antigen in the kidney biopsy specimens. Second, since mouse passage or repeated subcultures appear to result in the loss of the NSAP, antisera raised against these strains (commonly used in immunization procedures) might not contain antibodies to the NSAP. Finally, it is conceivable that more than one streptococcal antigen could be involved in the pathogenesis of APSGN. This might explain the apparently controversial results of different investigators (Seegal *et al.*, 1965; Lange *et al.*, 1976) with respect to the localization of the antigens in the streptococcal cell. Along these lines, it is also tempting to speculate that, depending on the strain which causes nephritis ("skin" versus "throat" strains), the protein could be either primarily excreted into the tissues or remain attached to the cell. Thus, the same antigen would be "localized" in two different sites, depending on the strain examined.

3. *The Role of Altered GBM and Cross-Reactive Streptococcal Antigens in Progressive Glomerulonephritis*

3.1. *Introduction*

While controversy exists as to the exact incidence of APSGN cases that progress to chronic disease (Jennings and Earle, 1961; Baldwin *et al.*, 1974), most investigators do agree that chronic glomerulonephritis may occur after the acute episode. As mentioned earlier, the unanswered question is, how does the disease progress in the absence of a continued exogenous antigenic stimulus?

3.2. *Background*

To begin with, several investigators (Markowitz and Lange, 1964; Holm, 1967) have established that there is a serological cross-reaction between group A streptococci and antigens in the renal glomerular tissue. While it was originally suggested that only certain "nephritogenic" strains were capable of exhibiting the cross-reactions (Markowitz and Lange, 1964), other evidence suggests that many group A streptococcal strains possess these cross-reactive antigens (Holm, 1967). Experimental evidence also supports the concept that these cross-reactive antigens play a biological role. Antiserum to group A streptococcal membranes binds to renal glomerular antigens and induces nephritis in experimental animals (Rapaport *et al.*, 1969). Prior immunization with streptococcal antigens results in accelerated rejection of both skin

(Rapaport and Markowitz, 1969) and renal homografts (Rapaport *et al.*, 1971). Finally, a clinical report (First *et al.*, 1977) has indicated that streptococcal infections may induce a rapid homograft rejection.

The possibility that cellular reactions could play a role in the progression of glomerulonephritis has its roots both in experimental data and observations in human disease. For example, Fig. 7 is a photomicrograph of an H & E

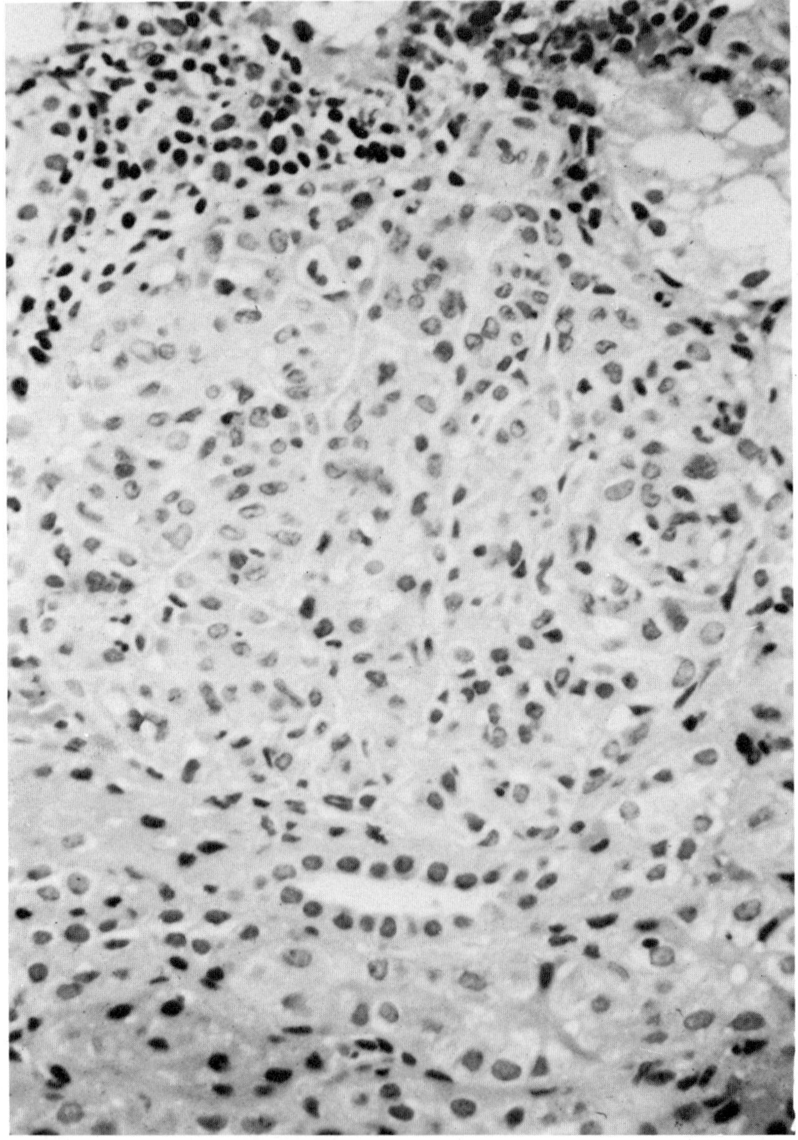

Figure 7. Glomerulus of a renal biopsy from a patient with idiopathic proliferative glomerulonephritis, showing marked cellular infiltration. H & E; × 384.

Table 2. Migration Inhibition Studies to Streptococcal and Renal Antigens in Patients with Progressive Glomerulonephritis

Subjects	Antigens[a]					
	GBM[b]	SCM[b]	GBM[c]	SCM[c]	FK[d]	GBM[e]
Normals	0/21	0/21	0/21	0/21	2/23	0/16
Minimal change	0/9	0/19	0/12	0/12	8/8	0/8
Proliferative glomerulo-	16/16	18/23	7/17	11/17	8/11	9/29
nephritis	0/8	0/8	0/6	0/6	3/6	0/8
Membranous	NT	NT	2/7	4/7	1/2	0/8
Membranoproliferative	2/4	3/6	6/6	0/6	NT	NT
Goodpasture's	NT	NT	0/11	0/11	NT	0/8
Pyelonephritis						

[a] Abbreviations used: GBM, glomerular basement membrane (adult); SCM, streptococcal cell membrane; FK, fetal kidney; NT, not tested.
[b] Macanovic *et al.* (1972).
[c] Dardenne *et al.* (1972).
[d] Mallick *et al.* (1972).
[e] Mahieu *et al.* (1972).

section from a patient with chronic idiopathic proliferative glomerulonephritis. Recent evidence both in experimental models and in humans has demonstrated that a number of the proliferating cells seen during glomerulonephritis (originally thought to be of glomerular endothelial or mesangial origin) are in reality macrophages or monocytes (i.e., the effector arm of cell-mediated immunity) (Atkins *et al.*, 1976; Schreiner *et al.*, 1978).

Turning to the human disease, many investigators have demonstrated that there is increased cellular reactivity to renal and streptococcal antigens in patients with progressive glomerulonephritis (Mahieu *et al.*, 1972; Macanovic *et al.*, 1972; Dardenne *et al.*, 1972; Rocklin *et al.*, 1970; Mallick *et al.*, 1972; Bendixen, 1968) (Table 2). Of interest is the observation that this reactivity was primarily confined to the group of chronic nephritics who had been classified as having proliferative lesions. It is also emphasized that these patients had heightened cellular reactivity to streptococcal antigens (walls or membranes) of at least two different streptococcal strains (Zabriskie *et al.*, 1970) (Fig. 8).

A review of the type of renal antigens used in these studies indicated that the cellular reactivity was most pronounced when fetal renal antigens were used (Rocklin *et al.*, 1970). Since one study suggested that fetal GBM have less sialic acid content when compared to adult GBM (Blue and Lange, 1976a), the heightened cellular reactivity observed in these patients could be due to a cellular reaction to GBM antigens which were exposed after removal of the peripheral carbohydrate residues; i.e., "altered" membrane antigen. Furthermore, it was suggested that the cross-reaction between renal and streptococcal antigens might be enhanced following removal of the carbohydrate residues of the renal antigens (Blue and Lange, 1976b). Quish and Lange (1973) have shown that immunization with glycosidase-treated GBM results in heightened antigenicity. If one thinks in terms of actually how

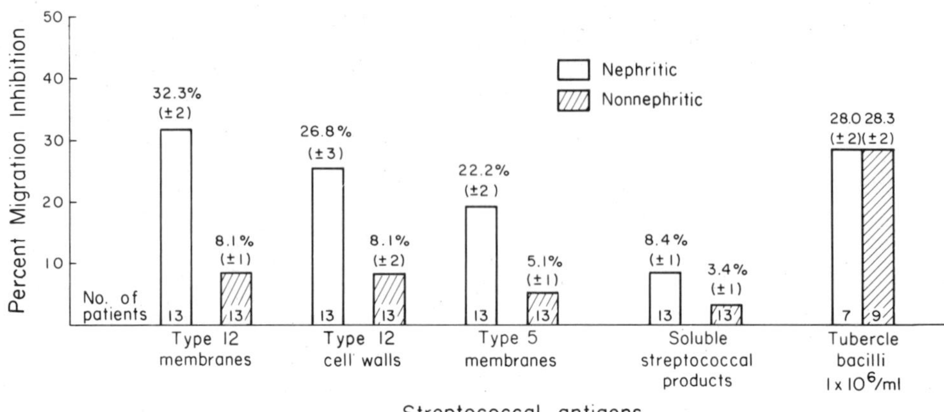

Figure 8. Cellular reactivity to streptococcal antigens in patients with chronic glomerulonephritis as measured by the migration inhibition assay.

these antigens might be uncovered in the disease state, *in vivo*, the release of lysosomal hydrolases during phagocytosis of immune complexes could be the mechanism resulting in the alteration of glomerular antigens (Weissman *et al.*, 1971).

3.3. Methods of Isolation of GBM and Enzymatic Alteration

Proceeding on this basis, experiments were designed to selectively remove terminal carbohydrate residues via enzymatic treatment of human GBM preparations. GBM antigens were isolated by standard molecular sieving techniques (Misra, 1972) followed by ionic detergent extractions (Meezan *et al.*, 1975). These preparations were then treated with glycosidases and the various membrane preparations were tested in the lymphocyte blastogenesis assay in a group of chronic nephritis patients (Fillit *et al.*, 1978).

3.4. Cellular Immune Studies in Patients with Progressive Glomerulonephritis

Table 3 demonstrates that 12 of 24 patients with different histologic forms of chronic nephritis had cellular reactivity to glycosidase-treated GBM. Little or no reactivity was seen to the native or collagenase-treated membrane antigens. In addition, these patients were also tested for their reactivity to streptococcal membranes. It was found that patients with high reactivity to the glycosidase-treated membrane antigens also exhibited heightened cellular reactivity to the streptococcal antigens (Fillit *et al.*, 1978).

In order to further explore the specificity of this reaction, a separate group of chronic nephritis patients were tested with a newly prepared batch of renal antigens. Once again (and in confirmation of our previous findings), the predominant reactivity was seen in patients with proliferative disease (Table 4). It should be emphasized that in the second study, our criterion

Table 3. Cellular Reactivity to GBM Antigens[a]

Antigen	Group	Nonreactors	Reactors[b]	*p*
Native GBM	GN	21	3	
	NC	16	2	NS
	NGRD	6	1	NS
Collagenase-treated GBM	GN	15	3	
	NC	12	1	NS
	NGRD	7	0	NS
Glycosidase-treated GBM	GN	12	12	
	NC	17	1	0.012
	NGRD	8	0	0.002

[a] Abbreviations used: GN, glomerulonephritis; NC, normal controls; NGRD, nonglomerular renal disease; NS, not significant.
[b] Result greater than two standard deviations above mean control.

for determining increased cellular reactivity was quite strict. Only those individuals who exhibited a stimulation index of greater than 3.0 were considered to be reactors. Although the other histologically defined groups did not differ significantly from the normals, certain individuals within these groups did show heightened reactivity to altered membrane antigens. This finding may have diagnostic or prognostic implications for these particular individuals within the focal segmental or membranous group of patient. The specificity of the reaction to streptococcal antigens was again attested to in this group by the fact that at least three different streptococcal preparations exhibited this heightened stimulation (Table 5) while reactivity to BCG and PHA was not significantly different between controls and nephritics.

3.5. Biochemical Studies of Altered GBM

Preliminary biochemical data illustrated in Table 6 indicate that the amino acid composition of the human GBM preparations agree quite well

Table 4. Responses to Altered GBM by Histologic Type

	Stimulation index > 3	Fisher's exact test
Normal controls	4/27	—
Glomerulonephritis		
Proliferative	6/7	0.00094
Focal segmental sclerosis	2/10	NS[a]
Membranous	3/7	NS
Other (including minimal change, membrano-proliferative, and global sclerosis)	1/7	NS

[a] NS, not significant.

Table 5. Response to Streptococcal Antigens in Glomerulonephritis

	Normal controls	Gly reactors[a]
S43	15.05 ± 1.77[b] (26)	25.8 ± 3.78 (20) $p < 0.01$[c]
T49	19.31 ± 4.40 (9)	31.93 ± 6.20 (12) $0.05 < p < 0.10$
SKSD	3.27 ± 0.81 (15)	10.2 ± 3.63 (9) $p < 0.05$
BCG	3.45 ± 1.04 (15)	4.82 ± 1.69 (9) NS
PHA	114.7 ± 8.5 (42)	98.6 ± 10.1 (17) NS

[a] Patients with stimulation index > 3.0 in response to glycosidase-treated GBM.
[b] Mean stimulation index ± standard error. Numbers in parentheses represent number of individuals studied.
[c] Student's *t* test; gly reactors vs. normal controls.

with those described by Westberg and Michael (1970) with a characteristically high content of glycine and hydroxyproline. After treatment with glycosidases, one can see that there is no significant change in the amino acid composition. This suggests that glycosidase treatment per se does not alter the amino acid composition of the GBM and speaks against the presence of

Table 6. Amino Acid Analysis of Native and Altered Human GBM

	Human GBM[a]	Human GBM[b]	Altered human GBM[b]
Aspartic acid	67.7	63	66
Threonine	36.7	30	33
Serine	48.9	51	56
Glutamic acid	91.3	90	91
Proline	57.9	91	84
Glycine	221	264	262
Alanine	59.8	64	64
Valine	35.6	22	19
Methionine	13.2	15	15
Isoleucine	31,3	26	27
Leucine	65.3	50	55
Tyrosine	15.3	14	16
Phenylalanine	24.9	24	25
Hydroxylysine	26.1	24	24
Lysine	19.5	18	18
Histidine	14.2	11	12
Arginine	38.0	52	52
3-Hydroxyproline	22.2	—	—
4-Hydroxyproline	81.3	72	75

[a] Prepared by extensive sonication: data of Westberg and Michael (1970).
[b] Prepared by detergent extraction: current study.

any contaminating proteins. Table 7 demonstrates that the glycosidase treatment does remove approximately 70% of the sialic acid residues on the membrane.

3.6. Discussion

In this work it has been shown that GBM altered by glycosidases but not native GBM reproducibly results in cellular reactivity as measured by the blast transformation assay in patients with progressive glomerulonephritis, predominantly those in the proliferative group. Several other investigators have shown similar cellular reactivity using the migration inhibition assay and different preparations of GBM (Mahieu *et al.*, 1972; Macanovic *et al.*, 1972; Dardenne *et al.*, 1972; Rocklin *et al.*, 1970; Mallick *et al.*, 1972; Bendixen, 1968). Thus, the evidence for cellular reactivity to GBM in glomerulonephritis is well documented and clearly reproducible. Not only does GBM induce lymphocyte transformation, but it also results in macrophage migration inhibition, an effect thought to be mediated by lymphokines released by specific antigen-stimulated lymphocytes. Since cellular reactivity to GBM in progressive glomerulonephritis is demonstrable using both assays, it seems unlikely that such reactivity is purely an *in vitro* phenomenon.

Long-term investigations on the diagnostic and prognostic value of cellular reactivity to GBM in glomerulonephritis may help to define a primary immunopathologic role for the observed phenomenon in the disease process. In addition, *in vitro* investigations of cellular reactivity to altered GBM in relationship to the process of proliferation and sclerosis may also help to define a primary role for such reactivity in the disease process. Finally, though cellular reactivity to altered GBM may be an epiphenomenon, such reactivity may nevertheless prove to be a useful diagnostic and prognostic marker in correlation with the clinical state.

Cellular reactivity was observed exclusively with altered and not native GBM. Morphologic and biochemical alteration of GBM has been observed in glomerulonephritis in man and animals (Hawkins and Cochrane, 1968; Burkholder, 1969). Thus, that altered GBM has immunologic reactivity as well is consistent with these observations. The biochemical basis for reactivity to GBM glycoproteins with altered carbohydrates is found in the growing literature on the role of carbohydrates in a number of immunologic and

Table 7. Sialic Acid Content of Native and Altered Human GBM

	% sialic acid
Native GBM[a]	0.88
Native GBM[b]	0.81 ± 0.031 (n = 4)
Altered GBM[b]	0.25 ± 0.031 (n = 3)

[a] Prepared by extensive sonication: data of Westberg and Michael (1970).
[b] Prepared by detergent extraction: current study.

nonimmunologic phenomena, such as the regulation of the life span of circulating glycoproteins (Ashwell and Morell, 1974), and the activation of complement (Fearon, 1978). In addition, loss of negative charges (including sialic acid) from the glycoprotein filtration barrier of the glomerulus is a likely cause for proteinuria, and other morphologic phenomena seen *in vivo* during glomerulonephritis (Brenner *et al.*, 1978).

Finally, it has been confirmed that patients with progressive glomerulonephritis have heightened cellular reacitivty to streptococcal antigens, as found previously by a number of other investigators (Macanovic *et al.*, 1972; Dardenne *et al.*, 1972; Zabriskie *et al.*, 1970). Since it is unlikely that most patients with progressive glomerulonephritis have a primary streptococcal etiology, the most likely explanation for this observation is based on the observed cross-reaction between streptococcal and glomerular antigens. The role of streptococcal and other microbial organisms with possible cross-reactive antigens to glomerular structures on the predisposition, exacerbation, and progression of progressive glomerulonephritis clearly demands further investigation.

References

Ashwell, G., and Morell, A. G., 1974, The role of surface carbohydrates in the hepatic recognition and transport of circulating glycoproteins, *Adv. Enzymol.* **41:**99.

Atkins, R. C., Holdsworth, S. R., Glasgow, E. F., and Matthews, F. E., 1976, The macrophage in human rapidly progressive glomerulonephritis, *Lancet* **2:**830.

Baldwin, D. S., Gluck, M. C., Schacht, R. G., and Gallo, G., 1974, The long-term course of poststreptococcal glomerulonephritis, *Ann. Intern. Med.* **80:**342.

Bendixen, G., 1968, Organ specific inhibition of the *in vitro* migration of leucocytes in human glomerulonephritis, *Acta Med. Scand.* **184:**99.

Blue, W. T., and Lange, C. F., 1976a, Age related carbohydrate content of mouse kidney glomerular basement membrane and its reactivity to anti-streptococcal membrane antisera, *Immunochemistry* **13:**295.

Blue, W. T., and Lange, C. F., 1976b, Immunologic cross-reactivity between antisera to group A type 12 streptococcal cell membrane and human glomerular basement membrane: The effect of age and carbohydrate content, *Mech. Ageing Dev.* **5:**209.

Brenner, B. M., Hostetter, T. H., and Humes, H. D., 1978, Molecular basis of proteinuria of glomerular origin, *N. Engl. J. Med.* **298:**826.

Burkholder, P. M., 1969, Ultra-structural demonstration of injury and perforation of glomerular capillary basement membrane in acute proliferative glomerulonephritis, *Am. J. Pathol.* **56:**251.

Dardenne, M., Zabriskie, J. B., and Bach, J.-F., 1972, Streptococcal sensitivity in chronic glomerulonephritis, *Lancet* **1:**126.

Fearon, D. T., 1978, Regulation by membrane sialic acid of B1H dependent decay dissociation of amplification C3 convertase of the alternative complement pathway, *Proc. Natl. Acad. Sci. USA* **75:**1971.

Feldman, J. O., Mardiney, M. R., and Shuler, S. E., 1966, Immunology and morphology of acute poststreptococcal glomerulonephritis, *Lab. Invest.* **15:**283.

Fillit, H. M., Read, S. E., Sherman, R. L., Zabriskie, J. B., and van de Rijn, I., 1978, Cellular reactivity to altered glomerular basement membrane in glomerulonephritis, *N. Engl. J. Med.* **298:**891.

First, M. R., Linnemann, C. C., Jr., Munda, R., McConnell, C. M., Ramundo, N., Alexander, J.

W., and Nathan, P., 1977, Transmitted streptococcal infection and hyperacute rejection, *Transplantation* **24:**400.

Fox, E. N., 1974, M Proteins of group A streptococci, *Bacteriol. Rev.* **38:**57.

Halbert, S. P., and Keatinge, S. L., 1961, The analysis of streptococcal infections, VI. Immunoelectrophoretic observations on extracellular antigens detectable with human antibodies, *J. Exp. Med.* **113:**1013.

Hawkins, D., and Cochrane, C. G., 1968, Glomerular basement membrane damage in immunological glomerulonephritis, *Immunology* **14:**665.

Holm, S. E., 1967, Precipitinogens in beta-hemolytic streptococci and some related human kidney antigens, *Acta Pathol. Microbiol. Scand.* **70:**79.

Jennings, R. B., and Earle, D. P., 1961, Post-streptococcal glomerulonephritis: Histopathological and clinical studies of the acute, subsiding acute and early chronic latent phases, *J. Clin. Invest.* **40:**1525.

Krause, R. M., 1958, Studies on the bacteriophages of hemolytic streptococci, II. Antigens released from the streptococcal cell wall by a phage associated lysin, *J. Exp. Med.* **108:**803.

Lange, K., Ahmed, U., Kleinberger, H., and Treser, G., 1976, A hitherto unknown streptococcal antigen and its probable relation to acute poststreptococcal glomerulonephritis, *Clin. Nephrol.* **5:**207.

Macanovic, M., Evans, D. J., and Peters, D. K., 1972, Allergic response to glomerular basement membranes in patients with glomerulonephritis, *Lancet* **2:**207.

McCarty, M., 1964, *The Streptococcal Cell Wall and Its Biologic Significance in the Streptococcus; Rheumatic Fever and Glomerulonephritis* (J. Uhr, ed.), Williams & Wilkins, Baltimore.

McCluskey, R. S., Vassali, P., Gallo, G., and Baldwin, D. S., 1966, An immunofluorescent study of pathogenic mechanisms in glomerular diseases, *N. Engl. J. Med.* **274:**695.

Mahieu, P., Dardenne, M., and Bach, J.-F., 1972, Detection of humoral and cell-mediated immunity to kidney basement membranes in human renal diseases, *Am. J. Med.* **53:**185.

Maizel, J. B., 1971, Polyacrylamide gel electrophoresis of viral proteins, *Methods Enzymol.* **5:**179.

Mallick, N. P., Williams, R. J., McFarlane, H., Orr, W. M., Taylor, G., and Williams, G., 1972, Cell-mediated immunity in nephritic syndrome, *Lancet* **1:**507.

Markowitz, A. S., and Lange, C. F., Jr., 1964, Streptococcal related glomerulonephritis, *J. Immunol.* **92:**565.

Meezan, E., Hjelle, J. T., and Brendel, K., 1975, A simple, versatile, non-disruptive method for the isolation of morphologically and chemically pure basement membranes from several tissues, *Life Sci.* **17:**1721.

Misra, R. P., 1972, Isolation of glomeruli from mammalian kidneys by graded sieving, *Am. J. Clin. Pathol.* **58:**135.

Noble, R. C., and Vosti, K. L., 1973, Biological and immunologic comparison of nephritogenic and non-nephritogenic strains of group A, M-type 12 streptococcus, *J. Infect. Dis.* **128:**761.

Quish, T. B., and Lange, C. F., Jr., 1973, Increased antigenicity of glycoproteins after carbohydrate treatment, *Res. Commun. Chem. Pathol. Pharmacol.* **5:**473.

Rammelkamp, C. H., Jr., 1954, Acute hemorrhagic glomerulonephritis, in: *Streptococcal Infections* (McCarty, ed.), Columbia University Press, New York.

Rapaport, F. T., and Markowitz, A. S., 1969, Streptococcal antigen and antibodies in transplantation, *Transplant. Proc.* **1:**638.

Rapaport, F. T., Markowitz, A. S., McCluskey, R. T., Hanaoka, T., and Shimada, T., 1969, Induction of renal disease with antisera to group A streptococcal membranes, *Transplant. Proc.* **1:**981.

Rapaport, F. T., Chase, R. M., Jr., Markowitz, A. S., McCluskey, R. T., Shimada, T., and Watanabe, K., 1971, Cross-reactions in mammalian transplantation with particular reference to streptococcal antigens and andtibodies, *Transplant. Proc.* **3:**89.

Rocklin, R., Lewis, E. J., and David, J. R., 1970, *In vitro* evidence for cellular hypersensitivity to glomerulonephritis, *N. Engl. J. Med.* **283:**498.

Schreiner, G. F., Cotran, R. S., Pardo, V., and Unanue, E. R., 1978, A mononuclear cell component in experimental immunological glomerulonephritis, *J. Exp. Med.* **147:**369.

Seegal, B. C., Andres, G. A., Hsu, K. C., and Zabriskie, J. B., 1965, Studies on the pathogenesis of acute and progressive glomerulonephritis in man by immunofluorescence and immunoferritin techniques, *Fed. Proc.* **24:**100.

Todd, E. W., and Lancefield, R. C., 1928, Variants of hemolytic streptococci; their relation to type specific substance, virulence and toxin, *J. Exp. Med.* **48:**751.

van de Rijn, I., Zabriskie, J. B., and McCarty, M., 1977, Group A streptococcal antigens cross-reactive with myocardium: Purification of heart-reactive antibody and isolation and characterization of the streptococcal antigen, *J. Exp. Med.* **146:**579.

Wannamaker, L. W., 1958, The differentiation of three distinct desoxyribonucleases of group A streptococci, *J. Exp. Med.* **107:**797.

Weissman, G., Zurier, R. B., Spieler, P. J., and Goldstein, J. M., 1971, Mechanisms of lysosomal enzyme release from leukocytes exposed to immune complexes and other particles, *J. Exp. Med. S.* **134:**1495.

Westberg, N. G., and Michael, A. F., 1970, Human glomerular basement membrane preparation and composition, *Biochemistry* **9:**3837.

Zabriskie, J. B., Lewshenia, R., Moller, G., Wehle, B., and Falk, R. E., 1970, Lymphocytic responses to streptococcal antigens in glomerulonephritis patients, *Science* **168:**1105.

31

The Contact (Hageman Factor) System in Inflammation

Charles G. Cochrane, Susan D. Revak, and Roger C. Wiggins

1. Introduction

Injury of the glomerulus results from the accumulation of immunologic reactants along the basement membrane. Intermediate factors exist that interact after antigen and antibody combine that produce injury. These intermediates are the humoral and cellular mediators that are activated either directly or indirectly by the interaction of antigen and antibody at the site. Several of these mediator pathways have been uncovered. One involves the activation of the complement system along the glomerular basement membrane(GBM), followed by the accumulation of circulating neutrophils. The neutrophils are stimulated to release injurious constituents such as proteolytic enzymes and basic proteins by the discharge of lysosomal granules, which induce injury of the structure of the GBM. The neutrophilic constituents and fragments of the GBM appear in the urine during the development of injury and proteinuria (reviewed by Cochrane, 1968).

Since proteolytic enzymes derived from the lysosomal granules could be shown to hydrolyze GBM *in vitro* (Cochrane and Aikin, 1966), it would appear that the complement–neutrophil–protease system may be responsible for at least one form of glomerular injury.

A second mediation system (Unanue *et al.*, this volume) results from the accumulation of mononuclear leukocytes, which are, probably, mono-

---

Charles G. Cochrane, Susan D. Revak, and Roger C. Wiggins · Department of Immunopathology, Scripps Clinic and Research Foundation, La Jolla, California 92037. This work was supported in part by NIH Grants HL 16411, AI 07007, HL 21544, the Council for Tobacco Research, Office of Naval Research Contract 207-027, and Biomedical Research Support Program Grant 1 S07 RR 05514.

cytes.Using rats immunized to rabbit IgG, followed by injection of rabbit anti-rat GBM, a mononuclear cell infiltrate appeared between 48 and 96 hr after injection of the nephrotoxic antibody. Injury was apparent at this time.

A third form of mediation of immunologic glomerular injury is a catchall, since many different mediator systems could be involved. Defined in a negative sense, one can say only that this injury does not require the humoral and cellular factors noted in the first two forms of injury. Thus, despite marked diminution of the third and terminal components of complement, or in the absence of neutrophils, this injury in the form of proteinuria still develops following binding of antibody, to the GBM or following deposition of circulating immune complexes. A discussion of the mediator systems potentially involved in this injury has been published recently (Cochrane, 1979).

A fourth mechanism of mediation was described by Salant *et al.*, (1980) in which antibodies to renal tubular antigen were injected I.V. in rats. The proteinuria that resulted required the presence of complement, but was not affected by depletion of neutrophils.

Another plasma system of proteins, which bears similarities in many respects to the complement system, may have relevance to the complement- and neutrophil-independent glomerulonephritis. This is the Hageman factor (HF) system of plasma proteins, a system that has come under a great deal of experimental scrutiny in the past several years. It is of interest to review the biochemistry of the early, contact phase of the HF system with the thought that a strong likelihood exists that one or more of the components may participate in the mediation of this form of glomerular injury. Certain features of the contact system suggest its participation in glomerular injury. Hageman factor binds to isolated glomerular basement membrane where it is rapidly activated by kallikrein (Cochrane and Wuepper, 1972); activated Hageman factor in minute quantities (2ng, or 1/10,000th of the Hageman factor in 1 ml of plasma) is capable of inducing increased vascular permeability (Yamamoto and Cochrane, 1981); and Hageman factor undergoes cleavage associated with activation in the kidney during the development of anti-GBM-induced glomerulonephritis (Wiggins and Cochrane, 1982).

In recent years the biochemical features of the HF system have been brought into focus through a considerable amount of experimental effort. This system, consisting of a group of plasma proteins, stands out with the complement proteins as a major system in plasma possessing inflammatory capacities. Far less is known of the role of the components of the HF–kallikrein system in inflammatory disease since it has been only in the past few years that precursor components have been isolated and purified so as to allow these studies to be performed. Nevertheless, with knowledge of some of the basic biochemical parameters now available, information is being obtained on the role of this system in inflammatory disease.

The components of the HF–kallikrein system are illustrated in Fig. 1. Three molecules are assembled when plasma contacts a negatively charged surface, generating activity of the system. The molecules involved are HF

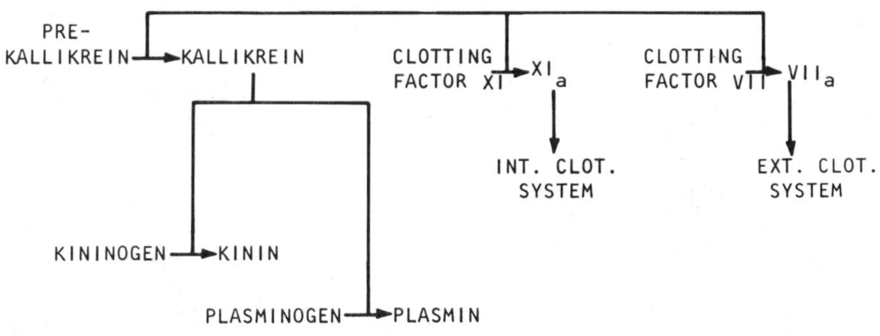

Figure 1. Protein components of the contact phase of the Hageman factor system.

(clotting Factor XII), prekallikrein, and high-molecular-weight (HMW) kininogen. The approximation of HF and prekallikrein leads to a reciprocal activation of the two molecules, and this action in turn initiates activity of the system. Other enzymes, derived from stimulated cells, may substitute for kallikrein in activating HF, as will be noted later in this chapter, and the same may be true for kallikrein. Once activated, HF is capable of activating additional prekallikrein and clotting Factor XI of the intrinsic clotting system and Factor VII of the extrinsic clotting system. Kallikrein, in turn, in its capacity as an endopeptidase, cleaved bradykinin from HMW kininogen and activates plasminogen.

The molecules of this system are capable of rendering many features of the inflammatory process. Principal among these is the peptide bradykinin, which evokes increased vascular permeability, hypotension, and contraction of smooth muscle, elicits pain after pretreatment of the tissues with prostaglandin, and stimulates the generation of arachadonate and thereby synthesis of prostaglandins. Activated HF, when injected intradermally, produces an increased vascular permeability in the guinea pig, although the mechanism of its action is unclear. Plasmin activates C1 of the complement system as well as being able to cleave C3 to yield active fragments. Plasmin also liberates from both fibrinogen and fibrin, fragments that are capable of increasing vascular permeability and eliciting a chemotactic response to neutrophils. Finally, the coagulation process itself is an almost constant feature of inflammation, and at times the most detrimental element in an inflammatory reaction. Knowledge of the biochemistry and biologic activities of the components of the HF system may be of fundamental importance in a complete understanding of the inflammatory process.

Four of the principal molecules that initiate activity of the HF system are listed in Table 1. As noted, the components are present in human (and rabbit) plasma in low concentrations. HF, prekallikrein, monomeric clotting

Table 1. Protein Components of the Hageman Factor Activated Systems

Component	Molecular weight	Plasma concn (μg/ml)	Structure
Hageman factor	80,000	24	Single chain
Prekallikrein	80,000	50	Single chain
Factor XI	160,000	4	Dimer
High-molecular weight kininogen	110,000	70	Single chain

Factor XI, and plasminogen each have molecular weights of approximately 80,000, while HMW kininogen has a molecular weight of 110,000. Upon activation, each of the first three molecules becomes an active serine protease with high substrate specificity.

As noted in Fig. 1, the molecules that generate activity of this system are assembled on a negatively charged surface. A variety of surfaces have been found that serve this function. Glass or kaolin, the agents commonly used in laboratories, serve this function. Several biologically important substances also may allow a fruitful assembly of the molecules. Substances associated with collagen (Niewiarowski *et al.*, 1965; Wilner *et al.*, 1968), possibly glycosaminoglycans, and vascular basement membrane (Cochrane and Wuepper, 1972) can bring about activation of HF. Bacterial lipopolysaccharides (Morrison and Cochrane, 1974) and urate crystals (Kellermyer and Breckenridge, 1965) also have been shown to subserve this purpose. The surface with its negative charges is thought to function in two ways as demonstrated to date. It serves to bind and thereby assemble HF, HMW kininogen, prekallikrein, and clotting Factor XI. It also induces changes in HF rendering the molecule far more susceptible to the action of proteolytic enzymes (Griffin, 1978) and induces changes in the conformation of HF (Fair *et al.*, 1977).

2. Molecules Involved in the Activation of the Contact System in Plasma

That generation of activity of the system is fulfilled by the interaction of three molecules, HF, prekallikrein, and HMW kininogen, along a negatively charged surface, is shown in Table 2. For the experiments summarized in this table, HF, prekallikrein, and HMW kininogen were mixed in concentrations similar to those found in normal human plasma. Then kaolin was added to provide a surface and, after incubation, precursor Factor XI was added. If HF is activated, it converts Factor XI to its active form which is then assessed in Factor XI-deficient plasma. In the top row of Table 2, it can be seen that a combination of kaolin with HF, prekallikrein, and HMW kininogen activated Factor XI to yield 0.34 clotting unit (one clotting unit being equal to the total amount of Factor XI activity in 1.0 ml normal

Table 2. Activation of Factor XI by Mixtures of HF, HMWK, Prekallikrein (PK), and Kaolin[a]

Reagent				Factor XI_a generated (clotting unit/ml)
Kaolin	HF	HMWK	PK	
+	+	+	+	0.34
+	−	−	−	0[b]
−	+	+	+	0.001
+	−	+	+	0.001
+	+	−	+	0.026
+	+	+	−	0.030

[a] The + or − sign indicates the presence or absence of the indicated reagent in a mixture containing Factor XI at 0.83 unit/ml which was incubated 8 min at 37°C and then assayed for Factor XI_a activity. The concentrations of HF, HMWK, and PK, when present in the mixture, were 18, 14, and 6 μg/ml, respectively. Kaolin concentration was 3.6 mg/ml. The solution contained 0.10 M NaCl, 0.05 M Tris–Cl at pH 7.4. The observed clotting times varied from > 300 sec for Factor XI alone to 118 sec for 0.34 clotting unit/ml.

[b] The background activity for Factor XI alone plus kaolin was 0.006 clotting unit/ml and this value was subtracted from each value in order to define the net activation of Factor XI.

plasma). When any one or a combination of the proteins was omitted, the amount of Factor XI that was activated was reduced greatly. Other experiments (Griffin and Cochrane, 1976) have shown that the rate of activation of Factor XI using the three purified components, HF, prekallikrein, and HMW kininogen, is closely comparable to that when Factor XI in whole plasma is activated. It would appear that the three molecules are sufficient to bring about the generation of HF activity at a rate that allows full expression of at least one of its functions, namely the activation of Factor XI. In whole plasma, the rate of activation takes on considerable importance in that inhibitors constantly damp enzyme activities. If the rate were too slow, the cascading development of zymogen to enzyme conversion in the subsequent generation of molecules would not occur.

3. *The Association of Activation of Molecules with Limited Proteolytic Cleavage*

Upon activation, HF, prekallikrein, and Factor XI undergo limited proteolytic cleavage when normal plasma is exposed to a negatively charged surface. Data indicate an association of cleavage of the molecules with acquisition of enzymatic activity. Cleavage generally occurs initially at one site, and yields two fragments held together by a disulfide linkage. Such a cleavage is illustrated in Fig. 2. In this figure, radiolabeled prekallikrein and Factor XI were added to whole plasma which was then exposed to a glass surface. After a short incubation period (30 sec to 5 min), the radiolabeled proteins can be examine in polyacrylamide gel electrophoresis in SDS and

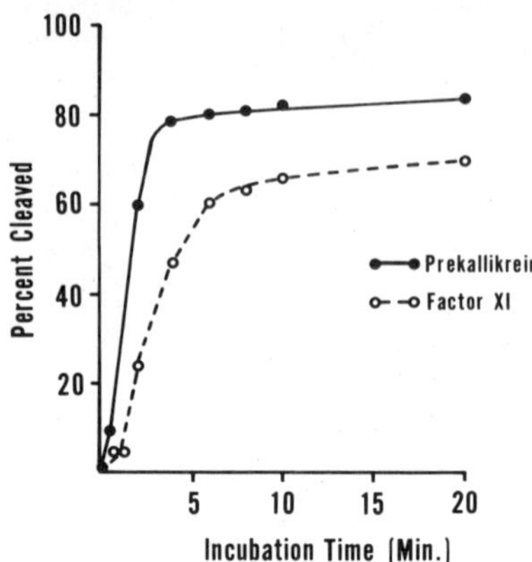

Figure 2. Cleavage of radiolabeled prekallikrein and Factor XI in whole plasma exposed to glass. 127I-labeled prekallikrein or Factor XI was added to whole plasma. The plasma was then incubated in glass tubes at 22°C for the times indicated. SDS with 2-mercaptoethanol was then added at 100°C and the samples assayed in SDS–polyacrylamide gel electrophoresis. (From Revak, *et al.*, 1974.)

in the presence or absence of reducing agent (2-mercaptoethanol). In the absence of reducing agent, kallikrein and Factor XI retain their native molecular weight. But upon reduction, the activated molecules become dissociated into two fragments. The active enzyme site resides in the light chain in each case. The molecular weight of the light chain generally is 25,000 to 35,000. That activity of the molecule is associated with cleavage has been shown both by comparison of cleavage and acquisition of proteolytic capacity as a function of time, and by the binding of [^{3}H]diisopropylphosphofluoridate (DPF) into the light chain of the cleaved molecules at a rate several orders of magnitude faster than into the uncleaved molecule.

Activation of HF when plasma contacts a negatively charged surface is predominantly associated with cleavage of the HF into heavy (54,000 molecular weight) and light (26,000) chains as depicted in Fig. 3 (Revak *et al.*, 1974, 1977; Revak and Cochrane, 1976). In this case, an active fragment of HF has appeared even in the absence of reduction. As shown in the upper panel, radiolabeled HF, added to whole human plasma which was then exposed to glass, underwent partial cleavage into fragments of 54,000 and 26,000 molecular weight. When such a preparation was reduced, as shown in the lower panel, it was seen that far more of the protein had undergone cleavage, as much of the molecule at the native molecular weight was dissociated by reduction into fragments of 52,000 and 28,000 molecular weight. The site responsible for binding HF to the negatively charged surface lies in the 54,000-molecular-weight fragment, while the enzyme site lies in the 26,000-molecular-weight fragment (Revak *et al.*, 1977).

Activation of HF is accompanied by cleavage inside and outside of a disulfide loop as shown in Fig. 4. The two points of cleavage are shown as site 1 and 2. When cleavage occurs at site 1, only the active HF molecule remains surface-bound by virtue of the positively charged amino acid residues present in the heavy chain. When cleavage then occurs at site 2, the light chain bearing the enzymatic site dissociates from the surface. This phenomenon of a second point of cleavage, with release of the active fragment, took

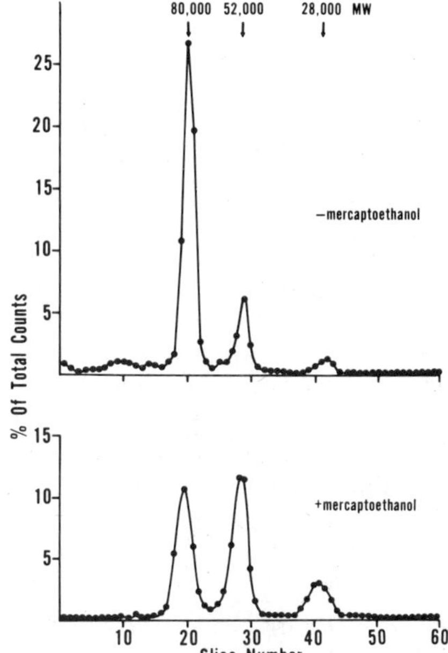

Figure 3. Cleavage of radiolabeled Hageman factor in whole plasma exposed to glass. [^{125}I]-HF was added to plasma and incubated in glass tubes for 2 min at 22°C. SDS in the absence (top panel) or presence (bottom panel) of 2-mercaptoethanol was added at 100°C and the mixture then assayed for cleavage on SDS–polyacrylamide gels. (From Revak *et al.*, 1974.)

on biologic importance when it was found that only the HF cleaved at site 1 and remaining surface-bound was capable of activating both prekallikrein and clotting Factor XI. The fragment, released into the supernatant after cleavage occurs at site 2, possessed prekallikrein-activating but only a slight and probably insignificant amount of activity for Factor XI (Revak *et al.*, 1978). Thus, generation of activity of the kallikrein–kinin system, but not of the intrinsic clotting system, might be expected to be disseminated in the fluid phase.

It has been contended that HF might become activated upon a negatively charged surface without proteolytic cleavage (Cochrane *et al.*, 1972; Ratnoff and Saito, 1977). Presumably, conformational changes in the molecule, developing upon contact with the surface, would allow expression of an enzymatically active site. To support this, studies employing spectroscopic techniques have been conducted. Changes in the molar ellipticity of HF upon contact with quartz or another negatively charged material, ellagic acid, were observed in studies using circular dichroism spectroscopy (McMillan *et al.*, 1974). Exposure of hydrophobic sites on the HF upon exposure

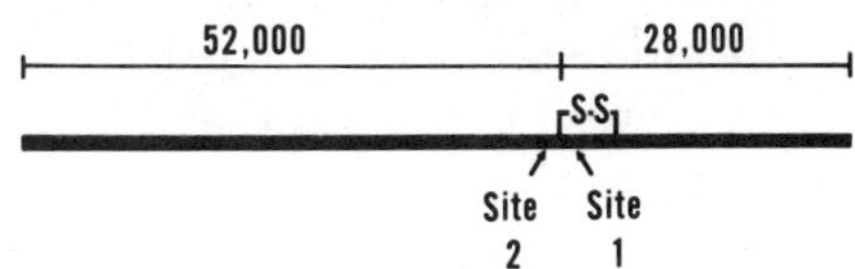

Figure 4. The structure of Hageman factor. Preferred cleavage sites in the polypeptide chain, in the presence of plasma, are noted by arrows. (From Revak *et al.*, 1974.)

to negatively charged substances has been suggested (Fair *et al.*, 1977). Whether cleavage of the molecule had occurred was not demonstrable in the studies. It was not possible to relate unequivocally changes in the molecular configuration of HF in the absence of cleavage with the acquisition of enzymatic activity.

Support for the theory that proteolytic cleavage of HF is required for its activation is derived from: (1) the close association of cleavage with activation in whole plasma and with purified components; and (2) the finding that in plasma deficient in prekallikrein or HMW kininogen, HF neither activates within 2–5 min nor undergoes cleavage even though it binds normally to a negatively charged surface (Revak *et al.*, 1977). Addition of prekallikrein or HMW kininogen restores both the observed cleavage of HF and the normal expression of HF activities. Purified HF either in solution or on a surface failed to enhance the uptake of [^{3}H]-DPF, while HF cleaved by kallikrein or trypsin readily incorporated [^{3}H]-DPF into the light chain (Griffin, 1977; Meier *et al.*, 1977; Claeys and Collen, 1978).

4. *A Role of Prekallikrein in the Activation of HF*

The enzyme in whole plasma responsible for cleavage of the HF was sought in extensive studies. In examining several likely enzymes, it became apparent that kallikrein was at least 10-fold more active than plasmin or Factor XI in activating HF in fluid (Cochrane *et al.*, 1972), or on a surface (Griffin, 1978). In purified systems, kallikrein cleaved HF into the same fragments as the enzyme in whole plasma (Revak *et al.*, 1977). Strong evidence for a role of kallikrein also was obtained by Dr. Kirk Wuepper in this laboratory. He found that Fletcher trait plasma which had been shown to be deficient in developing activity of HF when the plasma contacted a surface was actually deficient in prekallikrein (Wuepper, 1973). Thus, a plasma with a genetic deficiency of prekallikrein did not support the rapid activation of HF in the presence of a surface. Addition of purified prekallikrein restored the normal rate of activation of HF. Strong evidence supported the conclusion that prekallikrein is essential for the activation and cleavage of HF when plasma contacts an appropriate surface. Further studies by Weiss *et al.* (1974) showed that addition of activated HF to the prekallikrein-deficient plasma restored normal functions of the HF-contact system. In other studies, radiolabeled HF added to prekallikrein-deficient plasma failed to undergo cleavage for several minutes after contact with a surface, while radiolabeled HF in normal plasma was cleaved maximally (Revak *et al.*, 1977). HF in the prekallikrein-deficient plasma after 5 min contact with the activating surface, slowly underwent cleavage into its two fragments (Revak *et al.*, 1977). This corresponds to the slow activation of HF that is known to occur in such plasma after addition of a surface. The factors responsible for the slow cleavage of HF on the surface in the absence of prekallikrein remained unknown.

5. *A Role of HMW Kininogen in the Activation of HF and Prekallikrein*

It appears that HF and prekallikrein undergo reciprocal activation during surface-dependent activation of HF in normal plasma. It became apparent, however, that a cofactor was involved in this reaction. Schiffman and Lee (1974) observed a deficiency in the activation of partially purified Factor XI by active HF. The deficiency was corrected by addition to the reaction mixture of an α-globulin fraction of normal plasma containing what was described as "contact activation cofactor." Additional studies also indicated that another factor is essential for contact activation. Human plasma, bearing a new and distinct defect in the early stages of coagulation, was described (Waldman and Abraham, 1974). Soon, similar plasmas were observed in several laboratories and the missing factor was determined to be HMW kininogen (Wuepper *et al.*, 1975a,b; Saito *et al.*, 1975; Donaldson *et al.*, 1976; Colman *et al.*, 1975; Lutcher, 1976). HMW kininogen restored full activity of the contact system to the deficient plasma. The identity of HMW kininogen and Schiffman's contact activation cofactor was made (Schiffman *et al.*, 1975). Bovine HMW kininogen previously had been isolated and much of the amino acid sequence was known (Han *et al.*, 1976).

The means by which HMW kininogen acts to augment the contact activation of plasma was examined. It was observed that the molecule enhanced the activation of prekallikrein by HF (Griffin and Cochrane, 1976). In addition, it augmented cleavage of HF by kallikrein in the presence of a negatively charged surface (Griffin and Cochrane, 1976; Meier *et al.*, 1977). A much smaller effect of HF on prekallikrein was found in the absence of a surface (Lin *et al.*, 1977). The rate of activation of Factor XI in the presence of physiologic concentrations of purified HF, prekallikrein, HMW kininogen, and a surface was found to correspond to the rate of Factor XI activation in plasma (Griffin and Cochrane, 1976). It appeared that the three molecules, HF, prekallikrein, and HMW kininogen, suffice to bring about the full rate of activation of the contact system in plasma.

The mechanism by which HMW kininogen acts in its capacity as cofactor remained to be determined. It was observed that stoichiometric quantities of HMW kininogen and HF acted on the surface to induce optimal activation of HF (Griffin and Cochrane, 1976). There was no evidence that HMW kininogen possessed enzymatic activity. It was then observed that prekallikrein and HMW kininogen exist as a bimolecular complex in plasma (Mandle *et al.*, 1976); and later, that Factor XI and HMW kininogen also exist as a complex (Thompson *et al.*, 1977). These observations then acquired meaning when it was found that HMW kininogen served to bind both prekallikrein and Factor XI to the surface where interaction with HF could take place (Wiggins *et al.*, 1977). Radiolabeled prekallikrein or Factor XI was added to normal plasma, to HMW kininogen-deficient plasma, or to HF-deficient plasma, and then exposed to a negatively charged surface. After an incubation period, the supernatant fluid was separated from the negatively charged surface. The radiolabeled prekallikrein or Factor XI was examined to determined the quantity remaining surface-bound and the extent of cleavage (representing activation). The results of the experiment, shown in Fig. 5, indicate that the radiolabeled Factor XI in plasma failed to bind to the surface in the absence of HMW kininogen. Addition of the purified HMW kininogen to the deficient plasma restored the surface-binding of Factor XI and allowed cleavage to take place as it did in normal plasma. In HF-deficient plasma, binding took place, but cleavage did not result. Most of the cleaved, radiolabeled Factor XI remained surface-bound. When radiolabeled prekallikrein was substituted for radiolabeled Factor XI, similar results were obtained except that the majority of kallikrein, in cleaved form, appeared in the supernatant. The data suggest that HMW kininogen might be directly responsible for bringing about surface-binding of Factor XI and prekallikrein (Wiggins *et al.*, 1977).

A postulated mechanism of activation of HF, prekallikrein, and Factor XI is shown in Figs. 6 and 7.

6. *Dissemination of Activity into the Fluid Phase*

While a negatively charged surface augments activation of the components manifold (Griffin, 1978), it has become clear that activity of both HF

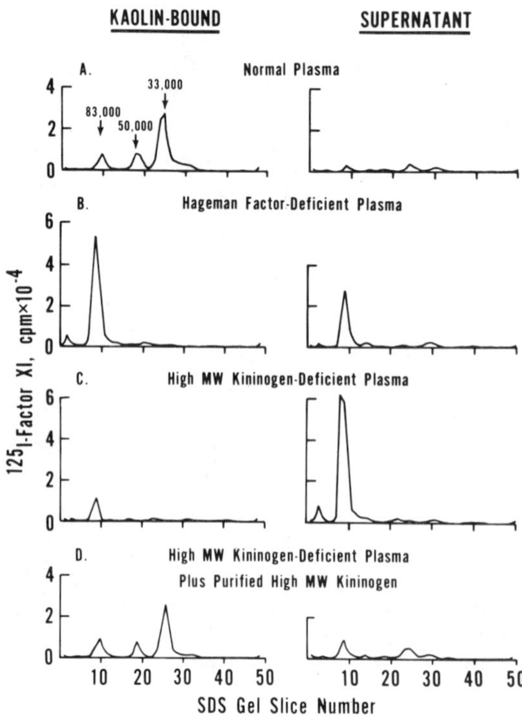

Figure 5. The binding and cleavage of [125I]-Factor XI in various plasmas after the addition of kaolin and incubation for 2 min at 27°C. The kaolin-bound and supernatant proteins were separated by centrifugation and analyzed on SDS–polyacrylamide gels in the presence of mercaptoethanol. A, normal plasma; B, HF-deficient plasma; C, HMW kininogen-deficient plasma; D, same as C, but reconstituted with purified HMW kininogen to a final concentration corresponding to 1 clotting unit/ml undiluted plasma. (From Schiffman *et al.*, 1975.)

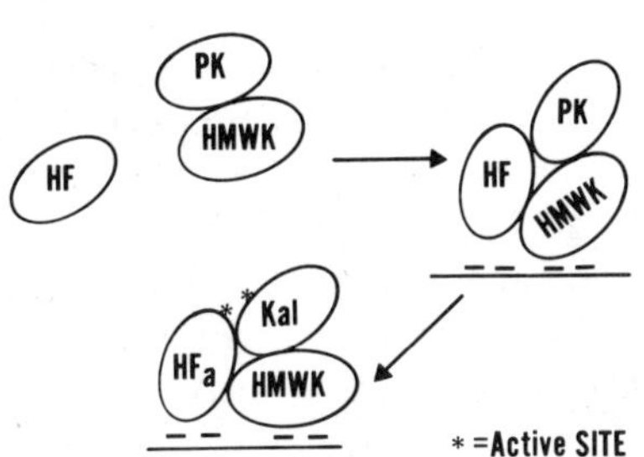

Figure 6. Postulated mechanism of the activation of HF and prekallikrein (PK) on a negatively charged surface. The molecules in solution are shown in the upper left, with PK and HMW kininogen (HMWK) in complexed form. In the presence of a negatively charged surface, shown at the upper right, the molecules assemble with apposition of HF to both HMWK and PK. HF and PK then undergo proteolytic cleavage leading to activation. It is unclear whether HF or PK becomes activated initially or whether the majority of HF molecules are activated by kallikrein (Kal) previously released into solution after activation on the surface.

and kallikrein are given off into the fluid phase. The release of the 28,000-molecular-weight form of active HF (HF_a) from the surface after exposure to kallikrein follows cleavage outside of the disulfide loop (site 2) in the HF molecule (see Fig. 4). The released HF_a fragment can rapidly activate prekallikrein in solution, but is extremely poor at cleaving and activating Factor XI whether it be in solution or on a surface (Revak *et al.*, 1978). HF_a that is cleaved only within the disulfide loop (at site 1), remains surface-bound, and activates both Factor XI and prekallikrein. Cleavage of HF at site 2 converts HF_a to a selective activator of the kallikrein pathway in solution, while the activation of the intrinsic clotting system is primarily a surface phenomenon. The fact that Factor XI, upon activation, remains bound predominantly to the surface (probably to the HMW kininogen), underscores this (see Fig. 5).

Recent studies have shed light on a second means by which active components are disseminated into the soluble phase. As noted above, kallikrein is released readily from the surface during the activation of the contact system (Wiggins *et al.*, 1977; Revak *et al.*, 1978). The rapidity with which kallikrein is released in active form is remarkable. When radiolabeled prekallikrein was added to normal plasma at 22°C with an activating surface (kaolin), incubation of the mixture for 40 sec revealed that 78% of the prekallikrein in the supernatant and 75% of the prekallikrein on the surface was cleaved. Ninety percent of the radiolabeled molecules were in the supernatant. In addition, over 90% of the HMW kininogen in the supernatant and on the surface had been cleaved (unpublished observations). About 40%

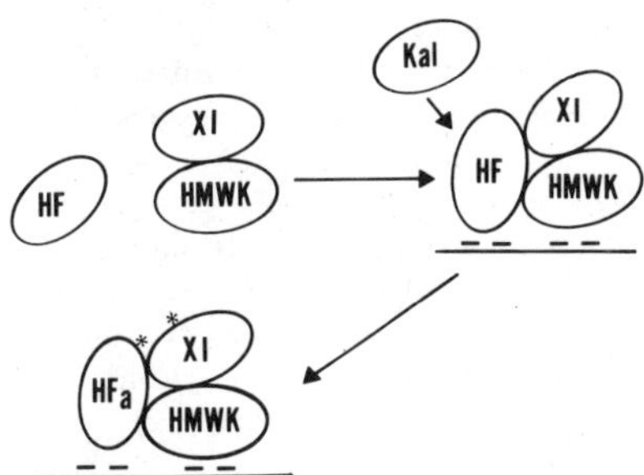

Figure 7. Postulated activation of Factor XI by HF on a negatively charged surface. The assembly of molecules occurs as in Fig. 6, but the HF is activated by kallikrein (Kal) which has been released from the generating group of molecules shown in Fig. 6. The activated Factor XI remains bound and does not readily dissociate as does kallikrein.

of the HMW kininogen was surface-bound. The amount of HF_a appearing in the supernatant even at 4°C over the short time span was constant and only represented a few percent of the total (Cochrane and Revak, unpublished observations). The experiments have suggested that a higher concentration of kallikrein is produced rapidly around the generating unit of surface-bound HF_a and HMW kininogen. The number of molecules of prekallikrein that are converted to kallikrein on the generating unit appears to be enormous. The effect of this phenomenon in biological systems will be a focus for future study.

7. *Cleavage and Activation of HF by Cellular Enzymes*

It has become apparent that enzymes released from cells upon stimulation cleave and activate surface-bound HF. Peripheral leukocytes from allergic individuals release a kallikrein-like enzyme upon contact with antigen or with antibody to IgE (Newball *et al.*, 1975). The enzymes so released rapidly cleave surface-bound HF (Newball *et al.*, 1978). Cleavage of HF occurs at both site 1 and site 2 (Fig. 4), with a marked preference for the latter.

In additional studies in this laboratory, Dr. R. Wiggins has observed that an enzyme present in cultured rabbit endothelial cells cleaves and activates HF (Wiggins *et al.*, 1979).

The role of these cellular proteases in the generation of inflammatory reactions will necessitate further study, but the association of these cells and activation of the HF system may well prove to be of considerable significance.

References

Claeys, H., and Collen, D., 1978, Purification and characterization of bovine factor XII, *Eur. J. Biochem.* **87:**69.

Cochrane, C. G., 1968, Immunologic tissue injury mediated by neutrophilic leukocytes, in: *Advances in Immunology* (F. J. Dixon and H. G. Kunkel, eds.), pp. 97–162, Academic Press, New York.

Cochrane, C. G., 1979, Mediation systems in neutrophil-independent immunologic injury of the glomerulus, in: *Contemporary Issues in Nephrology-3; Immunologic mechanisms of renal disease* (C. B. Wilson, B. M. Brenner and J. H. Stein, eds.), Churchill Livingston, Edinburgh.

Cochrane, C. G., and Aikin, B. S., 1966, Polymorphonuclear leukocytes in immunologic reactions: The destruction of vascular basement membrane *in vivo* and *in vitro, J. Exp. Med.* **124:**733.

Cockrane, C. G., and Wuepper, K. D., 1972, The kinin-forming system: Delineation and activation, in: *Immunopathology* (P. A. Miescher, ed.), pp. 220–235, Schwabe, Basel.

Cochrane, C. G., Revak, S. D., Aikin, B. S., and Wuepper, K. D., 1972, The structural characteristics and activation of Hageman factor, in: *Inflammation: Mechanisms and Control* (I. H. Lepow and P. A. Ward, eds.), pp. 119–138, Academic Press, New York.

Cochrane, C. G., Revak, S. D., and Wuepper, K. D., 1973, Activation of Hageman factor in solid and fluid phases: A critical role of kallikrein, *J. Exp. Med.* **138:**1564.

Colman, R. W., Bagdasarian, A., Talamo, R. C., Scott, C. F., Seavey, M., Guimaraes, J. A., Pierce, J. V., Kaplan, A. P., and Weinstein, L., 1975, Williams trait: Human kininogen deficiency with diminished levels of plasminogen proactivator and prekallikrein associated with abnormalities of the Hageman factor-dependent pathways, *J. Clin. Invest.* **56:**1650.

Donaldson, V. H., Glueck, H. I., Miller, M. A., Movat, H. Z., and Habal, F., 1976, Kininogen deficiency in Fitzgerald trait: Role of high molecular weight kininogen in clotting and fibrinolysis, *J. Lab. Clin. Med.* **87:**327.

Fair, B. D., Saito, H., Ratnoff, O. D., and Rippon, W. B., 1977, Detection by fluorescence of structural changes accompanying the activation of Hageman factor (factor XII), *Proc. Soc. Exp. Biol. Med.* **155:**199.

Griffin, J. H., 1978, The role of surface in the surface-dependent activation of Hageman factor (factor XII), *Proc. Natl. Acad. Sci. USA* **75:**1998.

Griffin, J. H., 1977, Molecular mechanism of surface-dependent activation of Hageman factor (coagulation factor XII), *Fed. Proc.* **36:**329.

Griffin, J. H., and Cochrane, C. G., 1976, Mechanisms for involvement of high molecular weight kininogen in surface-dependent reactions of Hageman factor (coagulation factor XII), *Proc. Natl. Acad. Sci. USA* **73:**2554.

Han, Y. N., Kato, H., Iwanaga, S., and Suzuki, T., 1976, Primary structure of bovine plasma high molecular weight kininogen, *J. Biochem.* **79:**1201.

Kellermyer, R. W., and Breckenridge, R. T., 1965, The inflammatory process in acute gouty arthritis. I. Activation of Hageman factor by sodium urate crystals, *J. Lab. Clin. Med.* **65:**307.

Lin, C. Y., Scott, C. F., Bagdasarian, A., Pierce, J. V., Kaplan, A. P., and Colman, R. W., 1977, Potentiation of the function of Hageman factor fragments by high molecular weight kininogen, *J. Clin. Invest.***60:**7.

Lutcher, C. L., 1976, Reid trait: A new expression of high molecular weight kininogen deficiency, *Clin. Res.* **24:**440A.

McMillan, C. R., Saito, H., Ratnoff, O. D., and Walton, A. G., 1974, The secondary structure of human Hageman factor (factor XII) and its alteration by activating agents, *J. Clin. Invest.* **54:**1312.

Mandle, R. J., Colman, R. W., and Kaplan, A. P., 1976, Identification of prekallikrein and high molecular weight kininogen as a complex in human plasma, *Proc. Natl. Acad. Sci. USA* **11:**4179.

Meier, H. L., Pierce, J. V., Colman, R. W., and Kaplan, A. P., 1977, Activation and function of human Hageman factor: The role of high molecular weight kininogen and prekallikrein, *J. Clin. Invest.* **60:**18.

Morrison, D. C., and Cochrane, C. G., 1974, Direct evidence for Hageman factor (factor XII) activation by bacterial lipopolysaccharides, *J. Exp. Med.* **140:**797.

Newball, H. H., Talamo, R., and Lichtenstein, L. M., 1975, Release of leukocyte kallikrein mediated by IgE, *Nature (London)* **254:**635.

Newball, H. H., Revak, S. D., Cochrane, C. G., Griffin, J. H., and Lichtenstein, L. M., 1978, Cleavage of Hageman factor by a basophil kallikrein of anaphylaxis, *Clin. Res.* **26:**519A.

Niewiarowski, S., Bankowski, E., and Fiedoreck, T., 1964, Adsorption of Hageman factor (factor XII) on collagen, *Experientia* **20A**367.

Niewiarowski, A. Bankowski, E., and Rogowicka, I., 1965, Studies on the adsorption and activation of the Hageman factor (factor XII) by collagen and elastin, *Thromb. Diath. Haemorrh.* **14:**387.

Ratnoff, O. D., and Saito, H., 1977, Activation of Hageman factor by Sephadex-ellagic acid mixtures, *Thromb. Hemostasis* **38:**12.

Revak, S. D., and Cochrane, C. G., 1976, The relationship of structure and function in human Hageman factor: The association of enzymatic and binding activities with separate regions of the molecule, *J. Clin. Invest.* **57:**852.

Revak, S. D., Cochrane, C. G., Johnston, A. R., and Hugli, T. E., 1974, Structural changes accompanying enzymatic activation of human Hageman factor, *J. Clin. Invest.* **54:**619.

Revak, S. D., Cochrane, C. G., and Griffin, J. H., 1977, The binding and cleavage characteristics of human Hageman factor during contact activation: A comparison of normal plasma with plasmas deficient in factor XI, prekallikrein, or high molecular weight kininogen, *J. Clin. Invest.* **58:**1167.

Revak, S. D., Cochrane, C. G., Bouma, B. N., and Griffin, J. H., 1978, Surface and fluid phase activities of two forms of activated Hageman factor produced during contact activation of plasma, *J. Exp. Med.* **58:**719.

Saito. H., Ratnoff, O. D., Waldman, R., and Abraham, J. P., 1975, Fitzgerald trait: Deficiency of a hitherto unrecognized agent, Fitzgerald factor, participating in surface-mediated reactions of clotting, fibrinolysis, generation of kinins, and the property of diluted plasma enhancing vascular permeability (PF/DIL), *J. Clin. Invest.* **55:**1082.

Salant, D. J., Belok, S., Madaio, M. P., and Couser, W. C., 1980, A new role for complement in experimental nephropathy in rats, *J. Clin. Invest.* **66:**1339.

Schiffman, S., and Lee, P., 1974, Preparation, characterization and activation of a highly purified factor XI: Evidence that a hitherto unrecognized plasma activity participates in the interaction of factors XI and XII, *Br. J. Haematol.* **27:**101.

Schiffman, S., Lee, P., and Waldman, R., 1975, Identity of contact activation cofactor and Fitzgerald factor, *Thromb. Res.* **6:**451.

Thompson, R., Mandle, R., Jr., and Kaplan, A. P., 1977, Association of factor XI and high molecular weight kininogen in human plasma, *J. Clin. Invest.* **60:**1376.

Waldman, R., and Abraham, J., 1974, Fitzgerald factor: A heretofore unrecognized coagulation factor, *Blood J. Haematol.* **44:**934.

Weiss, A. S., Gallin, J. I., and Kaplan, A. P., 1974, Fletcher factor deficiency: A diminished rate of Hageman factor activation caused by absence of prekallikrein with abnormalities of coagulation, fibrinolysis, chemotactic activity and kinin generation, *J. Clin. Invest.* **53:**622.

Wiggins, R. C., and Cochrane, C. G., 1982, Hageman factor in acute nephrotoxic nephritis in the rabbit. Submitted for publication.

Wiggins, R. C., Bouma, B. N. Cochrane, C. G., and Griffin, J. H., 1977, Role of high molecular weight kininogen in surface-binding and activation of coagulation factor XI and prekallikrein, *Proc. Natl. Acad. Sci. USA* **74:**4636.

Wiggins, R. C., Loekntoff, D. J., Cochrane, C. G., Griffin, J. H., and Edgington, T. E., 1979, Activation of Hageman factor by endothelial cells of the rabbit, *J. Clin. Invest.* **65:**197.

Wilner, G. D., Nossel, H. L., and Leroy, E. C., 1968, Activation of Hageman factor by collagen, *J. Clin. Invest.* **47:**2608.

Wuepper, K. D., 1973, Prekallikrein deficiency in man, *J. Exp. Med.* **138:**1345.

Wuepper, K. D., Miller, D. R., and LaCombe, M. J., 1975a, Flaujeac trait: Deficiency of kininogen in man, *Fed. Proc.* **34:**859 (abstract).

Wuepper, K. D., Miller, D. R., and LaCombe, M. J., 1975b, Flaujeac trait: Deficiency of human plasma kininogen, *J. Clin. Invest.* **56:**1663.

Yamamoto, T., and Cochrane, C. G., 1981, Guinea pig Hageman factor as a vascular permeability factor, *Am. J. Path.,* **105:**164.

32

The Function of the Reticuloendothelial System in Autoimmune Disease

Michael M. Frank

1. Introduction

For the past 4 or 5 years, a new methodology for assessing the functional status of membrane receptors on the fixed macrophages of the reticuloendothelial system (RES) which recognize immunologically active materials and mediate their removal from the bloodstream (Frank *et al.*, 1977; Jaffe *et al.*, 1976; Atkinson and Frank, 1974a,b,c; Atkinson *et al.*, 1973; Schreiber and Frank, 1972a,b) has been developed. This account of the current status of that work is not meant to be a definitive statement of the role of the reticuloendothelial membrane receptors in the clearance of immunologically active materials from the blood in patients with nephritis. There are some data on patients with nephritis, but these questions are not definitively answered. However, this methodology holds potential promise for development of an understanding of the pathophysiologic basis of a number of perplexing autoimmune diseases.

2. Hepatic Clearance of Erythrocytes Coated with IgM and Complement via C3b Receptors

The methods used were developed originally to assess the functions that antibody and complement serve when deposited on erythrocyte surfaces to cause those erythrocytes to be removed from the circulation and destroyed (Jaffe *et al.*, 1976; Atkinson and Frank, 1974a,b,c; Atkinson *et al.*, 1973;

Michael M. Frank · Laboratory of Clinical Investigation, National Institute of Allergy and Infectious Diseases, National Institutes of Health, Bethesda, Maryland 20205.

Schreiber and Frank, 1972a,b). There was interest in learning how antibody and complement on an erythrocyte surface lead to shortened survival and destruction of the circulating cell. The conclusions of those earlier studies were several. First, it was found that IgM antibody of a number of different types (rabbit anti-guinea pig erythrocyte IgM, human anti-A blood group substance IgM, and human cold-agglutinin IgM) all required complement to produce their biologic effects, and in the absence of activation of the classical complement pathway, coating of erythrocytes with these IgM antibodies did not lead to shortened survival of the cells. When cells coated with IgM antibody were injected into the circulation of animals or man, they were rapidly cleared and, in fact, were gone from the circulation within minutes of the time of injection (Fig. 1). The site of clearance of these antibody coated cells was the liver. A series of experiments was performed to elucidate the pathophysiologic basis of this interesting sequestration pattern. It was possible to show that the injection of the IgM coated cells led to rapid activation of the complement cascade via the classic complement pathway. In the absence of classic complement pathway activity the cells survived normally, even if the alternative complement pathway was intact. Activation of complement led to the very rapid deposition of the early components C1, C4 and C2 as well as C3 on the erythrocyte surface. The key complement fragment deposited on the erythrocyte surface was the opsonic fragment of C3, C3b. As the erythrocytes coated with antibody and complement filtered through the sinusoids of the liver, they adhered to Kupffer cells, macrophages with C3b receptors which line the hepatic sinusoids, by virtue of the C3b receptors. The red cells were efficiently removed from the circulation as they traversed the liver. Since a major portion of the cardiac output passes through the liver, the cells were rapidly cleared from the circulation. The

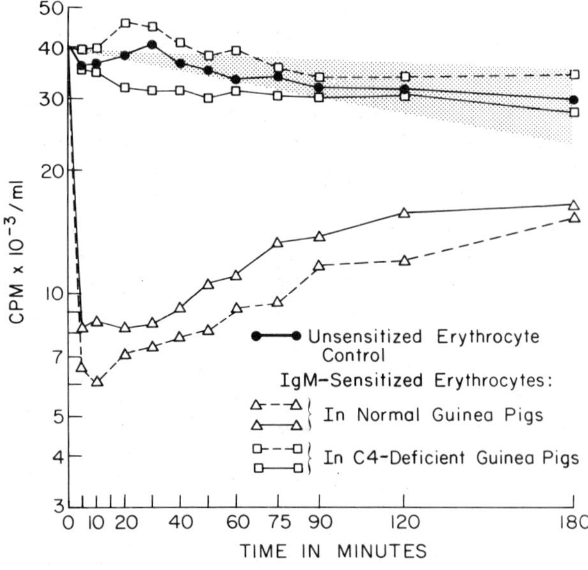

Figure 1. Clearance of IgM-sensitized erythrocytes in normal and C4-deficient guinea pigs. Similar patterns are obtained in man. The cells are rapidly cleared by the liver, and a portion of the cells reappear in the circulation over a period of hours. There is no clearance at all in C4-deficient guinea pigs. (From Schreiber and Frank, 1972a)

erythrocytes, now adherent to Kupffer cell membranes because of the attachment to the C3b receptors, underwent one of two fates. A small proportion of the cells were phagocytosed. In human studies this amounted to about one of three adherent red cells. The majority of the cells, however, were not phagocytosed because the adherence of the C3b coated erythrocyte to the Kupffer cell membrane surface was not a good stimulus for phagocytosis (Montovani *et al.*, 1972; Frank *et al.*, 1977; Jaffe *et al.*, 1976; Atkinson and Frank, 1974c). The adherent erythrocytes had an opportunity to interact with the C3 inactivator system in the blood plasma. This series of inactivator proteins acts on C3b to produce stepwise cleavage which results in two fragments, C3c and C3d (Gaither *et al.*, 1978; Gitlin *et al.*, 1975; Ruddy and Austen, 1971). If the C3b is cell bound as it was in the erythrocyte clearance studies, the cleavage reaction leads to the release of fluid-phase C3c and retention of C3d on the erythrocyte surface. The cells no longer interacted with the C3b receptor on Kupffer cell membranes and were released back into the circulation where they survived normally (Frank *et al.*, 1977; Reynolds *et al.*, 1975). Thus, the effect of complement in this model was not to cause membrane damage directly, but to lead to the deposition of an active immunologic complement fragment on the erythrocyte surface which could interact with receptors for that specific fragment, thereby mediating removal of the cells from the circulation. It was possible to study the quantitative aspects of this phenomenon, and it was shown that 60 molecules of IgM antibody on the erythrocyte surface was sufficient to cause clearance of erythrocytes in guinea pigs and 20 molecules of IgM antibody on the erythrocyte surface was sufficient to cause clearance of IgM-coated erythrocytes in man.

3. *Splenic Clearance of Erythrocytes Coated with IgG via Fc Receptors*

The situation with regard to IgG antibody was quite different (Atkinson and Frank, 1974a; Schreiber and Frank, 1972a,b). Coating erythrocytes with IgG antibody led to the progressive removal of the antibody-coated erythrocytes from the circulation (Fig. 2). The shape of the clearance curve was quite different from that of IgM. There was no clearance and release pattern but a monoexponential decay of cells from the circulation when plotted as a semilogarithmic function. The cleared cells were phagocytosed efficiently and never released back into the circulation to survive normally. The site of sequestration and phagocytosis was the spleen rather than the liver except at very high doses of antibody. Complement augmented IgG clearance in situations in which complement was activated, but the clearance of the IgG-coated erythrocytes was still mediated by the spleen. Thus, in one situation complement mediated clearance via hepatic Kupffer cells and in a second situation augmented clearance via phagocytic cells within the spleen. In the case of IgG antibody, there are Fc receptors on the membranes of fixed

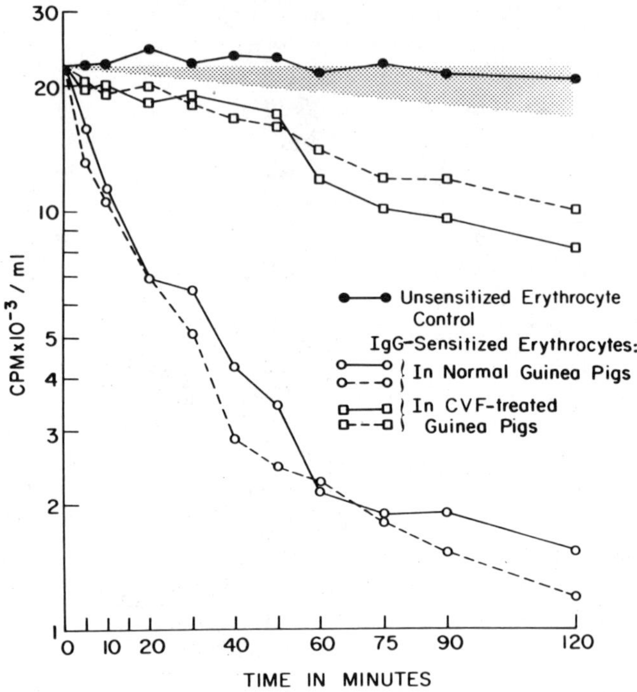

Figure 2. Clearance of IgG-sensitized erythrocytes in normal and cobra venom factor-treated animals. The latter group of animals has normal levels of serum C4 but markedly depressed levels of C3–9. There is some clearance in the complement-deficient animals, but it is markedly depressed. Similar curves showing progressive erythrocyte removal from the circulation can be obtained in man. (From Schreiber and Frank, 1972a)

macrophages of the RES, and clearance can be mediated in the absence of complement activation, although complement increases the efficiency of clearance enormously.

During the course of these studies, it became evident that a technology which allowed one to approach the question of the functional status of receptors for IgG antibody and complement on the fixed phagocytic cells of the RES had been developed. These receptors were important for the clearance of cells in normal individuals and had developed values for clearance in normal individuals as part of the hemolytic anemia studies. It was evident that one could take the same cellular preparations into various patient groups and determine if the receptors were behaving normally. This was begun in an extensive series of studies over the last several years. What has emerged is the fact that the activity of the Fc receptors and C3b receptors may vary in different disease states and that the usual test for RES function, the test that examines the ability of the RES to remove aggregated human serum albumin from the circulation, measures something different from tests that examine the receptor-specific clearance of sensitized erythrocytes. The ability to determine whether the Fc receptors and C3b receptors are functioning normally in various kinds of autoimmune disease may be of major interest. For example, it is known that the Fc receptors are of prime importance in removing immune complexes from the circulation and it is also known that when immune complexes are injected into the circulation of a normal animal, they are rapidly cleared (Mannik *et al.*, 1971). Under most experimental circumstances, injected immune complexes are not deposited in the kidneys. Moreover, it is known that in order to induce renal deposition of immune complexes, one must inhibit the interaction of immune complexes with the RES so that the complexes are not cleared and continue to circulate to be deposited in renal tissue (Haakenstad and Mannik, 1974). Thus, one can modify the complexes themselves so that they no longer interact efficiently with phagocytic cell receptors. One can also alter the functional status of the RES by one of a number of methods that cause an overload of the RES clearance mechanisms. In these cases, the immune complexes are not removed efficiently, continue to circulate, and are deposited in various tissue sites.

Fairly extensive studies of certain types of liver disease as well as of certain types of rheumatologic conditions such as systemic lupus erythematosus (SLE) and Sjögren's syndrome (Jaffe *et al.*, 1978; Frank *et al.*, 1977) have been completed. The functional status of these receptors in various kinds of renal disease is being examined and a number of interesting points already have emerged from these studies.

4. Studies in Human Disease

Patients with three types of hepatic disease were evaluated (Jaffe *et al.*, 1978). These included patients with primary biliary cirrhosis, chronic active hepatitis, and alcoholic cirrhosis. The latter group served as controls. In brief, these studies demonstrated that patients with hepatitis B-antigen-negative, chronic active hepatitis had no abnormalities of receptor function by these methods leading to a delay in clearance. Similarly, patients with alcoholic cirrhosis had no abnormalities of these receptors by these methods. However, patients with primary biliary cirrhosis all had an abnormality in function of the C3b receptors when tested (Fig. 3). Their Fc receptors were normal as well as their ability to clear aggregated albumin. On the other hand, it was found that patients with active SLE all have a marked defect in Fc receptor function (Frank *et al.*, 1977). The defect is at times quite striking, and patients with severe SLE may be completely unable to clear IgG-coated erythrocytes from the circulation. Although no correlation was shown between the levels of circulating immune complexes and receptor defects in the patients with primary biliary cirrhosis and chronic active hepatitis, it was found that there was a correlation between the presence of circulating immune complexes and the inability to clear IgG-coated erythrocytes from the circulation in patients with SLE. Thus, these patients had a profound defect in the activity of Fc receptors which correlated directly with the

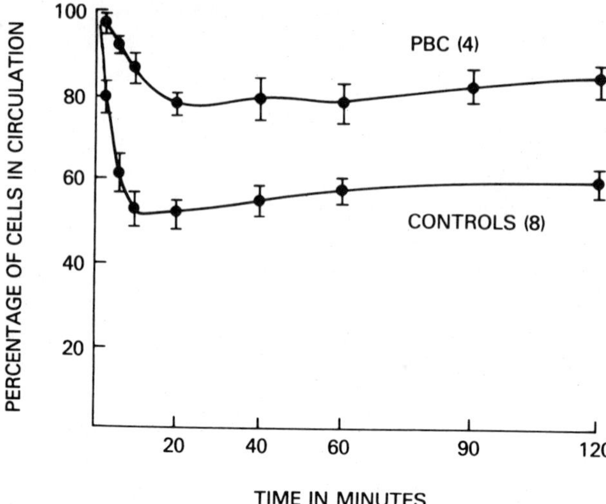

Figure 3. Clearance of IgM anti-A-isoagglutinin-sensitized erythrocytes in eight normal individuals and in four patients with primary biliary cirrhosis. (From Jaffe *et al.*, 1978, *J. Clin. Invest.*)

immune complex levels. It is tempting to speculate that the Fc receptor defect in these patients leads to continued circulation of complexes, allowing these complexes to be deposited in various tissue sites where they can produce considerable tissue injury.

The reason for this Fc receptor defect in patients with SLE is unknown. It may be that these patients develop large amounts of circulating immune complexes which effectively compete for and neutralize receptor function. It may also be that these patients have an underlying defect in receptor function which allows normally formed complexes to circulate and thereby leads to the disease state. The data do not allow for a choice between these two hypotheses at the present time. However, serial studies and family studies should allow these two possibilities to be separated. This is the first clear-cut defect in RES function demonstrated in patients with SLE. Interestingly, the patients showed normal clearance of aggregated human serum albumin, again underlining the fact that these tests measure different parameters.

There have been found some diseases like SLE in which there is a clear-cut close association between the presence of circulating complexes as detected by the method used, the Clq-binding assay, and a clearance defect. There are many other diseases, however, where this association does not hold up. Primary cirrhosis and chronic active hepatitis are such examples. In these two situations, there is no correlation between circulating immune complex levels and Fc receptor function. The situation is even more striking in the case of Sjögren's syndrome. In this situation, almost all patients have circulating immune complexes by our assays. However, only a subset of these patients have Fc receptor defects. It is interesting that the vast majority of patients in this subset have the various signs and symptoms of immune complex-like diseases. Thus, it is the patients with the clearance defects who have rheumatoid arthritis, interstitial nephritis, interstitial pulmonary lung disease, etc. In this situation, then, there is a total disassociation between the presence of immune complexes by this assay and the presence of a clearance defect. The clearance defect, however striking, correlates with the type and extent of disease present in the various patient groups.

Evaluation of patients with various kinds of renal disease (Fig. 4) has been started recently. In general, there is a striking correlation between the presence of immune complexes, Fc receptor defects, and the presence of renal disease in the patients with SLE. In a number of other diseases in which immunologic renal damage occurs, there is a correlation between clearance defects and the presence of renal disease. In many cases, there is a total disassociation between the presence of circulating complexes and Fc receptor function. One example of that is Sjögren's syndrome. A second example is mixed cryoglobulinemia. These patients all have large amounts of circulating immune complexes. Nevertheless, most of the patients do not have renal disease and do not have an Fc receptor defect. The three patients studied who developed renal disease all manifest an Fc receptor defect.

As shown by these examples, there is a correlation between renal disease and clearance defects. Depending on the kind of disease one chooses to study, there may be a correlation between circulating immune complexes and clearance defects as well. These data suggest that different types of circulating complexes exist in a variety of clinical diseases, and it is these differences in the type and composition of the complexes which determine in part the way they are handled in the patient and whether they cause renal disease. This approach to the study of renal disease in man will offer a great

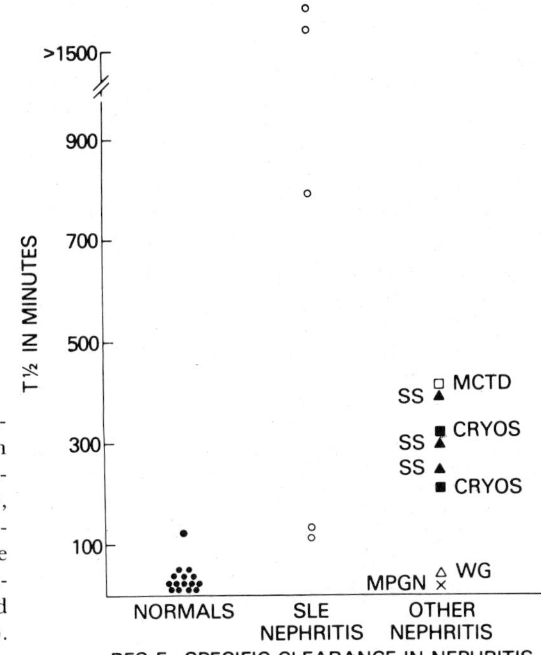

Figure 4. Clearance of anti-Rh-IgG antibody-coated erythrocytes in patients with a number of types of renal disease including systemic lupus erythematosus (SLE), Sjögren's syndrome (SS), Wegener's granulomatosis (WG), membranoproliferative glomerulonephritis (MPGN), mixed connective tissue disease (MCTD), and mixed essential cryoglobulinemia (CRYOS). (From Frank *et al.*, 1979)

deal of new and important information into the mechanisms of renal deposition of immune complexes and, hopefully, will provide further insight into both the causation of these diseases and their treatment.

ACKNOWLEDGMENTS. A great many individuals have contributed importantly to these studies. The original animal studies were performed in collaboration with Drs. Alan Schreiber and John P. Atkinson. The human clearance studies were done in collaboration with Drs. Atkinson and C. J. Jaffe. The studies of patients with hepatic disease were performed with Drs. E. A. Jones, J. M. Vierling, C. Jaffe, and T. J. Lawley. Those of systemic lupus erythematosus were done in collaboration with Drs. R. P. Kimberly, M. Hamburger, T. Lawley, and P. H. Plotz. Those of Sjögren's syndrome were performed with Drs. H. Moutsopoulos, M. Hamburger, T. Lawley, and T. Chused. Those on mixed cryoglobulinemia were done with Drs. M. Hamburger, T. Lawley, P. Gorevic, and E. C. Franklin. The patients with Wegener's granuloma and membranoproliferative glomerulonephritis were studied in collaboration with Drs. A. Fauci and J. Balow, respectively.

References

Atkinson, J. P., and Frank, M. M., 1974a, Complement-independence clearance of IgG-sensitized erythrocytes: Inhibition by cortisone, *Blood* **44:**629.

Atkinson, J. P., and Frank, M. M., 1974b, The effect of bacillus Calmette-Guerin-induced macrophage activation on the *in vivo* clearance of sensitized erythrocytes, *J. Clin. Invest.* **53:**1742.

Atkinson, J. P., and Frank, M. M., 1974c, Studies on the *in vivo* effects of antibody: Interaction of IgM antibody and complement in the immune clearance and destruction of erythrocytes in man, *J. Clin. Invest.* **54:**339.

Atkinson, J. P., Schreiber, A. D., and Frank, M. M., 1973, Effects of corticosteroids and splenectomy on the immune clearance and destruction of erythrocytes, *J. Clin. Invest.* **52:**1509.

Frank, M. M., Jaffe, C. J., Kimberly, R. P., Lawley, T. J., and Plotz, P. H., 1977, An immunospecific clearance defect in patients with systemic lupus erythematosus (SLE) related to the levels of circulating immune complexes (IC), *Clin. Res.* **25:**357A (abstract).

Frank, M. M., Schreiber, A. D., Atkinson, J. P., and Jaffe, C. J. 1977, Pathophysiology of immune hemolytic anemia, *Ann. Intern. Med.* **87:**210.

Frank, M. M., Hamburger, M. I., Lawley, T. J., Kimberly, R. P., and Plotz, P. H., 1979, Defective reticuloendothelial system Fc-receptor function in systemic lupus erythematosus, *New Engl. J. Med.* **300:**518.

Gaither, T. A., Gadek, J., and Frank, M. M., 1978, C3b inactivator: The effect on cell bound C3b and a simplified functional assay, *J. Immunol.* **120:**1774.

Gitlin, J. D., Rosen, F. S., and Lachmann, P. J., 1975, The mechanism of action of the C3b inactivator (conglutinogen-activating factor) on its naturally occurring substrate, the major fragment of the third component of complement (C3b), *J. Exp. Med.* **141:**1221.

Haakenstad, A. O., and Mannik, M., 1974, Saturation of the reticuloendothelial system with soluble immune complexes, *J. Immunol.* **112:**1939.

Jaffe, C. J., Atkinson, J. P., and Frank, M. M., 1976, The role of complement in the clearance of cold agglutinin-sensitized erythrocytes in man, *J. Clin. Invest.* **58:**942.

Jaffe, C. J., Vierling, J. M., Jones, E. A., Lawley, T. J., and Frank, M. M., 1978, Receptor specific clearance by the reticuloendothelial system in chronic liver diseases: Demonstration of defective C3b specific clearance in primary biliary cirrhosis, *J. Clin. Invest.* **62:**1069.

Mannik, M., Arend, W. P., Hall, A. P., and Gilliland, B. C., 1971, Studies on antigen–antibody complexes. I. Elimination of soluble complexes from the rabbit circulation, *J. Exp. Med.* **133:**713.

Montovani, B., Rabinovitch, M., and Nussenzweig, V., 1972, Phagocytosis of immune complexes by macrophages: Different role of the macrophage receptor sites for complement (C3) and for immunoglobulin (IgG), *J. Exp. Med.* **135:**780.

Reynolds, H. Y., Atkinson, J. P., Newball, H. H., and Frank, M. M., 1975, Receptors for immunoglobulin and complement on human alveolar macrophages, *J. Immunol.* **114:**1813.

Ruddy, S., and Austen, K. F., 1971, C3b inactivation of man. II. Fragments produced by C3b inactivator cleavage of cell bound or fluid phase C3b, *J. Immunol.* **108:**742.

Schreiber, A. D., and Frank, M. M., 1972a, Role of antibody and complement in the immune clearance and destruction of erythrocytes. I. *In vivo* effects of IgG and IgM complement-fixing sites, *J. Clin. Invest.* **51:**575.

Schreiber, A. D., and Frank, M. M., 1972b, Role of antibody and complement in the immune clearance and destruction of erythrocytes. II. Molecular nature of IgG and IgM complement-fixing sites and effects of their interaction with serum, *J. Clin. Invest.* **51:**583.

33

A Role of Mononuclear Phagocytes in Immunologically Induced Glomerulonephritis

Emil R. Unanue, George F. Schreiner, and Ramzi S. Cotran

1. Introduction

This chapter summarizes a study on a model of immunological renal injury in which a prominent mononuclear cell component infiltrating the glomerulus has been identified (Schreiner *et al.*, 1978). The evidence indicates that the mononuclear cell component contributes to the glomerular injury. The experimental model is an accelerated form of nephrotoxic serum nephritis (NTN).

It is well established that glomerular renal injury can be produced by an immunological antigen–antibody reaction at the level of the glomerular capillary wall (reviewed by Unanue and Dixon, 1967; Dixon, 1968). The immune reaction is brought about either by direct binding of anti-glomerular basement membrane (GBM) antibodies to antigens of the GBM or, as occurs more frequently, by deposition of phlogogenic antigen–antibody complexes. Either immune reaction at the level of the GBM can cause injury by the fixation of complement, a process which then leads to the accumulation of polymorphonuclear neutrophils (Hammer and Dixon, 1963; Cochrane *et al.*, 1965). The neutrophils are directly responsible for the complement-dependent injury, perhaps by secretion of proteases that affect critical molecules of the GBM. Aside from this well-characterized complement–neutrophil-mediated injury, it is known that immune reactions also can cause pathologic

---

Emil R. Unanue, George F. Schreiner, and Ramzi S. Cotran · Departments of Pathology, Harvard Medical School and Peter Bent Brigham Hospital, Boston, Massachusetts 02115. This work was supported by NIH Grants AI 14732, CA 14723, and HL 08251.

changes through complement–neutrophil-unrelated mechanisms. For example, in the model of NTN, which has been an invaluable tool for analyzing the problems of immunologically mediated glomerulonephritis, the anti-GBM antibodies rapidly bind to the glomerulus, fix complement, and induce proteinuria. This is the heterologous phase, as in the commonly used model in which rats are injected with rabbit anti-rat GBM antibodies. Proteinuria persists for long periods of time as a result of the host initiating an immune response to the nephrotoxic antibody planted in the glomerulus, which behaves as a glomerulus-planted antigen (the autologous phase) in this example. The subsequent stage classically has been ascribed solely to the host's production of antibody. Although complement may be fixed during the early part of the autologous phase, neutrophils in glomeruli are not a conspicuous feature of this later phase (Unanue and Dixon, 1965). More relevant are the studies utilizing noncomplement-fixing antibodies. Several years ago, Seegal and associates showed that duck anti-rat GBM antibodies injected into rats induced acute nephrotoxic nephritis (Hasson *et al.*, 1957). These antibodies did not fix complement in the glomerulus (Hammer and Dixon, 1963; Hasson *et al.*, 1957), nor did they result in neutrophil infiltration (Cochrane *et al.*, 1965). The conclusion was inescapable that antigen–antibody reactions in the GBM could produce an increase in permeability without the aid of a neutrophil infiltrate. The mechanisms of glomerular injury not involving complement and neutrophils are unknown.

These studies were directed toward whether mononuclear phagocytes could be an important cellular component in immunological injury. Cells resembling macrophages had been described in glomeruli in various experimental models, particularly in NTN (for example, Kondo *et al.*, 1972; Shigematsu, 1976). Prominent "proliferative" component with cells resembling monocytes and macrophages is a conspicuous element of rapidly progressive glomerulonephritis in man.

2. An Accelerated Model of NTN with a Mononuclear Cell Component

2.1. Experimental Design

The experimental model developed is that of an accelerated form of NTN using the rat (Schreiner *et al.*, 1978). Rats are immunized with rabbit IgG in Freund's complete adjuvant and 5 days later are injected intravenously with a subnephritogenic dose of rabbit anti-rat anti-GBM antibody (nephrotoxic antibody, NTAb). Daily 24-hr collection of urine is examined for proteinuria. A representative experiment is shown in Fig. 1. The dose of NTAb by itself is insufficient to cause proteinuria. Rats immunized with adjuvant alone (without rabbit IgG) and then given NTAb do not develop renal disease. The rats immunized with rabbit IgG develop a glomerulonephritis that peaks in intensity from 2 to 4 days after injection of NTAb

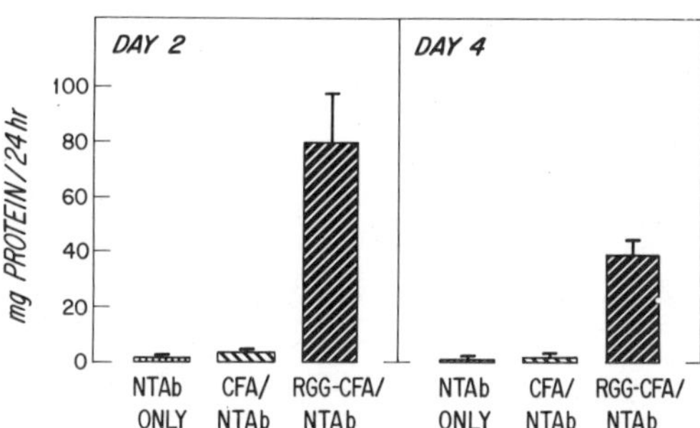

Figure 1. Rats were immunized as indicated with complete Freund's adjuvant (CFA) or with adjuvant containing rabbit IgG (RGG-CFA); some were not immunized at all. Five days after immunization, a subnephritogenic dose of NTAb was given intravenously. (From Unanue and Dixon, 1964.)

and then slowly regresses. In many rats, there is a mild proteinuria during the first 24 hr. This mild proteinuria is accompanied by neutrophil infiltration (by 2 hr after injection) and disappears if the rat is treated with cobra venom factor. Thus, the 24-hr proteinuria is related to the classical complement–neutrophil injury brought about as a summation of the subnephritogenic dose of NTAb with small amounts of rat anti-rabbit IgG. By 5 days after rabbit IgG immunization, most rats have no detectable antibody in serum but do show a very small amount in the glomeruli.

The stage of this accelerated NTN, the focus of these studies, starts at 48 hr. It is characterized by a conspicuous presence of mononuclear cells in the glomerulus. These cells were depicted by ultrastructural analysis in the original paper (Schreiner *et al.*, 1978). Several cell types were observed. The most frequent was a cell with morphological characteristics identical to monocytes. These monocytes were present in the lumen with cytoplasmic extensions that adhered to the GBM or were adherent to the GBM more extensively, displacing endothelial cells. Cells resembling macrophages containing many dense vacuoles also were found well attached to the GBM and on peripheral areas of the capillary loops separated from the mesangium. Finally, a minor cellular component was comprised of cells resembling lymphocytes of various sizes.

The mononuclear cells were most prominent in glomeruli up to 96 hr after NTAb injection and then slowly disappeared. At the time of appearance of the mononuclear phagocytes, frequent mitoses were found in glomerular cells, particularly in the endothelial cells. About four to nine mitoses per 10 glomeruli were found in the nephritic rats in contrast to less than one per 10 glomeruli in control rats.

This accelerated model of NTN permitted analysis of the nature of the mononuclear cells and their possible role in producing an increase in glomerular permeability, as well as examination of the factor(s) leading to their appearance in glomeruli.

2.2. *Effect of X-Irradiation*

One experimental manipulation that was employed was to determine if X-irradiation could help in analysis of the role of the mononuclear infiltrate.

Table 1. Effect of X-Irradiation on Proteinuria[a]

	Experimental manipulations			Proteinuria			Glomerular cell counts
Group[b]	RGG-CFA	X-Ray	NTS	Day 1	Day 2	Day 4	(Day 2)[c]
1	–	–	+	2.4 (± 5.2)	2.5 (± 4.5)	0.5 (± 2.3)	51.6 (± 7.4)
2	+	–	+	14.6 (± 3.3)	20.3 (± 3.2)	28.7 (± 5.5)	74.8 (± 13.8)
3	+	+	+	14.9 (± 3.4)	6.8 (± 3.9)	3.9 (± 4.8)	52.3 (± 5.8)

[a] From Schreiner *et al.* (1978).

[b] Each group consisted of four to six rats, some of which were immunized with 1 mg of rabbit IgG in adjuvant (RGG-CFA) 5 days before injection of 0.8 ml of NTS. Three days after immunization, one group of rats received 800 R of whole-body X-irradiation but with the area of kidney protected by a lead shield. Differences between proteinuria of Groups 2 and 3 vs. 1 on Day 1 and between Group 2 vs. 1 and 3 on Days 2 and 4 all statistically significant ($p < 0.05$ by t test).

[c] Glomerular cell counts were made on two rats sacrificed on Day 2. Counts were made on a 1- to 2-μm methacrylate section. Differences in glomerular cell counts of Group 2 vs. 1 and 3 are also significant ($p < 0.05$).

It was thought most likely that the mononuclear cells were monocytes originating from proliferating bone marrow precursors. If this were the case, it might be possible to eliminate the precursor cells on the basis of their known radiosensitivity. Rats were immunized with rabbit IgG in Freund's adjuvant and 3 days later were irradiated with 900 R of systemic irradiation but with the kidneys protected by a lead cuff. After 2 days, NTAb was injected. Under this protocol, X-irradiation was given after immunization with rabbit IgG. The reasoning behind this was to minimize effects of X-irradiation on the immune response. It was found that the proteinuria during the 48- to 96-hr period and the mononuclear cell infiltrate were abolished. However, the early 24-hr proteinuria related to complement and neutrophils was not affected. To evaluate the extent to which the anti-rabbit IgG response of the rat is affected during the early period following NTAb injection, the amounts of rat IgG found in the glomeruli by immunofluorescence were titrated. X-irradiated rats showed rat IgG in a linear pattern along the GBM as did the control rats not given X-irradiation, albeit in a somewhat lower amount. The significance of mild variations in the fixation of host immunoglobulin was felt to be minimal on the basis of simultaneous experiments described later. These demonstrated that passive administration of host-anti-NTAb to unprimed animals prior to NTAb injection could not mimic the mononuclear hypercellularity. Table 1 shows the results of this experiment. It was concluded that the mononuclear cell infiltrate was radiosensitive and responsible for producing an increase in glomerular permeability.

In the next experiment, the radiosensitive cells were studied by systemic injection of [^{3}H]thymidine and examination of glomeruli by autoradiography. The experimental manipulations and results are shown in Table 2. Group 1 shows that rats immunized with rabbit IgG and given thymidine 4 days later and immediately sacrificed contained very few weakly labeled glomerular cells by autoradiography. Thus, it was apparent that only an occasional glomerular cell was involved in DNA synthesis. If the rats were sacrificed 3 days after thymidine, then one found a definite number of labeled cells (about one to two per glomerulus, Group 2). Such cells were not found if

Table 2. Autoradiographic Studies in Rats with NTN[a,b]

Group	Experimental manipulation				Labeled cells per glomerulus
	Day 0	Day 4	Day 5	Sacrifice	
1	RGG-CFA	[^{3}H]-TdR	—	½ hr after [^{3}H]-TdR	0.20–0.50
2	RGG-CFA	[^{3}H]-TdR	—	Day 7	1.10–2.10
3	RGG-CFA	X-ray + [^{3}H]-TdR	—	Day 7	0.05–0.25
4	RGG-CFA	[^{3}H]-TdR	NTS	Day 7	8.40–11.60
5	RGG-CFA	X-ray + [^{3}H]-TdR	NTS	Day 7	0.05–0.30

[a] From Schreiner *et al.* (1978).

[b] Protocol is described in the text. RGG-CFA refers to the immunization with rabbit IgG in adjuvant. The kidneys were processed for autoradiography and counts made of labeled cells in glomeruli. Figures in last column represent number of labeled cells per glomerulus.

the rats were given systemic irradiation with the kidneys protected by the lead cuff just prior to thymidine administration (Group 3). A possible conclusion is that a small number of mononuclear cells from a rapidly dividing precursor in the marrow do lodge in the glomeruli normally.

Group 4 shows the results of rats immunized with rabbit IgG, injected 4 days later with [^{3}H]thymidine, 5 days later with NTAb, and then sacrificed at Day 7 (i.e., 3 days after thymidine). In this group, most of the increase in cellularity is explained by radiolabeled cells in glomeruli. Rats under the same protocol but given systemic irradiation at the time of [^{3}H]thymidine injection contained no radiolabeled cells (Group 5). The obvious conclusion from these results is that the mononuclear cells in glomeruli are derived from radiosensitive, dividing precursors located outside the kidney. On the basis of the morphological analysis and the autoradiographic studies and from the information that is known with regard to origins and kinetics of mononuclear phagocytes, it is reasonable to conclude that monocytes infiltrate the glomeruli following an immunological insult in response to an as yet unknown stimulus.

2.3. *Pathogenesis of the Mononuclear Infiltrate*

The point under investigation relates to the nature of the process that results in monocyte infiltration of glomeruli. It is possible that monocytes enter the glomerulus in response to: (1) any nonspecific inflammatory damage; (2) an antigen–antibody reaction, possibly complement fixing; (3) a cellular-immunity type of reaction; and (4) combinations of the three. One approach taken is to reduce serum complement levels by injection of cobra venom factor. Rats were immunized with rabbit IgG and then given NTAb 5 days later. Cobra venom factor was administered during the day preceding NTAb injection and at the time of its injection. The results depicted in Table 3 show that the early 24-hr proteinuria, which was quite high in this particular experiment, was abolished in the treated rats. These treated rats had minimal neutrophil infiltration in their glomeruli and no fixation of C3 by immunofluorescence. These same rats exhibited proteinuria by Day 2 to Day 4 after NTAb comparable to that of the controls. Their glomeruli at Days 2 and 4 exhibited hypercellularity without fixation of rat C3. This experiment

Table 3. Effect of Injection of Cobra Venom Factor[a]

Experimental manipulations			Proteinuria		
Day 0	Day 4	Day 5	Day 5	Day 7	Day 8
RGG-CFA	CVF	CVF + NTS	5.9	31	23.5
RGG-CFA	—	NTS	77.9	47	36.7

[a] Each group, made up of eight rats, was preimmunized with rabbit IgG in CFA and given a subnephritogenic amount of NTS 5 days later. One group received cobra venom factor starting 24 hr before NTS. Each rat received a total of 130 μg of cobra venom protein. Treated rats, sacrificed from 24 hr to 4 days, showed no significant amounts of glomerular-bound C3. Glomerular cell mononuclear infiltrate was identical in both groups.

Table 4. Effects of Transferring Rabbit IgG Immune T Cells[a]

Lymph node cells	Kidneys with hypercellularity	% increase in cells	% hypercellular glomeruli	Proteinuria
RGG	8/11	12.4	37 (10/11)	4/11
CFA	0/9	—	9 (5/9)	0/9

[a] On Day 0, Lewis rats received adjuvant with or without rabbit IgG; 5 days later, the rats were sacrificed and lymphocytes harvested from lymph nodes; 10^8 were injected into recipients, intravenously. The next day all rats received a subnephritogenic dose of NTAb. Proteinuria was determined during the first 48 hr after injection, at which time the rats were sacrificed. This table summarizes two experiments.

strongly suggests that the mononuclear infiltration is a complement-independent process unrelated to the early 24-hr lesion.

A different experimental approach is to try to passively transfer the lesion either with antiserum or with immune lymphocytes. The experimental approach was to administer Freund's adjuvant not containing rabbit IgG first and 5 days later administer the subnephrotoxic dose of NTAb. In one set of experiments, a group of rats received various amounts of sera from rats immunized with rabbit IgG. In a second set of experiments, the rats received lymph node cells from the rabbit IgG immune rats.

The administration of rat antibodies to rabbit IgG induced proteinuria during the first 24 hr. This proteinuria, which was comparable to that present in the basic protocol, declined from Day 2 to Day 4 and was accompanied by a variable and mild mononuclear cell infiltrate. The florid mononuclear infiltration caused by administration of antibodies alone was not reproduced.

The results of transfer of lymphocytes are shown in Tables 4 and 5. Out of 11 rats that received 10^8 immune lymph node cells, four developed mild proteinuria. None of nine rats that received lymph node cells from rats given Freund's adjuvant alone showed proteinuria. More striking were the morphological results in that 8 of the 11 rats that received immune lymph node cells had hypercellular glomeruli. The hypercellularity was focal, and

Table 5. Transfer of Rabbit IgG Immune T Cells[a]

RGG				CFA			
Glomerular cells	S.D.	% > 2 S.D.	Proteinuria	Glomerular cells	S.D.	% > 2 S.D.	Proteinuria
74.0	10.7	0	2.5	65.4	7.3	0	1.7
80.0	12.8	12	2.8	70.9	9.9	0	9.2
86.2	14.1	28	37.1	71.2	8.9	0	1.5
87.0	11.0	24	4.4	72.4	9.0	4	3.7
87.5	14.8	32	0.8	78.3	12.2	8	0.6
89.3	13.1	32	57.3	79.6	11.0	4	6.7

[a] In this experiment, two sets of Lewis rats received lymphocytes immune from rats immunized to rabbit IgG (RGG) or adjuvant (CFA) in a protocol identical to that of Table 4. The table shows results of glomerular counts, with standard deviations and percentage of glomeruli with cellular content over 2 S.D.; mean counts of normal glomeruli were 73 cells with S.D. of 10.8. Each count represents one rat.

consisted of mononuclear cells only in some glomeruli. This could be ascertained clearly by doing glomerular cell counts. While the control rats that received Freund's adjuvant immune lymph node cells showed only 9% of their glomeruli with a cell count which was greater than two standard deviations above the mean of control glomerular cell counts, 37% of the glomeruli in the experimental groups showed hypercellularity as defined above. Earlier, McCluskey and associates reported that transfer of T cells in a similar model resulted in transfer of hypercellularity, but no mention was made of proteinuria (Bhan *et al.*, 1978).

This last series of experiments suggests but does not prove that a cellular immune reaction may be one factor responsible for the presence of monocytes in the glomeruli. Further experiments are required to establish this last point firmly.

3. Conclusions

Using the accelerated model of autologous NTN, several important points have been established. It is clearly apparent that mononuclear phagocytes infiltrate the glomerulus and that this infiltration is accompanied by functional derangement of glomerular function. This is the first clear demonstration that a cellular element other than the neutrophil can participate in glomerular injury. Autoradiographic analysis and the experiments involving X-irradiation provided solid evidence about the origin and role of these cells.

The manner by which monocytes induce injury is unknown, but it may be the release of enzymes by a process similar to that believed to take place in the neutrophil-dependent injury. Attention has been directed to the conspicuous proliferation of intrinsic glomerular cells that accompanies the mononuclear infiltrate. Previous studies of delayed hypersensitivity lesions in the skin also had shown a marked proliferation of endothelial cells at the time when large numbers of macrophages infiltrated the skin. It is possible that the cellular proliferation is caused by the release of biologically active molecules from macrophages. A number of these have been identified in culture fluids of monocytes. In another series of studies, it has been shown that macrophages in culture release a molecule that induces neovascularization (Polverini *et al.*, 1977). Angiogenesis was assayed *in vivo* in the guinea pig cornea by implanting the culture fluids near the limbus and observing the growth of new blood vessels.

The stimulus that induces the monocytes to infiltrate glomeruli is not elucidated completely. The possibility that part of the infiltrate may be a cellular response to T-cell stimulation as takes place in classical delayed reactions is of note. Support for this comes from the preliminary cell transfer experiments. The experiments decomplementing rats with cobra venom factor (Table 3) or transferring antibody described above suggest minimal participation of antibody and complement.

References

Bhan, A. K., Schneeberger, E. E., Collins, A. B., and McCluskey, R. T., 1978, Evidence for a pathogenic role of a cell-mediated immune mechanism in experimental glomerulonephritis, *J. Exp. Med.* **148:**246.

Cochrane, C. G., Unanue, E. R., and Dixon, F. J., 1965, A role of polymorphonuclear leukocytes and complement in nephrotoxic nephritis, *J. Exp. Med.* **122:**99.

Dixon, F. J., 1968, The pathogenesis of glomerulonephritis, *Am. J. Med.* **44:**493.

Hammer, D. K., and Dixon, F. J., 1963, Immunologic events in the pathogenesis of nephrotoxic serum nephritis in the rat, *J. Exp. Med.* **117;**1019.

Hasson, M. W., Bevan, M., and Seegal, B. C., 1957, Immediate or delayed nephritis in rats produced by duck anti-rat kidney sera, *Arch. Pathol.* **64:**192.

Kondo, Y., Shigematsu, H., and Kobayashi, Y., 1972, Cellular aspects of rabbit Masugi nephritis, *Lab. Invest.* **27:**620.

Polverini, P. J., Cotran, R. S., Gimbrone, M. A., Jr., and Unanue, E. R., 1977, Activated macrophages induce vascular proliferation, *Nature (London)* **269:**804.

Schreiner, G. F., Cotran, R. S., Pardo, V., and Unanue, E. R., 1978, A mononuclear cell component in experimental immunological glomerulonephritis, *J. Exp. Med.* **147:**369.

Shigematsu, H., 1976, Glomerular events during the initial phase of rat Masugi nephritis, *Virchows Arch. B* **5:**187.

Unanue, E. R., and Dixon, F. J., 1964, Experimental glomerulonephritis. IV. Participation of complement in nephrotoxic nephritis, *J. Exp. Med.* **119:**965.

Unanue, E. R., and Dixon, F. J., 1965, Experimental glomerulonephritis. V. Studies of the interaction of nephrotoxic antibodies with tissues of the rat, *J. Exp. Med.* **121:**697.

Unanue, E. R., and Dixon, F. J., 1967, Experimental glomerulonephritis: Immunologic events and pathogenetic mechanisms, *Adv. Immunol.* **6:**1.

34

Genetic Structure of the HLA Region and Implication for Function

Charles B. Carpenter

A number of human disease processes are strongly associated with certain antigens of the HLA system. Although HLA antigens, expressed on most body tissues, are the "strong" barriers to tissue transplantation, their role outside of the medical artifacts of transplantation and transfusion has not been clearly appreciated. Review of this area requires first an outline of what is known of the genes and gene products of the HLA major histocompatibility complex (MHC), followed by a summary of some of the principal disease relationships and discussion of the potential mechanisms of such associations in relation to the immunobiological role of the MHC.

1. The Major Histocompatibility Complex

In every species studied so far, there exists a group of "strong" transplantation antigens which account for most of the rejection reaction to transplanted tissues. Although weaker antigenic systems may account for some rejections, especially when the graft recipient has been immunized previously with the same antigens, matching for the major antigens minimizes the intensity of immunological rejection. It is now established that a single genetic region, encompassing a number of closely linked genes on a single chromosome (No. 6 in humans), codes for several major histocompatibility antigens. Some of these are identifiable by serological means, and others by their ability to induce a proliferative response by lymphocytes in tissue culture. The human MHC, analogous to H-2 in the mouse and RT1 in the

Charles B. Carpenter · Immunogenetics Laboratory, Renal Division, Department of Medicine, Brigham and Women's Hospital, Boston, Massachusetts 02115.

rat, is called HLA, and consists at present of three serologically defined loci (sometimes abbreviated as SD, old nomenclature) and one locus for the mixed lymphocyte culture (MLR or LD locus, old nomenclature). Serologically detectable antigens closely associated with MLR-stimulating antigens have been defined recently. The number of possible alleles (Table 1) make HLA the most polymorphic genetic system known in man. Phenotypic expression of antigens follows a simple Mendelian codominant pattern. The antigens inherited from a given parent are referred to as a haplotype (Bach and van Rood, 1976; van Rood *et al.*, 1976a; Götze, 1977; Carpenter, 1978a; Kissmeyer-Nielsen, 1975; Bodmer, 1978).

1.1. HLA-A,B,C

HLA serologically defined (SD) antigens usually are detected by alloantibodies reacting with lymphocytes in a lymphocytotoxic (complement-dependent) reaction. Women immunized in the course of pregnancy are the usual sources of typing antisera. These classical HLA antigens are present on the surface of all nucleated cells, and are known to be glycoproteins, each consisting of a heavy and a light chain. The molecules of the three Class I loci (A, B, C) consist of β_2-microglobulin as the light chain, while the heavy chain contains the variable conformation unique to the antigen specificity (Table 2). The products of each locus can move independently in the lipid membrane, as shown by capping studies. Certain structural homologies exist among the heavy chains of the antigens of the three loci. This lends weight to the hypothesis that they represent evolutionary duplications of a more primitive gene. The HLA-A,B,C, antigens alone comprise a highly polymorphic system, whereas a given individual can have but two codominantly expressed antigens for each locus, one from each parental haplotype. A number of racial variations in antigen frequencies are known, and such data are available in the referenced publications. The alleles of the HLA-C locus have not been defined completely as yet.

Table 1. HLA Antigens—(8th International Workshop—1980)

Locus A	A1, 2, 3, 9 (w23, w24)[a], 10(w25, w26), 11, 28, 29, w19, (w30, w31, w32, w33), w34, w36, w43.
Locus B	B5 (w51, w52, w53), 7, 8, 14, 27, w35, 37, 16(w38, w 39), 40(w60, w61), w41, w42, 12(w44, w45), w47, w48, 21, (w49, w50), 22(w54, w55, w56), 17(w57, w58), 15(w62, w63).
Locus C	Cw1, w2, w3, w4, w5, w6, w7, w8
Locus D	Dw1, 2, 3, 4, 5, 6, 7, 8, 9, 10, 11, 12
Locus DR[b]	DR1, 2, 3, 4, 5, w6, 7, w8, w9, w10,

[a] "w" means a provisional workshop designation. Parentheses enclose splits of the originally defined antigen.
[b] HLA-D and DR are well correlated for D/DR 1, 2, 3, 5, 7, 8. DR4 includes both Dw4 and Dw10, while D/DRw6 are poorly correlated. Though bearing the same numbers, DRw9 and DRw10 are not at all related to Dw9 and Dw10. (Dupont et al, 1980).

Table 2. Gene Products of the Major Histocompatibility Complex

	Class I	Class II
Structure	β_2-Microglobulin (11,600 mw) + heavy chain (44,000 mw)	α chain (34,000 mw) + β chain (26,000–29,000 mw)
Tissues	Virtually all cells, excepting human red blood cells	Absent on platelets, T cells, red blood cells
Identification	Serology	Mixed lymphocyte response (MLR) and serology (Ia)
Nomenclature		
Mouse (H-2)	D, K	I (LAD, Ia)
Rat (RT1)	Ag-B (A region)	MLR/Ia (B region)
Human (HLA)	A, B, C	D, DR (Ia)
Function(s)	Targets for effector antibodies and killer cells	Key role in initiation of immune response (Ir genes)

1.2. Mixed Lymphocyte Response: HLA-D

It has been well established that the gene product(s) responsible for stimulation of lymphocytes in the allogeneic mixed lymphocyte culture (MLC) is different from the HLA-A,B,C antigens, and this locus is now established as the HLA-D locus. So far, 11 D locus determinants have been recognized clearly. Table 3 provides population data for the D locus as defined by homozygous (for HLA-D) typing cells.

There are two approaches to definition of HLA-D at this point. The formal definition of D locus determinants is accomplished by use of homozygous typing cells (HTC). The HLA region alleles inherited from one of an individual's parents constitute a *haplotype*. Each individual has two, usually different, HLA haplotypes. If there has been consanguinity in a family background (e.g., first-cousin marriage), it is possible to have an individual homozygous for all HLA antigens. If a capital letter is used to designate an

Table 3. HLA-D Locus Antigen and Gene Frequencies (P) in Caucasians[a]

	Percentage	P
Dw1	19.3	0.102
Dw2	15.2	0.078
Dw3	16.4	0.085
Dw4	15.6	0.082
Dw5	14.6	0.075
Dw6	10.5	0.054
Dw7	18.6	0.098
Dw10	6.9	0.035
	$\sum P$	0.609

[a] Extensive racial population studies have yet to be performed.

HLA haplotype, then such a homozygous individual will be an "A/A." Such cells can respond in mixed lymphocyte response (MLR) to A/B cells, but cannot stimulate them. Individuals who happen to be homozygous for HLA-D, but not HLA-A,B,C, also can be used for HTC. Such HTC when used as stimulating cells against a random population can be used to define the presence or absence of a similar D locus determinant (Dupont *et al.*, 1976). A positive "typing response" occurs when the degree of stimulation is extremely small, indicating that the heterozygote being tested does not respond to the homozygous D locus antigen shared with the typing cell. The second approach to D locus definition is the use of lymphocytes which have been primed *in vitro* by prior exposure to a known D locus incompatibility. When confronted with cells sharing this specificity, they produce an accelerated DNA synthetic response, whereas cells not sharing antigens with the original stimulating cell produce a more slowly evolving primary proliferative response. This primed lymphocyte test (PLT) is currently under intensive evaluation for its value in D locus typing. In addition, PLT reagents have revealed the existence of a second Class II locus, centromeric to DR, called SB (Shaw *et al.*, 1980).

Figure 1 illustrates the inheritance of HLA antigens as haplotypes in families, a matter of simple Mendelian co-dominant expression of all alleles, one set (haplotype) from each parent.

1.3. HLA-DR, The Human "I" Region

Although there is as yet no clear evidence for immune response (Ir) genes in man, analogous to the Ir genes of the H-2 MHC in the mouse, the serologically definable Ia antigens, determined by genes of the I region in the mouse, do have analogies in man (van Rood *et al.*, 1976b; Bodmer, 1978). These antigens are expressed very poorly, if at all, on platelets and peripheral T cells, but are present on peripheral blood B cells and at least some monocytes. A large number of human allo-antisera exist which have such preferential B cell reactivity, and which do not correlate with HLA-A,B,C specificities. In fact, exhaustive absorption of all anti-HLA antibodies with platelets is one approach to producing pure anti-B cell ("Ia") antibodies in man. There is firm evidence that some of these sera recognize a locus or loci closely related to the D region. Hence, they are called "HLA-DR", for "D-related". HLA-DR gene products do not contain a β_2-microglobulin subunit. These "Ia" antigens appear to be topographically related to receptors for the Fc portion of IgG (FcR), whereas HLA-A,B,C determinants are not. These characteristics have been useful in analysis of alloantibodies present in human sera.

1.4. CML Typing

Analysis of the specificities of "killer cells" (cytotoxic lymphocytes) obtained after MLR proliferation shows a close preference of Class I antigens

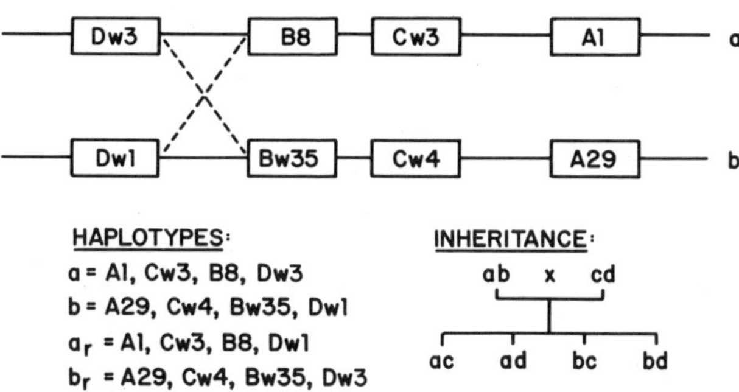

Figure 1. Inheritance of HLA haplotypes. Each chromosomal segment of linked genes is termed a haplotype, and each individual inherits one haplotype from each parent. The A, B, C, D antigens of haplotypes A and B are shown for this hypothetical individual in chromosomal order on the diagram, and also below as they would be written in text. If individual ab were to marry cd, their offspring would be of four types only, as far as HLA is concerned. Occasionally (dotted cross), recombination occurs in the germ line (meiosis) of a parent, resulting in an altered haplotype. The frequency of recombinant children is a measure of the map distance (1% recombination frequency = 1 cM; see Fig. 2). (From Carpenter, 1978b, with permission.)

as targets for cell-mediated lympholysis (CML); however, there are now data which show that the CML targets are closely associated with Class I determinants, but are not identical (Bradley and Festenstein, 1978). Whether Class I and CML determinants are different portions of the same molecule, or are products of different but closely linked genes remains to be established. In population studies, sufficient numbers of discrepancies exist between the two approaches to typing to justify the development of separate definitions for CML antigen systems, defined by the primed cytotoxic cell.

1.5. *Population Studies*

Not only are the individual HLA antigens not distributed randomly in various populations, but there are common associations of alleles in the haplotypes of certain populations. This phenomenon is termed *linkage disequilibrium* because the alleles in question are present in the same haplotype more often than would be predicted by random association. The mathematical expression of this excess, or disequilibrium, is the difference between the observed haplotype frequency and the product of the population frequencies of the two antigens in question. This value is called delta (Δ), and has been calculated for a number of racial populations. The highest Δ value is seen for the A1, B8 haplotype in Caucasoids, and ranges from 0.04 to 0.09.

Among the highest statistically significant Δ values are the following pairs:

Caucasoids	Blacks	Mongoloids
A1, B8	Aw30, B8	A9, B15
A2, B12	A9, B14	A9, B40
A3, B7	B9, B17	A9, Bw35

In addition, linkage disequilibria have recently been appreciated for B12, Cw5; Cw35, Cw4; A10, Cw3; B15, Cw3; Bw22, Cw3; B27, Cw1; and B27, Cw2. Furthermore, the D locus specificities are commonly associated with B locus antigens as follows: Dw1 with Bw35; Dw2 with B7; Dw3 with B8; and Dw4 with B15 and B12.

1.6. Chromosomal Order of Genes (Short Arm of Chromosome 6:6p)

Figure 2 shows the relative positions of the A, B, and C and D HLA loci as defined by a large number of family studies in which intra-HLA recombinations have been documented. B and C are very closely linked with only two well-documented examples of recombinations, whereas the recombination fractions between A–B and B–D are about 0.8 centimorgans (cM); that is, in less than 1% of informative meioses has recombination been documented among these loci. In comparing this arrangement with that of H-2 in the mouse, one can say that A and B are analogous to the D and K loci of H-2 and that the D locus (MLR) is analogous to the lymphocyte activating determinant (LAD_1) in the mouse, with the exception that LAD_1 is mapped between D and K, rather than outside of this region.

Shown also in this schematic diagram are four complement components.

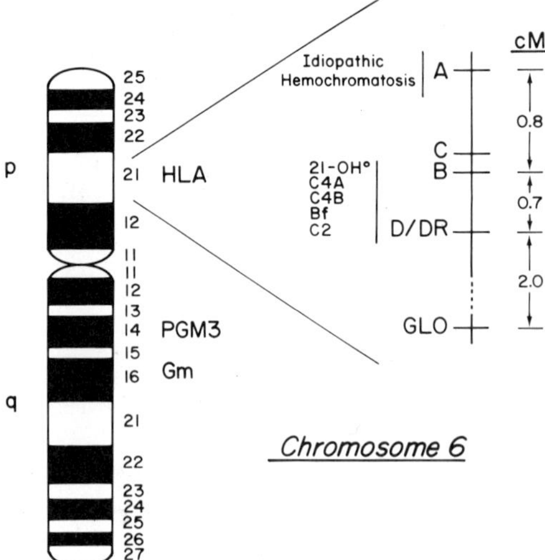

Figure 2. Short arm of human chromosome No. 6. The relative positions of HLA loci are shown. A centimorgan (cM) indicates cross-over frequency. (See text.) (From Carpenter, 1982, with permission.)

It is well established now that a gene for the structural polymorphism of factor B (Bf) of the alternative pathway of complement activation is linked to HLA (Jersild *et al.*, 1976; Carpenter *et al.*, 1977). C2 deficiency, a "blank" gene resulting in absent production of C2 (homozygous), or approximately 50% serum levels of C2 (heterozygous), and structural polymorphism of C2, are very closely mapped to Bf. Since C2 and Bf are structurally and functionally analogous, it is likely that they represent reduplication of a more primitive gene, or that one is the archetype of the other. C4, encoded by 2 loci C4A and C4B, has recently been shown to have polymorphisms linked to HLA, and these markers turn out to be the same as the red blood group antigens, Chido and Rodgers, previously shown to be HLA-linked. C3 is not HLA-linked but the lymphocyte/monocyte *receptor* for activated C3, (C3b/d) is dependent upon a 6th chromosome gene(s) (Curry *et al.*, 1976).

Other markers on chromosome 6 have been mapped in relation to HLA. Phosphoglucomutase-3 (PGM-3) has been assigned to this chromosome by somatic cell hybrid studies. Observations of recombinations within the HLA region have proved the orientation of PGM-3 to the q side of HLA. Glyoxylase-1 (GLO) is clearly linked to chromosome 6, and is centromeric to HLA, and 21-hydroxylase maps between HLA-B and D (Yang *et al.*, 1978).

2. *HLA and Disease*

It should be apparent from the above that the HLA antigen region is not only complex in itself, but there exist other closely linked genes, such as those for some of the complement components. The observed facts of linkage disequilibrium for certain allelic combinations immediately suggest the possibility that closely linked gene clusters may account for a variety of cell interaction phenomena, rather than the observed disease susceptibilities being necessarily related to the function of an HLA antigen per se. In fact, several diseases of unknown etiology have been shown to have varying degrees of association with HLA antigens, with none of them approaching the diagnostically useful 90% frequency of B27 in ankylosing spondylitis (Möller, 1975).

2.1. *Statistical Considerations*

Whenever an association is only partial, it becomes critical to evaluate the following: Controls (ethnicity, age), diagnostic criteria, and conservative correction of "p" value. One should not confuse "association" with "linkage." Linked traits do not necessarily show an HLA association at all; e.g. atopy in a general population shows no HLA antigen association. *Relative risk* (RR) is a convenient expression for comparing studies and population groups:

$$\text{RR} = \frac{(\text{No. patients positive for antigen}) \times (\text{No. controls negative for antigen})}{(\text{No. patients negative for antigen}) \times (\text{No. controls positive for antigen})}$$

2.2. *Ankylosing Spondylitis*

The RR of 87 in Table 4 is for Caucasians, and means that a B27-positive person has 87 times the chance of developing ankylosing spondylitis than one lacking this antigen. The RR for Blacks is considerably less, but is still highly significant. Among Japanese, the antigen B27 is extremely rare, but is present in 77% of ankylosing spondylitis patients. In surveys of B27 positive "healthy" individuals, a frequency as high as 20% of early changes

Table 4. Association between HLA Antigens and Disease (Partial list)

Disease	Antigen	Relative risk
Rheumatic		
Ankylosing spondylitis	B27	87
Reiter's syndrome	B27	37
Acute anterior uveitis	B27	10.3
Psoriatic arthritis, central	B27	10.7
Reactive arthritis (yersinia, salmonella, gonococcus)	B27	18
Rheumatoid arthritis	Dw4	6.1
	DRw4	6.0
Juvenile rheumatoid arthritis, (pauciarticular)	DR5	5.2
Gastrointestinal		
Gluten-sensitive enteropathy	DR3	21
	B8	9.5
Chronic active hepatitis	DR3	6.8
	B8	3.6
Hemochromatosis	A3	8.2
	B14	26.7
	A3, B14	90
Skin		
Dermatitis herpetiformis	Dw3	13.5
Psoriasis vulgaris	Cw6	4.8
Pemphigus	DR4	32
Endocrine		
Juvenile diabetes mellitus	B8	3.3
	B15	3.0
	DR3	2.8
	DR4	5.3
Graves' disease	B8	3.6
	Dw3	3.7
Addison's disease	B8	6.4
	Dw3	10.5
Neurologic		
Myasthenia gravis	B8	4.4
Multiple sclerosis	Dw2	5.0
	DR2	3.9
Renal		
Idiopathic membranous glomerulonephritis	DR3	5.7
Goodpasture's Syndrome (anti-GBM)	DR2	15.9
IgA Nephropathy	DR4	4.1
Minimal change (steroid responsive)	B12	3.5

of ankylosing spondylitis has been reported. Hence, B27-testing has some value in diagnostic evaluation of patients, and correlates extremely well with precise historical data obtained from the patient.

2.3. *Other Arthritides*

These include Reiter's and post-infectious "reactive" arthritis (salmonella, yersinia, and probably gonococcus). RRs are less, and relationship to ankylosing spondylitis unclear, as long-term follow-ups are needed. Juvenile rheumatoid arthritis has only a slight increase in B27 frequency, unless spondylitis is also present. Pauciarticular juvenile rheumatoid arthritis is associated with HLA-DR5. Adult R.A. shows *no* HLA-A,B,C association, but does have a RR of 6.1 for HLA-Dw4.

2.4. *The HLA-B8-DR3 Group (Table 4)*

Juvenile diabetes mellitus (JDM), insulin-dependent, and *not* maturity onset disease, shows an increase in B8, and in some series, B15. DR4 is in linkage disequilibrium with B15. An even greater frequency of Dw3/DR3 in linkage disequilibrium with B8 has been noted. Could the diabetes gene itself be in disequilibrium with Dw3 or Dw4? Current studies are aimed at discovering putative markers which show even higher associations, but also at studies in families in which more than one sibling is affected. Thus far, HLA identical siblings, as well as identical twins, have a less than 50% concordance rate, implicating an additional environmental (?) factor. In contrast, HLA nonidentity results in only 4–7% concordance (25% frequency expected). Hence, juvenile diabetes mellitus appears to be HLA-linked, as well as HLA-associated, but the precise genetics are unknown, and more than one gene may be involved.

Graves' disease illustrates a critical point. The RR of 3.6 for Caucasians with B8 and Dw3 is statistically significant, but what of the Japanese in whom B8 is absent? In this race Graves' disease is associated with a different antigen, Bw35 (RR = 5). In other words, the HLA antigens appear to serve as markers within racial populations for chromosomal regions which carry the true susceptibility genes. Note that this situation contrasts sharply from ankylosing spondylitis in which B27 does maintain an association in Japanese.

Celiac disease (gluten-sensitive enteropathy) has a striking HLA-B8 association (RR = 9.5), as does chronic active hepatitis, but more significant is the DR3 association.

2.5. *Multiple Sclerosis*

Multiple sclerosis is another example of a much closer association with a D locus antigen (Dw2) than a B locus antigen. In this case, a slightly increased frequency of B7 is clearly attributable to linkage disequilibrium of B7 with Dw2, and not to any role for B7 itself.

2.6. *Malignancy*

In general, no striking HLA associations have been discerned. However, a phenomenon of HLA-associated enhanced survival in acute lymphatic leukemia (↑ A2) and in acute myelogenous leukemia (↑ B12) has been reported. Whereas no HLA association exists for breast cancer incidence in the general population, there are data showing an increased frequency of certain HLA-A,B haplotypes in kindreds with multiple cases of breast cancer. Nasopharyngeal carcinoma in Chinese does show a striking increased frequency of a D locus antigen not present in Caucasians.

2.7. *Idiopathic Hemochromatosis*

Idiopathic hemochromatosis shows an increased frequency of both A3 and B14, which in family studies appears to be as the HLA-A3, B14 haplotype. The RR is higher for both A3 and B14, than either alone. There is therefore a strong degree of linkage disequilibrium for the A3, B14 haplotype and the gene(s) related to this defect in iron absorption which is inherited as a recessive trait.

2.8. *Congenital Adrenal Hyperplasia (C.A.H., 21-OH deficiency)*

Recently, analysis of families affected with this autosomal recessive disease shows a clear linkage to the HLA region, with informative recombinant families placing the gene between HLA-B and D.

2.9. *Rheumatic Diseases and C2 Deficiency*

Heterozygous C2 deficiency is present in 1–2% of normal individuals, whereas it is present in 3–5% of patients with SLE or juvenile rheumatoid arthritis (JRA), (but not adult rheumatoid arthritis). Though not striking, this finding shows some disease prediposition when partial C2 deficiency (C2d) is present. Although complement activity per se could be a factor, the striking degree of linkage disequilibrium of *HLA-A10, B18, Dw2, C2d, BfS* indicates that C2d may be a marker for other relevant genes. This cluster of linked genes may be seen in as many as 75% of SLE/JRA families in which C2d is first identified.

2.10. *Renal Disease*

Data for renal disease show associations with anti-GBM (Goodpasture's) (DR2), idiopathic membranous glomerulonephritis (DR3) and some indication of an association of IgA nephropathy with HLA-Bw35 and DR4. HLA-B12 is noticeably increased in minimal change nephrotic syndrome (Table 4).

2.11. Recombination

An increased rate of intra-HLA recombination has been observed in one study of juvenile diabetic families, suggesting that disruption of the phase relationships of alleles within a haplotype may add to the risk of disease manifestation. However, other series have been unconfirmatory, and this hypothesis of HLA-related disease predisposition is without firm support.

2.12. Reflections on the Current Disease Association Data

1. Most clinically definable diseases have shown statistical associations, suggesting an important role for immune response genes in pathogenesis.
2. Large population studies need to be emphasized less than studies in families having more than one affected member in order to establish *linkage* to the HLA chromosome.
3. Clinical usefulness is limited at present, other than in ankylosing spondylitis. Classification of some disease entities may be modified by careful clinical subgrouping along with HLA antigen clusters. There is some indication that Dw2 confers a greater risk for a more fulminant clinical course in multiple sclerosis, for example. Although HLA-B8, Dw3, and Dw4 cluster in juvenile but not maturity onset diabetes, B8-positive patients are not clinically distinguishable from B8-negative patients, with the possible exception of a greater persistence of anti-islet cell antibodies in the former group.

3. Mechanisms

The unprecedented association of a number of apparently different disease processes with cell surface markers coded for by a relatively small gene region, one which is important in at least some aspects of the immune response, has led to the hypothesis that these diseases are dependent upon abnormalities in immune regulation. Precisely how this is expressed is still obscure, and one has some difficulty conjuring up immunological factors in hemachromatosis, and congenital adrenal hyperplasia, for example. Other concepts have been proposed: (1) cell surface structures, coded for by this region, act as receptors for viruses or other environmental agents, or (2) they resemble antigenically the putative pathogen, resulting in a depressed immune response because of tolerance to self. There are no clear examples as yet of these possibilities. The limitations, of course, are in not knowing what pathogen to study in these idiopathic diseases. In this regard, there has been some excitement about epidemiologic evidence for seasonal clustering of new cases of juvenile diabetes mellitus with outbreaks of coxsackie B virus infections. However, these associations are not found uniformly, and the serologic responses of newly discovered diabetics to such viruses are not different from controls.

The recent observations on the association of virus-induced antigens on cell surfaces with H-2D/K antigens, showing that cytolysis of the infected cell by "killer" cells requires compatibility of the histocompatibility antigens of attacking and target cells, indicates that histocompatibility antigens do play some role in body defense against some viruses (Doherty *et al.,* 1976). In other words, killer T cells appear to require a double specificity, one for the foreign antigen, and the other for the relevant MHC-coded self marker. The degree to which self recognition is essential may vary with the virus systems used, but it is at least possible that some disease processes involve alterations in host appreciation of virus–HLA interactions.

Clearly, the possibility of linkage of immune regulatory genes ("Ir") to certain HLA antigens, as previously mentioned, remains of great interest. However, it must be emphasized that there is much more speculation than fact at this point. An example of how this might work comes from the possibility that juvenile diabetes mellitus, Addison's disease, and Graves' disease (all B8-associated) result from an autoimmunity against these endocrine tissues, and that the control system for this is what is HLA-linked.

It has been estimated that there could be several hundred genes yet to be defined in the entire MHC region, and since the sum total of the immune response includes an extraordinary array of humoral and cellular recognition and effector processes, it is likely that workers will be busy for quite some time in this area of immunobiology. Finally, linkage of two apparently nonimmunological diseases, hemochromatosis and congenital adrenal hyperplasia, to HLA shows that some genes may be fortuitously present in the HLA region. Therefore, some of the HLA and disease associations may be shown not to relate to the immune system.

References

Alper, C. A. 1981, Complement and the MHC *in* The role of the major histocompatibility complex in immunobiology. (M. E. Dorf, ed.) pp 173–220, Garland STPM Press, New York.

Bach, F. H., and van Rood, J. J., 1976, The major histocompatibility complex: Genetics and biology, *N. Engl. J. Med.* **295:**806.

Bach, F. H., Bradley, B. A., and Yunis, E. J., 1977, Response of primed LD typing cells to homozygous typing cells, *Scand. J. Immunol.* **6:**277.

Bodmer, W. (ed.), 1978, *Histocompatibility Testing 1977,* Munksgaard, Copenhagen.

Bradley, B. A. and Festenstein, H., 1978, Cellular typing. *Brit. Med. Bull.* **34:**223.

Carpenter, C. B. (ed.), 1978a, *Clinical Histocompatibility Testing 2,* Grune & Stratton, New York.

Carpenter, C. B., 1978b, Transplant rejection in HLA-identical recipients, *Kidney Int.* **14:**283.

Carpenter, C. B., 1982, The major histocompatibility gene complex, in: Harrison's Principles of Internal Medicine, 10th Edition (Petersdorf, R. G., ed.), in press, McGraw-Hill, New York.

Carpenter, C. B., Raum, D., Glass, D., and Schur, P. H., 1977, Ordering of genes for HLA antigens and complement components on the human 6th chromosome, in: *HLA and Malignancy* (E. Cohen, ed.), p. 9, Liss, New York.

Curry, R. A., Dierich, M. P., Pellegrino, M. A., and Hock, J. A., 1976, Evidence for linkage between HLA antigens and receptors for complement components C3b and C3d in human–mouse hybrids, *Immunogenetics* **3:**465.

Doherty, P. C., Götze, D., Trinchieri, G., and Zinkernagel, R. M., 1976, Models for recognition of virally modified cells by immune thymus-derived lymphocytes, *Immunogenetics* **3:**517.

Dupont, B., Hansen, J. A., and Yunis, E. J., 1976, Human mixed lymphocyte culture reaction: Genetics, specificity and biological implications, *Adv. Immunol.* **23:**107.

Dupont, B., Braun, D. W. Yunis, E. J. and Carpenter, C. B. 1980, HLA-D by cellular typing. *in* Histocompatibility Testing 1980, (P. I. Terasaki, ed.). UCLA Press, Los Angeles, pp. 229–267.

Götze, D. (ed.), 1977, *The Major Histocompatibility System on Man and Animals,* Springer-Verlag, Berlin.

Jersild, C., Rubinstein, P., and Day, N. K., 1976, The HLA system and inherited deficiencies of the complement system, *Transplant. Rev.* **32:**43.

Kissmeyer-Nielsen, F. (ed.), 1975, *Histocompatibility Testing 1975*, Munksgaard, Copenhagen.

Möller, G. (ed.), 1975, HLA and Disease, *Transplant Rev.* **22**.

Shaw, S, Pollack, M. S., Payne, S. M., Johnson, A. H., 1980, HLA-linked B cell alloantigens of a new segregant series: population and family studies of the SB antigens. *Human Immunology* **1:**177.

van Rood, J. J., de Vries, R. R. P., and Bradley, B. A., 1981, Genetics and biology of the HLA system, in: *The Role of the Major Histocompatibility Complex in Immunobiology*, (Dorf, M. E., ed.), Garland STPM Presss, New York, p. 59.

van Rood, J. J., Van Leeuwen, A., Termijtelen, A., and Keuning, J. J., 1976b, B cell antibodies, Ia-like determinants in man, *Transplant. Rev.* **30:**122.

Yang, S. Y., Levine, L. S., Zachmann, M., New, M. I., Prader, A., Oberfield, S. E., O'Neill, G. J., Pollack, M. S., and Dupont, D., 1978, Mapping of the 21-hydroxylase deficiency gene within the HLA linkage group, *Transplant. Proc.* **10:**753.

35

Genetic Defects of the Complement Pathways: Relationship to HLA and Disease

Peter H. Schur

1. Introduction

There are known and theoretical defects in the immune response system which might make an individual susceptible to the development of nephritis. Certainly the various deficiencies of immunoglobulins, B and T lymphocytes are well known, and are clinically characterized by recurrent infections. They are not known to be associated with renal diseases, other than perhaps urinary tract infections. Increasing interest has focused lately on inherited, isolated deficiencies of components of the complement system. While first recognized in otherwise normal individuals (reviewed in Jersild *et al.*, 1976; Carpenter *et al.*, 1977; Schur, 1977, 1978; Agnello, 1978), there have recently been numerous reports of their association with disease.

2. Association between Complement Deficiencies and Disease

The associations between complement deficiencies and diseases, including renal diseases, are summarized in Table 1 (references for these can be found in the review articles cited above). Low levels of Clq have frequently been noted in patients with combined immunodeficiency and probably represents decreased Clq synthesis in response to low IgG levels. Two families

---

Peter H. Schur · Divison of Rheumatology and Immunology, Brigham and Women's Hospital, Harvard Medical School, Boston, Massachusetts 02115. This work was supported by NIH Grants AM 11414, AM 05577, AI 00366, AM 07031, RR 05669, The New England Peabody Foundation, and The Gebbie Foundation.

Table 1. *Hereditary Complement Deficiencies in Man—Clinical Associations*

Component	No. of cases	Clinical features	Renal disease
Clq	Many	Combined immunodeficiency	—
Clr	1	LE	Focal glomerulonephritis
	1	Infections and arthritis (sibling)	None
	1		Chronic glomerulonephritis
Cls	3	LE	None
	2	Normal	None
C4	2	LE	Glomerulonephritis (both)
	1	Normal	—
C2	Many	Normal	—
	29	LE	—
	7	LE	Nephritis
	11	JRA	—
	10	Intrinsic asthma	—
	4	Vasculitis, purpura	Nephritis (2)
	2		Membranoproliferative glomerulonephritis
	1	Hypertension with nephritis	
	5	Infections	
	2	Rheumatoid arthritis	
	1	Osteoarthritis	
	1	Dermatomyositis	
	1	Hodgkins	
	1	CLL, dermatitis herpetiformis	
	1	Multiple sclerosis	
	1	Hypogammaglobulinemia	
C3	5	Infections	
C5	1	LE	Nephritis
	1	Recurrent infections	
C6	3	Infections	
	1	Normal	
C7	4	Normal	
	2	Infections	
	1	Raynauds	
	1	Ankylosing spondylitis	
C8	1	Gonorrhea	
	1	Xeroderma pigmentosum	
	1	LE	Nephritis
C1 1NH	Many	Hereditary angioedema	
	6	Angioedema and LE	Nephritis (1)
C3b inactivator	2	Infections	

with inherited Clr deficiency have been described. In one family, one individual has lupus erythematosus (LE); although renal function was normal, a renal biopsy showed focal glomerulonephritis. A sibling with Clr deficiency has arthritis and repeated infections. In another family with Clr deficiency, the propositus had chronic glomerulonephritis with hematuria, proteinuria, and hypertension. The first individual described with Cls deficiency had LE without clinical nephritis. Another family with four siblings with Cls deficiency has been described. Two had lupus, two were normal. Three unrelated individuals with C4 deficiency have been described. One is otherwise normal. The other two have LE, and both have nephritis.

By far the most common form of complement component deficiency is that of C2, being found in approximately 1 in 10,000 individuals in the general population (Stratton, 1974). After the initial description of this inherited C2 deficiency (C2d) in otherwise normal individuals, there have been numerous reports of the association between C2d and immune disorders. Prominent in this association have been LE, renal disease, and vasculitis (see Table 1). Of the 29 patients with LE and C2d (on whom there is adequate information available), seven were found to have renal disease (Wild *et al.*, 1976; Osterland *et al.*, 1975; Day *et al.*, 1973, 1975; Pickering *et al.*, 1971; Roberts *et al.*, 1978; Glass *et al.*, 1976; Schur, 1978; Angello, 1978; R. I. Rynes, personal communication; K. Fraser and S. Ruddy, personal communication). Of the four patients with vasculitis and/or purpura, two had the nephritis of Henoch–Schönlein purpura (Gelfand *et al.*, 1975; Einstein *et al.*, 1975). Two patients have been noted to have C2d and membranoproliferative glomerulonephritis (Friend *et al.*, 1975; Jersild *et al.*, 1976; Kim *et al.*, 1977). Additional associations with C2d have been made, but the number of cases reported have been small (see Table 1).

Regarding the terminal complement sequence, C3–9, few immune or renal defects have been noted, but repeated infections have been noted in patients with deficiencies of either C3, C5, C6, C7, C8, and C3b inactivator (see Table 1). Of the LE cases associated with C5 and C8 deficiencies, both had renal disease. Of the five cases of LE associated with C1 inhibitor deficiency and hereditary angioedema, one had renal disease (Kohler *et al.*, 1976).

Another type of complement abnormality associated with renal disease is found in patients with partial lipodystrophy and mesangiocapillary glomerulonephritis. In some of these patients, C3 deficiency may antedate the development of overt nephritis (Sissons *et al.*, 1976). This deficiency reflects activation by C3 nephritic factor, an immunoglobulin. These data suggest that the nephritis may develop in part because of this complement abnormality, rather than being a consequence of complement activation.

3. Role of Inherited Complement Deficiencies in Disease

An important factor in considering the possible role of inherited complement deficiencies in these immune disorders is to determine whether these are simply chance associations. After all, serum complement levels frequently are measured in patients with these disorders because of their known high frequency of acquired complement disorders. As noted, however, these deficiencies may occur in normal individuals. The best epidemiological data available are those regarding C2d. Homozygous C2d exists in about 1 in 10,000 (Stratton, 1974) and heterozygous C2d in about 1 in 100 individuals

(Glass *et al.*, 1976). Therefore, the finding of heterozygous C2d in nearly 6% of LE patients (Glass *et al.*, 1976) and in addition that 37% of homozygous C2d individuals in 38 kindreds suffered from LE (Agnello, 1978) suggests that this is more than just a chance association ($p < 0.001$ for heterozygous C2d). These C2d LE patients appear to be similar to other LE patients in all respects except that they tend to have a paucity of antinuclear antibodies. These may represent an (Ir gene related) immune defect. Furthermore, renal disease is uncommon in the homozygous C2d LE patient, but can be exacerbated severely by transfusion (Roberts *et al.*, 1978). Such epidemiological or gene frequency studies have not been done regarding other complement components, but present data suggest that these deficiencies are far rarer. The increasing availability of assays for total hemolytic complement in serum (CH_{50}) will undoubtedly result in the detection of more such cases when one finds a zero CH_{50} level and then determines which component is missing.

What is the clinical role of these inherited complement component deficiencies? The association of deficiency of either C3, C5, C6, C7, C8, or C3b inactivator with repeated infections is perhaps easy to understand in view of the importance of these complement components in chemotaxis and phagocytosis, thus participating in the normal immune clearance of bacteria. The mechanism of the association between the inherited complement component deficiency, particularly of the early complement components, and immune or hypersensitivity diseases is not as clear. These components, including C4 and C2, do play a role in the immune clearance of complexes (Mannik *et al.*, 1971) and in viral neutralization (Daniels *et al.*, 1969). However, not all individuals with C4d and C2d appear to be afflicted by recurrent infections. Furthermore, the association of immune disease with heterozygous C2d, where there is adequate complement to participate in the usual complement-dependent reactions, suggests that the C2d represents primarily a genetic rather than a biological marker, and that the association between C2d and LE is due to some other factor(s). The association between C4d and C2d and HLA (reviewed in Jersild *et al.*, 1976; Carpenter *et al.*, 1977; Schur, 1977, 1978) provides a clue to another possible interrelationship. There is now ample evidence from these and other observations of the strong linkage disequilibrium between the loci for C2d and the HLA haplotype A10 B18 (Jersild *et al.*, 1976; Carpenter *et al.*, 1977; Schur, 1977, 1978) (Fig. 1). In some families, the association has been with another haplotype, but often

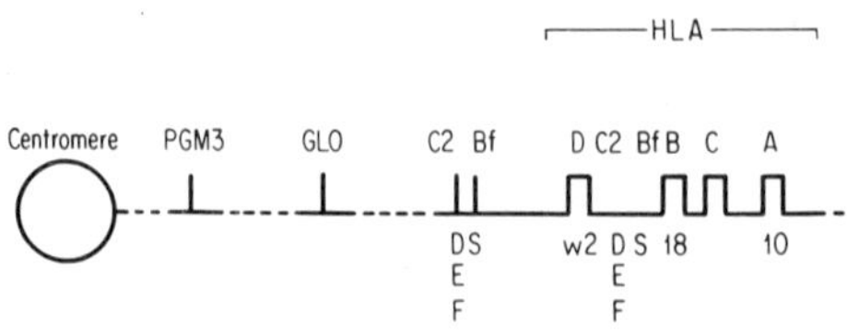

Figure 1. An area of the short arm of the sixth chromosome in C2d individuals indicating that most such individuals are HLA-A10, HLA-B18, HLA-Dw2, and properdin factor B allotype "S." GLO is glyoxalase; PGM3 is phosphoglucomutase-3—both are controlled by genes on this chromosome.

including either A10 or B18 in the haplotype. These differences are probably the result of crossovers (Gibson *et al.*, 1976; Glass *et al.*, 1976; Raum *et al.*, 1976). In addition, C2d is in strong linkage disequilibrium with HLA-Dw2 (Fu *et al.*, 1975a,b; Friend *et al.*, 1975; Hauptmann *et al.*, 1977; Jersild *et al.*, 1976; Opelz and Glovsky, 1976; Day *et al.*, 1976), and another sixth chromosomal marker, Bf-S (the properdin factor B allotype) (Glass *et al.*, 1976; Raum *et al.*, 1976; Hauptmann *et al.*, 1977; Day *et al.*, 1976; Schur, 1978) (Fig. 1). Therefore, C2d appears to be part of a "super-gene" complex (linkage group).

C4d appears to be linked to varying haplotypes, in one family with A2, Bw40 (Rittner *et al.*, 1975); in another with A2, B12; and in the third with A2, B15 (Ochs *et al.*, 1976). There are little if any firm data on associations between other complement component deficiencies or allotypes and HLA (Jersild *et al.*, 1976).

4. *Summary*

Since there is increasing evidence that Ir genes may be closely linked to those of HLA (see Table 2), the HLA-linked complement deficiencies also may be linked to Ir genes which may express themselves as immunologically mediated disease. In a sense, then, C2d may be only a marker gene for a subset of patients with LE, although C2d may in itself magnify clinical expression of disease. Observations have been made in other rheumatic diseases where for instance a number of different microorganisms can trigger spondyloarthritis in the genetically susceptible HLA-B27 individual. If one then proposes that SLE or lupus-like disease is triggered by an abnormal immune response to exogenous factors, such as various viral infections, altering the balance between B- and T-cell function, then patients with inherited deficiencies of C2 may be particularly susceptible to such an infection leading either to SLE or active disease (with depletion of other components). The meaning of the relationship between inherited complement defects, disease, HLA genes, susceptibility to infection, and Ir genes

Table 2. Ir Genes in Man Linked to HLA

Associations
Ragweed IgE Ab—segregate with HLA within families
Low Ab response to live influenza vaccine—B16
Ab to measles—A3
In vitro response to strep Ag—Bw35
Ab to gluten—B8
In vitro response to trichophyton—B8
No associations
DTH: *Candida*, mumps, TB
Ab: polio, diphtheria toxoid, rubella, influenza (killed)

and immune regulation is not yet understood fully. Further study should lead to a better understanding of the role of the HLA region in immunity and of the mechanism whereby environmental factors can affect genetically susceptible individuals.

ACKNOWLEDGMENTS. Dr. Glass' contribution to these studies is greatly appreciated.

References

Agnello, V., 1978, Complement dificiency states, *Medicine* **57:**1.

Carpenter, C. B., Raum, D., Glass, D., and Schur, P. H., 1977, Ordering of genes for HLA antigens and complement components on the human sixth chromosome, in: *HLA and Malignancy* (G. P. Murphy, ed.), pp. 9–20, Liss, New York.

Daniels, C. A., Borsos, T., Rapp, H. J., Synderman, R., and Notkins, A. L., 1969, Neutralization of sensitized virus by purified components of complement, *Proc. Natl. Acad. Sci. USA* **65:**528.

Day, N. K., Geiger, H., McLean, R., Michael, A., and Good, R. A., 1973, C2 deficiency: Development of lupus erythematosus, *J. Clin. Invest.* **52:**1601.

Day, N. K., L'Esperance, P. L. L., Good, R. A., Michael, A. F., Hansen, J. A., Dupont, B., and Jersild, C., 1975, Hereditary C2 deficiency: Genetic studies and association with the HL-A system, *J. Exp. Med.* **141:**1464.

Day, N. K., Rubinstein, P., Case, D., Hansen, J. A., Good, R. A., Walker, M. E., Tulchin, N., Dupont, B., and Jersild, C., 1976, Linkage of gene for C2 deficiency and the major histocompatibility complex (MHC) in man: Family study of a further case, *Vox Sang.* **31:**96.

Einstein, L. P., Alper, C. A., Bloch, K. J., Herrin, J. T., Rosen, F. S., David, J. R., and Colten, H. R., 1975, Biosynthetic defect in monocytes from human beings with genetic deficiency of the second component of complement, *N. Engl. J. Med.* **292:**1169.

Friend, P. S., Handwerger, B. S., Kim, Y., Michael, A. F., and Yunis, E. J., 1975, C2 deficiency in man, genetic relationship to a mixed lymphocyte reaction determinant (7a*), *Immunogenetics* **2:**569.

Fu, S. M., Stern, R., Kunkel, H. G., Dupont, B., Hansen, J. A., Day, N. K., Good, R. A., Jersild, C., and Fotino, M., 1975a, LD-7a association with C2 deficiency in five of six families, in: *Histocompatibility Testing* (F. Kissmeyer-Nielsen, ed.), pp. 933–936, Munksgaard, Copenhagen.

Fu, S. M., Stern, R., Kunkel, H. G., Dupont, B., Hansen, J. A., Day, N. K., Good, R. A., Jersild, C., and Fotino, M., 1975b, Mixed lymphocyte culture determinants and C2 deficiency in four families, *J. Exp. Med.* **142:**495.

Gelfand, E. W., Clarkson, J. E., and Minta, J. O., 1975, Selective deficiency of the second component of complement in a patient with anaphylactoid purpura, *Clin. Immunol. Immunopathol.* **4:**269.

Gibson, D. J., Glass, D., Carpenter, C. B., and Schur, P. H., 1976, Hereditary C2 deficiency: Diagnosis and HLA gene complex associations, *J. Immunol.* **116:**1065.

Glass, D., Raum, D., Gibson, D., Stillman, J. S., and Schur, P. H., 1976, Inherited deficiency of the second component of complement: Rheumatic disease associations, *J. Clin. Invest.* **58:**853.

Hauptmann, G., Tongio, M. M., Gross-Wilde, H., and Mayer, S., 1977, Linkage between C2 deficiency and the HLA-A10, B18, Dw2/Bf S haplotype in a French family, *Immunogenetics* **4:**447.

Jersild, C., Rubinstein, P., and Day, N. K., 1976, The HLA system and inherited deficiencies of the complement system, *Transplant. Rev.* **32:**43.

Kim, Y., Friend, P. S., Dresner, I. G., Yunis, E. J., and Michael, A. F., 1977, Inherited deficiency of the second component of complement (C2) with membranoproliferative glomerulonephritis, *Am. J. Med.* **62:**765.

Kohler, P. F., Percy, J., Campion, W. M., and Smyth, C., 1976, Hereditary angioedema and 'familial' lupus erythematosus in identical twin boys, *Am. J. Med.* **56:**406.

Mannik, M., Arond, W. P., Hall, A. P., and Gilliland, B. C., 1971, Studies on antigen–antibody complexes. I. Elimination of soluble complexes from rabbit circulation, *J. Exp. Med.* **133:**713.

Ochs, H., Rosenfield, S. I., Thomas, E. D., Giblet, E. R., Alper, C. A., Dupont, B., Schaller, J. G., Gilliland, B. C., Hansen, J. A., and Wedgewood, R. J., 1977, Linkage between the gene or genes controlling synthesis of the fourth component of complement and the major histocompatibility complex, *N. Engl. J. Med.* **296:**470.

Opelz, G., and Glovsky, M. M., 1976, HLA antigen studies in a family with C2 deficiency, *J. Immunogenet.* **3:**303.

Osterland, C. K., Espinoza, L., Parker, L. P., and Schur, P. H., 1975, Inherited C2 deficiency and systemic lupus erythematosus: Studies on a family, *Ann. Intern. Med.* **82:**323.

Pickering, R. J., Michael, A. F., Herdman, R. C., Good, R. A., and Gewurz, H., 1971, The complement system in chronic glomerulonephritis in three newly associated aberrations, *J. Pediatr.* **78:**30.

Raum, D., Glass, D., Carpenter, C. B., Alper, C. A., and Schur, P. H., 1976, The chromosomal order of genes controlling the major histocompatibility complex, properdin factor B, and deficiency of the second component of complement, *J. Clin. Invest.* **58:**1240.

Rittner, C., Hauptmann, G., Gross-Wilde, H., Grosshans, E., Tongio, M. M., and Mayer, S., 1975, Linkage between HLA (major histocompatibility complex) and genes controlling the synthesis of the fourth component of complement, in: *Histocompatibility Testing* (F. Kissmeyer-Nielsen, ed.), pp. 945–953, Munksgaard, Copenhagen.

Roberts, J. L., Schwartz, M. M., and Lewis, E. J., 1978, Hereditary C2 deficiency and systemic lupus erythematosus associated with severe glomerulonephritis, *Clin. Exp. Immunol.* **31:**328.

Schur, P. H., 1977, Complement testing in the diagnosis of immune and autoimmune diseases, *Am. J. Clin. Pathol.* **68:**647.

Schur, P. H., 1978, Genetics of complement deficiencies associated with lupus-like syndromes, *Arthritis Rheum.* **21:**5153.

Sissons, J. G. P., West, R. J., Fallow, J., Williams, D. G., Boucher, B. J., Amos, N., and Peters, D. K., 1976, The complement abnormalities of lipodystrophy, *N. Engl. J. Med.* **294:**461.

Stratton, F., 1974, cited by Lachmann, P. J., Genetic deficiencies of the complement system, *Boll. Ist. Sieroter. Milan.* **53**(Suppl. I)**:**195.

Wild, J. H., Zvaifler, N. J., Mauuller-Eberhard, H. J., and Wilson, C. B., 1976, C3 metabolism in a patient with deficiency of the second component of complement (C2) and discoid lupus erythematosus, *Clin. Exp. Immunol.* **24:**238.

36

Complement Abnormalities in Allergy and the Nephrotic Syndrome

J. F. Soothill

1. Introduction

The role of antigen-nonspecific defective antigen handling (immunodeficiency) in immunopathology arising from contact with foreign antigens, is an ongoing study in the author's laboratory (Soothill, 1976). It has been shown that genetic (immunodeficiency and other) and environmental factors predispose to atopy. Following the demonstration that steriod-responsive nephrotic syndrome may be provoked by allergen contact (Hardwicke *et al.*, 1959), it was found that these factors may predispose to this syndrome in many patients and for IgA deposit disease (Berger *et al.*, 1971). This work on atopy must be summarized if this extrapolation is to be understood.

2. Atopy, Complement, and Glomerular Disease

Atopy is a familial, antigen-nonspecific predisposition to react with an immediate (IgE) response to common inhalant and food antigens. It is associated with many syndromes (e.g., eczema and asthma, hay fever, etc.) which may be expressed differently in members of the same family. Concordance is not perfect in indentical twins. The influence of season and place of birth on the prevalence of disease suggests that neonatal environmental factors are important also.

Atopy is associated significantly, although only occasionally, with sustained IgA deficiency (Kaufman and Hobbs, 1970). The implication of this finding was emphasized by the demonstration that transient IgA deficiency commonly precedes the development of much childhood atopy (Taylor *et*

J. F. Soothill · Institute for Child Health, London WC1N 1EH, England.

al., 1973). This supports the view that adverse neonatal contact with antigen in the vulnerable individual is important in sustained sensitization. The similarity of syndromes of infection in children with defects of either antibody, complement, or phagocytes suggests that these mechanisms act as a chain. Similarly, defects (homozygote or heterozygote) of C2 deficiency (Turner *et al.*, 1978), neutrophil mobility (Hill and Quie, 1974), and yeast opsonization (Turner *et al.*, 1978) as well as cystic fibrosis (Warner *et al.*, 1976) are associated with atopy. All of these mutant genes except that of the neutrophil mobility defect are common (> 1% of the population), and, along with transient IgA deficiency, probably account for the majority of atopy (Turner *et al.*, 1978).

Yeast opsonization is considered to be a function of the alternative pathway of complement by Soothill and Harvey (1977). Complement component concentrations may be low, not only because they are potential primary deficiency causes of a disease, but also because they may be consumed as a result of it; also they may rise as acute–phase reacting proteins. If a number of different defects are capable of predisposing to the same disease, the postulated distribution concentrations of each potentially defective substance in the disease is bizarre: there will be too many patients with abnormally low levels and too many with abnormally high levels even though the mean might be the same as the control mean, as was observed with IgA in atopics by Kaufman and Hobbs (1970). If all the low values of complement components were secondary to consumption, the different components would be expected to be down together. However, in atopics, Soothill and colleagues found that low-levels of C2 and low yeast opsonization were virtually mutually exclusive which strongly suggested that the defects were primary.

The recognition that steroid-responsive relapsing nephrotic syndrome (SRRNS) may result from antigen contact in an atopic (Hardwicke *et al.*, 1959), established that this disease can have an immunopathogenetic cause. The mechanism of renal damage remains unknown, but the unique form of noncomplement-fixing IgG-containing antigen–antibody complex detected in their blood (Levinsky *et al.*, 1978) may play a part. A systematic study of atopy and of tissue type in SRRNS has shown that there was a small increase of prevalence of atopy and of tissue type HLA B12, but these two features were related. This study suggested that an atopic patient with HLA B12 has a considerably greater chance of developing this disease (Thompson and Soothill, 1970). This suggests the possibility of an immunodeficiency basis. Of the defects associated with atopy, described above, only the yeast opsonization defect and C2 can be studied at the time of the overt illness.

In a second series of patients with SRRNS (Trompeter *et al.*, 1980), the excess of HLA B12 was confirmed. The yeast opsonization was defective in 1 in 6 of the patients studied in remission, off all treatment. This is significantly more common than the 1 in 20 of the population, but neither it nor the HLA B12 was closely linked to atopy in this series. Therefore, it seems that this defect can predispose to the presumed common pathway of immunopathological injury, either in association with its atopy effects, or independently of them. The concept of continued vulnerability to environmental triggers, which could include allergens, due to continuing abnormal immunological responsiveness, led to the demonstration that cyclophosphamide, given during steroid-maintained remission, prevented relapse on steroid withdrawal (Barratt and Soothill, 1975). It is interesting that SRRNS patients with HLA B12 are significantly more liable to relapse following cyclophosphamide than those without HLA B12 (Trompeter *et al.*, 1980). This fact could be useful in assessing indications for such treatment and is perhaps the first useful therapeutic deduction from tissue typing other than for grafts.

The mechanism of the defective yeast opsonization is still uncertain. All known complement components are present and functional. Miller and Nilsson (1970) suggested that C5 was functionally defective. It has been shown that inulin or *E. coli* endotoxin activation of complement may be defective in these sera, suggesting that the alternative pathway may be defective (Soothill and Harvey, 1977). It is likely that there is more than one defect, since there are three peaks on the distribution curve of yeast opsonization in atopics of which two are low, but only one (the lowest) is associated with tissue type HLA Bw35 (Turner *et al.*, 1977). This form was not observed in Soothill's small series of SRRNS. In the families studied thus far, it appears that these defects may be inherited by an unusual form of dominant inheritance (Soothill and Harvey, 1977).

In the recurrent hematuria syndrome of childhood, IgA is deposited in the glomeruli (Berger *et al.*, 1971). IgA deposits also occur, with IgG, in Henoch–Schönlein purpura nephritis. Levinsky and Soothill (1978) have shown that IgA-containing antigen–antibody complexes are detected in the serum in most patients with the latter disease, but those with nephritis have IgG complexes too. It has been suggested that chronic soluble complex disease results from defective clearance of the complexes from the blood (Soothill and Steward, 1971). It is likely that diseases associated with circulation of complexes of different types will be caused by different defects of clearance. Studies with the MOPC 315 mouse myeloma protein suggest that IgA complexes are cleared quickly from the blood (Stokes *et al.*, 1980). Presumably, the alternative pathway of complement is involved. Therefore, yeast opsonization was measured in patients with recurrent hematuria syndrome but was found to be normal. Measurement of complement fixation by inulin or by *E. coli* endotoxin, using a simple complement fixation titration method, gave low values in patients with recurrent hematuria syndrome, and intermediate values in their parents (obligate heterozygotes), which is suggestive of yet another defect of the alternative pathway of complement that is apparently inherited as an autosomal recessive.

3. Conclusion

These studies support the general view that many immunopathologic diseases result from defective antigen clearance, and that different defects of the antibody–complement–phagocyte pathway (which achieves this clearance) often cause different diseases. However, each one also may cause the same set of diseases, the specific diseases being determined by an interacting mechanism such as tissue type. The wide role of complement defects in immunopathology is reviewed by Schur in this volume. The role of defects of phagocytes is confined to the lupus (ANF negative as in complement deficiencies) of heterozygotes for chronic granulomatous disease (Thompson and Soothill, 1970) and the atopic diseases with defective neutrophil mobility (Hill and Quie, 1974).

The immunodeficiency hypothesis for immunopathology gives rise to the possibility of positive treatment (active or passive immunization) rather than of immunosuppression. The latter has been achieved in renal disease only in SRRNS with allergy to grass pollens (Hardwicke *et al.*, 1959) and possibly with plasma exchange. The concept that genetically vulnerable persons are at special risk in the neonatal period and the demonstration that neonatal environmental factors, especially infant feeding, influence subsequent development of eczema (Matthew *et al.*, 1977) permits optimism that, in some renal disease, too, neonatal environmental factors contributing to disease in the genetically vulnerable, may be susceptible to modification, and, so, to disease prevention.

ACKNOWLEDGMENT. I am very grateful to my colleagues whose work I have referred to for this collaborative program of team work.

Reference

Barratt, T. M., and Soothill, J. F., 1970, Controlled trial of cyclophosphamide treatment in steroid sensitive relapsing nephrotic syndrome of childhood, *Lancet* **2:**479.

Berger, J. G., Yaneva, I. H., and Hinglais, N., 1971, Immunohistochemistry of glomerulonephritis, *Adv. Nephrol.* **1:**11.

Hardwicke, J., Soothill, J. F., Squire, J. R., and Holti, G., 1959, The nephrotic syndrome with pollen hypersensitivity, *Lancet* **1:**500.

Hill, H. R., and Quie, P. G., 1974, Raised serum IgE levels and defective neutrophil chemotaxis in three children with eczema and recurrent bacterial infections, *Lancet* **1:**183.

Kaufman, H. S., and Hobbs, J. R., 1970, Immunoglobulin deficiencies in an atopic population, *Lancet* **2:**1061.

Levinsky, R. J., and Soothill, J. F., 1978, The heterogeneity of immune complexes in disease, in: *Protides of the Biological Fluids*, 26th Colloquium (H. U. B. Peeters, ed.), Pergamon Press, Elmsford, N. Y.

Levinsky, R. J., Malleson, P. N., Barratt, T. M., and Soothill, J. F., 1978, Circulating immune complexes in steroid responsive nephrotic syndrome, *N. Engl. J. Med.* **298:**126.

Matthew, D. J., Taylor, B., Norman, A. P., Turner, M. W., and Soothill, J. F., 1977, Prevention of eczema, *Lancet* **1:**321.

Miller, M. E., and Nilsson, V. R., 1970, A familial deficiency of the phagocytosis-enhancing activity of serum related to a dysfunction of the fifth component of complement (C5), *N. Engl. J. Med.* **282:**354.

Soothill, J. F., 1976, Some intrinsic and extensive factors predisposing to allergy, *Proc. R. Soc. Med.* **69:**439.

Soothill, J. F., and Harvey, B. A. M., 1977, A defect of the alternative pathway of complement, *Clin. Exp. Immunol.* **27**:30.

Soothill, J. F., and Steward, M. W., 1971, The immunopathological significance of the heterogeneity of antibody affinity, *Clin. Exp. Immunol.* **9**:193.

Stokes, C. R., Swarbrick, E., and Soothill, J. F., 1980, Immune elimination and enhanced antibody responses: functions of circulating IgA, *Immunology* **40**:455.

Taylor, B., Norman, A. P., Orgel, H. A., Stokes, C. R., Turner M. W., and Soothill, J. F., 1973, Transient IgA deficiency and the pathogenesis of infantile atopy, *Lancet* **2**:111.

Thompson, E. M., and Soothill, J. F., 1970, Chronic granulomatous disease—Quantitative clinicopathological relationships, *Arch. Dis. Child.* **45**:24.

Thomson, P. D., Barratt, T. M., Stokes, C. R., Turner, M. W., and Soothill, J. F. 1976, HLA antigens and atopic features in steroid responsive nephrotic syndrome of childhood, *Lancet* **2**:765.

Trompeter, R. S., Barratt, T. M., Kay, R., Turner, M. W., and Soothill, J. F., 1980, HLA, Atopy and cyclophosphamide in steroid-responsive childhood nephrotic syndrome, *Kidney Int.* **17**:113.

Turner, M. W., Brostoff, J., Wells, R. S., Stokes, C. R., and Soothill, J. F., 1977, HLA in eczema and hay fever, *Clin. Exp. Immunol.* **27**:43.

Turner, M. W., Mowbray, J. F., Harvey, B. A. M., Brostoff, J., Wells, R. S., and Soothill, J. F., 1978, Defective yeast opsonization and C2 deficiency in atopic patients, *Clin. Exp. Immunol.* **34**:253.

Warner, J. O., Norman, A. P., and Soothill, J. F., 1976, Cystic fibrosis heterozygosity in the pathogenesis of allergy, *Lancet* **1**:990.

37

Immunogenetic Aspects of Glomerulonephritis

Peter S. Friend

1. Development of Immune Complex Glomerulonephritis

Experimental and correlative human studies have shown that the development of immune complex glomerulonephritis is a consequence of: (1) the immune or antibody response to exogenous and certain host antigens; (2) the localization of the complexes so formed in glomeruli and vessels by a mechanism which has not been defined in humans; (3) the participation of effector mechanisms and of mediators of the inflammatory response, which are in part related to the complement system; and (4) injury to the glomerular capillary filter.

2. Immune Responsiveness in the Mouse

Immune responsiveness in the mouse and other experimental animals is under genetic control. Specificity is conferred at the level of antigen recognition by immune response genes (Benacerraf and McDevitt, 1972). Irrespective of the specificity of antibody produced in a given responder, a group of genes may regulate the general level of antibody synthesis. Mice selectively bred for quantitative differences in the level of antibody response to heterologous erythrocytes (Biozzi *et al.*, 1972) will exhibit the same discrepant responsiveness when challenged with a variety of other unrelated complex immunogens. No significant differences in antibody affinity are observed in high and low lines of antibody-producing mice (Katz and Steward,

---

Peter S. Friend · Balboa Internal Medicine Group, 306 Walnut Avenue, Suite 38, San Diego, California 92102. The author is a recipient of a Clinical Investigator Award (1 K08 AM 00445 01) from the NIAMDD.

1976), demonstrating that antibody affinity and antibody levels are under independent genetic control. The demonstration of differential susceptibility to viral oncogenesis (Lilly *et al.*, 1964) which mapped toward the K end of the H-2 complex (Lilly, 1970) was the first suggestion that Ir genes might play an important role in natural populations in disease resistance. The demonstration of an Ir gene controlling susceptibility to autoimmune thyroiditis (Vladutiu and Rose, 1971) suggested a biologic role for such genes in autoimmune reactions.

The (NZB × NZW)F_1 hybrid mouse manifests an aggressive glomerulonephritis analogous to human lupus nephritis. Since neither the NZB nor the NZW parental strain manifests an early florid glomerulonephritis with renal failure, the occurrence of lupus nephritis in the hybrid heterozygote would appear to depend on the expression of at least two dominant or codominant genes, each parent contributing at least one gene. Genetic studies of spontaneous autoantibody production in gonadectomized NZB and DBA/2 offspring (Raveche *et al.*, 1978) have suggested that a single dominant gene is reponsible for anti-single-stranded DNA production with the quantity of antibody in positive mice being determined either by a gene dosage effect or a regulatory gene. Inasmuch as NZB and DBA/2 share the same H-2 type and all NZB but no DBA/2 mice produced anti-single-stranded DNA antibody, the locus of antibody production control appeared to reside outside of H-2.

3. Genetics of Nephritis in Experimental Models

A genetic dependency upon the expression of autologous immune complex glomerulonephritis has been demonstrated by the susceptibility of certain strains of inbred rats but not of others under a specified set of experimental conditions (Strenglein *et al.*, 1975). Since the highly susceptible Lewis and Lewis/BDV as well as the poorly susceptible Lewis/Brown-Norway rats share the same genetic background and differ only in respect to the major histocompatibility complex, the possibility of an H-1-linked genetic factor controlling susceptibility to autologous immune complex disease was suggested. This conclusion is qualified with the observation (Sugisaki *et al.*, 1973) that even the supposedly highly resistant Brown-Norway strain can develop autologous immune complex disease under conditions of more aggressive immunization. In a rat model of toxin-induced anti-GBM antibody, histocompatibility-linked genetic restriction has been demonstrated (Druet *et al.*, 1977). Under a specified set of experimental conditions, mercuric chloride induces anti-GBM antibody in Brown-Norway rats but not in various other inbred rat strains. Hybrid breeding experiments with Brown-Norway and with Lewis rats have demonstrated the production of anti-GBM antibody only in those rats bearing the H-1^n haplotype either in the homozygous or heterozygous state.

4. *Hypothesis*

Given the high degree of analogy between the histocompatibility systems of man and of experimental animals, the hypothesis to be entertained is that the immune response of the human host is a critical determinant in development of complex disease or autoantibody formation and may be to a great extent genetically determined. In this context, chronic glomerulonephritis might result from exposure to a variety of different antigens each leading to a unique response with complex formation, glomerular deposition, and injury. At this primitive stage of understanding, any such hypothesis is tendered with the recognition that determinants other than immune responsiveness may be responsible for the unique association of glomerulonephritis, complement deficiency, and the major histocompatibility complex.

5. *Immunogenetic Aspects of Human Nephritis*

Deficiency of the second component of complement is the single most common component deficit, occurring with a gene frequency of 1% in the population at large. Greater than one-half of individuals with complete absence of C2 have an associated autoimmune disease and/or glomerulonephritis. Individuals with a partial absence of C2 may have increased incidence of systemic lupus erythematosus (SLE) or of juvenile rheumatoid arthritis (Glass *et al.*, 1976). Our own studies (Friend *et al.*, 1975) demonstrated that three unrelated individuals with, respectively, membranous lupus nephropathy, chronic membranoproliferative glomerulonephritis, and polyarteritis, and totally deficient in C2 were mutually poorly reactive in mixed lymphocyte culture and homozygous for the MLC determinant HLA-Dw2. Genetic linkage disequilibrium was strongly suggested between C2 deficiency and the HLA markers A10, B18, Dw2. The gene controlling the elaboration of C2 in man was shown to be separate from and to map outside of the D locus of HLA, based on the observation of an HLA-D-C2 deficiency recombinant. The precise relationship of glomerular disease to C2 deficiency and/or possibly unique HLA Ir genes is unknown (Dupone *et al.*, 1977). Observations such as these plus the previously alluded to conjunction in the mouse of histocompatibility, immune responsiveness, resistance to viral oncogenesis, and susceptibility to autoimmunity provided support for the notion that immunogenetic factors might play a role in the development of glomerulonephritis in man.

In a separate investigation (Friend *et al.*, 1977a; Friend and Michael, 1978), 13 individuals with systemic lupus, a disease offering the spectrum of chronic immune injury in man, were studied to discern whether or not distinct patterns of renal histopathology could be correlated with discrete serologic antibody profiles. In contrast to individuals with either diffuse proliferative nephritis or active lupus without renal disease, those with pure membranous lupus nephropathy were found to be characterized by a unique immune response in that their sera contained only small quantities of antibody to native DNA essentially all of which was nonprecipitating.

Recalling that Ir genes in the mouse are operationally defined by quantitative differences in the level of antibody produced in response to a given antigen and that human B lymphocytes selectively express a unique set of alloantigens possibly analogous to the murine Ia antigens, these observations in lupus nephritis suggested studies to further examine other well-characterized glomerulopathies to ascertain whether genetic similarities might obtain among unrelated individuals with a discrete glomerulopathy. Accordingly, patients with chronic membranoproliferative glomerulonephritis, a common form of identifiable chronic progressive glomerular destruction in man, were investigated for B-cell antigen associations. Reacting sera derived from multiparous mothers of membranoproliferative patients with a panel of patient B cells, showed a reagent which was highly discriminative for a B-cell antigen present in 77% of membranoproliferative patients and in only 17% of a normal population and in none of a disease control group comprised of patients with polycystic kidneys, a hereditary and presumably nonimmune-mediated progressive interstitial renal disease. The risk of developing membranoproliferative nephritis was estimated to be 17 times greater in the presence of the discriminative antigen than in its absence. This was the first demonstration in man of the association of an immune-mediated glomerulonephritis with a specific B-lymphocyte determinant (Friend *et al.*, 1977b). Subsequently, in another study utilizing currently available B-cell alloantisera of defined specificity, others have examined biopsy-proven and radiommunoassay-positive anti-GBM-mediated Goodpasture's syndrome and have found the B-lymphocyte specificity DRW2 to be present in 88% of the patients so examined and in only 32% of the normal population. The relative risk was calculated to be 16 (Rees *et al.*, 1978). Utilizing a panel of pregnancy sera as well as a panel of HLA-D-related sera from the 7th International Histocompatibility Workshop (Reinertsen *et al.*, 1978), the B-lymphocyte alloantigens HLA-DRw2 and HLA-DRw3 have been found to be increased in SLE. In addition, one pregnancy serum was found to react with B lymphocytes from 76% of lupus patients and only 14% of normal controls, yielding a calculated relative risk of 19. The association of SLE with at least two independent HLA-DRw specificities may be analogous to the demonstration in murine systems that more than one Ir gene regulates the immune response to complex antigens and that at least two independent genes specify spontaneous autoantibody production in the NZB mouse.

IgA-IgG nephropathy or Berger's disease (Berger, 1969) is a relatively discrete clinical entity with a generally favorable prognosis, although a minority of Berger's patients develop terminal renal failure. In those undergoing renal transplantation, recurrence of IgA deposition is observed frequently in the grafted kidney, suggesting that systemic abnormalities of the host may be involved in the pathogenesis of the disease. A proportion of patients with Berger's disease manifest elevated levels of serum, nasal, or salivary IgA. The role of IgA in relation to the pathogenesis of the glomerulonephritis, however, remains obscure, and significant glomerular deposits of IgA may be observed in nephritides of anaphylactoid purpura and systemic lupus. In anaphylactoid purpura, an association of HLA-Bw35 and nonstreptococcal-related nephritis has been reported (Nyulassy *et al.*, 1977). Similarly, in two reports of the French population (Noël *et al.*, 1978; Berthoux *et al.*, 1978), HLA-Bw35 was found to be increased significantly in patients with IgA-IgG nephropathy. Interestingly, although not correlated with the Bw35 marker per se, the risk of recurrence of IgA disease in the renal transplant was higher in a related HLA-identical or haplo-identical kidney than in a kidney from a cadaver. In contrast to these findings, those from the United Kingdom (Brettle *et al.*, 1978) did not demonstrate an HLA-A, B, or DRw association with IgA-IgG nephropathy. Parenthetically, it should be noted that whereas in France IgA nephropathy is the most common form of nephritis seen, it is a relatively uncommon entity in the United Kingdom.

An investigation of the association of the HLA markers Bw35, Dw1, and B-lymphocyte determinants identified by three alloantisera (L, B, and F) with IgA-IgG nephropathy has been made in Minnesota Caucasians (Friend *et al.*, 1979). Among a control panel of 50 healthy Minnesota Caucasians, HLA-Bw35 is associated significantly with HLA-Dw1, and Dw1 with the B-lymphocyte determinants identified by the three alloantisera. Serum to serum correlations among the alloantisera are strong. Among a patients panel of 18 Minnesotans with Berger's disease, however, Bw35 is not associated with Dw1 and the correlation of sera L and B with Dw1 lessened (Table 1). In the disease state, B-lymphocyte reactivities are significantly increased to sera L and B with relative risks of 5 and 4, respectively (Table 2). That the discordance between HLA-D and B-cell typings in the disease state is not a simple function of the differing methodologies employed is suggested by serum F which maintains a strong association with Dw1 in health and disease and does not increase in frequency in the disease state. The number of patients is small and the inferences statistical; however, the increased frequency of B-cell typing reactions in IgA nephropathy identified by sera B and L, either unassociated or loosely associated with DW1, suggests the

Table 1. Correlation between Lymphocyte Surface Antigens in Patients with IgA Nephropathy and in Normal Controls[a]

	IgA nephropathy		Normals	
	r	p	r	p
Bw35 vs. Dw1	0.06	> 0.1	0.47	< 0.005
Dw1 vs. L	0.40	> 0.05	1.00	< 0.005
Dw1 vs. B	0.28	> 0.1	0.50	< 0.005
Dw1 vs. F	0.84	< 0.01	0.82	< 0.005

[a] The highly significant associations in the normal population between Bw35, Dw1, L, and B are lessened or eradicated in patients with IgA nephropathy.

Table 2. Frequency, Relative Risk, and Significance of Markers in IgA Nephropathy[a]

	Bw35	Dw1	B-Cell sera L	B-Cell sera R	B-Cell sera F
% positive, IgA/normals	21/16	17/20	56/20	72/40	22/22
Relative risk	1.38	0.80	5.0	3.9	1.0
p	NS	NS	< 0.05	< 0.05	NS

[a] Controls = 50 healthy, unrelated Minnesota Caucasians. IgA = 24 patients Bw35 typed; 18 patients Dw1 and B-cell sera typed.

possible existence of additional disease-associated B-cell antigens and emphasizes the possible informativeness of defining B-cell alloantisera on disease panels.

6. Summary

In summary: (1) structural genes for certain serologic components of the inflammatory response, such as C2 and factor B, are HLA-linked and map closely to HLA-D; (2) discrete patterns of immune complex injury in the kidney, such as membranous lupus nephropathy, may be associated with unique serologic antibody profiles or levels of autoresponsiveness; (3) specific genetically stipulated B-lymphocyte cell surface determinants may be correlated with greatly increased susceptibility of unrelated individuals to certain immune-mediated glomerulonephritides, such as membranoproliferative nephritis with serum MCG-3; and (4) some nephritis-associated B-cell antigens may be peculiar to the disease state and possibly distinct from HLA-D, such as alloantisera L and B in IgA nephropathy.

Limitations of Human Studies

The limitation of these human studies and of those of others in this particular endeavor is that although they point out certain provocative associative or phenomenologic relationships between complement deficiency, possibly unique Ir genes, and/or antibody response with injury to the glomerular filter, they do not address the mechanisms underlying such injury. A major problem in the study of susceptibility to nephritis is the lack of definition of a causative agent or specific antigen in the vast majority of glomerulonephritides including those associated with glomerular annihilation leading to renal failure. Clearance, localization, and effector mechanisms are also suspect in the genesis of chronic nephritis. No highly satisfactory way exists to approach the role of renal clearing and localization mechanisms in human nephritis. For example, the assessment of mesangial function is not approachable in humans.

To conduct a worthwhile study of mechanisms underlying disease susceptibility, the ideal model is one in which there is a specific etiologic agent, measurable immune response(s), and a clinically manifest disease. Acute poststreptococcal glomerulonephritis potentially represents such a model. The etiologic agents (nephritogenic streptococci) are known. A measure of immunologic responsiveness or lack thereof to some constituent or product of the causative organism may derive *in vivo* from quantitating the serologic antibody response to several specific extracellular or cellular streptococcal antigens and *in vitro* by lymphocyte blastogenesis (Greenberg *et al.*, 1975) to a crude preparation of streptococcal antigens. Finally, studies of families with one or more affected individuals could determine whether responsiveness could be correlated with histocompatibility markers and protection from or liability to clinical disease.

ACKNOWLEDGMENTS. The author gratefully acknowledges the friendship and guidance of Drs. Alfred Michael and Edmond Yunis during the course of these studies.

References

Benacerraf, B., and McDevitt, H. O., 1972, Histocompatibility-linked immune response genes, *Science* **175:**273.

Berger, J., 1969, IgA glomerular deposits in renal disease, *Transplant. Proc.* **1:**939.

Berthoux, F. C., Gagne, A., Sabatier, J. C., Ducret, F., LePetit, J. C., Marcellin, M., Mercier, B., and Brizard, C. P., 1978, HLA-BW35 and mesangial IgA glomerulonephritis (Letter), *N. Engl. J. Med.* **298:**1034.

Biozzi, G., Stiffel, C., Mouton, D., Bouthillier, Y., and Decreusefond, C., 1972, Cytodynamics of the immune response in two lines of mice genetically selected for "high" and "low" antibody synthesis, *J. Exp. Med.* **135:**1071.

Brettle, R., Peters, D. K., and Batchelor, J. R., 1978, Mesangial IgA glomerulonephritis and HLA antigens (Letter), *New Engl. J. Med.* **298:**200.

Druet, E., Sapin, C., Günther, E., Feingold, N., and Druet, P., 1977, Mercuric chloride-induced anti-glomerular basement membrane antibodies in the rat: Genetic control, *Eur. J. Immunol.* **7:**348.

Dupont, B., Good, R. A., Hauptmann, G., Schrueder, I., and Seligmann, M., 1977, Immunopathology, immunodeficiencies, and complement deficiencies, in: *HLA and Disease* (J. Dausset and A. Svejgaard, eds.), Munksgaard, Copenhagen, pp. 233–248.

Friend, P. S., Handwerger, B. S., Kim, Y., Michael, A. F., and Yunis, E. J., 1975, C2 deficiency in man. Genetic relationship to a mixed lymphocyte reaction determinant (7a*), *Immunogenetics* **2:**569.

Friend, P. S., Kim, Y., Michael, A. F., and Donadio, J. V., 1977a, Pathogenesis of membranous nephropathy in systemic lupus erythematosis; possible role of nonprecipitating DNA antibody, *Brit. Med. J.* **1:**25.

Friend, P. S., Yunis, E. J., Noreen, H. J., and Michael, A. F., 1977b, B-cell alloantigen associated with chronic mesangiocapillary glomerulonephritis, *Lancet* **1:**562.

Friend, P. S., and Michael, A. F., 1978, Hypothesis: Immunologic rationale for the therapy of membranous lupus nephropathy, *Clin. Immunol. Immunopathol.* **10:**35.

Friend, P. S., Yunis, E. J., Noreen, H., Reinsmoen, N., Dubey, D., and Michael, A. F., 1979, B-lymphocyte determinants in immunoglobulin A nephropathy, *J. Immunol.* **123:**2182.

Glass, D., Raum, D., Gibson, D., Stillman, J. S., and Schur, P. H., 1976, Inherited deficiency of the second component of complement: Rheumatic disease associations, *J. Clin. Invest.* **58:**853.

Greenberg, L. J., Gray, E. D., and Yunis, E. J., 1975, Association of HL-A5 and immune responsiveness in vitro to streptococcal antigens, *J. Exp. Med.* **141:**935.

Katz, F. E., and Steward, M. W., 1976, Studies on the genetic control of antibody affinity: The independent control of antibody levels and affinity in Biozzi mice, *J. Immunol.* **117:**477.

Lilly, F., 1970, The role of genetics in Gross virus leukemogenesis, *Bibl. Haematol. (Basel)* **36:**213.

Lilly, F., Boyse, E. A., and Old, L. J., 1964, Genetic basis of susceptibility to viral leukemogenesis, *Lancet* **2:**1207.

Noël, L. H., Descamps, B., Jungers, P., Bach, J.-F., Busson, M., Suet, C., Hors, J., and Dausset, J., 1978, HLA antigen in three types of glomerulonephritis, *Clin. Immunol. Immunopathol.* **10:**19.

Nyulassy, S. Buc, M., Sasinka, M., Pavlovic, M., Slugen, I., Hirschova, V., Kaisenova, M., Menkyna, R., and Stefanovic, J., 1977, The HLA system in glomerulonephritis, *Clin. Immunol. Immunopathol.* **7:**319.

Raveche, E. S., Steinberg, A. D., Klassen, L. W., and Tjio, J. H., 1978, Genetic studies in NZB mice. I. Spontaneous autoantibody production, *J. Exp. Med.* **147:**1487.

Rees, A. J., Peters, D. K., Compston, D. A. S., and Batchelor, J. R., 1978, Strong association between HLA-DRW2 and antibody-mediated Goodpasture's syndrome, *Lancet* **1:**966.

Reinertsen, J. L., Klippel, J. H., Johnson, A., Steinberg, A. D., Decker, J. L., and Mann, D. L., 1978, B-Lymphocyte alloantigens associated with systemic lupus erythematosus, *N. Engl. J. Med.* **299:**515.

Stenglein, B., Thoenes, G. H., and Günther, E., 1975, Genetically controlled autologous immune complex glomerulonephritis in rats, *J. Immunol.* **115:**895.

Sugisaki, T., Klassen, J., Milgrom, F., Andres, G. A., and McCluskey, R. T., 1973, Immunopathologic study of an autoimmune tubular and interstitial renal disease in Brown-Norway rats, *Lab. Invest.* **28:**658.

Vladutiu, A. O., and Rose, N. R., 1971, Autoimmune murine thyroiditis relation to histocompatibility (H-2) type, *Science* **174:**1137.

38

Autoantibodies in Systemic Lupus Erythematosus

Eng M. Tan

1. Introduction

Systemic lupus erythematosus (SLE) is a disease which has engaged the clinical and research efforts of many groups of investigators, including rheumatologists, nephrologists, dermatologists, and hematologists. In addition, many immunologists interested in mechanisms underlying autoimmunity have studied patients with SLE and models of this disease in experimental animals. There is abundant evidence showing that immune complexes are involved in the generalized vasculitis and more specifically in the nephritis seen in patients with SLE. The immune complex disease is known to be related to circulating autoantibodies, and in this chapter we shall discuss the current information available concerning autoantibodies to intracellular antigens in SLE.

Tables 1–3 present the current information available on the types of autoantibodies to intracellular antigens which have been identified in the sera of patients with SLE. This is not a commplete list of autoantibodies, even to intracellular antigens. In addition, autoantibodies to surface or membrane antigens have been characterized as well as autoantibodies to red cells, platelets, and components of the coagulation system (Kunkel, 1977). The types of autoantibodies have been divided into those directed against nucleic acids, histones or DNA–histone complexes, and nonhistone components. These subjects will be discussed in this sequence.

Eng M. Tan · Autoimmune Disease Center, Scripps Clinic and Research Foundation, La Jolla, California 92037. Supported by NIH Grant AM 20705 and by a grant from the Kroc Foundation for the Advancement of Medical Science.

Table 1. Autoantibodies to Intracellular Antigens: Antibodies to Nucleic Acid Antigens

Antigenic specificity	Serological and clinical characteristics of antibody
Double-stranded DNA (double helix)	Does not cross-react with single-stranded DNA. Few reported cases in SLE.
Double- and single-stranded DNA	Antibodies cross-react with double- and single-stranded DNA. Commonly referenced as antibody to native DNA. Present in 70% of SLE
Single-stranded DNA	Antibodies reactive with purines and pyrimidines. Some cross-react with single-stranded RNA. Not reactive with double-stranded DNA. Present in SLE and many other diseases
Single-stranded RNA, double-stranded RNA	Antibodies reactive with native RNA and synthetic RNA polymers

2. *Autoantibodies to Nucleic Acids*

Antibodies to DNA are of three major types (Stollar, 1975; Tan *et al.*, 1966; Wold *et al.*, 1968). There have been a number of reports concerning antibodies which react only with double-stranded DNA, i.e., the antigenic determinant is related to the double-helical conformation of DNA. This type of antibody does not cross-react with single-stranded DNA. It appears that antibodies of this specificity are relatively unusual. On the other hand, antibodies which recognize antigenic determinants present in common or shared between double- and single-stranded DNA are relatively common in SLE, approaching 70% in many reported studies. Since these antibodies cross-react in immunological identity between double- and single-stranded DNA, the determinant is presumed to be the polydeoxyribose-phosphate backbone of DNA. However, this has not been demonstrated clearly and it is not known whether the purines and pyrimidines of DNA are part of the antigenic determinant. In the literature, it is this type of antibody which is usually referred to as antibody to native DNA. The important feature is that the majority of these antibodies cross-react in immunological identity between double- and single-stranded DNA. Antibodies of this specificity were the

Table 2. Autoantibodies to Intracellular Antigens: Antibodies to Histones and DNA–Histone Complexes

Antigenic specificity	Serological and clinical characteristic to antibody
Deoxyribonucleoprotein (soluble nucleoprotein and DNA–histone)	Antibody is LE cell factor of serum
Histones (H1, H2A, H2B, H3, H4)	Antibodies present in 25% of SLE but in >90% of drug-induced LE

Table 3. Autoantibodies to Intracellular Antigens: Antibodies to Nonhistone Components

Antigenic specificity	Serological and clinical characteristics of antibody
Sm antigen	Antibody is serological marker for SLE. Also present in MRL mouse. Antigen is DNA-binding protein
Nuclear RNP	Present in 30–40% of SLE, 90% in mixed connective tissue diseases
Cytoplasmic RNP	Present in 10% of SLE
SS-A (Ro) antigen	Present in 25–30% of SLE, 70% of Sjögren's syndrome
SS-B (Ha, La) antigen	Present in 10–15% of SLE, 40–50% of Sjögren's syndrome
PCNA (proliferating cell nuclear antigen)	Present in 5% of SLE

first to be recognized as playing a role in immune complex formation in patients with SLE (Tan *et al.*, 1966). Antigen–antibody complexes of this immune system have been identified in serum and have been eluted from the kidneys of patients (Koffler *et al.*, 1967; Krishnan and Kaplan, 1967).

Antibodies which react only with single-stranded DNA and do not cross-react with double-stranded DNA are also present in high incidence in SLE. In one study, this was reported to be 87% (Koffler *et al.*, 1971). This type of antibody reacts with the purine and pyrimidine determinants present on single-stranded DNA. Many of these antibodies also cross-react with purine and pyrimidines present on single-stranded RNA. It has been shown clearly that antibodies reactive only with single-stranded DNA are not restricted to patients with SLE but are also present in patients with many other diseases, including chronic active hepatitis, rheumatoid arthritis, infectious mononucleosis, and chronic bronchitis.

Antibodies to single-stranded RNA and to double-stranded RNA also have been identified in SLE (Eilat *et al.*, 1978; Koffler *et al.*, 1971). Antibodies to single-stranded RNA also are involved in the immune complex nephritis of patients with SLE, since antibodies and antigens of these specificities have been identified in kidneys and isolated from eluates (Andres *et al.*, 1970).

3. Antibodies to Histones and DNA–Histone Complexes

Antibodies to DNA–histone complexes can be demonstrated by several techniques including immunodiffusion, precipitation, and radioimmunoassay (Holman and Deicher, 1959; Tan, 1967). The antigenic reactivity of this complex requires both the DNA and the histone moieties. It is clear that DNA alone is not the antigenic determinant, since antibodies to DNA can be distinguished from those which react with the DNA–histone complex.

Antibodies reacting with this complex were shown to be the serum factors responsible for production of the LE cell. It also has been shown that most sera containing antibodies to the DNA–histone complexes concomitantly have antibodies reactive with native DNA.

Antibodies which are reactive only with histones also are present in the sera of patients with SLE. This was initially demonstrated with the micro-

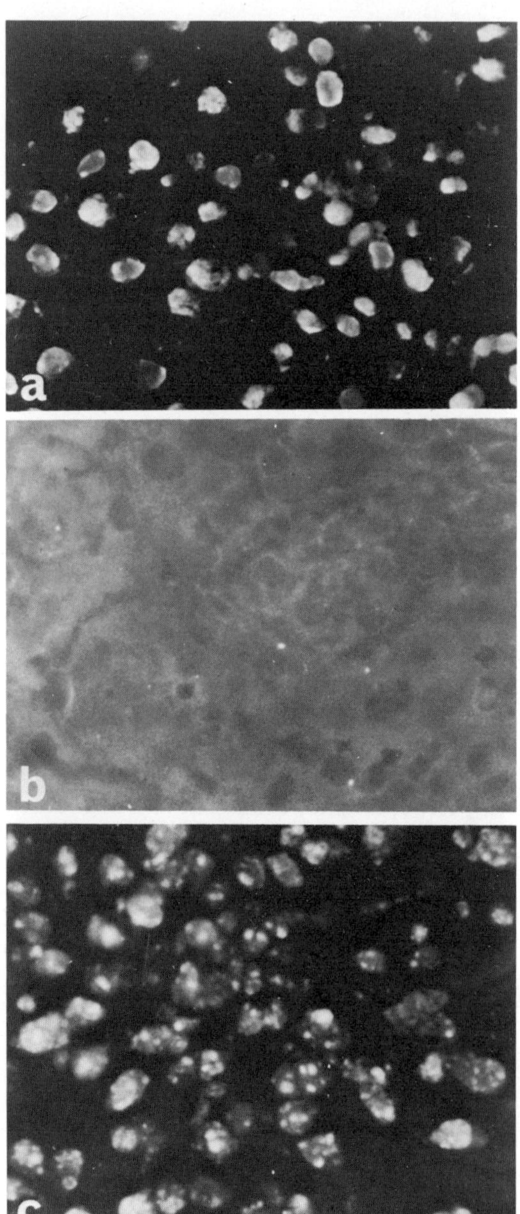

Figure 1. Immunofluorescent method for the detection of autoantibodies to nuclear histones. On untreated tissue section (a), serum containing autoantibodies to histones produced a patchy to homogeneous pattern of nuclear staining. On acid-extracted section (b), histones and other nonhistone proteins have been extracted by this treatment and the serum was negative for any nuclear staining. When the acid-extracted section was reconstituted with purified nuclear histones (c), the serum became positive again for nuclear staining, showing a more clumpy pattern than in the untreated section (a).

complement fixation method (Stollar, 1971). An immunofluorescent technique has been developed which can be used readily for the determination of antibodies to histones (Tan *et al.*, 1976). This involves the use of tissue sections which have been extracted with 0.1 N HC1. This treatment removes histones and many other nonhistone proteins from the nucleus. After acid extraction, the tissue section can be reconstituted with purified histones, which complex to the DNA remaining in the extracted nuclei. Thus, a substrate is created containing histones to the exclusion of nonhistone nuclear proteins. An example of this immunofluorescent method is presented in Fig. 1. Sera containing antibodies to histones generally produce a homogeneous or patchy nuclear staining on unextracted tissue sections, become negative on acid-extracted tissue sections because the antigen has been removed by such treatment, and finally become positive again for nuclear staining on the histone-reconstituted section. With this method of analysis, it was determined that antibodies to histones were present in 25% of all patients with idiopathic SLE. In contrast, 90% or more of patients with drug-induced (procainamide or hydralazine) lupus have antibodies to nuclear histones (Fritzler and Tan, 1978). This technique of reconstitution of nuclear components which bind to DNA can be used as an assay system for the detection of other antinuclear antibodies. Klein and his co-workers have used a similar system in studies of the Epstein–Barr virus nuclear antigen (EBNA) and antibody (Ohno *et al.*, 1977).

4. Antibodies to Nonhistone Components

The identification of antibodies to nonhistone components of the nucleus was facilitated greatly by the combination of immunodiffusion and immunofluorescent techniques. Many nonhistone antigens of the nucleus are soluble in saline and extracts of nuclei can be used as sources of soluble nuclear antigens. In the immunodiffusion system, one can demonstrate several precipitating antibodies as illustrated in Fig. 2. Although SLE sera generally contain antinuclear antibodies of many specificities, including antibodies to nucleic acids, histones, and nonhistone proteins, careful search will reveal certain sera which are relatively monospecific and contain one type of antinuclear antibody in high titer. These sera can then be used as useful reagents for characterizing the precipitating antigen–antibody systems. The identification of a specific precipitating antigen–antibody system has been helped by the observation that antibodies to nonhistone components generally give a speckled nuclear staining pattern on immunofluorescence (Northway and Tan, 1972). These speckled staining patterns are produced by antibodies to Sm antigen, nuclear ribonucleoprotein (RNP), the SS-A and SS-B antigens, and an antigen present in the nuclei of proliferating cells (PCNA).

Antibody to the Sm antigen was one of the first precipitating antigen–antibody systems described (Tan and Kunkel, 1966). It has been increasingly

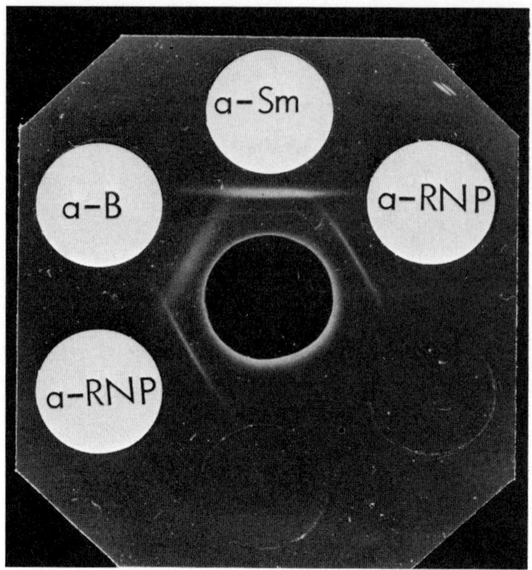

Figure 2. Immunodiffusion study showing the presence of multiple nonhistone protein antigens in a saline extract of rabbit thymus nuclei (center well). In the surrounding wells, various sera containing antibodies to Sm antigen, nuclear RNP, and SS-B antigen show precipitin lines against the nuclear extract. The three precipitin systems show immunological nonidentity.

apparent after several years of investigation that antibody to the Sm antigen is highly specific for SLE and might constitute a serological marker for this disease. The antigen is a nonhistone protein which has the capacity to bind to DNA. There is a preferential binding for single-stranded DNA compared to double-stranded DNA (Reyes and Tan, 1977). Antibody to the Sm antigen has been shown to be present in the sera of the MRL strain of mice with lupus erythematosus. Interestingly, this antibody which is a serological marker for human lupus erythematosus was not detected in the New Zealand or in the BXSB strains of mice, both of which are also considered to be models of human lupus (Eisenberg *et al.*, 1978).

Antibodies to nuclear RNP are present in approximately 30 to 40% of patients with SLE. In another connective tissue disease called mixed connective tissue disease, this antibody is present in almost all patients and is characterized by extremely high titers and by absence of antinuclear antibodies of other specificities (Sharp *et al.*, 1972). In the past, the nuclear RNP antigen also was called extractable nuclear antigen (ENA). Since many nonhistone nuclear components are extracted readily from nuclei, this terminology is no longer appropriate.

The SS-A and SS-B antigen–antibody systems initially were identified with the sera of patients with Sjögren's syndrome and hence the terminology assigned to these systems (Alspaugh *et al.*, 1976).In Sjögren's syndrome, antibody to SS-A antigen is present in 70% and antibody to SS-B in approximately 50%. In SLE, these are present in lower percentage, 25 to 30% for SS-A antibody and 10 to 15% for SS-B antibody. Akizuki and associates have described an autoantibody system which they have called Ha (Akizuk, *et al.*, 1977). Immunologically, there is no difference between the SS-B and the Ha system. In terms of the prevalence of this autoantibody in connective tissue diseases, the results are also identical (Tan *et al.*, 1977).

Previously, Reichlin and associate described presumed cytoplasmic antigens (Ro and La) which precipitated with antibodies in sera of patients with lupus (Mattioli and Reichlin, 1974). Now it has been shown that the Ro antigen is immunologically identical with SS-A and the La antigen with SS-B (Alspaugh and Maddison, 1979). Still to be resolved are questions concerning why the Ro and La antigens were thought to be cytoplasmic antigens whereas the SS-A and SS-B antigens are intranuclear antigens.

An interesting autoantibody in systemic lupus is directed against a nuclear antigen present in proliferating cells (Miyachi *et al.*, 1978). By immunofluorescence, it can be detected as an antibody reacting selectively with certain cells and not with others as illustrated in Fig. 3. This autoantibody does not stain nuclei of normal peripheral lymphocytes, but after stimulation with mitogens such as PHA, Con A, and pokeweed mitogen, approximately 20% of cells show positive nuclear staining (Table 4). Autoantibody of this specificity was detected in three of 70 patients with SLE. This antibody may be a useful reagent for identifying proliferating or "blastoid" cells.

Antibodies to cytoplasmic antigens also have been characterized and include antibodies which are reactive with cytoplasmic RNP and with ribosomes (Koffler *et al.*, 1977; Miyachi and Tan, 1979). Some reports show a relationship between antibodies to cytoplasmic antigens and renal disease in patients with SLE.

5. Discussion

SLE is characterized by an exuberant production of autoantibodies as described above. In general, autoantibodies in other diseases are less heterogeneous in specificities. It is becoming clear that different connective tissue diseases are characterized by different sets of autoantibodies. Some, like antibody to the Sm antigen, are highly specific for one disease (SLE), whereas others, like antibody to nuclear RNP, are present in several diseases but are most prevalent in one particular disease (mixed connective tissue disease). This observation has led to the concept of the presence of different profiles of autoantibodies in different connective tissue diseases (Notman *et al.*, 1975).

Table 4. Indirect Immunofluorescence Showing Percent Staining for PCNA in Human Lymphocytes after Mitogen Stimulation

Mitogen	Before stimulation	After stimulation
PHA[a]	0%	20%
Con A[b]	0%	20%
PWM[c]	0%	20%

[a] Phytohemagglutinin, 10 μl/ml.
[b] Concanavalin A, 24 μl/ml.
[c] Pokeweed mitogen, 50/ml.

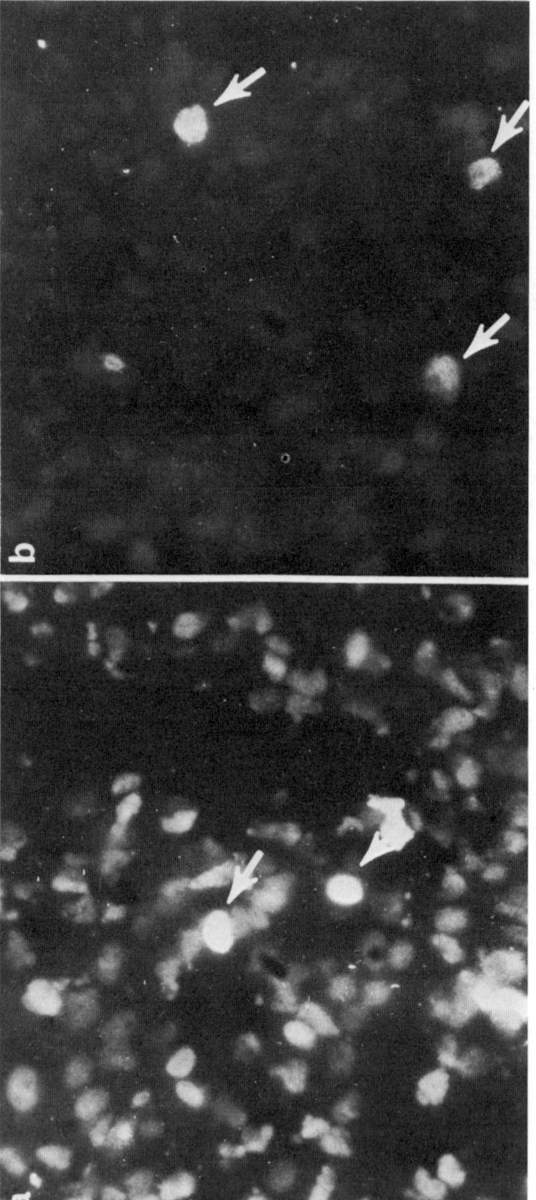

Figure 3. Serum from a patient with antibody against proliferating cell nuclear antigen (PCNA) was reacted with a section of mouse kidney. At a low dilution of serum (a), many nuclei in the mouse kidney section showed nuclear staining. It could be observed, however, that a few nuclei (arrows) showed stronger nuclear staining. At a higher dilution of serum (b), the majority of cells in the kidney section were negative for nuclear staining. The nuclei of three cells (arrows), however, continue to show strong nuclear staining. This was produced by antibody to PCNA. These three cells were not glomerular or tubular cells but were cells in the interstitial areas of the kidney.

These profiles of autoantibodies have been very useful in differential diagnosis and in classification.

The presence of autoantibodies in the circulation of patients with SLE results in a situation where antigen–antibody complexes can form if homologous antigens gain entry into the circulation. Immune complexes involving double-stranded DNA, single-stranded DNA, and certain nonhistone nuclear components have been clearly implicated in immune complex disease (Andres *et al.*, 1970; Koffler *et al.*, 1967, 1971; Krishnan and Kaplan, 1967; Nydegger *et al.*, 1974; Tan *et al.*, 1966). It is highly probable that other nuclear/cytoplasmic antigen–antibody complexes might also be implicated. The reasons why intracellular antigens become available as extracellular macromolecules and gain entry into the circulation are unknown. This intriguing question as well as the disturbed immune regulation resulting in autoantibody production remain challenging areas of investigation.

6. Summary

SLE is an autoimmune disease characterized by a complex array of circulating antibodies to nuclear and cytoplasmic antigens. There are antibodies which are reactive with nucleic acids, deoxyribonucleoprotein, histones, and nonhistone components. Some of these autoantibodies can be involved in immune complex formation with autologous antigens and have been implicated in immune complex disease in the kidneys.

References

Akizuki, M., Powers, R., Jr., and Holman, H. R., 1977, A soluble acidic protein of the cell nucleus which reacts with serum from patients with systemic lupus erythematosus and Sjögren's syndrome, *J. Clin. Invest.* **59:**264.

Alspaugh, M. A., and Maddison, P., 1979, Resolution of the identity of certain antigen–antibody systems in systemic lupus erythematosus and Sjögren's syndrome: An interlaboratory collaboration, *Arthritis Rheum.* **22:**796.

Alspaugh, M. A., Talal, N., and Tan, E. M., 1976, Differentiation and characterization of autoantibodies and their antigens in Sjögren's syndrome, *Arthritis Rheum.* **19:**216.

Andres, G. A., Accinni, L., Beiser, S. M., Christian, C. L., Cinotti, G. A., Erlanger, B. F., Hsu, K. C., and Seegal, B. C., 1970, Localization of fluorescein-labeled antinucleoside antibodies in glomeruli of patients with active systemic lupus erythematosus nephritis, *J. Clin. Invest.* **49:**2106.

Eilat, D., Steinberg, A. D., and Schechter, 1978, The reaction of SLE antibodies with native, single-stranded RNA: Radioassay and binding specificities, *J. Immunol.* **120:**550.

Eisenberg, R. A., Tan, E. M., and Dixon, F. J., 1978, Presence of anti-Sm reactivity in autoimmune mouse strains, *J. Exp. Med.* **147:**582.

Fritzler, M. J., and Tan, E. M., 1978, Antibodies to histones in drug-induced and idiopathic lupus erythematosus, *J. Clin. Invest.* **62:**560.

Holman, H., and Deicher, H. R., 1959, The reaction of the lupus erythematosus (L.E.) cell factor with deoxyribonucleoprotein of the cell nucleus, *J. Clin. Invest.* **38:**2059.

Koffler, D., Schur, P. H., and Kunkel, H. G., 1967, Immunological studies concerning the nephritis of systemic lupus erythematosus, *J. Exp. Med.* **126:**607.

Koffler, D., Carr, R., Agnello, V., Thoburn, R., and Kunkel, H. G., 1971, Antibodies to polynucleotides in human sera: Antigenic specificity and relation to disease, *J. Exp. Med.* **134:**294.

Koffler, D., Faiferman, I., and Gerber, M. A., 1977, Radioimmunoassay for antibodies to cytoplasmic ribosomes in human serum, *Science* **198:**741.

Krishnan, C., and Kaplan, M. H., 1967, Immunopathologic studies of systemic lupus erythematosus. II. Antinuclear reaction of gammaglobulin eluted from homogenates and isolated glomeruli of kidneys of patients with lupus nephritis, *J. Clin. Invest.* **46:**569.

Kunkel, H. D., 1977, The immunologic approach to SLE, *Arthritis Rheum.* **20:**5139.

Mattioli, M., and Reichlin, M., 1974, Heterogeneity of RNA protein antigens reactive with sera of patients with systemic lupus erythematosus: Description of a cytoplasmic nonribosomal antigen, *Arthritis Rheum.* **17:**421.

Miyachi, K., and Tan, E. M., 1979, Antibodies reacting with ribosomal ribonucleoprotein in connective tissue diseases, *Arthritis Rheum.* **22:**87.

Miyachi, K., Fritzler, M. J., and Tan, E. M., 1978, Autoantibody to a nuclear antigen in proliferating cells, *J. Immunol.* **121:**2228.

Northway, J. D., and Tan, E. M., 1972, Differentiation of antinuclear antibodies giving speckled staining patterns in immunofluorescence, *Clin. Immunol. Immunopathol.* **1:**140.

Notman, D. D., Kurata, N., and Tan, E. M., 1975, Profiles of antinuclear antibodies in systemic rheumatic diseases, *Ann. Intern. Med.* **83:**464.

Nydegger, U. E., Lambert, P. H., Gerber, H., and Miescher, P. A., 1974, Circulating immune complexes in the serum in systemic lupus erythematosus and in carriers of hepatitis B antigen, *J. Clin. Invest.* **54:**297.

Ohno, S., Luka, J., Lindahl, T., and Klein, G., 1977, Identification of a purified complement-fixing antigen as the Epstein–Barr virus-determined nuclear antigen (EBNA) by its binding to metaphase chromosomes, *Proc. Natl. Acad. Sci. USA* **74:**1605.

Reyes, P. A., and Tan, E. M., 1977, DNA-binding property of Sm nuclear antigen, *J. Exp. Med.* **145:**749.

Sharp, G. C., Irwin, W., Gould, G., and Holman, H. R., 1972, Mixed connective tissue disease—An apparently distinct rheumatic disease syndrome associated with a specific antibody to an extractable nuclear antigen (ENA), *Am. J. Med.* **52:**148.

Stollar, B. D., 1971, Reactions of systemic lupus erythematosus sera with histone fractions and histone–DNA complexes, *Arthritis Rheum.* **14:**485.

Stollar, B. D., 1975, The specificity and applications of antibodies to helical nucleic acids, *Crit. Rev. Biochem.* **3:**45.

Tan, E. M., 1967, An immunologic precipitin system between soluble nucleoprotein and serum antibody in systemic lupus erythematosus, *J. Clin. Invest.* **46:**735.

Tan, E. M., and Kunkel, H. G., 1966, Characteristics of a soluble nuclear antigen precipitating with sera of patients with systemic lupus erythematosus, *J. Immunol.* **96:**464.

Tan, E. M., Carr, R. I., Schur, P. H., and Kunkel, H. G., 1966, DNA and antibody to DNA in the serum of patients with systemic lupus erythematosus, *J. Clin. Invest.* **45:**1732.

Tan, E. M., Robinson, J., and Robitaille, P., 1976, Studies on antibodies to histones by immunofluorescence, *Scand. J. Immunol.* **5:**811.

Tan, E. M., Christian, C., Holman, H. R., Homma, M., Kunkel, H. G., Reichlin, M., Sharp, G. C., Ziff, M., and Barnett, E. V., 1977, Anti-tissue antibodies in rheumatic diseases, *Arthritis Rheum.* **20:**1419.

Wold, R. T., Young, F. E., Tan, E. M., and Farr, R. S., 1968, Deoxyribonucleic acid antibody: A method to quantitate its primary interaction with deoxyribonucleic acid, *Science* **161:**806.

39

Serological Studies of Antibodies Reactive with RNA and RNA–Protein Antigens

David Koffler, Thomas E. Miller, and Robert G. Lahita

1. Introduction

Antibodies reactive with nuclear and cytoplasmic ribonucleoproteins and with RNA have received increasing attention as a result of the detection of antibodies which are helpful for the identification of subpopulations of patients with rheumatoid disease. In contrast to the DNA and DNA–protein systems, relatively little is known about the pathogenetic role of these antibodies in the induction of tissue injury. The development of sensitive and reproducible assays for these antibodies should enhance understanding of this potentially important system. The major antibodies which have been identified and the primary techniques utilized for their demonstration are indicated in Table 1. Immunological evaluation of these antibodies has been complicated by the lack of a standardized nomenclature similar to that in usage for antibodies reactive with DNA and DNA–protein antigens. Difficulties inherent in the preparation of purified antigens which are stable and resistant to serum and tissue ribonucleases have further complicated attempts to define antibodies associated with RNA antigens. Each of the major antibodies will be reviewed with respect to method of assay, clinical correlation, and potential pathogenetic importance in rheumatoid disease.

2. Antiribosomal Antibodies

Antibodies reactive with ribosomes have been detected by a variety of tests including complement fixation (Deicher *et al.*, 1960), bentonite floccu-

David Koffler and Thomas E. Miller · Department of Pathology and Laboratory Medicine, Hahnemann Medical College and Hospital, Philadelphia, Pennsylvania 19102. ***Robert G. Lahita*** · The Rockefeller University, New York, New York 10021.

Table 1. Serological Studies of Antibodies Reactive with RNA and RNA–Protein Antigens

	Hemagglutination	Agar gel precipitation	Radioimmunoassay	Immunofluorescence	Complement fixation
Nuclear RNP	Akizuki, and Steinberg (1977), Koffler *et al.* (1971, 1974), Notman *et al.* (1975), Reichlin and Mattioli (1974), Sharp *et al.* (1972, 1976), Winfield *et al.* (1975b)	Akizuki and Steinberg (1977), Gaudreau *et al.* (1978), Koffler *et al.* (1971), Mattioli and Reichlin (1971, 1973), Northway and Tan (1972), Notman *et al.* (1975), Peltier *et al.* (1977), Sharp *et al.* (1972, 1976)		Gaudreau *et al.* (1978), Mattioli and Reichlin (1971), Northway and Tan (1972), Sharp *et al.* (1972)	Akizuki and Steinberg (1977), Maddison and Reichlin (1977), Mattioli and Reichlin (1971, 1973), Sharp *et al.* (1972)
Nucleolar RNP		Miyawaki, *et al.* (1978), Pinnas *et al.* (1973)		Miyawaki and Richie (1973), Miyawaki *et al.* (1978), Pinnas *et al.* (1973), Ritchie (1970), Watanabe *et al.* (1969), Winfield *et al.* (1975b)	Watanabe *et al.* (1969)
Cytoplasmic RNP Ribosomes		Koffler *et al.* (1978), Lamon and Bennett (1970), Schur and Monroe (1969), Schur *et al.* (1967), Sturgill and Preble (1967)	Cavanagh (1977), Koffler *et al.* (1977, 1978)	Homberg *et al.* (1974), Watanabe *et al.* (1969)	Deicher *et al.* (1960), Homberg *et al.* (1974), Sturgill and Preble (1967)

La		Mattioli and Reichlin (1974), Provost *et al.* (1977)			
RNA Single-stranded		Koffler *et al.* (1971), Lamon and Bennett (1970), Miyawaki and Ritchie (1973), Pinnas *et al.* (1973), Schur and Monroe (1969)	Eilat *et al.* (1976, 1977, 1978), Miller *et al.* (1975)	Miyawaki and Ritchie (1973)	
Double-stranded	Koffler *et al.* (1969, 1971, 1974), Schur and Monroe (1969), Thoburn *et al.* (1971), Winfield *et al.* (1975b)	Miyawaki and Ritchie (1973), Schur and Monroe (1969), Schur *et al.* (1971)	Attias *et al.* (1973), Miller *et al.* (1975), Miyawaki and Ritchie (1973), Pillarisetty and Talal (1976), Pillarisetty *et al.* (1977), Schur *et al.* (1971), Talal *et al.* (1971, 1976)	Miyawaki and Ritchie (1973)	Schur *et al.* (1971)
Poly A	Koffler *et al.* (1971)	Koffler *et al.* (1971), Schur and Monroe (1969)	Pillarisetty and Talal (1976), Pillarisetty *et al.* (1975, 1977), Talal *et al.* (1976)		

lation (Sturgill and Carpenter, 1965), indirect immunofluorescence with tissue sections (Homberg *et al.*, 1974),fluorescent spot tests (Sturgill and Preble, 1967), agar gel diffusion (Schur *et al.*, 1967; Sturgill and Preble, 1967), and most recently by radioimmunoassay (Cavanagh, 1977; Koffler *et al.*, 1977, 1978). Precipitating antibodies to ribosomes were found in 15% of sera of systemic lupus erythematosus (SLE) patients closely associated with the occurrence of renal disease (Schur *et al.*, 1967). Neither the RNA nor the protein components of ribosomes alone showed precipitating activity. Utilizing a more sensitive radioimmunoassay system with intrinsically labeled ribosomes, antibodies were demonstrated in 70% of SLE sera in approximately equal incidence in patients with active disease with or without renal involvement and in patients with inactive disease (Koffler *et al.*, 1978). In addition, these antibodies were found in 30% of patients with rheumatoid arthritis, in 28% of those with chronic active hepatitis, and appear to have a distribution similar to antibodies reactive with single-stranded DNA (see DNA) (Koffler *et al.*, 1977).

On the basis of studies using purified ribosomal RNA for the inhibition of the binding of antiribosomal antibodies to labeled ribosomes, SLE sera could be segregated into three groups: (1) sera containing only anti-ribosomal RNP (rRNP) antibodies (no inhibition by rRNA); (2) sera containing only anti-RNA antibodies (complete inhibition by rRNA) (Fig. 1); (3) sera containing both antiribosomal and anti-RNA antibodies (partial inhibition by rRNA)(Fig. 2). Sera containing antibodies restricted to anti-rRNP uniformly came from patients with active disease, half of whom had renal disease. Sera from 7 of 20 patients with high titers of antiribosomal antibodies showed precipitin reactions with cytoplasmic ribosomes, which were eliminated by ribonuclease treatment.

A solid-phase radioimmunoassay was used to study antibodies with specificity for the protein moiety of ribosomes (Cavanagh, 1977). In this study, a homogeneous subgroup of antiribosomal antibodies detected by immunofluorescence in less than 1% of SLE sera was assayed. These antibodies were unaffected by treatment of tissue sections with ribonuclease, but were eliminated by trypsin treatment. As previously demonstrated, spleen phosphodiesterase was capable of destroying antigenicity of ribonuclease-resistant preparations. This suggested the possibility of persistence of antigenic sites in the "core" RNA oligonucleotide rich in purine bases (Lamon and Bennett, 1970). It was not completely demonstrated that solid-phase-bound ribosomes are susceptible to ribonuclease, whereas trypsin treatment would most likely dissociate the ribosomal preparation from the polystyrene tubes. Therefore, the evidence for antibody to a protein determinant of ribosomes based on the available data appears to be inconclusive.

Further investigation of subpopulations of antiribosomal antibodies is required to assess the clinical and diagnostic value of these antibodies in addition to the previously cited evidence for an association of these antibodies with active disease, especially with renal disease. Serial studies suggest that these antibodies may correlate with episodes of disease activity in selected

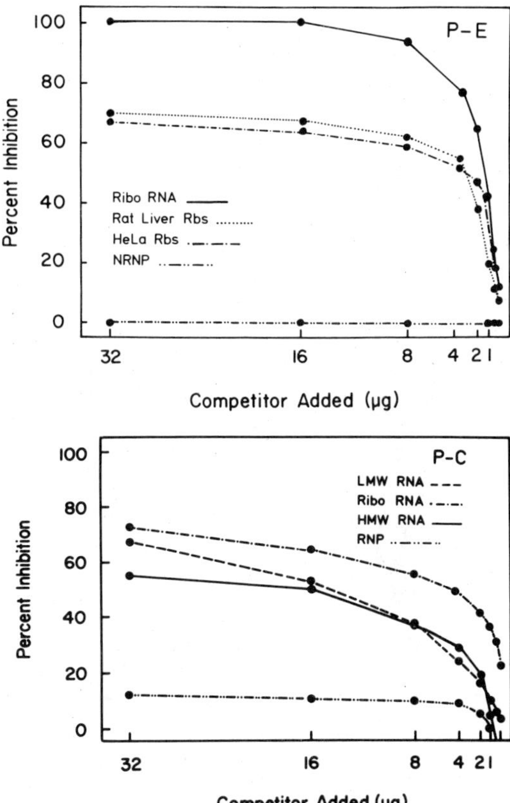

Figures 1 and 2. Radioimmunoassay with labeled cytoplasmic ribosomes showing complete inhibition with rRNA (P-E) and partial inhibition by rRNA (P-C). No significant inhibition is observed for nuclear RNP in either serum.

patients (Fig. 3). This suggests a possible pathogenetic role in the formation of circulating immune complexes, although they may be elevated also during periods of inactive disease in association with increased titers of anti-ssDNA antibodies. The correlation between these antibodies in individual sera (93% of sera positive for antiribosomal antibodies are positive for anti-ss DNA antibodies), in serial studies, and the similar distribution in disease states suggest that immunogens for these antibodies are released simultaneously, perhaps as a result of tissue breakdown.

3. Anti-RNA Antibodies

Antibodies reactive with rRNA were first demonstrated in several SLE sera using RNA-coated latex particles and agar gel precipitation (Lamon and Bennett, 1970). Utilizing a nitrocellulose filter assay (Eilat *et al.*, 1978) with MS [^{125}I]-RNA antigen, approximately 50% of SLE sera were found to contain anti-RNA antibodies, whereas sera from patients with rheumatoid arthritis, Sjögren's syndrome, and progressive systemic sclerosis did not demonstrate significant titers of anti-RNA antibodies. Inhibition of a radioim-

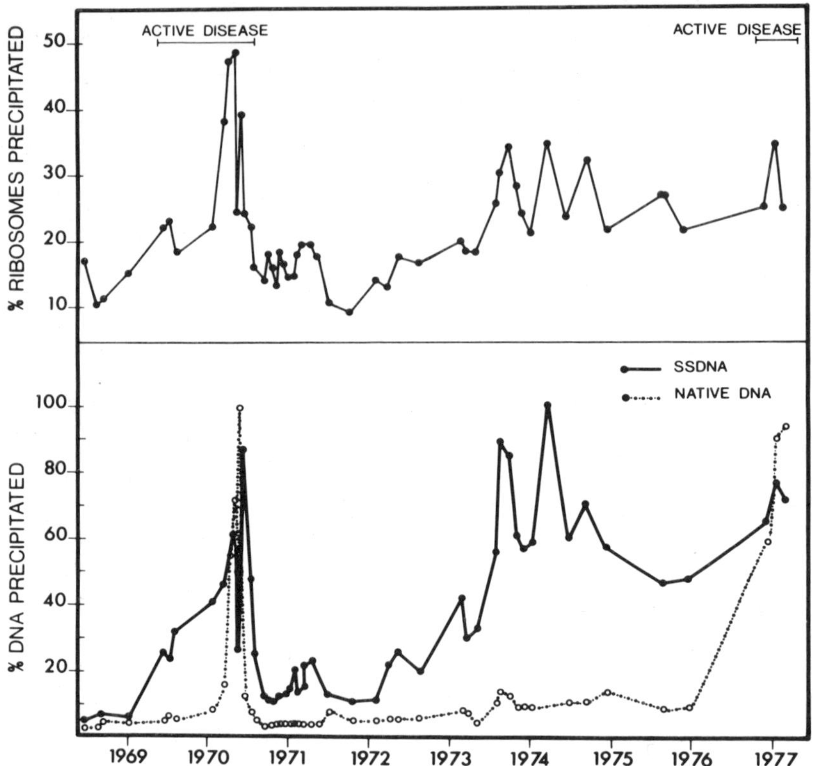

Figure 3. Serial study of patient P-JH showing the titers of antibodies reactive with ribosomes, ssDNA, and native DNA during periods of active disease and in the absence of clinical symptoms. Note the elevation of antibodies to all three antigens during both periods of clinical activity although antibodies to ribosomes and ssDNA were also elevated during inactive periods. The titers of these antibodies were closely correlated throughout the clinical course.

munoassay for antiribosomal antibody (Koffler *et al.*, 1978) indicated that 80% of sera containing antibodies reactive with cytoplasmic ribosomes had specificity for rRNA. The filter assay, in contrast to the Farr-type radioimmunoassay, demonstrated a significant relationship between disease activity in SLE and the presence of anti-RNA antibodies, whereas anti-RNA antibodies detected by inhibition of ribosomal binding showed no selective occurrence in patients with active disease.

The anti-RNA antibody population is heterogeneous and reactive with determinants of high-molecular-weight RNA (structural RNA), low-molecular-weight RNA (tRNA), and isolated nuclear RNA. The failure of nuclear RNA to react with anti-RNA antibodies when RNA is incorporated as a component of nuclear RNP may be related to steric inhibition of RNA determinants inasmuch as nuclear RNP consists of 90% protein and 10% RNA. In contrast, NZB–NZW mice have a unique population of antibodies reactive with tRNA (Eilat *et al.*, 1976, 1977). No significant cross-reactivity was noted for anti-RNA antibodies with ssDNA, native DNA, or poly A.

Both radioimmunoassay procedures had comparable results in regard to the specificity of RNA antibodies. The differences in incidence observed in patients with active and inactive disease may be related to differences in the sensitivity of the assays for detection of subpopulations of antibody. Therefore, the pathogenetic and diagnostic significance of these antibodies remain to be clarified by further investigation.

4. *Anti-Poly A Antibodies*

Antibodies reactive with poly rA were first detected by a hemagglutination assay in 25% of SLE sera (Koffler *et al.*, 1971) and subsequently in approximately 75 to 90% of SLE sera by a sensitive radioimmunoassay employing tritiated poly rA (Pillarisetty and Talal, 1976). In addition, precipitin reactions have been demonstrated with poly rA by agar gel diffusion (Koffler *et al.*, 1971; Schur and Monroe, 1969). These antibodies were found in 50% of sera from patients with discoid LE and in low incidence (less than 10%) in rheumatoid arthritis, Sjögren's syndrome, and normal sera (Pillarisetty and Talal, 1976). Approximately half of the antibody population reactive with dsRNA (polyA·polyU) demonstrated by hemagglutination showed complete or partial inhibition by single-stranded poly rA (Koffler *et al.*, 1971). Studies of the inhibition of the interaction of tritiated poly rA with anti-poly rA using 100% inhibition for poly rA as a standard in this system gave the following results: polyA·polyU 50% inhibition; poly dT–poly rA, 35% inhibition; no significant inhibitory activity was observed for native DNA or ssDNA. Poly rA is a relatively ribonuclease-resistant polynucleotide which is associated with mRNA in nuclei and cytoplasm and with viral nucleic acids. The propensity of this molecule to retain its structural integrity may facilitate immunogenicity. Although the serological significance of these antibodies has not been assessed, increased binding activity mainly of IgG has been observed in patients with active disease. Serum levels of anti-poly rA in SLE are twice the levels found in patients with discoid LE (Pillarisetty and Talal, 1976; Pillarisetty *et al.*, 1975). IgM anti-poly A antibodies, correlated with milder disease, occur in increased incidence in asymptomatic relatives of SLE patients.

5. *Anti-dsRNA Antibodies*

Antibodies reactive with synthetic dsRNA have been demonstrated in 50% of SLE patients using agar gel precipitation (Schur and Monroe, 1969), radioimmunoassay (Schur *et al.*, 1971), or hemagglutination assay (Koffler *et al.*, 1971). A more sensitive filtertype radio immunoassay (Attias *et al.*, 1973) with reovirus RNA detection antibodies reactive with dsRNA in 70% of SLE sera. They have been observed in low incidence (less than 20%) in patients with other rheumatoid diseases. One-fourth of sera positive by radioimmunoassay have demonstrated precipitating antibodies with dsRNA. Several populations of antibodies in this group have been identified by precipitin studies, namely antibodies reactive with poly rA, poly rI, and poly rG (Schur and Monroe, 1969). Strong reactivity of these antibodies with viral dsRNA obtained from reovirus and mycophage dsRNA and a lower degree of reactivity with ribosomal and tRNA was observed. It has been found that single-stranded poliovirus RNA reacts less well than the replicative form of the virus, further indicating the preferential requirement for the double-stranded configuration of RNA (Miller *et al.*, 1975). Although antibodies reactive with dsRNA are heterogeneous, it has been suggested that viral dsRNA may be a possible immunogen for these antibodies. The occurrence of these antibodies, therefore, may provide a clue to the ubiquitous nature of one type of virus in patients with SLE. These antibodies do not appear to have pathogenetic importance since they are not well correlated with disease activity nor are they selectively concentrated in cryoglobulins or in glomerular eluates.

6. Anti-Nuclear RNP Antibodies

Anti-nuclear RNP (nRNP) antibodies require both RNA and a nuclear protein complex for reactivity. The hemagglutination assay utilizing red blood cells coated with crude extracts of rabbit or calf thymus nuclei is a sensitive method for the detection and quantitation of these antibodies (Sharp *et al.*, 1972). Agar gel diffusion reactions have been useful for assessing the specificity of these antibodies and for demonstrating the independence of anti-nRNP antibodies from anti-Sm antibodies, anti-cytoplasmic ribosomal antibodies, and anti-La antibodies (Mattioli and Reichlin, 1973). Counter-immunoelectrophoresis has been employed as a sensitive method for detection of precipitin antibodies (Peltier *et al.*, 1977). The indirect immunofluorescence technique has been used to demonstrate a speckled staining pattern for these antibodies in nuclei, although antibodies to non-RNP nuclear antigens give a similar staining pattern (Northway and Tan, 1972). Ribonuclease treatment of tissue sections is not a reliable method for identifying these antibodies since the titer of several antibodies directed against nuclear antigens decreases following ribonuclease treatment of tissue sections. Complement fixation, one of the earliest techniques used for detection of antibodies to nuclear antigens (Robbins *et al.*, 1957), has been shown to detect anti-nRNP antibodies with a sensitivity comparable to hemagglutination (Akizuki and Steinberg, 1977).

The preparations used for the demonstration of anti-nRNP antibodies, rabbit thymus extract (RTE) and calf thymus extract (ENA), contain a mixture of cytoplasmic and nuclear antigens. This conclusion is based on several observations: antibodies reactive with cytoplasmic ribosomes, which show no reactivity with nRNP, are partially inhibited by RTE or ENA extracts (Fig. 4); the hemagglutination reaction with anti-nRNP antibodies is partially

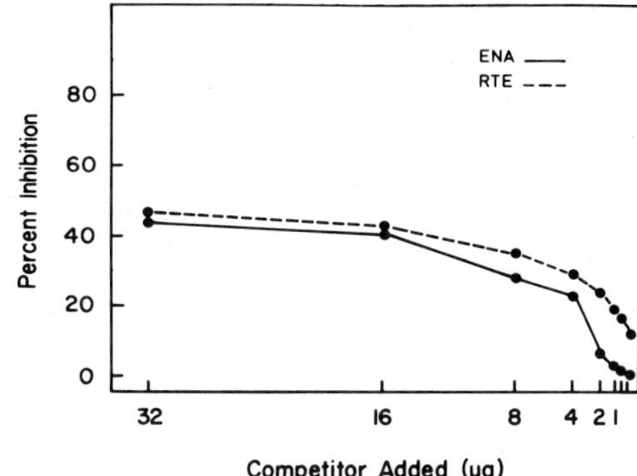

Figure 4. Radioimmunoassay of the mean inhibition of ENA and RTE antigens for the reaction of four SLE sera showing high binding activity with labeled ribosomes.

inhibited by purified cytoplasmic rRNP but not purified rRNA (Table 2); RTE is approximately 9% RNA, and ENA is approximately 1% RNA (Table 3). Inasmuch as 10–12% of RNA-to-protein ratio is characteristic of highly purified nuclear particles obtained by sucrose gradient centrifugation, it is evident that RTE which is a crude extract is contaminated by RNA and/or RNP of cytoplasmic origin. ENA appears to be more selective for nuclear material, but based on the hemagglutination and radioimmunoassay data, there is also cross-reactive material in ENA. Therefore, hemagglutination and agar gel diffusion studies, although primarily detecting antibodies reactive with purified nRNP, also may potentially detect antibodies of cytoplasmic origin.

Anti-nRNP antibodies, observed in approximately 30% of patients with

Table 2. Reactivity of Antibodies to Ribonuclease-Sensitive RTE Antigen (Nuclear RNP)

Serum	Dilution[a]	Cytoplasmic ribosomes[b]	nRNP[c]	RTE[d]	ENA[e]
A	17	0	5[f]	3	6
B	21	5	8	6	16
C	10	0	4	3	5
D	17	3	14	12	14
E	19	0	9	3	8
F	13	4	6	5	7
G	11	3	4	3	5
H	13	0	9	7	11
I	11	0	7	4	6
J	12	0	3	3	6

[a] Endpoint dilution used in the hemagglutination inhibition test expressed as $\log_2$.
[b] Cytoplasmic ribosomes showed no reactivity with anti-Sm antibodies and typical sucrose gradient profiles were obtained for ribosomes and rRna.
[c] Purified nuclear ribonucleoprotein.
[d] Rabbit thymus extract.
[e] Calf thymus nuclear extract.
[f] Inhibition titer of antigen–$\log_2$ titer. Reactivity of all inhibiting antigens eliminated by ribonuclease.

Table 3. Characterization of Antigens Used in Radioimmunoassay and Hemagglutination Studies

	260/280	% RNA	Reactivity with antibodies to: Sm[a]	Ribosomes[b]
ENA	—	1.4	+[c]	+
RTE	—	9.4	+	+
Cytoplasmic ribosomes	1.8	47.0	−[d]	+
Nuclear RNP	1.4	11.6	+	−
Ribosomal RNA	2.0	—	−	+
Nuclear RNA	2.0	—	−	+

[a] Antibodies to Sm antigen assayed by RTE hemagglutination.
[b] Antibodies to ribosomes determined by radioimmunoassay.
[c] Positive reactivity.
[d] No reaction.

active SLE and 10 to 15% with active SLE with renal disease, also occur in scleroderma (20%) and rheumatoid arthritis (10%) (Notman *et al.*, 1975). In all patients with mixed connective tissue disease (MCTD) overlap syndrome, anti-nRNP antibodies are demonstrable, by definition, frequently as a solitary antibody and in high titer. In contrast, patients with SLE commonly have coexistent anti-Sm and anti-nRNP antibodies. Increased titers of anti-nRNP antibodies also have been observed following the administration of procainamide in patients with myocardial infarction, and free nRNP antigen has been demonstrated in the serum of post-myocardial infarction patients without antibody formation in untreated patients (Winfield *et al.*, 1975b).

Quantitation of the amounts of anti-nRNP antibody using precipitin and quantitative complement fixation techniques indicates that these antibodies may comprise a significant portion of the IgG fraction and contribute to hypergammaglobulinemia (Maddison and Reichlin, 1977). Amounts ranging from 0.12 to 8.6 mg specific antibody/ml serum (constituting from 2 to 33% of the total IgG) have been demonstrated. Selected patients with large amounts of this antibody appear to have a vigorous immune response to nRNP, a phenomenon which appears to be linked to relatively low anti-DNA antibody titers. It has been suggested that anti-nRNP antibodies are minor participants in immune complexes (Cano *et al.*, 1977). They are present in low incidence in glomerular eluates (Koffler *et al.*, 1974) and cryoglobulins (Winfield *et al.*, 1975a), but unlike DNA antibodies, they usually do not fluctuate with disease activity. Therefore, the nRNP system does not appear to be prominently related to the induction of renal disease. Although the source of the immunogen for these antibodies has not been identified, the presence of these antibodies in a clinical setting of procainamide administration and circulating nRNPost-myocardial infarction raises the possibility that a haptene may enhance the immunogenicity of endogenous nRNP in hyperimmune SLE patients.

7. *Anti-La Antibodies*

A soluble cytoplasmic RNP nonribosomal antigen (La) present in low incidence (7%) has been described by agar gel precipitation as a system independent of cytoplasmic ribosomes and nRNP (Mattioli and Reichlin, 1974). These antibodies are correlated closely with the presence of antibodies to a non-nucleic acid cytoplasmic precipitating antigen (Ro) which is demonstrable in about 30% of SLE sera (Clark *et al.*, 1969). Eighty percent of sera containing anti-La antibodies contain anti-Mo antibodies in contrast to the negative association observed with anti-nRNP antibodies and anti-native DNA antibodies (Reichlin and Mattioli, 1974). Anti-La and anti-Ro antibodies are found in 25% of sera from patients with Sjögren's syndrome and in less than 2% of sera from patients with rheumatoid arthritis, progressive systemic sclerosis, and polymyositis and are not demonstrable in the sera of patients with discoid LE. They have been observed in a subgroup of antinuclear antibody-negative SLE patients with cutaneous lupus and in patients with a lupus-like syndrome without skin disease (Provost *et al.*, 1977). Therefore, these antibodies may have utility in identifying a subpopulation of SLE patients although their pathogenetic significance has not been clarified.

8. *Antinucleolar Antibodies*

Antinucleolar antibodies demonstrated by indirect immunofluorescence are found in 8 to 10% of patients with rheumatoid disease (Ritchie, 1970).When present in the absence of other antinuclear antibodies, they are highly suggestive of progressive systemic sclerosis, occurring in 50% of these patients. Low-molecular-weight RNA extracted from nucleoli inhibits the reactivity of one population of antinucleolar antibodies (Miyawaki and Ritchie, 1973; Pinnas *et al.*, 1973) which appear to have precipitating activity with nucleolar 7 S RNA (Miyawaki and Ritchie, 1973). A second specificity for antinucleolar antibodies, designated MU antigen, which is sensitive to ribonuclease and trypsin treatment, appears to be antigenically related to cytoplasmic ribosomes (Miyawaki *et al.*, 1978). A third specificity, TM antigen, is resistant to ribonuclease and trypsin treatment and is present both within the nucleolus as well as in extranucleolar material (Miyawaki *et al.*, 1978). No pathogenetic significance has been attributed to the occurrence of these antibodies, but their solitary occurrence in progressive systemic sclerosis is diagnostically useful.

ACKNOWLEDGMENTS. I should like to acknowledge the invaluable contribution of Henry G. Kunkel for his advice and guidance in many of the experimental studies summarized in this chapter, and also to my other colleagues at The Rockefeller University for their contributions to these studies.

References

Akizuki, M., and Steinberg, A., 1977, Demonstration of antibodies to soluble nuclear antigens by complement fixation test: An application of microtiter technique, *J. Immunol. Methods* **18:**295.

Attias, M. R., Sylvester, R. A., and Talal, N., 1973, Filter radioimmunoassay for antibodies to reovirus RNA in systemic lupus erythematosus, *Arthritis rheum.* **16:**719.

Cano, P. O., Jerry, L. M., Sladowski, J. P., and Osterland, C. K., 1977, Circulating immune complexes in systemic lupus erythematosus, *Clin. Exp. Immunol.* **29:**197.

Cavanagh, D., 1977, A solid-phase radioimmunoassay for the detection of antibodies to ribosomes, *Anal. Biochem.* **79:**217.

Clark, G., Reichlin, M., and Tomasi, T. B., 1969, Characterization of a soluble cytoplasmic antigen reactive with sera from patients with systemic lupus erythematosus, *J. Immunol.* **102:**117.

Deicher, H. R. G., Holman, H. R., and Kunkel, H. G., 1960, Anticytoplasmic factors in the sera of patients with systemic lupus erythematosus and certain other diseases, *Arthritis Rheum.* **3:**1.

Eilat, D., Schechter, A. N., and Steinberg, A. D., 1976, Antibodies to native tRNA in NZB/NZW mice, *Nature (London)* **259:**141.

Eilat, D., DiNatale, P., Steinberg, A. D., and Schechter, A. N., 1977, Properties of tRNA-specific antibodies from NZB/NZW mice, *J. Immunol.* **118:**1016.

Eilat, D., Steinberg, A. D., and Schechter, A. N., 1978, The reaction of SLE antibodies with native, single stranded RNA: Radioassay and binding specificities, *J. Immunol.* **120:**550.

Gaudreau, A., Amor, B., Kahn, M. F., Rychewaert, A., Sany, J., and Peltier, A. P., 1978, Clinical significance of antibodies to soluble extractable nuclear antigens (anti-ENA), *Ann. Rheum. Dis.* **37:**321.

Homberg, J. C., Rizzetto, M., and Doniach, D., 1974, Ribosomal antibodies detected by immunofluorescence in systemic lupus erythematosus and other collagenoses, *Clin. Exp. Immunol.* **17:**617.

Koffler, D., Carr, R. I., Agnello, V., Feizi, T., and Kunkel, H. G., 1969, Antibodies to polynucleotides: Distribution in human serums, *Science* **166:**1648.

Koffler, D., Carr, R., Agnello, V., Thoburn, R., and Kunkel, H. G., 1971, Antibodies to polynucleotides in human sera: Antigenic specificity and relation to disease, *J. Exp. Med.* **134:**294.

Koffler, D., Agnello, V., and Kunkel, H. G., 1974, Polynucleotide immune complexes in serum and glomeruli of patients with systemic lupus erythematosus, *Am. J. Pathol.* **74:**109.

Koffler, D., Faiferman, I., and Gerber, M. A., 1977, Radioimmunoassay for antibodies to cytoplasmic ribosomes in human serum, *Science* **198:**741.

Koffler, D., Miller, T. E., and Lahita, R. G., 1978, Studies on the specificity and clinical correlation of antiribosomal antibodies in SLE sera, *Arthritis Rheum.* **22:**463.

Lamon, E. W., and Bennett, J. C., 1970, Antibodies to ribosomal ribonucleic acid (rRNA) in patients with systemic lupus erythematosus (SLE), *Immunology* **19:**439.

Maddison, P. J., and Reichlin, M., 1977, Quantitation of precipitating antibodies to certain soluble nuclear antigens in SLE, their contribution to hypergammaglobulinemia, *Arthritis Rheum.* **20:**819.

Mattioli, M., and Reichlin, M., 1971, Characterization of a soluble nuclear ribonucleoprotein antigen reactive with SLE sera, *J. Immunol.* **107:**1281.

Mattioli, M., and Reichlin, M., 1973, Physical association of two nuclear antigens and mutual occurrence of their antibodies: The relationship of the Sm and RNAprotein (MO)systems in SLE sera, *J. Immunol.* **110:**1318.

Mattioli, M., and Reichlin, M., 1974, Heterogeneity of RNA protein antigens reactive with sera of patients with systemic lupus erythematosus: Description of a cytoplasmic nonribosomal antigen, *Arthritis Rheum.* **17:**421.

Miller, J. R., Caliguiri, L. A., and Tamm, I., 1975, Reaction of poliovirus RNAs with antibodies to double stranded RNA demonstrated by an immunochemical binding assay, *J. Virol.* **16:**290.

Miyawaki, S., and Ritchie, R. F., 1973, Nucleolar antigen specific for antinucleolar antibody in the sera of patients with systemic rheumatic disease, *Arthritis Rheum.* **16:**726.

Miyawaki, S., Kohmoto, K., Kurata, N., and Ofuji, T., 1978, Identification and characterization of two new soluble nuclear antigens reactive with sera of patients with connective tissue diseases, *Arthritis Rheum.* **21:**803.

Northway, J. D., and Tan, E. M., 1972, Differentiation of antinuclear antibodies giving speckled staining patterns in immunofluorescence, *Clin. Immunol. Immunopathol.* **1:**140.

Notman, D. D., Kurata, N., and Tan, E. M., 1975, Profiles of antinuclear antibodies in systemic rheumatic diseases, *Ann. Intern. Med.* **83:**464.

Peltier, A. P., Aussel, T., Haim, T., and Cyna, L., 1977, Ribonucleoprotein (RNP) soluble nuclear antigen: Demonstration of its reaction with serum antibodies by counter-immunoelectrophoresis and further partial characterization, *J. Immunol. Methods* **16:**153.

Pillarisetty, R. J., and Talal, N., 1976, Clinical studies of antibodies binding polyriboadenylic acid in systemic lupus erythematosus, *Arthritis Rheum.* **19:**705.

Pillarisetty, R. J., Becker, M. J., Palmer, D. W., and Talal, N., 1975, Antibodies binding polyriboadenylic acid in systemic lupus erythematosus, *Clin. Exp. Immunol.* **22:**419.

Pillarisetty, R. J., Block, S. R., and Talal, N., 1977, Discordant distribution of IgM and IgG antibodies to DNA and RNA in monozygotic twins with systemic lupus erythematosus, *Arthritis Rheum.* **20:**1314.

Pinnas, J. L., Northway, J. D., and Tan, E. M., 1973, Antinucleolar antibodies in human sera, *J. Immunol.* **111:**996.

Provost, T. T., Razzaque Ahmed, A. R., Maddison, P. J., and Reichlin, M., 1977, Antibodies to cytoplasmic antigens in lupus erythematosus: Serologic marker for systemic disease, *Arthritis Rheum.* **10:**1457.

Reichlin, M., and Mattioli, M., 1974, Antigens and antibodies characteristic of systemic lupus erythematosus, *Bull. Rheum. Dis.* **24:**756.

Ritchie, R. F., 1970, Antinucleolar antibodies: Their frequency and diagnostic association, *N. Engl. J. Med.* **282:**1171.

Robbins, W. C., Holman, H. R., Deicher, H., and Kunkel, H. G., 1957, Complement fixation with cell nuclei and DNA in lupus erythematosus, *Proc. Soc. Exp. Biol. Med.* **96:**575.

Schur, P. H., and Monroe, M., 1969, Antibodies to ribonucleic acid in systemic lupus erythematosus, *Proc. Natl. Acad. Sci. USA* **63:**1108.

Schur, P. H., Moroz, L. A., and Kunkel, H. G., 1967, Precipitating antibodies to ribosomes in the serum of patients with systemic lupus erythematosus, *Immunochemistry* **4:**447.

Schur, P. H., Stollar, B. D., Steinberg, A. D., and Talal, N., 1971, Incidence of antibodies to double stranded RNA in systemic lupus erythematosus and related diseases, *Arthritis Rheum.* **14:**342.

Sharp, G. C., Irvin, W. S., Tan, E. M., Gould, R. G., and Holman, H. R., 1972, Mixed connective tissue disease—An apparently distinct rheumatic disease syndrome associated with a specific antibody to an extractable nuclear antigen (ENA), *Am. J. Med.* **52:**148.

Sharp, G. C., Irvin, W. S., May, C. M., Holman, H. R., McDuffie, F. C., Hess, E. V., and Schmid, F. R., 1976, Association of antibodies to ribonucleoprotein and Sm antigens with mixed connective tissue disease, systemic lupus erythematosus and other rheumatic disease, *N. Engl. J. Med.* **295:**1149.

Sturgill, B. C., and Carpenter, R. R., 1965, Antibody to ribosomes in systemic lupus erythematosus, *Arthritis Rheum.* **8:**213.

Sturgill, B. C., and Preble, M. R., 1967, Antibody to ribosomes in systemic lupus erythematosus: Demonstration by immunofluorescence and precipitation in agar, *Arthritis Rheum.* **10:**538.

Talal, N., Steinberg, A. D., and Daley, G. G., 1971, Inhibition of antibodies binding polyinosinic polycytidylic acid in human and mouse lupus sera by viral and synthetic ribonucleic acids, *J. Clin. Invest.* **50:**1248.

Talal, N., Pillarisetty, R. J., DeHoratius, R. J., and Messner, R. P., 1976, Immunologic regulation of spontaneous antibodies to DNA and RNA. I. Significance of IgM and IgG antibodies in SLE patients and asymptomatic relatives, *Clin. Exp. Immunol.* **25:**377.

Thoburn, R., Koffler, D., and Kunkel, H. G., 1971, Distribution of antibodies to native DNA, single stranded DNA, and double stranded RNA in mouse serums, *Proc. Soc. Exp. Biol. Med.* **136:**711.

Watanabe, N., Fisher, H. M., and Epstein, W. V., 1969, Specificity and reactivity of cytoplasmic and nucleolar antibody in SLE sera, *Arthritis Rheum.* **12:**173.

Winfield, J. B., Koffler, D., and Kunkel, H. G., 1975a, Specific concentration of polynucleotide immune complexes in the cryoprecipitates of patients with systemic lupus erythematosus, *J. Clin. Invest.* **56:**563.

Winfield, J. B., Koffler, D., and Kunkel, H. G., 1975b, Development of antibodies to ribonucleoprotein following short-term therapy with procainamide, *Arthritis Rheum.* **18:**531.

40

Modulation of Autoimmunity by Sex Hormones

Norman Talal

1. Sexual Influence in Autoimmune Disease

It has been known for some time that females are more likely than males to have many autoimmune diseases. Patients with Klinefelter's disease [in which phenotypic males have an extra X chromosome (XXY) and fail to develop male secondary sexual characteristics] also are more likely to develop autoantibodies or autoimmune disease. These patients often have gynecomastia and an abnormality of hormone mechanism which results in hyperestrogenemia (Stern *et al.*, 1977).

Monozygotic twins with Klinefelter's syndrome were recently studied. Both had features of autoimmunity (Michalski *et al.*, 1978). One twin had clinical systemic lupus erythematosus (SLE) and the other had clinical myasthenia gravis (MG). Both had significant levels of antibodies to the acetylcholine receptor, but the twin with SLE also had high-titered antibodies to nucleic acids and to lymphocyte surface antigens. The twin with MG lacked these characteristic SLE findings. These observations support the hypothesis of an important environmental factor in the pathogenesis of autoimmunity, since the twins were identical genetically and hormonally.

No explanation for the female predominance of autoimmunity was forthcoming for many years, but it is now clear from animal studies that sex hormones significantly modulate the expression of autoimmunity. The most extensively studied animal model for lupus is the NZB/NZW F_1 (B/W) mouse, a hybrid of the NZB and NZW strains (Howie and Helyer, 1968). This mouse spontaneously develops an autoimmune disease which is similar to human

Norman Talal · Department of Medicine, University of Texas Health Sciences Center, San Antonio, Texas 78284.

SLE in three important respects: (1) the formation of antibodies to nucleic acids, particularly to double-stranded DNA; (2) the deposition of DNA-containing immune complexes in the kidney, which leads to renal insufficiency and death; and (3) a sex factor which is manifested in earlier onset of disease in females, who usually die before 1 year of age.

It is probable that normal mechanisms of immunologic regulation are disordered in NZB and B/W mice (Talal, 1976). Genetic and/or viral factors may contribute to this regulatory disturbance (Warner, 1973; Levy, 1974). B cells, T cells, macrophages, and thymic epithelial function are all abnormal in this condition. The loss of suppressor T cells with consequent escape of autoantibody-producing B-cell clones is of major interest.

In an attempt to determine the significance of this sex difference, B/W male mice were castrated at 2 weeks of age (prepuberty) (Roubinian *et al.*, 1977). These males, unlike the sham males, had a survival rate identical to that of the sham females (Fig. 1). The castrated females were no different from sham females. Most were dead by the age of 9 or 10 months. This experiment suggested that androgenic hormones have a protective effect.

In the second experiment, prepubertal castration was combined with the sustained administration of either male or female hormones (Roubinian *et al.*, 1978). As hypothesized, there was a prolongation of survival in mice given androgen. Female mice who were castrated and given androgen lived significantly longer than sham-operated females. By contrast, there was a significantly decreased survival time for animals given estrogen. These results suggested that the survival time of these experimental animals was dependent more upon the nature of the sex hormone administered than upon their genetic sex.

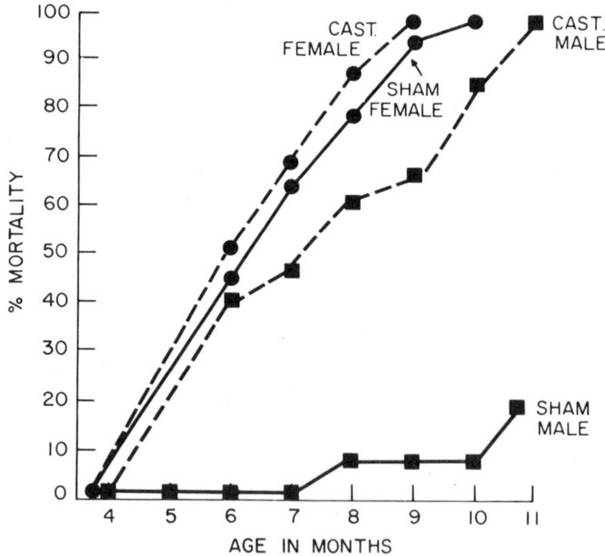

Figure 1. Effect of castration on cumulative mortality in B/W mice.

The sex hormone-dependent changes were reflected in other measurements of autoimmunity. One significant parameter is the amount of IgG antibodies to DNA present in serum. Estrogen accelerated, and androgen delayed, the development of IgG antibodies to DNA. Antibodies to RNA reacted similarly. Mice that received androgen showed less immune complex deposition in the kidneys than did mice that received estrogen, as determined by light, immunofluorescent, and electron microscopy.

Since therapy can be initiated only after signs of disease are present, it was important to study the effects of delayed androgen treatment, initiated at a time when autoimmune disease was more advanced. It was found that delayed androgen treatment (started at 3 and 6 months of age) also prolonged survival in female B/W mice (Roubinian *et al.*, 1979).

Interestingly enough, mice in these experiments had less immune complex nephritis, even though there was no significant reduction in levels of anti-DNA antibodies. Hormonal effects on the complement system or on the elimination of immune complexes may be responsible for prolonged survival despite high concentrations of antibodies to DNA. An effect on antibody formation itself seems unlikely.

The enhanced immunologic reactivity of female mice of many normal strains (compared to males) is observed with both thymus-dependent and thymus-independent antigens. This is also true of cell-mediated immune responses. Augmented immune reactivity comparable to the female response is seen in castrated male mice. The thymus is required for these effects, which may be explained by the action of sex hormones on T-lymphocyte subpopulations, possibly influencing the equilibrium between helper and suppressor cells.

Androgen also increases the concentration of several complement components in mice, including C4 and C5 and the binding protein for C4. The weakly androgenic compound danazol is useful in the treatment of hereditary angioneurotic edema because it increases the concentration of the C1 esterase inhibitor in humans.

2. *Summary*

There are many ways in which sex hormones can interact with the immune system to influence the expression of an autoimmune potential. Androgens suppress and estrogens accelerate the expression of murine lupus as determined by survival rates, concentration of antibodies to nucleic acids, and severity of immune complex nephritis. These results may help explain the female predominance of human lupus and the increased incidence of autoimmunity in patients with Klinefelter's syndrome. The immunoregulatory function of the thymus as well as the complement system may be involved in the action of male hormones. These results support the thesis that SLE is a disorder of immunologic regulation, and that the administration of androgens might create a more balanced immunologic equilibrium in humans.

References

Howie, J. B., and Helyer, B. J., 1968, The immunology and pathology of NZB mice, *Adv. Immunol.* **9:**215.

Levy, J. A., 1974, Autoimmunity and neoplasia: The possible role of C-type viruses, *Am. J. Clin. Pathol.* **62:**258.

Michalski, J. P., Snyder, S. M., McLeod, R. L., and Talal, N., 1978, Monozygotic twins with Klinefelter's syndrome discordant for systemic lupus erythematosus and symptomatic myasthenia gravis, *Arthritis Rheum.* **21:**306.

Roubinian, J. R., Papoian, R., and Talal, N., 1977, Androgenic hormones modulate autoantibody responses and improve survival in murine lupus, *J. Clin. Invest.* **59:**1066.

Roubinian, J. R., Talal, N., Greenspan, J. S., Goodman, J. R., and Siiteri, P. K., 1978, Effect of castration and sex hormone treatment on survival, anti-nucleic acid antibodies, and glomerulonephritis in NZB/NZW F_1 mice, *J. Exp. Med.* **147:**1568.

Roubinian, J. R., Talal, N., Greenspan, J. S., and Goodman, J. R., 1979, Delayed androgen treatment prolongs survival in murine lupus, *J. Clin. Invest.* **63:**902.

Stern, R., Fishman, J., Brusman, H., and Kunkel, H. G., 1977, Systemic lupus erythematosus associated with Klinefelter's syndrome, *Arthritis Rheum.* **20:**18.

Talal, N., 1976, Disordered immunologic regulation and autoimmunity, *Transplant. Rev.* **31:**240.

Warner, N. L., 1973, Genetic control of spontaneous and induced anti-erythrocyte autoantibody production in mice, *Clin. Immunol. Immunopathol.* **1:**353.

41

Thymic and T-Cell Function in Murine and Human Lupus

Marie-Anne Bach and Jean-Francois Bach

The relationship between the thymus and systemic lupus erythematosus (SLE) both in mice and in man has been the matter of extensive investigation and speculation over the last 10 years. Thymic and T-cell abnormalities may be demonstrated in lupus syndromes in association with (or even preceding) autoantibodies, especially antinuclear factors and immune complexes. This basic observation poses the following questions:

1. What is the spectrum of the T-cell deficiency in terms of more recent knowledge on markers and functions of T-cell subsets? Are data as convincing in man as in NZB or B/W mice?
2. What is the cause of the T-cell deficiency? What are the respective roles of thymic epithelial failure and thymocytotoxic autoantibodies which often are found in these disease states?
3. What is the relationship between the T-cell dysfunction and the pathogenesis of autoimmunity?
4. Do the above considerations lead to valid new therapeutic approaches? If so, what is the current status of research in this area?

All of these are important questions not only for systemic lupus but also for a number of other autoimmune diseases that may have similar pathogenetic mechanisms. These questions mentioned above will be reviewed. Data from our laboratories will be emphasized. The reader is referred to several recent general reviews for more extensive literature (Talal, 1976, 1977; Bach *et al.*, 1976).

Marie-Anne Bach and Jean-Francois Bach · INSERM U 25, Hôpital Necker, 75015 Paris, France.

1. Thymic and T-Cell Function in Lupus

1.1. NZB and B/W Mice

1.1.1. T-Cell Markers

The number of T cells evaluated by the theta (Thy-1) marker is not clearly abnormal in NZB and B/W mice until late in life (Waksman *et al.*, 1972). The earliest time when a significant decline has been reported is 10 months (Stutman, 1972). However, when one looks at T-cell subsets by use of their T-cell alloantigens, one may demonstrate a marked and early decrease in the Ly-123$^+$ cells (Cantor *et al.*, 1978) known to be immature T cells, and involved in various complex aspects of regulation of immune responses. One should note also that when combining the theta marker and rosette formation, one may show a premature decline of the theta$^+$ spleen and lymph node rosette-forming cells (Bach *et al.*, 1973). An increased number of theta$^+$ spleen cells binding peanut agglutinin (PNA) in young NZB mice (J.-F. Bach *et al.*, 1978b) has been reported. This observation is not fully understood since PNA is generally considered to be a marker of immature T cells (Ly 123$^+$) said above to be deficient in NZB mice.

1.1.2. Mitogen Responses

The response of spleen cells from NZB and B/W mice to phytohemagglutinin (PHA) and concanavalin A (Con A) is clearly depressed and this depression is seen early in life, at about 4–6 months (Niaudet and Bach, 1976; Leventhal and Talal, 1970).

1.1.3. Antibody Responses

NZB mice generally show increased antibody responses to most antigens. Such increased response is particularly obvious for thymus-independent antigens such as polyvinylpyrrolidone (Bach and Niaudet, 1976) or pneumococcus polysaccharide (Barthold *et al.*, 1974). It is also true for several thymus-dependent antigens (Cerottini *et al.*, 1969). However, the increased responses tend to diminish with age to levels even below responses of nonautoimmune strains. NZB mice also show a depressed capacity to generate the suppressor T-cell factors after activation by Con A, that are normally capable of depressing antibody formation *in vitro* (Krakauer *et al.*, 1976). Thymocytes show an abnormal difficulty in developing tolerance (Playfair, 1971; Staples *et al.*, 1970).

1.1.4. Cell-Mediated Immunity

NZB and B/W mice show depressed MLC reactivity (Rodey *et al.*, 1971) and a depressed capacity of inducing graft versus host reactions. After 1 year of age, they may show delayed rejection of skin allografts (Gelfand and

Steinberg, 1973). Their capacity for generating cytotoxic T cells has been interpreted in diverse ways (Falkoff *et al.*, 1978). In our experience, NZB mice tend to show an increased cytotoxic response to allogeneic cells.

1.1.5. *Thymic Epithelial Function*

The thymic epithelium of NZB mice involutes prematurely (De Vries and Hijmans, 1967). Parallel to this thymic atrophy, one notes an early decline in the serum level of thymic hormones (Bach *et al.*, 1973) as well as in the capacity of thymic epithelium to restore T-cell competence of nude mice (Gershwin *et al.*, 1978; Blankwater and Lia, 1974; Stutman, 1974).

1.2. Human Lupus

A considerable number of studies have been devoted recently to the evaluation of T-cell-mediated immunity in human lupus. Most markers and functions have been found to be depressed at least partially. SLE patients often show decreased E rosette levels (Messner *et al.*, 1973; Hill *et al.*, 1978), low mitogen resposes (Malave *et al.*, 1975), depressed MLC (Suciu-Foca *et al.*, 1974), and low degree of reactivity in delayed hypersensitivity reactions (Abe and Homa, 1971).This effect is not constant nor is it a major one. In the experience of this laboratory, the response to PHA is only moderately depressed (Table 1) and MLC's are subnormal. A selective and nearly complete deficiency of lupus patients in generating cytotoxic T cells after contact with xenogeneic mouse nucleated cells (Table 2) has been shown. This abnormality is reminscent of the observation in the mouse that adult thymectomy also selectively decreases cytotoxic reactions (Bach, 1977). As adult thymectomy induces a selective depletion of Ly-123^+ cells (Cantor and Boyse, 1975), the role of the loss of this population in NZB mice and of its putative equivalent in human lupus is suggested to explain the failure of lymphocytes from SLE patients to generate antixenogeneic cytotoxic T cells. These data emphasize the concept that the lupus syndromes are associated with a decline in certain T-cell subsets that may not be detected when looking at the whole T-cell population, as is done when using the E rosette test. It is interesting that a deficiency of suppressor T cells assessed after Con A

Table 1. PHA Responses of Lymphocytes from Patients with SLE and Rheumatoid Arthritis (RA)

	Peak response (cpm $\times$ 10^{-3})	Response to 100 μ g PHA (cpm $\times$ 10^{-3})
SLE (27)	45.6 ± 11.6[a]	59.1 ± 13.8
Controls (27)	53.4 ± 10.0	62.6 ± 14.6
RA (23)	23.4 ± 4.5	35.8 ± 12.6
Controls (23)	35.4 ± 10.8	48.2 ± 14.4

[a] Mean ± 2 S.E.

Table 2. Xenogeneic CML (Human PBL P-815 Mastocytoma Cells)

	% specific lysis Killer cell/target cell ratio			
	100 : 1	50 : 1	25 : 1	12.5 : 1
Lupus patients (16)	2.3 ± 0.8	2.4 ± 0.9	1.5 ± 0.7	0.7 ± 0.4
Normal subjects (16)	39 ± 5.5	35 ± 1	27 ± 5	19 ± 4
Renal failure (7)	33 ± 3	27 ± 2	17 ± 1.5	14 ± 4

activation has been reported recently in human lupus (Sagawa and Abdou, 1978).

2. *Mechanisms of T-Cell Abnormalities*

The most attractive hypothesis to link all the phenomena mentioned above relates to a primary dysfunction of the thymic epithelium regardless of its etiology, genetic programming for early aging, virus infection, etc. In this hypothesis, the thymus would not be capable of inducing normal T-cell differentiation. The premature cessation of thymic hormone secretion could explain in part or totally this incapacity. The correction of a number of the T-cell abnormalities mentioned above by thymic grafting (Niaudet and Bach, 1976; Gershwin and Steinberg, 1975) or injections of thymic factor (Bach and Niaudet, 1976; Dauphinee *et al.*, 1974) would fit with this hypothesis. An intrinsic deficiency of prothymocytes (or stem cells), which would also explain the recently described apparent intrinsic B-cell abnormalities, also could be taken into consideration. The incapacity of NZB thymic epithelium to restore T-cell function in nude mice, in contrast to the ability of epithelium of other strains to restore it (Blankwater and Lia, 1974; Stutman, 1974), favors the hormone hypothesis.

Alternatively, one might argue that the T-cell abnormalities are secondary to serum changes found in lupus syndromes: circulating immune complexes, known to depress several *in vitro* T-cell functions; anti-T-cell, antithymus antibodies; or other factors. The anti-T-cell antibody is a particularly interesting candidate. It is found with high frequency both in NZB mice (Shirai and Mellors, 1971) and in human lupus (Werner and Kunkel, 1973). Its T-cell specificity might explain its particular effect on T cells. Recent reports suggest that it is particularly active on the suppressor T cells (Klassen *et al.*, 1977).

It is apparent that the overall interpretation is probably intermediate between the two extreme hypotheses just presented. Serological factors probably play a role in mice by aggravating the immune deficiency. They have been shown to be responsible for the delay in allograft rejection (Gelfand *et al.*, 1974). They also may contribute, when present at high titer, to the decreased suppressor T-cell function. In man, they probably explain some of the decrease in E rosettes or delayed-type hypersensitivity reactions, as suggested by the normalization of these abnormalities often observed under steroid treatment and the good correlation found between low E rosette levels and low complement levels (Hill *et al.*, 1978). However, one cannot attribute the early thymic and T-cell changes to these serological factors, particularly to the antithymus antoantibodies. Thus, the kinetics of serum levels of thymic hormone are normal after injection of the circulating thymic hormones in old NZB mice (that show the antithymus antibodies) whereas accelerated hormone catabolism would be seen in the case of peripheral destruction (Bach and Niaudet, 1976). Thymic grafts may prevent some aspects of the autoimmune disease (see further) and, as already mentioned, correct several of the T-cell changes. Finally, the appearance of anti-T-cell anitbody is variable, and contrasts swith the regular onset of thymic changes. The induction of anti-T-cell autoantibody in nude mice after injection of lipopolysaccharide (Izui *et al.*, 1978) illustrates the possibility that the production of the antibodies can be stimulated by dysregulation of the immune system (polyclonal activation in the case of nude mice, loss of suppressor T cells in NZB smice).

3. Relationships between T-Cell Dysfunction and Pathogenesis of Autoimmunity

SLE is clearly a multifactorial autoimmune disease.

Nonimmunological factors intervene. These include: viruses which may be the cause of thymic epithelium infection, source of nuclear antigens, adjuvant of immune responses, or others; sex hormones that probably modulate the immune system; deficiency of certain complement components; extrinsic factors such as UV light or certain drugs. Some of these factors are genetically controlled as may be the immunologic factors described above. Much progress recently has been achieved in NZB mice in advancing our knowledge of genes involved in the control of autoimmunity (Knight *et al.*, 1977; Ratche *et al.*, 1978). Similarly, in man, the linkage of lupus to certain HLA phenotypes (Grumet *et al.*, 1971) has been made. The high frequency of hereditary transmission of the disease or of other related immunological abnormalities has been fully demonstrated (Brunges *et al.*, 1961).

The pathogenetic role of an abnormality of regulatory T cells represents an attractive hypothesis. T-Cell changes represent one of the earliest abnormalities detectable in NZB mice with the exception of the recently described increase of IgM production at birth that might eventually itself relate to the deficiency of maternal suppressor T cells. Treatment of NZB mice with thymocytes from newborn NZB mice or thymic factor protects from some manifestations of autoimmunity (Gershwin and Steinberg, 1975; M.-A. Bach *et al.*, 1978a) and normalizes antibody production against thymus-independent antigens (Bach and Niaudet, 1976; Barthold *et al.*, 1974). The aggravation of the autoimmune disease of both male and female NZB and male B/W mice after neonatal thymectomy fits well with this hypothesis (Roubinian *et al.*, 1977). The observation of prevention of the abnormal anti-DNA antibody production in female B/W mice is a priori more difficult to explain. This paradoxical effect of neonatal thymectomy could be due to a total eradication of helper T cells that are probably necessary for anti-DNA antibody production. In the latter case, the loss of suppressor T cells could not be expressed as it is in nonthymectomized B/W mice that lose thymic function after having built up a pool of long-lasting helper T cells.

The low level of Ly-123$^+$ cells could represent the selective absence of a regulatory cell, crucial to the generation of suppression. In fact, it has recently been shown (Cantor *et al.*, 1978) that Ly-123$^+$ cells are necessary for the expression of T-cell-mediated suppression according to a feedback circuit. Recent experiments show that NZB mice are probably normally capable of generating suppression but lack an intermediate cell necessary for the expression of this suppression (Bach and Bach, unpublished). When DBA/2 (H-2^d) mice are injected with sheep red blood cells (SRBC) and their spleen cells are transferred 14 days later into syngeneic, nonirradiated recipients, the second host shows suppressed capacity of producing anti-SRBC plaque-forming cells after administration of SRBC. NZB mice, in similar transfer experiments, do not show such suppression. However, when NZB spleen cells are transferred into H-2-compatible DBA/2 recipients, suppression is seen, whereas NZB recipients of immunized DBA/2 spleen cells are not suppressed (Table 3). Such intervention of two sets of cells in the development of suppression might explain why, in certain systems, NZB mice do not show any decreased suppressor activity, and may even present with increased suppressive activity (Roder *et al.*, 1977). They might then lack the induced cell population.

The abnormality in the suppressor T-cell system probably does not operate only at the B-cell level, that is, directly on antibody production. The *in vitro* IgM production by B cells from NZB mice has been shown to be normally suppressed by supernatants from activated T cells taken from nonautoimmune strains (Krakauer *et al.*, 1976),which demonstrates the ability of NZB "B" cells to receive suppressor signals. However, the abnormalities of T-cell-mediated suppressor cells could apply to the suppression of helper T cells as well as to that of B cells. In fact, the autoantibody-producing B cell is submitted to the dual action of Ly-1$^+$ helper cells and of Ly-23$^+$ suppressor cells. The Ly-123$^+$ cell, which is a putative precursor of such Ly-

Table 3. Transfer of Suppression in H-2-Compatible Mice

Origin of transferred cells	No. of transferred cells	PFC per spleen ± S.E.	
		DBA/2	NZB
DBA/2	10 × 10	28,714 ± 7,400 (7)	201,834 ± 28,304 (5)
NZB	10 × 10	38,056 ± 9,362 (6)	209,750 ± 32,540 (5)
—	0	175,833 ± 24,470 (9)	410,472 ± 52,144 (7)

1^+ and Ly-23^+ cells, is probably the most abnormally represented cell in NZB mice. It regulates in a complex way the other T-cell subsets and more particularly the Ly-23^+ suppressor T-cell functions.

These considerations are highly speculative. They represent a good working hypothesis which can be tested by therapeutic protocols. Extreme caution must be used before extrapolation of these ideas to human lupus, where far fewer data are available.

4. *Thymic Substitution or Stimulation in Lupus Syndromes*

The thymic and T-cell deficiency observed in NZB and, to a lesser degree, B/W mice has prompted several workers to evaluate various types of thymus-related treatment in NZB and B/W mice.

Thymic grafts or thymocyte injections from neonatal syngeneic donors have been performed successfully by Gershwin and Steinberg (1975) with respect to hemolytic anemia. One should note, however, that such grafts only worked when administered early in life and repeated in time, probably due to the rapid termination of thymus function in autoimmune mice. In older mice, one may see the reappearance of normal mitogen responsiveness (Niaudet and Bach, 1976) but no prevention of autoimmunity.

Suppressor T-cell factors such as the soluble immune response suppressor obtained from Con A-activated mouse spleen cells have been used successfully in B/W mice (Krakauer *et al.*, 1977). Both antinuclear factor production and onset of glomerulonephritis were prevented. However, late treatment did not provide protection any more and eventually aggravated the disease (Steinberg *et al.*, 1978). Presumed "T-cell-stimulating" drugs have also been used, such as levamisole. Partial but significant protection has been obtained in cyclophosphamide-treated B/W mice (Zulman *et al.*, 1978).

Thymic extracts and purified thymic hormones recently have been tested on NZB and B/W mice in several laboratories. Thymic extracts or purified thymic serum factor have been shown to prevent several changes associated with loss of suppressor T-cell activity such as alloantigen-induced thymocyte proliferation in irradiated recipients (Dauphinee *et al.*, 1974), or enhanced production of antibodies against the thymus-independent polyvinylpyrrolidone antigen (Bach and Niaudet, 1976).

More recently, the effects of FTS treatment on the manifestations of autoimmunity (J.-F. Bach *et al.*, 1978a; M.-A. Bach *et al.*, 1978b) have been tested. Several aspects of autoimmunity were considered: anti-DNA antibodies, immune complex glomerulonephritis, Coombs' test defined hemolytic anemia, and Sjögren's syndrome. Previous studies have shown that NZB mice present an autoimmune sialoadenitis (Sjögren's syndrome) which results in atrophy of the submaxillary glands (Kessler, 1968). This atrophy is reflected by a decreased technetium uptake by the submaxillary glands after an intravenous injection of technetium, which is selectively fixed by the exocrine tissues. The curve of the amount of radioactivity in the submaxillary region as a function of time was drawn, and its slope was measured. Anti-DNA antibodies were measured by the Farr technique. Glomerular immunoglobulin deposits were detected in renal biopsies by immunofluorescence technique and proteinuria was regularly measured (M.-A. Bach *et al.*, 1978b). When started at the age of 3 weeks in NZB mice, FTS treatment completely prevented the appearance of Sjögren's syndrome (Table 4) and of hemolytic anemia, whereas it did not prevent anti-DNA antibody production. At variance with these results, when male or female NZB mice were treated from the age of 25 weeks with FTS, male mice, after treatment for 1 month, showed increased anti-DNA antibody titers, whereas females, which present at the same age high anti-DNA antibody titers, were not apparently affected. However, in old female NZB mice (55 weeks) which present lower anti-DNA antibody titers than earlier in their life, FTS treatment restored their anti-DNA antibody production to its previous level. Syngeneic newborn thymic grafts showed the same effects as FTS treatment on anti-DNA antibody production.

B/W mice were treated from the age of 6 weeks (i.e., before the cessation of their endogenous thymic secretion) with synthetic FTS as described above. After 4 months of treatment, FTS-treated mice showed higher anti-DNA antibody levels than did control mice. In parallel, an early glomerulonephritis was observed in FTS-treated mice with proteinuria and with endomembranous glomerular deposits of IgG and IgM. In contrast to these observations, FTS treatment completely prevented Sjögren's syndrome.

In summary, FTS treatment appeared to have strong but somewhat paradoxical effects on the immunological abnormalities of the autoimmune NZB and B/W mice. Early treatment prevented several abnormal immune responses such as high anti-PVP antibody production, hemolytic anemia, or the autoimmune destruction of the salivary glands. On the other hand, anti-DNA antibody production was not prevented by such treatment in NZB mice and was even increased in B/W mice, leading to an accelerated onset of their autoimmune glomerulonephritis. Late treatment increased all immune responses tested, including anti-DNA and anti-PVP antibody production. The effect of such late treatment on the evolution of Sjögren's syndrome has not yet been evaluated. The most likely explanation of these results is that early FTS treatment prevented the disappearance of suppressor cells normally present, and simultaneously stimulated a subpopulation of FTS-dependent helper T cells. The "thymus-independent" immune responses

Table 4. Effect of FTS Treatment in Sjögren's Syndrome (Technetium Uptake by Submaxillary Glands)

	Slope	
FTS-treated NZB mice	136.5 ± 15.9	$p < 0.01$ (FTS-treated vs. control NZB)
Control NZB mice	64.6 ± 5.3	
Nonautoimmune mice (C57BL/6)	111.7 ± 21.2	

(i.e., those which do not require many helper T cells) such as anti-PVP antibody production and probably hemolytic anemia as well as autoimmune sialoadenitis were depressed by the suppressor cells maintained by FTS treatment, whereas the production of thymus-dependent IgG anti-DNA antibodies (Roubinian *et al.*, 1977) is increased by FTS-stimulated helper T cells. In this scheme, late and short-term FTS treatment seemed to restore or stimulate only helper activity.

These data fit with a selective effect of FTS on Ly-123$^+$ cells. These cells play a major role in the regulation of the immune responses, either enhancing or depressing them (Cantor *et al.*, 1978) according to the signals they receive from other T-cell subsets. This could explain the apparently discordant results obtained with FTS treatment. It is notable that a similar enhancement of antinuclear antibody production has recently been reported with thymosin fraction V (Mehta *et al.*, 1978).

In conclusion, thymic substitution or T-cell stimulation does influence the development of autoimmunity. It is apparent that when given alone, such treatment may induce adverse effects and caution is needed before envisaging clinical applications. The undesired effect of helper cells could be circumvented by increasing the hormone dose. Recent data obtained indicate that when given at high dose, FTS shows predominant effects on suppressor T cells (M.-A. Bach *et al.*, 1978a). The effects could be circumvented also by associating with FTS various treatments supposedly active on helper T cells, such as antilymphocyte serum, or eventually cyclosporin A. In any case, the complete alteration in the autoimmune pattern of NZB and B/W mice as shown by disappearance of some manifestations and appearance of others using less than 1 ng FTS, indicates the T-cell control of autoantibody production is central to the disease and a particularly attractive target for any treatment aimed at normalizing the impaired immune system.

References

Abe, T., and Homa, M., 1971, Immunological reactivity in patients with systemic lupus erythematosus, *Acta Rheum. Scand.* **17:**35.

Bach, J.-F., Dardenne, M., and Salomon, J. C., Studies on thymus pproducts. IV. Absence of serum "thymic activity" in adult NZB and (NZB × NZW) F_1 mice, *Clin. Exp. Immunol.* **6:**255.

Bach, J.-F., Bach, M.-A., and Tron, F., 1976, New conceptions of autoimmunity and of systemic lupus erythematosus, in: *Advances in Nephrology*, Vol. 6, p. 5, Year Book Medical Publishers, Chicago.

Bach, J.-F., Bach, M.-A., Charreire, J., Blanot, D., Bricas, E., Charreire, J., Dardenne, M., and Pleau, J. M., 1978a, Facteur Thymique Serique (FTS), *Bull. Inst. Pasteur Paris* **76:**325.

Bach, J.-F., Dardenne, M., London, J., and Pyke, K., 1978b, Studies on the first stages of T lymphocyte maturation, in: *Pharmacology of Immunoregulation* (G. H. Werner and F. Floch, eds.), Academic Press, New York.

Bach, M.-A., 1977, Lymphocyte-mediated cytotoxicity: Effects of aging, adult thymectomy and thymic factor, *J. Immunol.* **119:**641.

Bach, M.-A., and Niaudet, P., 1976, Thymic function in NZB mice. IV. Regulatory influence of a circulating thymic factor on antibody production against polyvinylpyrrolidone in NZB mice, *J. Immunol.* **117:**760.

Bach, M.-A., Fournier, C., and Bach, J.-F., 1978a, Biological activities and site of action of the circulating thymic factor in: *Proceedings, 12th Leukocyte Culture Conference* (M. R. Quastel, ed.),Academic Press, New York, p. 177.

Bach, M.-A., Dardenne, M., and Droz, D., 1978b, Effect of FTS on autoimmune disease in NZB and B/W mice, in: *Pharmacology of Immunoregulation* (G. H. Werner and P. Floch, eds.), pp. 201–205, Academic Press, New York.

Barthold, D. F., Kysela, S., and Steinberg, A. D., 1974, Decline in suppressor T cell function with age in female NZB mice, *J. Immunol.* **112:**9.

Blankwater, M. J., and Lia, P. H. C., 1974, The effect of irradiated thymus grafts from normal littermates, NZB and BALB/c mice on the immune response of nude mice, in: *Proceedings of the First International Workshop on Nude Mice* (J. Nygaard and C. O. Povlsen, eds.), Gustav Fischer Verlag, Stuttgart.

Brunges, S., Zike, K., and Julian, R., 1961, Familial systemic lupus erythematosus: A review of the literature, with a report of ten additional cases in four families, *Am. J. Med.* **30:**529.

Cantor, H., and Boyse, E. A., 1975, Functional subclasses of T lymphocytes bearing different Ly antigens. I. The generation of functionally distinct T cell subclasses is a differentiation process independent of antigen, *J. Exp. Med.* **141:**1276.

Cantor, H., McVay-Boudreau, L., Hugenberger, S., Naidorf, K., Shen, F. W., and Gershon, R. K., 1978, Immunoregulatory circuits among T cell sets. II. Physiological role of feedback inhibition in vivo: Absence in NZB mice, *J. Exp. Med.* **147:**1116.

Cerottini, J.-C., Lambert, P. H., and Dixon, F. J., 1969, Comparison of the immune responsiveness of NZB and NZB × NZW F_1 hybrid mice with that of other strains of mice, *J. Exp. Med.* **130:**1093.

Dauphinee, M. J., Talal, N., Goldstein, A. L., and White, A., 1974, Thymosin corrects the abnormal DNA synthetic response of NZB mouse thymocytes, *Proc. Natl. Acad. Sci. USA* **71:**2637.

De Vries, M. J., and Hijmans, W., 1967, Pathological changes in thymic epithelial cells and autoimmune disease in NZB, NZW and (NZB × NZW)F_1 mice, *Immunology* **12:**179.

Falkoff, R. A., Scavalli, J. F., and Dutton, R. W., 1978, Independent analysis of T helper and T killer cell functions in young and old NZB mice, *J. Immunol.* **121:**897.

Gelfand, M. C., and Steinberg, A. D., 1973, Mechanism of allograft rejection in NZB mice. I. Cell synergy and its age-dependent loss, *J. Immunol.* **10:**1652.

Gelfand, M. C., Parker, L. M., and Steinberg, A. D., 1974, Mechanism of allograft rejection in NZB mice. II. Role of a serum factor, *J. Immunol.* **113:**1.

Gershwin, M. E., and Steinberg, A. D., 1975, Suppression of autoimmune hemolytic anemia in NZB mice by syngeneic young thymocytes, *Clin. Immunol. Immunopathol.* **4:**38.

Gershwin, M. E., Ikeda, R. M., Kruse, W. L., Wilson, F., Shifrine, M., and Spangler, W., 1978, Age-dependent loss in NZB mice of morphological and functional characteristics of thymic epithelial cells, *J. Immunol.* **120:**971.

Grumet, C., Coukell, A., Bodmer, J. G., Bodmer, W. F., and McDevitt, H. O., 1971, Histocompatibility antigens (HL-A) associated with systemic lupus erythematosus, *N. Engl. J. Med.* **285:**193.

Hill, G. S., Hinglais, N., Tron, F., and Bach, J.-F., 1978, Systemic lupus erythematosus: Morphologic correlations with immunologic and clinical data at the time of biopsy, *Am. J. Med.* **64:**61.

Izui, S., Louis, J., and Lambert, P. H., 1978, The spontaneous development of thymocytotoxic antibodies in athymic nude mice and its suppression after transfer of syngeneic thymocytes, *Eur. J. Immunol.* **8:**221.

Kessler, H. S., 1968, A laboratory model for Sjögren's syndrome, *Am. J. Pathol.* **56:**571.

Klassen, L. W., Krakauer, R. S., and Steinberg, A. D., 1977, Selective loss of suppressor cell function in NZB mice induced by NTA, *J. Immunol.* **119:**830.

Knight, J. G., Adams, D. D., and Purves, H. D., 1977, The genetic contribution of the NZB mouse to the renal disease of the NZB × NZW hybrid, *Clin. Exp. Immunol.* **28:**352.

Krakauer, R. S., Waldmann, T. A., and Strober, W., 1976, Loss of suppressor T cells in adult NZB/NZW mice, *J. Exp. Med.* **114:**662.

Krakauer, R. S., Strober, W., Rippeon, D. L., and Waldmann, T. A., 1977, Prevention of autoimmunity in experimental lupus erythematosus by soluble immune response suppressor, *Science* **196:**56.

Leventhal, B. G., and Talal, N., 1970, Response of NZB and NZB/NZW spleen cells to mitogenic agents, *J. Immunol.* **104:**918.

Malave, I., Layrisse, Z., and Layrisse, M., 1975, Dose-dependent hyperreactivity to phytohemagglutinin in systemic lupus erythematosus, *Cell. Immunol.* **15:**231.

Mehta, J., Knotts, L., Craig, C., Brukholder, S., Miller, C., and Hahn, B., 1978, Effect of altered lymphocyte function on immunologic disorders in NZB/NZW mice. III. Acceleration of disease by thymosin, *Arthritis Rheum.* **21:**196.

Messner, R. P., Lindstrom, P. D., and Williams, R. C., Jr., 1973, Peripheral blood lymphocyte cell surface markers during the course of systemic lupus erythematosus, *J. Clin. Invest.* **52:**3046.

Niaudet, P., and Bach, M.-A., 1976, Thymic function in NZB mice. I. Duration of thymic function in New-Zealand Black (NZB) mice, *Clin. Exp. Immunol.* **23:**328.

Playfair, J. H. L., 1971, Strain differences in the immune response of mice. III. A raised tolerance threshold in NZB thymus cells, *Immunology* **21:**1037.

Raveche, E. S., Steinberg, A. D., Klassen, L. W., and Tjio, J. M., 1978, Genetic studies in NZB mice. I. Spontaneous autoantibody production, *J. Exp. Med.* **147:**1487.

Roder, O. C., Bell, D. A., and Singhal, S. K., 1977, Regulation of the immune response in autoimmune NZB/NZW F_1 mice. I. The spontaneous generation of splenic suppressor cells, *Cell. Immunol.* **29:**272.

Rodey, G. E., Yunis, E. J., and Good, R. A., 1971, Progressive loss of in vitro cellular immunity with ageing in strains of mice susceptible to autoimmune disease, *Clin. Exp. Immunol.* **9:**305.

Roubinian, J. R., Papoian, R., and Talal, N., 1977, Effects of neonatal thymectomy and splenectomy on survival and regulation of auto-antibody formation in NZB/NZW mice, *J. Immunol.* **118:**1524.

Sagawa, A., and Abdou, N. I., 1978, Suppressor cell dysfunction in systemic lupus erythematosus: Cells involved and in vitro correction, *J. Clin. Invest.* **62:**789.

Shirai, T., and Mellors, R. C., 1971, Natural thymocytotoxic autoantibodies and reactive antigens in NZB and other mice, *Proc. Natl. Acad. Sci. USA* **68:**1412.

Staples, P. J., Steinberg, A. D., and Talal, N., 1970, Induction of immunological tolerance in old New Zealand mice repopulated with young spleen, bone marrow, or thymus, *J. Exp. Med.* **131:**123.

Steinberg, A. D., Krakauer, R. S., Reinertsen, J. L., Klassen, L. W., Ufeld, D., Reeves, J. P., Williams, G. W., and Antonovich, T., 1978, Therapeutic studies in NZB/NZW mice. VI. Age-dependent effects of concanavalin A-stimulated spleen cell supernate, *Arthritis Rheum.* **21:**204.

Stutman, O., 1972, Lymphocyte subpopulations in NZB mice: Deficit of thymus-dependent lymphocytes, *J. Immunol.* **109:**602.

Suciu-Foca, N., Buda, J., Theim, J., and Reemstma, K., 1974, Impaired responsiveness of lymphocytes in patients with systemic lupus erythematosus, *Clin. Exp. Immunol.* **18:**296.

Talal, N., 1976, Disordered immunological regulation and autoimmunity, *Transplant. Rev.* **31:**240.

Talal, N. (eds.) 1977, *Autoimmunity: Genetic, Immunologic, Virologic, and Clinical Aspects*, Academic Press, New York.

Waksman, B. H., Raff, M. C., and East, J., 1972, T and B lymphocytes in NZB mice: An analysis of the theta, TL, and MBLA markers, *Clin. Exp. Immunol.* **11:**1.

Werner, P., and Kunkel, H., 1973, Antibodies to a specific surface antigen of T cells in human sera inhibiting mixed leukocyte culture reactions, *J. Exp. Med.* **138:**1021.

Zulman, J., Michalski, J., McCombs, C., Greenspan, J., and Talal, N., 1978, Levamisole maintains cyclophosphamide-induced remission in murine lupus erythematosus, *Clin. Exp. Immunol.* **31:**321.

42

Immune Regulatory Abnormalities in Systemic Lupus Erythematosus

Alfred D. Steinberg, Josef S. Smolen, Tsuyoshi Sakane, Shunichi Kumagai, Chicao Morimoto, Thomas M. Chused, Ira Green, Fusao Hirata, Katherine A. Siminovitch, and Robert T. Steinberg

1. Introduction

Systemic lupus erythematosus (SLE) is a multisystem autoimmune disease characterized by B-cell hyperactivity, autoantibody formation, and by antibody-mediated tissue damage which leads to tissue inflammation in many organs. Genetic factors have been shown to play a role in the disorder on the basis of both family studies and associations with particular immune-associated antigens coded for in the major histocompatibility complex (Benacerraf and McDevitt, 1972; Decker *et al.*, 1979). However, multiple genes and multiple factors appear to modify the expression of illness (see Table 1). Moreover, the multiplicity of immune defects in patients with SLE and the differences among patients have complicated establishment of abnormalities which underlie the illness and those which result therefrom.

The working hypothesis for the last 10–15 years has been that SLE is a multifactorial disease (Table 1) both in humans and in mice (Steinberg *et al.*, 1969, 1981). Some factors may be necessary but not sufficient for disease expression. Different factors may carry different weight in different individuals. Thus, a strong environmental insult may induce disease in many, but not all, genetic types. Alternatively, in some individuals a sufficient genetic predisposition may allow rather trivial environmental insults of many diverse types to induce disease.

Alfred D. Steinberg, Josef S. Smolen, Tsuyoshi Sakane, Shunichi Kumagai, Chicao Morimoto, Thomas M. Chused, Ira Green, Fusao Hirata, Katherine A. Siminovitch, and Robert T. Steinberg · Section on Cellular Immunology, Arthritis and Rheumatism Branch, National Institute of Arthritis, Metabolism and Digestive and Kidney Diseases, NIH, Bethesda, Maryland 20205.

Table 1. Pathogenic Factors in SLE

Genetic	It appears that more than one gene is necessary for the development of SLE in humans and in mice. In the presence of appropriate background genes, a single accelerating gene may be sufficient to induce a severe disease which otherwise might be mild or asymptomatic. As a result of the interaction of several genes in order to bring about illness, patients with SLE may have normal parents or parents with other autoimmune problems. Nevertheless, family and twin studies show a clear-cut, though complex, pattern of inheritance. In mice, individual genes appear to predispose to particular autoimmune features (Raveche *et al.*, 1981).
Immune	Excessive B-cell activity includes generalized B-cell hyperactivity as well as a selective increase in particular autoantibodies.
	T-Cell abnormalities are complex. Defects in both helper and suppressor function are present. Different patients may have different defects. In mice, stem cells appear to be defective (Morton and Siegel, 1974; Eisenberg *et al.*, 1980; Laskin *et al.*, 1982).
Environmental	In mice, administration of polyclonal immune activators can accelerate disease or bring it about in mice that are not destined to get ill (Steinberg *et al.*, 1969; Smathers *et al.*, 1982). Viruses can accelerate or retard SLE in mice (Tonietti *et al.*, 1970; Oldstone and Dixon, 1972).
	It is known that sun exposure may accelerate disease in some patients with SLE. It is likely that a variety of environmental factors, especially infectious agents, may modify the pace of illness in patients.
Dietary	Recent studies have suggested that drastic alterations in diet may markedly influence the pace of illness in mice (Fernandes *et al.*, 1976; Prickett *et al.*, 1981). Such an effect has not yet been found in humans.
Hormonal	It appears that estrogens accelerate and androgens retard SLE. This hormonal effect is suggested by the predominance of SLE in humans during the child-bearing years. (NZB × NZW)F_1 mice have been shown experimentally to have marked retardation of disease when androgen treatment is initiated before weaning. Such an approach helps us to understand pathogenetic factors in SLE, but may not be useful as therapy. In addition, hormonal effects are not found in the BXSB mouse model of SLE (in fact, the males have accelerated illness relative to the females) and they are only minimal in NZB mice.

We have taken clues from studies with mice with SLE-like illnesses in our studies of patients with SLE. The present paper summarizes a great number of studies which were designed to shed light upon the cellular basis for human SLE. We are forced to conclude that multiple factors may underlie SLE and that the cellular basis may be different in individual patients.

2. Materials and Methods

Patients. Patients with SLE were seen in the outpatient or inpatient services of the Arthritis and Rheumatism Branch, NIADDK at the Clinical Center of the National Institutes of Health. All patients satisfied preliminary ARA criteria for SLE except for a rare patient in whom a high serum anti-DNA level was substituted for a positive LE cell test. Whenever possible, patients were studied prior to the onset of treatment with corticosteroids. In patients already receiving corticosteroids, blood was obtained at least 24 hr after the last dose. All blood was obtained in the morning in order to avoid variations in results due either to exertion or to endogenous hormone secretion.

Isolation of Peripheral Blood Mononuclear Cells. Peripheral blood was diluted in Hanks' balanced salt solution (HBSS) and separated over Ficoll–Hypaque or lymphocyte separation medium (Litton Bionetics, Rockville, Md.). The Interface cells were washed twice with HBSS and adherent cells removed on plastic petri dishes (Sakane *et al.*, 1978a; Smolen *et al.*, 1981a). The adherent cells were recovered later. Nonadherent cells were separated into T-cell and (B + null)-cell populations by rosetting with neuraminidase-treated sheep red blood cells (Sakane *et al.*, 1978a) or with a 5% suspension of untreated sheep red cells (Smolen *et al.*, 1981a). T cells were further separated into $T4^+$ and $T8^+$ subsets by killing with monoclonal antibodies + C (Smolen *et al.*, 1981b).

Study of Con A-Activated Suppressor Cells. T cells, 5×10^6, were incubated for 3 days with 50 μg Con A (Pharmacia Fine Chemicals, Piscataway, N.J.). To guarantee sufficient macrophage function, 3×10^5 macrophages (MØ), previously treated with mitomycin C, were added to the cultures. The Con A-activated cells were harvested, washed, treated with mitomycin C, and added to new cells obtained from the same donor which were stimulated in different ways in several assay systems. Control T cell were incubated without added Con A.

Autologous Mixed Lymphocyte Reaction. The AMLR was performed as described previously (Sakane *et al.*, 1978b; Smolen *et al.*, 1981a). This reaction consists of the proliferation of T cells in response to stimulation with equal numbers of autologous non-T cells or separated subsets of non-T cells. Equivalent results were obtained when the studies were performed in autologous serum, Ab serum, or selected fetal calf serum; however, the magnitude of the responses differed from assay to assay as well as from day to day.

Enrichment in Autologous Rosette-Forming T Cells. Although it has been shown that rosetting with autologous RBC does not provide a T-cell subset that is different from that obtained by rosetting with unrelated human RBC (Smolen *et al.*, 1981c), such rosetting cells provide a T-cell subset with special properties functionally. The ARFT were obtained by mixing 4×10^8 RBC/2 ml and 10^7 T cells/1 ml as described previously (Kumagai *et al.*, 1981a).

Studies of TNP-Modified Cells. The AMLR using TNP-modified autologous cells as well as the studies of killing of TNP-labeled cells were carried out as recently described (Kumagai *et al.*, 1981a).

Antibody-Dependent Direct Cellular Cytotoxicity. The ability of antibodies to T cells to kill T cells by ADCC was determined as recently described (Kumagai *et al.*, 1981b).

T-Cell Phenotyping. T cells from patients with SLE and controls were analyzed by flow cytometry as described (Smolen *et al.*, 1982).

3. Results

3.1. B-Cell Studies

3.1.1. Numbers of B and T Cells in the Blood of Patients with SLE

Patients with inactive SLE had near-normal numbers of B and T cells in the peripheral blood (approximately 60 to 85% of normal). In contrast, patients with active SLE had a marked reduction in numbers of both B and T cells to approximately 15 to 30% of normal.

3.1.2. Spontaneous Proliferation of B-Cell-Enriched Fraction in SLE

Peripheral blood mononuclear cells were obtained and the B-cell-enriched fraction studied for spontaneous incorporation of tritiated thymidine into cellular DNA during the first 16 hr of culture. It was found that cells from patients with SLE, regardless of disease activity, had significantly greater proliferation than did control cells. The magnitude of the increase was approximately 10-fold (Table 2).

3.1.3. Spontaneous Production of Antibodies by Cells from Patients with SLE

It is well known that patients with SLE produce autoantibodies. However, the increased proliferation of the B cells of patients suggested that a generalized B-cell hyperactivity might be present, rather than one just involving cells destined to make autoantibodies. In order to determine whether or not cells were making nonautoantibody antibody, numbers of cells producing antibodies to irrelevant haptens (to which the patients had not been exposed) were determined. It was found that with increasing disease activity there were increasing antihapten antibody-forming cells (Table 2).

3.1.4. Relationship between Disease Activity in SLE and Various Laboratory Measures

Antibodies to DNA and serum C are commonly used clinically to help in the assessment of disease activity of patients with SLE. Twenty-four

Table 2. Spontaneous Proliferation and Spontaneous Production of Antihapten Antibodies by B-Cell-Enriched Fractions from Patients with SLE

Patient group[a]	Proliferation[b]	Antihapten PFC[c]
Controls	0.4 ± 0.1	2
Inactive SLE	3.8 ± 1.1	8
Mildly active SLE	4.6 ± 1.0	26
Active SLE	4.4 ± 1.0	109

[a] Between 23 and 28 individuals in each group.
[b] Tritiated thymidine incorporation ($\times 10^{-3}$) during a 16-hr culture initiated immediately after isolation of the cells.
[c] IgG plaque-forming cells per 10^5 B cells.

Table 3. Correlations among Various Laboratory Measures and Disease Activity in 24 Patients with SLE[a,b]

	IgG	IgM	Anti-DNA	C3	ESR	IgG AFC
Disease activity	0.644	0.539	0.711*	−0.562	0.611	0.777*
Serum IgG	—	NS	0.735*	NS	0.863*	0.722*
Serum IgM	—	—	0.700*	NS	NS	NS
Anti-DNA	—	—	—	NS	0.687	0.591
C3	—	—	—	—	NS	NS
ESR	—	—	—	—	—	0.683
WBC	NS	NS	NS	NS	NS	NS

[a] All numbers listed are correlation coefficients obtained by Spearman rank order analysis. NS, not significant at $p = 0.01$; number without asterisk, significant between 10^{-2} and 10^{-4}; asterisk, $p < 10^{-5}$.
[b] AFC, numbers of antibody-forming cells producing IgG by reverse plaque assay; C3, the third component of complement determined by radial immunodiffusion; ESR, erythrocyte sedimentation rate (Westergren); WBC, white blood cell count; anti-DNA was determined by a modified Farr assay; serum IgG and IgM concentrations were determined by radial immunodiffusion disease activity was determined at the time of blood drawing by ADS.

patients were graded by ADS on a 0–10 scale with regard to disease activity as determined by history and physical exam immediately prior to blood drawing at 8 AM. This activity score was then compared with several laboratory studies determined on the basis of blood drawn at that time. It was found that anti-DNA, measured by the Farr assay, strongly correlated with disease activity ($p < 10^{-5}$). C3 levels correlated negatively with disease activity. Additional measures also were found to correlate with disease activity: serum IgG concentration and erythrocyte sedimentation rate correlated very well (Table 3). However, the best correlate of disease activity was the number of IgG antibody-forming cells in the blood (Blaese *et al.*, 1980).

3.2. T-Cell Studies

Patients with active SLE were found to have a fourfold reduction in numbers of peripheral blood T cells. In addition, we have consistently noted that patients with active SLE have large numbers of autologous erythrocytes in the mononuclear cell layer during Ficoll–Hypaque separation. These autologous erythrocytes appear to be attached to mononuclear cells.

3.2.1. Studies of Helper Function

We have repeatedly observed a marked helper cell impairment in the peripheral blood of patients with SLE. This is true of help for *in vitro* immunoglobulin synthesis as well as help for specific immune responses. An *in vivo* correlate may be the observation we have made that patients with active SLE have very poor primary immune responses to immunization. They also have markedly impaired skin test responses to recall antigens.

Recently we have found that patients with SLE have a marked impairment of T-cell help for B-cell colony formation (Kumagai *et al.*, 1982). This T-cell helper defect was especially noteworthy in view of the observation in the same study that SLE patients had an abnormally great ability to produce B-cell colonies.

3.2.2. *Studies of Suppressor Cell Function*

Our initial studies involved the analysis of Con A-activated T cells. Such cells had previously been shown to suppress various immune responses in an antigen-nonspecific manner. In our studies, Con A-activated T cells were added to a second culture in which the responder cells were autologous to the Con A-activated cells. In such studies, it was found that patients with SLE had a marked functional defect in their ability to suppress the B-cell proliferative response to pokeweed mitogen (Table 4). However, there was considerable variability among the various patients and with the T cells from a single patient with regard to suppression of different responses. The study of Con A-activated T cells from 10 individuals with SLE on four different responses is shown in Table 5. Most, but not all, patients had a defect in suppression of the PWM response and in the MLR; however, most had normal suppression of the proliferative response to PHA. About half were abnormal in their ability to suppress the proliferative response to Con A. Therefore, among SLE patients generally and in a given patient there is not a global defect in suppressor cell function. Rather, selective abnormalities are observed.

3.2.3. *The Autologous MLR in Patients with SLE*

The ability of T cells to respond to autologous non-T cells has been termed the AMLR. This reaction was studied in patients with SLE and in normal controls (Sakane *et al.*, 1978b). It was found that patients with active SLE were markedly defective in this form of cellular intercourse (Table 6). Moreover, the patients with active disease were much more defective than were those with inactive disease.

3.2.4. *Serial Studies of T-Cell Functions in Patients with SLE*

In order to determine whether or not the differences noted above were, in fact, attributable to disease activity, individual patients were studied when

Table 4. Con A-Activated T Cells from Normals, but Not SLE Patients, Suppress the Proliferative Response of Autologous B cells to Pokeweed Mitogen

Group[a]	Mean % suppression ± S.E.M.
Controls	40.6 ± 3.1
Active SLE	3.8 ± 5.9

[a] Ten individuals per group.

Table 5. Variability of Con A-Induced Suppressor Function among Patients with Active SLE[a]

	Percent suppression of the indicated immune response of autologous cells			
Patient	Proliferation to PHA (normal, 39–77)	Proliferation to Con A (normal, 60–78)	Proliferation to PWM (normal, 23–58)	Proliferation to allogeneic cells (normal, 35–92)
1	46	63	0	51
2	97	72	18	7
3	58	36	29	13
4	29	0	6	3
5	88	60	0	10
6	56	34	17	17
7	48	58	2	15
8	62	78	0	56
9	65	31	0	7
10	62	60	56	63

[a] After culture for 3 days, Con A-activated cells were treated with mitomycin C and added to autologous cells freshly drawn for the indicated assays all of which were performed in the optimal dosages and for the optimal periods of time. Patient 4 was subnormal for every response—her cells did not suppress normally any of the responses. Patient 10 suppressed all normally. The other patients had defects in one or two assays except for patients 3 and 6 who were defective in three of the four assays.

their disease was active and remotely when the disease was quiescent (Table 7). It was found that Con A-induced suppressor function was markedly impaired during active disease, but that it returned to normal during remission. This was true of Con A-induced suppression of the MLR (the proliferative response to allogeneic cells) and of the proliferative response of B cells to PWM (Table 7). In addition, patients with very defective AMLR activity during active disease had normal AMLR activity when their disease was inactive (Table 7).

3.2.5. *Ability of SLE T Cells to Differentiate into Killer T Cells*

In view of the marked impairment of the AMLR in active SLE, additional studies were performed. We believed that studying modified self determinants on lymphocytes might help us to understand losses of self tolerance in association with autoimmunity. As a result, an AMLR culture was per-

Table 6. The AMLR in Patients with SLE

		Tritiated thymidine incorporation $\times 10^{-3}$ cpm	
Group	Number	Mean	Range
Normal controls	38	9.5	5.1–27.5
Inactive SLE	15	5.0	1.6–11.4
Active SLE	18	0.9	0.0–2.2

Table 7. Effect of Disease Activity on the Generation of Con A-Induced Suppressor Function and AMLR in Individual Patients

Patient	Percent suppression					
	MLR		PWM		AMLR (cpm × 10^{-3})	
	Active	Inactive	Active	Inactive	Active	Inactive
1	14	63	28	81	0.5	10.5
2	9	66	16	70	0.7	10.0
3	17	62	17	74	0.8	12.1
4	3	66	6	80	1.1	7.7

formed, not just with autologous non-T cells, but also with TNP-modifed autologous cells. It was found that during such cultures, cytotoxic T cells were generated which could kill TNP-modified autologous cells (Kumagai *et al.*, 1981a). Moreover, cells from patients with active SLE, which failed to mount a proliferative response in the AMLR, mounted an abnormally high cytotoxic response to TNP-self cells (Table 8).

3.2.6. *Studies of Antibodies to T Cells Produced by Patients with SLE*

In a series of studies, it has become apparent that patients with SLE produce antibodies which interfere with normal T-cell function. Of particular interest was the observation that such antibodies could interfere with suppressor T-cell function (Twomey *et al.*, 1978). That would provide a possible explanation for the defect in suppressor T-cell function observed in such patients. However, as noted above, the defects in suppressor function were inconstant. As a result, it appeared that a much more selective effect of anti-T must occur or that there were both intrinsic defects in T-cell function and superimposed antibody effects. In addition, some SLE anti-T-cell antibodies killed only a very small fraction of all T cells, 5–10%, and yet abolished all suppressor function (Sakane *et al.*, 1979; Smolen *et al.*, 1981a). Since T cells which form rosettes with human erythrocytes (ARFT) are thought to represent an important T-cell subset, we studied the ability of SLE anti-T to kill

Table 8. Dissociation of the AMLR and the Generation of Cytotoxic T Cells against Hapten-Modified Targets[a]

Group	AMLR (cpm × 10^{-3})	% killing of TNP-target
Inactive SLE	5	4
Mildly active SLE	2	9
Active SLE	0	16

[a] SLE T cells were cultured with autologous non-T cells which had been modified with TNP. They were then tested for their ability to either proliferate in response to stimulation by autologous non-T cells (AMLR) or to kill TNP-modified autologous cells labeled with ^{51}Cr.

Table 9. Ability of SLE Anti-T-Cell Antibodies to Selectively Kill Autologous Rosette-Forming T Cells (ARFT)

	Percent killed at indicated dilution of antibody				
Cells	1:5	1:10	1:20	1:40	1:80
ARFT	84	81	79	76	70
T cells	32	30	18	15	7
Non-ARFT	28	19	15	9	1

ARFT and non-ARFT. Such studies were performed with several SLE anti-T. It was consistently found that the ARFT were killed selectively (Table 9).

3.2.7. *Demonstration of Suppressor Cells without the Requirement for Con A Induction as well as the Selective Killing of Such Cells by SLE Anti-T*

The AMLR and the TNP-AMLR were established with normal T cells and normal autologous non-T cells. An aliquot of the responder T cells was first treated with SLE anti-T-cell antibody + C. Such pretreated T cells mounted a much more vigorous AMLR, suggesting that the SLE anti-T had killed off suppressor cells selectively (Table 10, lines 1 and 2). Addition of ARFT autologous to the responder cells restored the normal suppressor function and overcame the SLE anti-T pretreatment (Table 10, line 3). Control non-ARFT failed to suppress (Table 10, line 4).

We took advantage of the availability of identical twins with SLE, one of which was active and one of which was inactive, to further study this exciting finding. T cells from the inactive twin mounted a good TNP-AMLR (Table 11, line 1) whereas T-cells from the twin with active SLE responded less vigorously (Table 11, line 2). Plasma from the active twin plus C pretreatment of the inactive twin's T cells caused a significant increase (Table (Table 11, line 3), whereas pretreatment with plasma from the inactive twin

Table 10. Ability of SLE Anti-T-Cell Antibodies to Selectively Kill Cells Which Suppress the AMLR and the TNP-AMLR

Treatment with SLE anti-T[a]	Addition of ARFT[b]	Addition of non-ARFT[b]	% of control response: AMLR	% of control response: TNP-AMLR
0	0	0	100	100
+	0	0	255[c]	240[c]
+	+	0	120[d]	110[d]
+	0	+	250[e]	255[e]

[a] Control non-SLE antibody and inactive SLE antibody had no effect.
[b] 2.5×10^4 cells added to 1×10^5 responder T cells.
[c] Increase in response by elimination of suppressor T cells.
[d] Addition of ARFT restores the normal AMLR. The SLE anti-T selectively kills ARFT which suppress the response.
[e] Non-ARFT are not able to suppress the response.

Table 11. Naturally Occurring (Noninduced) Suppressor T Cells Are Present in Inactive SLE, but Not Active SLE: A Study Using Identical Twins Discordant for Disease Activity[a]

T cells from inactive twin[b]	T cells from active twin	Active plasma	Fresh T cells added	TNP-AMLR (cpm $\times 10^{-3}$)
+	0	0	0	11.8 ± 1.0
0	+	0	0	4.3 ± 0.7
+	0	+	0	19.9 ± 1.1[c]
+	0	+	Active	21.8 ± 2.0
+	0	+	Inactive	10.1 ± 1.4[d]

[a] These twins were shown to be identical by both WBC and RBC typing at over 40 loci.
[b] A total of 1×10^5 responder cells were in each culture. When two sets of cells were added, 70% of the cells were from the first patient (anti-T-cell antibody + C pretreated) and 30% of the cells were from the second patient (fresh cells).
[c] Significant augmentation by pretreatment of T cells with anti-T-cell antibodies + C in the active twin's plasma.
[d] Significant suppression of the augmented response by suppressor T cells from the inactive twin, but failure of suppression by T cells from the active twin.

was ineffective (data not shown). Moreover, addition of fresh T cells from the inactive twin was able to suppress the response (Table 11, line 5); but fresh T cells from the active twin were not suppressive (Table 11, line 4). This study demonstrates the presence of suppressor T cells in a fresh T-cell population (not mitogen induced) from a patient with inactive disease, but their absence in a patient with active disease. It also shows that the patient without suppressor cell function had anti-T antibody which could eliminate suppressor function from her inactive identical twin.

3.2.8. *Antilymphocyte Antibodies of Patients with SLE Can Interact Specifically with a Membrane-Associated Modulator of Cellular Metabolism Necessary for Activation and Proliferation*

The antilymphocyte antibodies were further studied for their interaction with lipomodulin (Hirata *et al.*, 1981). Lipomodulin is a protein in the membranes of leukocytes which regulates—inhibits—the activity of the membrane-associated enzyme phospholipase A2. The enzyme cleaves phosphatidylcholine to liberate unsaturated fatty acids (mainly arachadonic acid) and lysophosphatidylcholine. Thus, by inhibiting the enzyme, lipomodulin inhibits the generation of arachadonic acid and the subsequent cellular processes dependent thereupon. This lipomodulin-mediated inhibition is removed by antibodies to lipomodulin. Such antibodies might thus serve to alter the ability of normal cellular regulation. A search for such antibodies was made. Indeed, they were found in the sera of many patients with SLE and also in the sera of (NZB $\times$ NZW)F_1 and MRL-lpr/lpr mice, both of which develop an illness resembling SLE. The MRL-lpr/lpr mice had higher titers of antibody to lipomodulin than did the (NZB $\times$ NZW)F_1. This result is consistent with their earlier onset of immune abnormalities, autoimmunity, and severe immunopathology as well as the unregulated lymphoproliferation observed in these mice. A total of 16 of 26 SLE sera were found to have antibodies to lipomodulin (Table 12). These antibodies were found to be of the IgM class in several of the patients.

3.2.9. *Ability of SLE Anti-T-Cell Antibodies to Mediate ADCC against T Cells: A Mechanism for in Vivo Destruction of T Cells or T-Cell Subsets*

Many, but not all, of the studies of anti-T-cell antibodies described to this point are most easily demonstrated in the IgM fraction of SLE sera. Moreover, the IgM antibodies are most easily demonstrated by reacting them with a target cell population and C at low temperatures. As a result, considerable doubt has been generated regarding the *in vivo* relevance of such antibodies. Although the antibodies could, of course, interact with T cells at higher temperatures and alter T-cell function in a more subtle manner than by C-mediated killing, we felt that it was important to demonstrate that anti-T could, in fact, mediate killing by a mechanism possible in the body. This led to a direct test of the ability of SLE anti-T-cell antibodies to mediate antibody-dependent, C-independent, direct cellular cytotoxicity (ADCC). This mechanism is a likely mode of tissue destruction in a variety of autoimmune diseases in a variety of organs. As a result, it would be especially suitable as a mechanism by which anti-T antibodies of patients with SLE interfered with normal T-cell function. Indeed, we found that SLE antibody could mediate ADCC against human T cells (first three lines of Table 13) and that such antibodies were present in active SLE but not inactive SLE or normal controls. Fractionation of the antibodies into IgG and IgM fractions indicated that IgG was mediating the ADCC. Much greater T-cell killing was observed with the IgG fraction than with the unseparated antibody (Table 13, lines 4 and 5). In addition, the IgG fraction of inactive SLE was positive (Table 13, line 6). Normal control IgG was not (Table 13, line 8). The cytotoxicity observed was inhibited by cold (unlabeled) antibody-coated target cells as well as by aggregated human IgG. Therefore, ADCC was, indeed, the mechanism of the killing. Antibodies obtained from patients during the active phases of their disease were able to kill freshly drawn T cells from the same individuals when their disease was quiescent. Therefore, these are truly autoantibodies; however, they cross-react widely with human T cells from other donors.

Table 12. Presence of Antilipomodulin Antibody in Sera of Patients with SLE

Group	Number with antilipomodulin/ total
Normal controls (HUMAN)	0/20
SLE	16/26[a]
MRL-*lpr*/*lpr* mice	14/14
(NZB × NZW) F_1 mice	15/18

[a] The antibody was found to be of the IgM class.

Table 13. Ability of IgG Anti-T-Cell Antibodies from Patients with Active SLE to Mediate the Killing of T Cells by Antibody-Dependent, C-Independent Direct Cellular Cytotoxicity (ADCC)

Source of antibody used to coat target T cells	% cytotoxicity (ADCC)[a]
Normal controls (total Ig)	1.4 ± 0.4
Inactive SLE (total Ig)	2.9 ± 0.5
Active SLE (total Ig)	15.8 ± 2.1
Active SLE IgG	26.7 ± 3.4
Active SLE IgM	2.8 ± 0.6
Inactive SLE IgG	12.6 ± 1.9
Inactive SLE IgM	2.2 ± 0.8
Normal control IgG	1.8 ± 0.5
Normal control IgM	0.8 ± 0.6

[a] The effector cells were unfractionated mononuclear cells. Cytotoxicity was inhibited by excess cold targets coated with the IgG fraction of SLE anti-T and by aggregated human IgG. The cytotoxicity was equivalent when autologous T-cell targets or unrelated human T-cell targets were used. Thus, the antibodies were truly autoantibodies, but recognized determinants shared by human T cells generally.

3.2.10. *T-Cell Phenotyping Suggests That SLE May Not Represent a Single Disease*

Over the years, a number of physicians have appreciated that the clinical and laboratory findings in individual patients with SLE vary greatly. Indeed, some patients have very different findings than do others. As a result, the variability of the expression of SLE has become well recognized. Nevertheless, it generally has been felt that SLE represents one disease, but that individual variability is due to differences in genetic backgrounds and environmental insults. In order to explore this problem, we studied the T-cell phenotypes of patients with SLE. In our initial studies we evaluated 29 patients with SLE (Morimoto *et al.*, 1980). Those patients were selected on the basis of drug therapy. As a result, patients with active renal disease and many patients with CNS disease were excluded by virtue of their therapy with immunosuppressive drugs or high doses of corticosteroids. That study concluded that patients with active SLE had a high ratio of $T4^+$ cells : $T8^+$ cells. That conclusion, however, results from patient selection. Patients with widespread multisystem disease were in the active group. The inactive group contained patients with more severe major organ involvement who were now in remission. The latter interpretation was possible because a second study was carried out without selection in an additional 32 patients (Smolen *et al.*, 1982). An additional group of patients has now been studied bringing the total close to 100. Table 14 summarizes the more recent data. Patients with a high R_T were found to differ from those with a low R_T with regard to certain clinical and laboratory features. They also shared certain abnormalities. For example, arthralgias and arthritis is widespread in patients with SLE and may be found in any group. Nevertheless, such abnormalities as Sicca syndrome, false-positive STS, muscle disease, and lymphadenopathy

Table 14. Separation of Patients with SLE on the Basis of T-Cell Phenotyping[a]

	Clinical and laboratory characteristics
Low R_T	Renal disease common, often severe
	Lymphopenia common
	Thrombocytopenia common
	Widespread multisystem disease uncommon
	Sicca syndrome uncommon
High R_T	Severe renal disease less common
	Widespread multisystem disease common
	Sicca syndrome common
	Lymphadenopathy common
	False-positive STS common
	Muscle disease common
Normal R_T	Most widespread disease
	Can have severe renal and CNS disease
	Features of high-R_T or low-R_T groups may occur

[a] Patients were divided into those with a subnormal R_T (< 1.04), a normal R_T (1.04–2.20), and a high R_T (> 2.20). R_T = % Leu 3a or OKT 4 cells/% Leu 2a or OKT 8 cells.)

are common in the high-R_T group, but not in the low-R_T group. Severe renal disease is more common in the low-R_T group, whereas widespread multisystem disease is more common in the high-R_T group. These differences are statistically highly significant by looking at the continuum of R_T and the presence of the clinical features as well as by X^2 analysis. The intermediate group with a normal R_T tends to share features of the other two groups. This group has many patients with CNS disease and patients may have renal disease as well as a widespread multisystem disorder. Patients with high R_T did not have a greater degree of disease activity nor a different treatment regimen, especially steroid dose, to explain their different T cell phenotypes.

4. *Discussion*

It is abundantly clear that patients with SLE produce autoantibodies. As a result, the proximate cause of their problems relates, in large measure, to those autoantibodies. However, many people, patients with SLE and others, produce large amounts of autoantibodies without associated symptomatology. As a result, the mere production of autoantibodies is not sufficient to bring about disease manifestations. Additional factors which lead to tissue injury are necessary. In addition, autoantibody production could be a primary event or it could result from more fundamental problems. However, the resolution of this chicken or the egg first question is very difficult in humans.

Despite the complexity of the problem and the inability to manipulate human lymphoid organs or perform the types of studies possible in experimental animals, study of immune abnormalities in SLE has shed considerable light upon the questions of pathogenesis of a variety of immune-related problems and has contributed to fundamental understanding in areas of immunobiology generally.

In this paper, we have presented evidence that SLE patients have B cells which proliferate excessively and which make too much immunoglobulin. However, it was noted that the proliferation, by itself, was not sufficient to result in illness. Inactive patients had proliferating B cells without excessive antibody or autoantibody production. As a result, it appears that a second signal—such as antigen or a helper T-cell signal—may be necessary to bring about excessive antibody or excessive autoantibody production. Alternatively, or in addition, a loss of T-cell suppressor function—in this case inhibition of differentiation into antibody secreting cells—may lead a patient from an inactive to an active state.

Of interest, there was a very strong correlation between clinical disease activity and antibody production whether measured by serum IgG concentration, serum anti-DNA, or total numbers of antibody-forming cells. However, since most antibody is not thought to be made in the blood, but in the lymphoid organs, and since patients with hypergammaglobulinemia associated with other illnesses may not have increased peripheral blood antibody-forming cells (such as some patients with Sjögren's syndrome), it is possible that the increased numbers of peripheral blood antibody-forming cells observed are secondary to an injury to endothelium or a derangement in the marrow or spleen so as to allow accelerated egress of such cells from their normal habitats into the blood.

Despite the mild uncertainty regarding the antibody-forming cells, patients with active SLE make much antibody and often make much anti-DNA. In fact, one of our patients made 3.94 mg anti-DNA/ml serum, an amount which represented one-quarter of all of her antibody (Steinberg *et al.*, 1972). The enormous amounts of antibody to a variety of self antigens found in this disease must have some explanation. We sought an explanation in the regulatory T cells which are thought normally to regulate the B cells. Before moving to the T cells, however, the very high anti-DNA deserves a comment. It is the clinical experience of one of us (A.D.S.) that patients with very high anti-DNA may be responsive to very vigorous therapy and, thereafter, run a benign course, even if renal disease was initially present. However, failure to vigorously treat such patients is often associated with progressive disease. In contrast, patients with lesser amounts of anti-DNA may respond less well to therapy. This paradox may be explained by the killing off of clones of B cells (or also helper T cells) which are necessary for anti-DNA production. This is not to say that all patients with very high anti-DNA always do well. The point is mentioned because it is widely thought that the higher the anti-DNA, the worse the prognosis. We are making the point that this may not always be the case and that there may be an exception at the extreme end of the spectrum.

In our attempt to understand the regulation of autoantibody production in patients with SLE, we carried out a series of studies of T-cell functions.

Very early studies, performed in collaboration with Dr. T. Waldmann, were performed in an attempt to analyze the suppressor functions of patients' T cells with regard to B-cell immunoglobulin production. We consistently found that SLE T cells has such a marked inability to help in immunoglobulin production that it was impossible to study the suppressor function in the assays. More recent studies have shown a defect in SLE T cells with regard to the ability to support the growth of B-cell clones. This has forced us to the conclusion that T cells from patients with active SLE do not function very well. However, the B cells from the patients are not wanting. They make much immunoglobulin despite inadequate help, and excessive B-cell colonies were produced despite inadequate T-cell help. In other words, the B cells appear to be semiautonomous. They are often hyperactive despite, rather than because, the inadequacy of the helper T cells.

In view of the difficulty in explaining B-cell hyperactivity on the basis of excessive helper function, we turned our full attention to suppressor function. The initial studies were a mixed blessing. Indeed, defects in Con A-induced suppressor function were found in many patients with SLE. However, the failure of suppression was present with regard to some immune functions and not others. The B-cell response to PWM could not be suppressed very well at all. In contrast, the T-cell response to PHA was usually quite well suppressed. That was not terribly discouraging since B-cell hyperactivity was the central problem in SLE. Therefore, defects in suppression of B cells, but not of T cells, would be quite consistent with the known abnormalities in SLE. However, individual patients differed markedly in their ability to suppress or not suppress various responses. This presented a degree of complexity which made study even more difficult. This difficulty was, in part, resolved by studying the same individuals serially. We found that an individual, when active, might have impaired suppressor cell function; but, when inactive, the same individual would be normal. Thus, there appeared to be a correlation between disease activity and excessive antibody production on the one hand and defective suppressor function on the other. However, there were considerable questions regarding the physiologic significance of Con A-induced suppressor cells. As a result, we devised a system to study suppressor function in an unmanipulated T-cell population. In such studies, we still found that when a patient had active disease there was impaired suppressor function, but that when the disease was inactive, suppressor function returned to normal. Moreover, the suppressor cells were enriched in a subset of T cells which form rosettes with human erythrocytes (ARFT).

The association between disease activity, excessive antibody production, and loss of suppressor function would be quite neat and complete were it not for one complicating factor. That was the recognition that anti-T-cell antibodies are produced by many patients with active SLE. As a result, we tried to determine whether or not the anti-T-cell antibodies produced might be responsible for the observed loss of suppressor cells. In fact, we found that IgM anti-T + C led to killing of T cells, including especially suppressor cell precursors, but not mature suppressor cells. Such antibodies could, therefore, reduce the pool of suppressor cell precursors and, thereby, reduce the ultimate expression of suppressor cell function. Moreover, some of the antilymphocyte antibodies were found to bind specifically to lipomodulin, a known regulatory protein in the lymphocyte membrane. The binding by such antibodies to lipomodulin would allow the dysregulation of the cellular metabolism and a predisposition to activation and proliferation. Such antibodies might lead to further B-cell proliferation, perhaps bypassing the need for helper or antigenic signals.

Two additional problems remained. The first was that anti-T-cell antibodies worked very well *in vitro* at low temperatures, but that patients' bodies were close to 37°. There was skepticism that such cold-reactive antibodies might interfere with normal immune factions at body temperature. We therefore carried out a study to determine if T-cell killing could occur by a mechanism commonly responsible for tissue destruction in autoimmune diseases: antibody-dependent, C-independent, direct cellular cytotoxicity (ADCC). We found that T cells from other humans, or even from the same patient, were killed at 37° by SLE IgG anti-T-cell antibodies by the mechanism of ADCC. Thus, it is possible that IgG anti-T-cell antibodies can exert their effects *in vivo*. In addition, the IgM anti-T-cell antibodies could alter recirculation patterns of T cells, without killing them, as has been found in mice (Gelfand *et al.*, 1974).

The second problem is more difficult: the chicken or the egg problem. That is, do the anti-T cell antibodies come first and interfere with regulatory T-cell function or vice versa. If the anti-T-cell antibodies come first, the T-cell regulatory defects would all be secondary to a B-cell product—an autoantibody. In that case, SLE would be a B-cell disorder with a variety of interesting T-cell epiphenomena. On the other hand, if the regulatory T-cell problem came first, it would help to explain the production of autoantibodies by B cells and their progeny. Unfortunately, this last question remains unanswered. However, we have observed examples of patients with regulatory T-cell abnormalities without large amounts of anti-T-cell antibodies and patients with large amounts of anti-T-cell antibodies without functional abnormalities. Therefore, it is possible that, in individual patients, the antibodies may come first in some, and the T-cell defects may come first in others. Perhaps very careful serial studies will allow a better answer in the future.

One of the common threads of our work has been the variability among patients with regard to immune functions. We asked directly whether or not individual patients might differ with regard to the two major T-cell subsets of humans, the OKT 4^+ or Leu $3a^+$ T cells, which include many (but not all) of the helper–inducer functions, and the OKT 8^+ or Leu $2a^+$ subset, which includes many of the suppressor and cytotoxic functions. We found that the ratio of these two populations, termed R_T, varied much more among patients with SLE than among normal controls. Indeed, there were approximately 50% of the SLE patients in the normal range and about 50% out of the normal range. Those patients who fell out of the normal range of R_T were evenly divided between abnormally low R_T and abnormally high R_T. There were marked differences in clinical and laboratory expressions of illness in the patients in the two groups of abnormal R_T. These differences were not, however, representative of a discrete subdivision of patients with SLE. Rather, there was a continuous spectrum from the lowest R_T to the highest R_T, through the normal range, of progressively increasing sicca syndrome, lymphadenopathy, muscle disease, false-positive STS, and widespread multisystem disease; there was progressively less lymphopenia, thrombocytopenia, and severe renal disease. Therefore, SLE represents not a single disease, but rather a symptom complex with variable expression and with some relationship between T-cell subsets and the expression of illness. However, the exact mechanism by which the T-cell subsets and the clinical and laboratory findings may be related is unknown at the present time.

During the course of our studies, we have emphasized experiments which might shed light upon self–self immune cell interactions. As a result, we have been especially hopeful that understanding of the AMLR might shed light upon the normal interactions between T cells and non-T cells and possible defects in those interactions in patients with SLE. Our initial studies indicated that patients with active SLE had a defect in the AMLR. Their T cells responded much less well to signals from autologous non-T cells than did normal T cells. However, we recently have found that macrophages (MØ) can suppress the AMLR (Smolen *et al.*, 1981a) and that the macrophage suppression takes precedence over stimulation by B cells. Moreover, addition of MØ as late as 48 hours after culture initiation still results in suppression of the (B + null) cell induced AMLR. As a result, patients with reduced numbers of B cells and relatively increased numbers of MØ might be expected to manifest suppression of the AMLR. Thus, the regulatory T cells of patients with SLE may be prevented by MØ from responding to signals from B cells. In addition, the T cells themselves appear to be hyporesponsive. Thus, the normal cellular intercourse is disrupted in SLE by defects in B-cell function, defects in T-cell function, and by anti-T-cell antibodies and by anti-B-cell antibodies.

Our studies of the AMLR have further indicated that organs rich in MØ, such as the spleen, would be expected to normally express much more stimulation of T cells by MØ, whereas organs depleted of MØ, relative to B cells (such as the lymph node), would manifest much more stimulation of T cells by B cells. In addition to the implication of these findings for normal immune responsiveness, there are implications for patients with SLE. Different subsets of T cells are stimulated by B cells and MØ (Hausmann and Stobo, 1979; Raff *et al.*, 1980; Hausmann *et al.*, 1981). As a result, different types of immune circuits would be expected to predominate in the spleen and lymph nodes. In patients with SLE, lymphadenopathy has been associated with a high R_T. This result provides a clue to the association between R_T and clinical expression of illness. Different immune circuits in different lymphoid organs may be expressed to varying degrees in different patients.

Further work on analyses of lymph node function in patients with SLE is in progress. We hope that such studies will allow for a more definitive picture of the immune defects in individual patients.

Although the precise cellular bases of SLE in different patients remain to be elucidated, it is clear that the immune abnormalities favor perpetuation of the initiated abnormal processes. Excessive proliferation of B cells serves as an underlying substratum for excessive antibody production. Antilipomodulin antibodies and other antibodies reactive with B cells serve to trigger B cells to further proliferate and differentiate. The anti-T-cell antibodies tend to eliminate suppressor T-cell precursors, thereby removing an important check upon unregulated B-cell hyperactivity. Thus, once started, the autoimmune process is self-perpetuating. It is apparent that avoiding the triggering of the process would be most desirable. Once started, suppression of the immune processes with drugs may allow the disease to be brought under control. Thereafter, however, there is no consensus regarding the means to prevent a subsequent disease flare. We believe that specific immune intervention as well as preventive practices should dominate thinking about therapeutic intervention. Until we are in a position to predict who is subject to developing SLE, such maneuvers would best be applied when the first remission is induced.

In summary, SLE is a multisystem disease which appears to be different in different individuals. As a result, it is possible that different approaches to therapy should be based not upon the details of the kidney biopsy but, rather, the immune profile of the patient. The drugs we give are still crude; however, they may be life-saving. We hope that further study of the immune system will allow specific defects to be uncovered in individual patients and for those to be corrected in a more specific and less toxic manner than is currently possible.

References

Benacerraf, B., and McDevitt, H. O., 1972, Histocompatibility-linked immune response genes, *Science* **175:**273.

Blaese, R. M., Grayson, J., and Steinberg, A. D., 1980, Elevated immunoglobulin secreting cells in the blood of patients with active systemic lupus erythematosus: Correlation of laboratory and clinical assessment of disease activity, *Am. J. Med.* **69:**345.

Decker, J. L., Steinberg, A. D., Reinertsen, J. L., Plotz, P. H., Balow, J. E., and Klippel, J. H., 1979, Systemic lupus erythematosus: Evolving concepts, *Ann. Intern. Med.* **91:**587.

Eisenberg, R. A., Izui, S., McConahey, P. J., Hang, L., Peters, C. J., Theofilopoulos, A. N. and Dixon, F. J., 1980, Male determined accelerated autoimmune disease in BXSB mice: Transfer by bone marrow and spleen cells, *J. Immunol.* **125:**1032.

Fernandes, G., Yunis, E. J., and Good, R. A., 1976, Influence of diet on survival of mice, *Proc. Natl. Acad. Sci. USA* **73:**1279.

Gelfand, M. C., Parker, L. M., and Steinberg, A. D., 1974, Mechanism of allograft rejection in New Zealand mice. II. Role of a serum factor, *J. Immunol.* **113:**1.

Hausmann, P. B., and Stobo, J. D., 1979, Specificity and function of a human autologous reactive T cell, *J. Exp. Med.* **149:**1537.

Hausmann, P. B., Stites, D., and Stobo, J. D., 1981, Antigen-reactive T cells can be activated by autologous macrophages in the absence of added antigen, *J. Exp. Med.* **153:**476.

Hirata, F., delCarmine, R., Nelson, C. A., Axelrod, J., Schiffman, E., Warabi, A., DeBlas, A. L., Nirenberg, M., Mangiello, V., Vaughan, M., Kumagai, S., Green, I., Decker, J. L., and Steinberg, A. D., 1981, Presence of autoantibody for phospholipase inhibitory protein, lipomodulin, in patients with rheumatic diseases, *Proc. Natl. Acad. Sci. USA* **78:**3190.

Kumagai, S., Steinberg, A. D., and Green, I., 1981a, Immune responses to hapten-modified self and their regulation in normal individuals and patients with SLE, *J. Immunol.* **127:**1643.

Kumagai, S., Steinberg, A. D., and Green, I., 1981b, Antibodies to T cells in patients with SLE mediated ADCC against human T cells, *J. Clin. Invest.* **67:**605.

Kumagai, S., Sredni, B., House, S., Steinberg, A. D., and Green, I., 1982, Defective regulation of B lymphocyte colony formation in patients with systemic lupus erythematosus, *J. Immunol.* **128:**258.

Laskin, C. A., Smathers, P. A., Reeves, J. P., and Steinberg, A. D., 1982, Studies of defective tolerance induction in NZB mice: Evidence for a marrow pre-T cell defect, *J. Exp. Med.* **155:**1025.

Morimoto, C., Reinherz, E. L., Schlossman, S. F., Schur, P. H., Mills, J. A., and Steinberg, A. D., 1980, Alterations of immunoregulatory T cell subsets in active systemic lupus erythematosus, *J. Clin. Invest.* **66:**1171.

Morton, J. I., and Siegel, B. V., 1974, Transplantation of autoimmune potential. I. Development of antinuclear antibodies in H-2 histocompatible recipients of bone marrow from New Zealand Black mice, *Proc. Natl. Acad. Sci USA* **71:**2162.

Oldstone, M. B. A., and Dixon, F. J., 1972, Inhibition of antibodies to nuclear antigen and to DNA in New Zealand mice infected with lactate dehydrogenase virus, *Science* **175:**784.

Prickett, J. D., Robinson, D. R., and Steinberg, A. D., 1981, Dietary enrichment with the polyunsaturated fatty acid eicosapentaenoic acid prevents proteinuria and prolongs survival in NZB × NZW F_1 mice, *J. Clin. Invest.* **68:**556.

Raff, H. V., Picker, L. J., and Stobo, J. D., 1980, Macrophage heterogeneity in man: A subpopulation of HLA-DR bearing macrophages required for antigen-induced T-cell activation also contains stimulators for autologous reactive T cells, *J. Exp. Med.* **152:**581.

Raveche, E. S., Novotny, E. A., Hansen, C. T., Tjio, J. H., and Steinberg, A. D., 1981, Genetic studies in NZB mice. V. Recombinant inbred lines demonstrate that separate genes control autoimmune phenotype, *J. Exp. Med.* **153:**1187.

Sakane, T., Steinberg, A. D., and Green, I., 1978a, Studies of immune functions of patients with SLE. I. Failure of suppressor T cell activity related to impaired generation of, rather than response to, suppressor cells, *Arthritis Rheum.* **21:**657.

Sakane, T., Steinberg, A. D., and Green, I., 1978b, Failure of autologous mixed lymphocyte reactions between T and non-T cells in patients with systemic lupus erythematosus, *Proc. Natl. Acad. Sci. USA* **75:**3464.

Sakane, Ts., Steinberg, A. D., Reeves, J. P., and Green, I., 1979, Studies of immune functions in patients with systemic lupus erythematosus: T cell subsets and antibodies to T cell subsets, *J. Clin. Invest.* **64:**1260.

Smathers, P. A., Steinberg, B. J., Reeves, J. P., and Steinberg, A. D., 1982, Effects of polyclonal immune stimulators upon NZB. *xid* congenic mice. *J. Immunol.* **128:**1414.

Smolen, J. S., Sharrow, S. O., Reeves, J. P., Boegel, W. A., and Steinberg, A. D., 1981a, The human autologous mixed lymphocyte reaction: Suppression by macrophages and T cells, *J. Immunol.* **127:**1987.

Smolen, J. S., Luger, T. A., Chused, T. M., and Steinberg, A. D., 1981b, Responder cells ins the human autologous mixed lymphocyte reaction, *J. Clin. Invest.* **68:**1601.

Smolen, J. S., Sharrow, S. O., and Steinberg, A. D., 1981c, Characterization of autologous rosette forming cells: A non-restricted phenomenon, *J. Immunol.* **127:**737.

Smolen, J. S., Chused, T. M., Leiserson, W. M., Reeves, Js. P., Alling, D. W., and Steinberg, A. D., 1982, Heterogeneity of immunoregulatory T cell subsets in systemic lupus erythematosus: Correlation with clinical features, *Am. J. Med.* **72:**783.

Steinberg, A. D., Baron, S., and Talal, N., 1969, The pathogenesis of autoimmunity in New

Zealand mice. I. Induction of anti-nucleic acid antibodies by polyinosinic·polycytidylic acid, *Proc. Natl. Acad. Sci. USA* **63:**1102.

Steinberg, A. D., Plotz, P. H., Wolff, S. M., Wong, W. G., Agus, S. G., and Decker, J. L., 1972, Cytotoxic drugs in treatment of non-malignant diseases, *Ann. Intern. Med.* **76:**619.

Steinberg, A. D., Huston, D. P., Taurog, J. D., Cowdery, J. S., and Raveche, E. S., 1981, The cellular and genetic basis of murine lupus, *Immunol. Rev.* **55:**121.

Tonietti, G., Oldstone, M. B. A., and Dixon, F. J., 1970, The effect of induced chronic viral infections on the immunological diseases of New Zealand mice, *J. Exp. Med.* **132:**89.

Twomey, J. J., Laughter, A. H., and Steinberg, A. D., 1978, A serum inhibitor of immune regulation in patients with systemic lupus erythematosus, *J. Clin. Invest.* **62:**713.

Index